AF214198

Introduction to Biological Imaging

Introduction to Biological Imaging

Manfred Auer, PhD
Department of Biomedical Engineering
Southeast University
Nanjing, Jiangsu
China

WILEY

This edition first published 2024

Registered Office(s)
John Wiley & Sons, Inc., 111 River Street, Hoboken, NJ 07030, USA
John Wiley & Sons Ltd, The Atrium, Southern Gate, Chichester, West Sussex, PO19 8SQ, UK

For details of our global editorial offices, customer services, and more information about Wiley products visit us at www.wiley.com.

Wiley also publishes its books in a variety of electronic formats and by print-on-demand. Some content that appears in standard print versions of this book may not be available in other formats.

Library of Congress Cataloging-in-Publication Data
Names: Auer, Manfred, author.
Title: Introduction to biological imaging / Manfred Auer.
Description: Hoboken, NJ : Wiley, 2024. | Includes index.
Identifiers: LCCN 2023052798 (print) | LCCN 2023052799 (ebook) | ISBN 9781119705949 (paperback) | ISBN 9781119705970 (adobe pdf) | ISBN 9781119705956 (epub)
Subjects: MESH: Diagnostic Imaging | Biological Phenomena | Diagnostic Techniques and Procedures | Image Processing, Computer-Assisted–methods
Classification: LCC RC78.7.D53 (print) | LCC RC78.7.D53 (ebook) | NLM WN 180 | DDC 616.07/54–dc23/eng/20231220
LC record available at https://lccn.loc.gov/2023052798
LC ebook record available at https://lccn.loc.gov/2023052799

Cover Design: Wiley
Cover Images: Courtesy of Manfred Auer; Courtesy of Ke Xu

Set in 9.5/12.5pt STIXTwoText by Straive, Pondicherry, India
Printed and bound by CPI Group (UK) Ltd, Croydon, CR0 4YY

C9781119705949_220324

To my children, my parents and Ulla. I am very grateful for your love and support.

Contents

Preface

Among the more ambitious goals in modern biology is our quest to find a link between (patho-) physiological state of an organism and the role that key molecules play in it, be that the process of tissue and organ development, the differentiation of individual cells, or the manifestation of disease.

However, biological systems are inherently complex with many components needed to sustain cellular function. In order to understand any complex system, one must determine its composition, i.e., identify the components it is made of, how each of these components carry out their specific task, and how they interact with one another to function together as an assembly of components. In other words, we need to determine the specific mechanism of function and its regulation for each relevant individual macromolecule, but we must also determine its interaction with other macromolecules. Therefore, detailed information is needed at different levels of scale and complexity, ranging from three-dimensional (3D) structure and function of individual macromolecules, which allows the determination of the reaction or interaction mechanisms at atomic scale, over the structural organization of such individual components into macromolecular and/or supramolecular complexes, as well as their spatiotemporal distribution and kinetics within organelles, cells, and tissues.

Furthermore, it is important to see how genetic modification or pharmacological intervention alters such macromolecular function, macromolecular interactions, and/or spatiotemporal distribution, and thus the overall supramolecular structural organization of organelles, cells, and tissues. Only when we understand holistically 3D structure, function, kinetics, and regulation of such macromolecules, molecular machines, and supramolecular complexes in their organelle-, cell-, and tissue-context will we be able to understand how such changes lead to physiological cell and tissue function and/or pathogenesis/disease progression.

The list of systems components can be determined by the various "-omics" approaches, with genomics and transcriptomics determining the nucleic acid sequences of genes and their transcribed messenger RNA, respectively, and thus link gene sequences and expression profiles to cellular behavior. Proteomics probes the translated gene products, i.e., proteins along with possible posttranslational modifications. Lipidomics studies cellular lipids and is a subset of metabolomics that aims to study all small molecules that are synthesized or broken down in any of the primary and secondary metabolic pathways of a cell. The presence and abundance of inorganic, small organic, and macromolecular components in cells and tissues can be detected by mass spectrometry approaches. Many of these aforementioned approaches are easily scalable, and in many cases the information can be obtained through the service of large regional or national centers, enabled by commercial vendors.

The "-omics" approaches often are nontargeted, collecting a vast amount of information about all present components. Targeted approaches that focus on the presence of a small subset of components are typically based on affinity probes with a reporter molecule that can be easily read out, e.g., with an optical light detector. Therefore, data collection and analysis is straightforward and lends itself to automation of the process and hence high throughput.

Not too surprisingly, the aforementioned tools of "-omics" for identification of components are widely used and can provide a large amount of information about a biological system, resulting in an ever-increasing parts list. However, knowing what components constitute such complex systems only gets one so far in understanding the inner workings of the system. A deeper understanding requires knowledge on how the parts fit together, in other words what their spatial and temporal relationship is, which components interact with other, and whether there are additional organizational levels that transcend the individual components. As an analogy, any complex machinery such as a car is more than the sum of all its constituent components (e.g., engine, wheels, brakes, a steering wheel, and power transmission). Thus, higher-level 3D organization of individual components can lead to new function, and 3D organization manifests itself at different levels. Naturally, it is not enough to understand the combustion engine; we also need to understand how this engine is connected to the wheels. Hence, we need to understand organization at different levels of scale and complexity, ranging from pistons and valves in the engine to the level of the entire car.

The biological equivalent is the anatomy of a living organism, which describes the system at the organ level, whereas histology examines the various tissue types that constitute the organs, and cell biology examines the complex system at the level of individual cells (and possibly a small group of individual cells), subcellular level of organelles, and supramolecular assemblies like the cytoskeleton. Determining the 3D structure of individual macromolecules (e.g., proteins and nucleic acids) and macromolecular machines (e.g., ribosomes and transcription machinery) typically falls into the repertoire of structural biology, which aims for atomic-resolution insight into the protein architecture of, e.g., an enzyme, and thus a chemical understanding of its enzymatic activity. There are good arguments to consider structural biology a part of bioimaging, and therefore the major techniques for structure determination are discussed in this volume, but a purist may point out that strictly speaking, techniques like NMR-spectroscopy and X-ray crystallography (and other scattering techniques) are not imaging techniques, at least not in a stricter sense of the word. Similarly, mass spectrometry in itself is not an imaging technique; however, images can be created from the information that is being recorded.

Layout of the Book

The layout of this book is guided by the idea that basic concepts, which typically have their home in disciplines like physics, (bio-)chemistry, biology, or computer science/mathematics need to be conquered first to truly appreciate how the different imaging disciplines are built on these basic concepts. We then examine how these basics concepts are used for each imaging approach.

A desired outcome would be for the reader to realize the many commonalities of different imaging techniques, which are often only separated from each other by the type of radiation that is used (e.g., particle radiation versus photons) or by which narrow band of the electromagnetic spectrum is being used for imaging. Ideally, the reader would also realize the common challenges that many imaging techniques are trying to overcome in their own way, be that with respect to signal detection, scale, complexity, and resolution.

Another important aspect in the layout of this book is the realization that different imaging techniques have substantially different goals. There are imaging techniques that provide information about the exact shape of individual macromolecules and supramolecular assemblies, where we aim for high-resolution 3D structures, whereas other approaches may not at all be interested in shape. Instead, they may be interested in spatiotemporal organization and macromolecular vicinity of such macromolecules.

Also, different levels of complexity exist: the most fundamental level of cellular function consists of small inorganic and organic molecules (e.g., metabolites) and macromolecules (e.g., proteins, nucleic acids, carbohydrates, and lipids). Thus, knowledge about their identity, presence, abundance, location, spatiotemporal distribution, and kinetics as well as regulation stands at the center of focus. 3D structural information may yield atomic-level insight about mechanisms of function.

The next higher level of organization are macromolecular machines and supramolecular complexes that typically underlie defined cellular function such as metabolism, replication, transcription and translation of genetic information, cell division, cell differentiation, signaling, and cell death, to name a few important cell biological phenomena.

Yet another level up; such processes often occur in defined cellular compartments. Hence, such processes ideally need to be studied in their native subcellular region and organelle context. However, such environments are often ill-defined with respect to the presence, abundance, and/or location of other macromolecules. For this reason, much progress of such cell biological processes has been made in reconstituted in vitro systems, where different parameters (such as composition and concentration) can be more easily controlled.

For some processes, e.g., cell–cell adhesion (to name an example), one may assume the presence of certain macromolecules based on the cell biological models that have been established for cell adhesion, but the presence of certain macromolecules known to be involved adhesion does not guarantee an intact, functional cell–cell adhesion complex. Hence, both the spatiotemporal localization of suspected cell–cell adhesion proteins to cell–cell adhesion sites and the actual ultrastructural organization of a cell–cell adhesion site need to be studied.

Therefore, regarding the layout of this book, the sequence of the chapters discussing the different imaging techniques also reflects differences in complexity when going from the level of macromolecular complexes to the levels of cellular organelles, cells, and ultimately tissues. We will briefly touch upon even higher organization of cells and tissues, when we acknowledge the presence of organs, yet the study of organs typically requires yet another set of bioimaging techniques, typically referred to as medical imaging. While medical imaging approaches also make an important contribution to the well-being of higher vertebrates (e.g., in veterinary medicine or vertebrate model systems for human health), it is typically not categorized as a bioimaging approach, but it is a category of imaging on its own. However, as will be discussed briefly, medical imaging techniques are based on the same foundational principles that are discussed in the beginning and deserve at least some space for discussion, even though they are the subject of their own specialized literature. The book ends with an outlook on where each of the disciplines may be heading to and a plea for the necessity and a possible path for a multiscale, multimodal integrated bioimaging future, perhaps building on the success that cosmology enjoyed, when combining and integrating various imaging techniques.

The reader may experience redundancy in terms of information, which to a large degree is intended, as first it allows a reader to read each chapter on their own, without the necessity of starting at the very beginning and read until the very end in a chronological order, but also because the desired effect is that the reader will come across information he/she already has learned in previous/other chapters and by coming across the same material possibly from a slightly different angle will hopefully reinforce the learning effect. At least that is the intention of the redundancy of various aspects of bioimaging.

This textbook aims for a broad readership ranging from the novice on bioimaging, who wants to get an overview, to professionals in bioimaging, who may have in-depth knowledge about their own discipline but may not be as well versed in other (neighboring) imaging techniques.

1

Introduction – A Brief History of Imaging

The 2011 News Focus section of one the leading science journals (Science 334: 1046–1051) identified fundamental questions remaining in biology. More than a decade later, many of these questions remain unsolved. The following bullet points list questions that will require imaging techniques as the key for answers:

Arranging the basic building blocks

- Does a gene's location in the nucleus matter? Genes on different parts of the chromosome and perhaps even on different chromosomes loop together in domains of active transcription. However, are there levels of organization beyond this?
- How does a cell position its proteins? With a typical cell making ~10,000 different types of proteins amounting to over a billion proteins altogether, protein distribution is far from random. How does the cell know where to position these proteins, and while eukaryotic cells employ organelles to compartmentalize metabolic pathways, and proteins often have sorting signals that will guide them to their final destination, "many proteins operate outside organelles and still need to find specific homes or molecular partners within the relatively vast spaces of a cell." mRNA is often non-stochastically distributed, and this observation may explain some of the protein's localization pattern but simply shifts the problem to how mRNA knows where to go.
- Are there specialized domains (c.g., lipid rafts) in cell membranes that allow the specific segregation of membrane proteins (e.g., into organized signaling platforms)?

Controlling cell differentiation

- What changes in cellular organization accompany cell differentiation?
- How do cells detect and migrate in response to tiny concentration gradients of chemicals in their environment?
- How do groups of cells migrate together (e.g., during development of the organism)?
- How does a cell or a tissue know its size and maintain it within the normal range? While cells can range in size from small to huge, for each cell type, a narrow range of dimensions is observed. So, while obviously small and large volumes are compatible with cellular function, how does each cell know when to stop growing? This question can be extended to tissues and organs. How is size so tightly controlled, and do these mechanisms act independently of each other?

Managing complex biological functions

- Can cells communicate over long distances (e.g., via membrane nanotubes)?
- How does the malfunction of a single protein lead to complex pathological phenotypes (e.g., cancer, neurodegenerative diseases, psychiatric diseases, organ failure, death)?
- Can we mathematically predict the behavior of cells and tissues/microbial communities in response to environmental challenges?
- Does the complexity of spatiotemporal organization of cells in the brain and the interplay of the separate components necessarily lead to conscience?
- Do microbial cells in a biofilm community coordinate behavior and how do they work together toward a sustainable lifestyle?

Other questions

- How do highly specialized cells and tissues know exactly where they are in the complex multicellular organism to behave appropriately? What is the underlying mechanism of their cellular GPS?
- What is the molecular mechanism of evolution? How does the mutation of single traits/protein sequences result in novel species?
- What did the first cell look like and how did it function? How was it possible for life as we know it to occur in the first place?

Introduction to Biological Imaging, First Edition. Manfred Auer.

As mentioned above, these questions have been formulated well over a decade ago, yet they essentially are still unanswered. Many questions point to the enigma of how biological processes are organized in space and time: it seems at this point unlikely that the sophisticated and often robust biological responses to any perturbations of the system are just the results of stochastic encounters of the constituent components. Hence, life is highly organized and structured, and it is these structural patterns that modern biology will need to elucidate.

1.1 Spatiotemporally Organization of Biological Processes

As is evident from the above-posed questions, one of the fundamental goals of biology is to understand how living organisms establish and maintain their spatiotemporal organization of the biochemical, cell biological and developmental biology processes that sustain life. Discussed below are a few examples of such spatiotemporal organization, such as the compartmentalization of cellular energy metabolism as well as the development and maintenance of tissues with the underlying differentiation of cells. Examples of cellular differentiation are the establishment of apical-basolateral polarity in epithelial cells or the unique organization of the cytoskeleton in such specialized cells such as muscle cells or neurons.

1.1.1 Metabolism

Long gone are the times in biology when cells were viewed as bags of enzymes. We now understand that cellular metabolism is organized by spatial compartmentalization of metabolic enzymes into specific cellular spaces. Different parts of the metabolic pathway take place in different organelles: Oxidative phosphorylation occurs in mitochondria, whereas most chemical reactions of glycolysis take place in the cytoplasmic space. Furthermore, enzymatic activity belonging to the same metabolic pathway often reside in close spatial proximity, which ensures highly efficient metabolism. Such chemical reactions are catalyzed by macromolecules (typically proteins), with many of these chemical reactions requiring a chemical energy source, such as adenosine-tri-phosphate (ATP). The phosphorylation of the substrate ADP to obtain ATP is catalyzed by the so-called F-type ATPase, a multi-protein complex that uses as energy a proton-gradient over the inner mitochondrial membrane, which is established by proteins of the respiratory chain. ATP generation occurs in mitochondria cristae, a three-dimensional membrane network continuous with the inner mitochondrial membrane. But even within this highly compartmentalized space of the mitochondria cristae, F-ATPases are not distributed randomly inside the cristae membrane but are found at locations of high membrane curvature at the end of mitochondria cristae.

1.1.2 Developmental Biology

Arguably one of the most intriguing examples of nature's ability for self-assembly and spatiotemporal pattern formation is the development of an organism starting with a single cell, the fertilized egg, to build the highly complex body of a vertebrate like zebrafish larvae or the human body. While developmental biologists have successfully determined the many transcription factors necessary for turning on the processes of tissue patterning and cell differentiation (e.g., into nerve, muscle, endothelial or epithelial cells), we do not have much information regarding the changes in cellular macromolecule abundance and distribution as well as changes in supramolecular 3D architecture inside cells that underlie morphogenesis and the formation of different tissue types. Highly specialized cells emerge from precursor stem cells, carrying out highly specialized functions. For example, vertebrate inner ear hair cells, the cells that underlie our senses of hearing and balance, display a highly prominent feature, known as the hair bundle, an F-actin-rich organelle, protruding from the apical surface of hair cells in the sensory epithelia. There are over 100 proteins that when mutated lead to loss of our senses of hearing and balance. Many gene products of known deafness genes localize to the hair bundle and play a role in either hair bundle formation, maintenance, or degeneration. This is a good example of where we stand for many topics in current biology, we have a reasonable idea of who is involved in a biological process, so we have a kind of parts list, but we do not know how the parts exactly fit together to sustain cellular function. Specifically, for the case of the hair bundle we do not know exactly how these over 100 proteins work together in a spatiotemporal pattern to form stereocilia, which are actin bundle-filled, finger-like membrane protrusions from the apical hair cell surface that collectively make up the hair bundle, the organelle of mechanoelectrical transduction. All we know is that genetic mutations in these over 100 deafness genes lead to hair bundle degeneration and thus hearing loss.

1.1.3 Disease Mechanisms

To truly understand pathogenesis and disease progression, it is not sufficient to identify a culprit mutation that alters the protein sequence of a key protein. Instead, we need to gain in-depth insight into what changes occur with respect to the spatiotemporal distribution of key proteins, and what are the resulting consequences for the overall subcellular morphology, behavior, and underlying 3D architecture. If cellular health is dependent on the presence and abundance of certain proteins, as well as their correct subcellular localization, we need to determine what constitutes a healthy range of abundance and distribution for each protein in a typical cell. Such parameters are largely unknown, as is the number, size and shape of organelles, cell–cell or cell–matrix junctions, the cytoskeleton, other key cellular machineries. Also, largely unknown is how the lack of expression or the malfunction at the level of a single protein can affect the rest of the cell, as disease typically manifests itself at the cell and tissue level.

1.2 Why Imaging?

From the sections above it should be obvious that completing a parts list, as is done by the various omics-efforts (e.g., genomics, transcriptomics, proteomics, and metabolomics), is only the starting point to understand biological processes. Imaging can turn a parts list into a wiring diagram by visualizing protein–protein interactions and thus to understand cellular function. From the very first days of cell biology, imaging played a major role in understanding cellular processes. Images of cells, first obtained by optical light microscopy and then later by electron microscopy, underscored the notion that cells are highly organized and contain many subcellular structures, such as the above-mentioned cellular powerhouses, also known as mitochondria. The nucleus stores and faithfully replicates the genetic information, transcribes DNA sequences into mRNA, some of which is transported into the ribosome-studded rough endoplasmic reticulum, where the mRNA sequence is translated by ribosomes into amino acid sequences that fold in 3D into functional proteins and protein complexes, some of which are then post-translationally modified, and ultimately secreted into the extracellular space via the Golgi apparatus. Other mRNA sequences are transported via the nuclear membrane into the cytoplasm, where they are translated into proteins by ribosomes, with the proteins being retained in the cytoplasm. It is increasingly clear that the high level of organization and the spatiotemporal separation of biochemical and cell biological processes are key to the proper function of cells, and thus ultimately to the health and survival of organisms.

1.2.1 A Very Brief History of Cellular Biological Imaging

A great deal of research over the last half century has been invested into studying spatiotemporally well-defined processes that underlie cellular function and the pathogenic consequences of a breakdown of this well-orchestrated macromolecular symphony. Apart from advances in cell culturing, cell sorting and cell fractionation, imaging arguably has played the most crucial role in cell biology by identifying the spatial location of subcellular components and their temporal changes of localization patterns. This is exemplified by the detailed description of cell division and the associated cytoskeletal changes. Microscopy marked the beginning of cell biological studies when Robert Hooke in 1655 looked at thin layer of cork and coined the word "cell," and when Anton van Leeuwenhoek in 1674 was the first to examine living cells, specifically green algae. They were helped by the intrinsic contrast of the cell wall compared to the empty cell interior of dead plant cells and the colored chloroplasts populating the cytoplasm, respectively. Hence the origin and infancy of cell biology was a search for structure and thus mostly descriptive, with thorough observation and description in form of manual drawings. Among the most famous cell biologists that used microscopy were Santiago Ramon y Cajal and Camillo Golgi, who were co-awarded the Nobel Prize in Physiology or Medicine in 1906 "in recognition of their work on the structure of the nervous system." Their discoveries relied on the development of microscopes based on the knowledge gathered by Joseph von Fraunhofer, Friedrich Adolph Norbert, and Ernst Abbe, operating close to the diffraction limit of light, as well as the development of staining protocols to enhance contrast, first introduced by Francois-Vincent Raspail in the middle of the 19th century.

Such stains, which included silver and gold salts, allowed the neuroanatomical drawings of neurons and their intercellular connections by Cajal and Golgi, and led to the discovery of the Golgi apparatus inside cells. However, the need for stains also meant that cells could not be studied in vivo but needed to be fixed and exposed to a variety of chemical reagents, limiting what could be accomplished by optical light microscopy. Around the middle of the 20th century, a new technology using electrons instead of photons emerged that had a two order of magnitude increased resolving power. The fact that electron microscopy revolutionized both material science and cell biology was recognized by the 1986 Nobel Prize in Physics, awarded to Dr. Ernst Ruska "for his fundamental work in electron optics, and the design of the first electron microscope."

Due to the strong interactions of electrons with matter, cells needed to be imaged in the vacuum of the electron microscope, and only very thin slices (typically 50–100 nm in thickness) could be imaged. This required the development of sample preparation techniques that allowed the cutting of vacuum-resistant ultra-thin sections, which led to tissue embedment into a plastic resin. The necessity for embedding cells and tissues into a plastic resin for the longest time resulted in sample preparation artifacts, such as aggregation and extraction, due to the prolonged exposure of biological material to organic solvents and the hydrophobic plastic resin needed to infiltrate cells prior to resin polymerization. Such sample preparation artifacts gave cellular electron microscopy (after its initial big success) a bad reputation, as it was unclear whether imaging results could be trusted, particularly if they showed unexpected imaging results. This skepticism has been partially overcome only in the two decades by cryogenic sample preparation techniques like high-pressure freezing and freeze-substitution, where the water-solvent is exchanged with an organic solvent well below 0 °C. While cryogenic sample preparation techniques have led to a significantly improved faithful preservation of cells and tissues, many researchers still will not trust the studying cellular volumes if any form of chemical fixation, staining, dehydration, or resin-embedding is used. They only accept the study of samples in their unstained, frozen-hydrated (vitreous) state, using cryo electron microscopy. This is widely considered as the gold standard of cellular imaging. However, this latest round of skepticism may be undeserved, as the use of cryogenic approaches such as high-pressure freezing followed by freeze-substitution and resin-based cellular electron microscopy yields excellent preservation. Furthermore, minor alterations of the macromolecular ultrastructure can be tolerated as cellular imaging does not aim for precise shape of macromolecules but examine larger-scaler organization that is not affected by heavy-metal staining.

Cellular resin-EM has yielded an enormous wealth of information regarding cellular architecture, which was recognized in the 1974 Nobel Prize of Physiology or Medicine for Albert Claude, Christian de Duve, and George Palade "for their discoveries concerning the structural and functional organization of the cell." Throughout the 1970s, 1980s, and early 1990s cellular electron microscopy remained a major tool in cell biology, however, most researchers used traditional resin sample preparation, that are known to lead to poor sample preservation, and only very few engaged in cryogenic approaches such as high-pressure freezing/freeze-substitution. From this era stems the often-undeserved reputation that resin-embedded samples are artifact-prone, and that only fully hydrated samples can be trusted.

By the mid 1980s, optical microscopy saw a revival, with the advent of fluorescent tags that could be genetically encoded, and thus no longer needed to be targeted to the candidate protein of interest via affinity probes. Affinity probe-based protocols that aimed at labeling a candidate protein with a synthetic fluorophore were typically not compatible with live cell imaging but requires a "light" chemical fixation and detergent-based penetration of the cells and tissues, which not only killed the cells but also could lead to extraction and possibly alteration of cellular ultrastructure. Even more importantly, several factors could influence labeling efficacy, such as the amount of penetration typically accomplished by the detergent, the crowdedness of the cell interior when retaining most of the cell's interior structure or the potential loss of the protein of interest when losing most of the cell's interior structure, the chemical alteration of the target protein by the chemical fixative and thus loss of affinity for the fluorescent probe as well as cross-reactivity of the affinity probe. Needless to point out that there were several possibilities for false negative and positive results. All this changed when fluorescent tags could be genetically encoded. Fusion proteins contained both the candidate protein of interest and a fluorescent protein that could be imaged. The earliest such fusion proteins were based on the naturally occurring green-fluorescent protein, whose sequence had been altered to enhance stability and fluorescence brightness, and subsequently for altered absorption and emission spectra (and thus altered color). The significance of this breakthrough in cell biological imaging was recognized in the 2008 Nobel Prize in Chemistry, awarded to Drs. Osamu Shimomura, Martin Chalfie, and Roger Y. Tsien "for the discovery and development of the green fluorescent protein, GFP."

Another technical advance that brought optical microscopy back to the limelight of cellular imaging was the addition of electronic equipment such as cameras and computers to optical microscopy, as such equipment allowed cells and their dynamics to be studied in their live state. This opened a new window on cells, as the dynamic properties of cells and their subcellular constituents could be observed, particularly when combining video microscopy with genetic encoding of fluorescent tags.

Breaking the diffraction limit barrier in optical microscopy in the early 2000s was another important milestone in cellular imaging, which was recognized by the 2014 Nobel Prize in Chemistry, awarded to Eric Betzig, Stefan Hell, and William E. Moerner for the "development of super-resolved fluorescence microscopy."

Over the last decade, both electron microscopy and optical microscopy overcame some of their respective limitations of their earlier days. Electron microscopy has overcome some of its narrow size limitations both in terms of field of view (XY) that could be imaged as well as the thickness (Z) of the sample, whereas optical microscopy overcame the resolution limits associated with diffraction-limited optical imaging. However, sample preparation challenges such as imaging in a vacuum or the need for specific tagging of molecules of interest remain. The advances in imaging in both fields have resulted in gigantic data sets that render their processing and analysis non-trivial. The advantage in interpretation of optical microscopy data sets is that each signal is specific, as the fluorophores were specifically targeted, hence only a few selected different macromolecules can be visualized at any given time. However, optical imaging data may also include time or spectral composition, and thus can be highly complex to analyze. In the absence of suitable macromolecule-specific tags, electron microscopy records every structure in the field of view, and not just a selected subset, which leads to the challenge of detecting and selecting features of interest within the entire 3D volume. Moreover, electron microscopy provides static yet comprehensive high-resolution ultrastructural information, whereas fluorescence light microscopy can yield static and/or dynamic information, but typically is limited to a few selected components. Hence, there is a desire to combine both optical and electron microscopy (also known as correlative light and electron microscopy – CLEM), by imaging the same sample sequentially first by optical microscopy to study the dynamics of biological processes, followed by a higher-resolution analysis of the cellular volume with increased resolution and subcellular context.

1.2.2 A Very Brief History of Macromolecular Biological Imaging

Structural biology is the logical endpoint of our millennia-old quest to understand the inner workings of the human body, from the anatomy of organs and the histology of cells and tissues to the study of the molecular and macromolecular building blocks of a living organism. Arguably, the oldest scientific discipline is anatomy, with the first documented scientific dissections being carried out in Alexandria in the 3rd century BCE. The tradition of dissection of corpses was taken up again in the 15th century and led to detailed drawings by Leonardo da Vinci and Michelangelo. Description of structure was seen as the key for understanding, both at the level of organs, and subsequently (from the 18th century onward) at the level of tissues. This quest was in part aided by the development of specific staining techniques and the availability of the compound microscope, and in the 19th century by the improvement of microscope through correction of spherical and chromatic aberrations. However, the world of macromolecules was beyond the diffraction limit of light microscopy and required an approach entirely different from the optical imaging that dominated biology in the 19th century. Progress in different disciplines in the 19th century such as mineralogy (determination of symmetry and space groups in mineral crystals), physics (the discovery of X-rays and their use for diffraction experiments in crystals, see also 1901 Nobel Prize in Physics for Wilhelm Röntgen, 1914 Nobel Prize in Physics for Max von Laue, 1915 Nobel Prize in Physics for William H. Bragg and William L. Bragg), organic chemistry and subsequent biochemistry (the isolation, purification, and crystallization of organic molecules and macromolecules) as well as mathematics (Fourier transform) culminated in the beginning of the 20th century in X-ray crystal diffraction studies and subsequent structure determination of small organic molecules such as cholesterol in 1937, penicillin in 1946 and vitamin B12 in 1956 (see 1964 Nobel Prize in Chemistry for Dorothy Crowfoot Hodgkin) as well as proteins like myoglobin in 1958 and hemoglobin in 1959 (see 1962 Nobel Prize in Chemistry for John Kendrew and Max Perutz). The importance of creating a model for the macromolecule that was consistent with the experimental data (rather than an actual visualization of the molecule itself) is most prominently evident for the double helix structure of DNA in 1953 (see 1962 Nobel Prize in Physiology or Medicine for Francis Crick, James Watson, and Maurice Wilkins). In the second half of the 20th century, X-ray crystallography dominated with an overwhelming number of high-resolution protein structures deposited into the protein databank. The success of X-ray crystallography for macromolecular structure determination also was the result of many small yet important technical innovations, such as overcoming the consequences of radiation damage by rapid freezing of the crystals, brighter radiation sources such as synchrotrons, and increased automation in data collection and data analysis.

A number of Nobel Prizes have been closely associated with the structure determination of proteins and other macromolecules by X-ray crystallography, including the 1988 Nobel Prize in Chemistry for Johann Deisenhofer, Robert Huber and Hartmut Michel for the determination of the three-dimensional structure of a photosynthetic reaction center, the 1997 Nobel Prize in Chemistry for Paul Boyer and John Walker for their elucidation of the enzymatic mechanism underlying the synthesis of adenosine triphosphate (ATP), the 2003 Nobel Prize in Chemistry for Peter Agre and Roderick MacKinnon for the discovery of water channels and the structural and mechanistic studies of ion channels, respectively, the 2006 Nobel Prize in Chemistry for Roger Kornberg for his studies on the molecular basis of eukaryotic transcription, and the 2009 Nobel Prize in Chemistry for Venkatraman Ramakrishnan, Thomas Steitz and Ada Yonath for studies of the structure and function of the ribosome, to name a few examples. Naturally, none of this would have been possible without the pioneering work of Sir John Kendrew and Max Perutz.

In the 1990s NMR spectroscopy started to contribute in a significant manner to the 3D high resolution structure models that have been entered in the protein data bank.

Initially, this method was restricted to protein domains and small proteins, given the size restrictions posed by early NMR spectrometers' magnetic field capacities, and the number of unique interactions in three-dimensions of functional groups in the protein amino acid sequence. But advances in biochemical site-specific labeling techniques, the use of higher field magnets and the development in solid state NMR spectroscopy have allowed since the structure determination of larger proteins. Two Nobel Prizes in Chemistry have been awarded since to Richard R. Ernst (in 1991) and Kurt Wüthrich (in 2002) for the "development of the methodology of high-resolution nuclear magnetic resonance (NMR) spectroscopy" and for the "development of nuclear resonance spectroscopy for determining the three-dimensional structure of biological macromolecules in solution," respectively.

Since the late 1960s electron microscopy has contributed to structural biology, with successful structure determination requiring either 2D crystalline, helical or icosahedral symmetry to allow implicit averaging of a large number of macromolecules in a defined and thus known orientation. To acknowledge the contribution of electron microscopy for structure determination of macromolecules, the 1982 Nobel Prize in Chemistry was awarded to Aaron Klug for "his development of crystallographic electron microscopy and his structural elucidation of biologically important nucleic acid-protein complexes." Only recently, symmetry and thus a periodic arrangement of macromolecules is no longer a prerequisite for high-resolution structure determination by electron microscopy. Cryo-electron microscopy of single particles without the exploitation of sample symmetry has since revolutionized structural biology, as indicated by the 2017 Nobel Prize in Chemistry, awarded to Jacques Dubochet, Joachim Frank, and Richard Henderson "for developing cryo-electron microscopy for the high-resolution structure determination of biomolecules in solution."

There were several challenges that electron microscopy needed to overcome before single-particle cryo-EM became the go-to method for structural biology:

First, as is implicated in the name transmission electron microscopy, all images of the macromolecules are projection views, which means in order to obtain a 3D image of the macromolecules a number of projection views of the macromolecules in different orientation need to be combined, which is most easily accomplished if the molecules either form regular arrays with helical symmetry such as tobacco mosaic virus, actin filaments, microtubules or 2D tubular crystals of the membrane protein acetylcholine receptor. Alternatively, specimen may adopt a spherical-like shape with icosahedral symmetry as many viruses naturally do, or arrange into a flat two-dimensional crystal, analogous to 3D crystals necessary for X-ray crystallography.

Second, due to the strong interaction of electrons with matter (including air), samples need to be studied in the vacuum of an electron microscope, which constitutes a particular problem for biological macromolecules that typically reside in an aqueous solution and thus require a hydration shell for the maintenance of a proper 3D structure. Stripping away such a hydration shell, as would happen in a vacuum, will effectively lead to a drying-out of the sample, which can denature macromolecules like proteins. Furthermore, the strong interaction of electrons with matter also leads to radiation damage and thus to the disintegration of the macromolecule(s) of interest. Early attempts in macromolecular EM imaging relied on exposure of the macromolecules, adhered to the support film of an electron microscope grid, to low concentration solutions of heavy metal salts such as uranyl acetate of phosphor-tungstic acid. After removing excess liquid, the grid was dried, resulting in a very thin layer of amorphous heavy metal, into which the macromolecule is embedded. As the electrons pass through the negatively stained sample, the macromolecules are destroyed, but the heavy metal cast remains largely intact, hence a negative imprint of the macromolecule can be visualized. Preservation of the samples was questionable when exposing the macromolecule to increasing salt concentrations during the drying process, in addition to flattening of the sample in the drying process and a possible collapse of the cast during the electron irradiation. Hence, 3D structures from negatively stained samples typically were limited to ~20 Å resolution. Electron microscopy experienced a significant boost with the development of cryogenic ultrafast sample preparation methods, with macromolecules localizing to small holes in a support film adsorbed to an electron grid. After removal of excess fluid, the grid containing macromolecules suspended in a very thin layer of buffer is plunged into liquid ethane held in a liquid state at liquid nitrogen temperature. This typically results in a thin layer of amorphous vitreous ice, in which the samples in their frozen-hydrated state can be imaged at low temperature in the electron beam at a minimal dose. This approach not only solved the issue of imaging in a vacuum but also minimized radiation damage. However, due to the low inherent signal of unstained specimen, elaborate methods for increasing the signal-to-noise ratio for each of the particles being imaged needed to be developed, either through implicit (such as exploiting symmetry) or through explicit averaging. Initially, throughput was low, and the task of structure determination was substantial, not unlike it was the case in the early days of X-ray crystallography. Just as it was the case for X-ray crystallography, cryo-EM tremendously benefitted from advances in sample preparation, automation for data collection, which allowed higher throughput, and advances in data processing, but the biggest leap was made by advances in detector technology that allowed to overcome one of the biggest challenges in cryo-EM, namely beam-induced specimen movement. Since the "resolution revolution" over the last decade, single particle cryo-EM has become the dominant force for structure determination to the point that many former X-ray crystallography lab have adopted cryo-EM as their primary approach for structure determination of proteins and macromolecular machines.

2

Basics of Atomic and Molecular Physics

2.1 Matter and Energy

2.1.1 Standard Model of Particle Physics

The standard model of particle physics distinguishes between fermions and bosons, with fermions being elementary particles (like quarks and leptons), the building blocks of atoms, and thus making up ordinary matter, whereas bosons carry a force and thus mediate the interactions between fermions. The most relevant boson for biology is the photon.

Quarks

With respect to fermions, only the up- and down-quarks with a $+2/3$ (positive) and a $-1/3$ (negative) charge, respectively, are relevant outside the realm of high-energy particle physics and thus to the chemistry of life. A combination of quarks constitutes baryons, with either two up- and one down-quark forming a proton or one up- and two down-quarks forming a neutron (Figure 2.1). Combinations of protons and neutrons form atomic nuclei with a net positive charge.

Protons have a slightly smaller mass than neutrons, and they are stable outside nuclei, whereas neutrons outside atomic nuclei are not stable, with a mean lifetime of ~15 minutes. Neutrons being by themselves (and thus outside the nucleus) decay into protons, electrons, and electron neutrinos. Quarks in the atomic nucleus are held together by the so-called strong force (strong interaction), mediated by gluons (which are members of the family of gauge bosons. Consequently, protons and neutrons are held together by the nuclear force and are stable inside the nucleus.

Leptons

Of the leptons, the negatively charged electron and to a much smaller degree its anti-material positively charged counterpart, the positron, are the only relevant ones as they are stable. They are both truly elementary particles with no internal structure. When electrons and positrons collide, they annihilate into two gamma-ray photons, whose detection is at the foundation of Positron Emission Tomography in medical imaging. Neutrinos hardly interact with matter and for this reason, they cannot be easily detected and are therefore irrelevant for biological imaging. Electrons are widely used in biological imaging (Figure 2.2). Electron microscopes fall into two categories, depending on how they are operated: In Transmission Electron Microscopy (TEM) electrons penetrate the sample, and thus the transmitted electrons are detected, whereas in Scanning Electron Microscopy (SEM), the detected electron signal can be thought of as being reflected from the surface of the samples. These two techniques will be discussed in much more detail later in the book.

Baryons/Hadrons

Protons and neutrons are baryons (subatomic particles) which are part of the hadrons.

Protons are rarely used as a particle source for direct imaging experiments, but they play a central role in Magnetic Resonance Imaging (MRI) and Nuclear Magnetic Resonance (NMR) spectroscopy. In NMR spectroscopy, changes of the nuclear spins in a magnetic field are detected and used for determining interactions and distances of atoms of functional groups in macromolecules (Figure 2.2).

Introduction to Biological Imaging, First Edition. Manfred Auer.

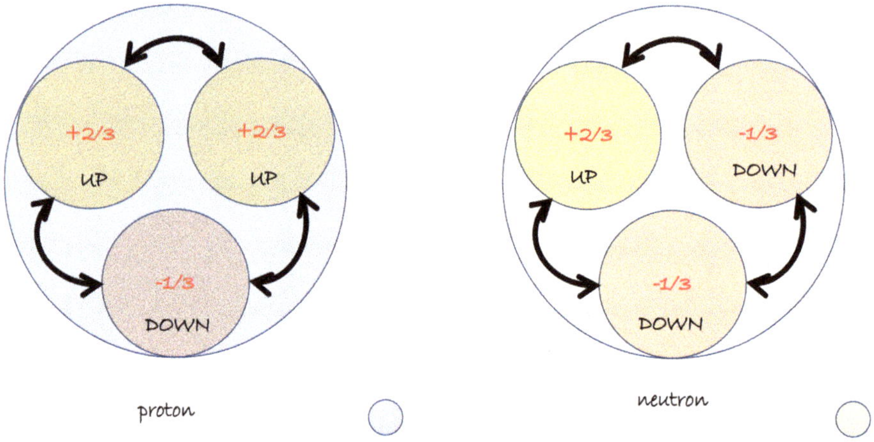

Figure 2.1 Protons and neutrons are the results of different combinations of quarks. According to the standard model of particle physics, quarks are considered elementary particle that do not have any substructure. Of all the quarks, the up-quark and the down-quark are the most relevant with respect to atomic nuclei. The up-quark can be thought of possessing a 2/3 positive charge, whereas the down-quark has a 1/3 negative charge. Both protons and neutrons are made of three quarks, with two up-quarks in combination with one down-quark results in a proton with a net positive charge, whereas the combination of one up with two down-quarks lead to the electroneutral neutron.

Neutrons can in principles be used for imaging, e.g., in small angle neutron scattering (SANS) but practical resolution limits, the challenges of beam collimation and refocusing and the requirement of rather unique facilities, such as a research reactor as a neutron source, limit the general impact of neutron imaging for biology.

Atoms/Ions

The combination of atomic nuclei and a surrounding electron cloud leads to atoms with a net neutral charge, but with a subatomic distribution of a positive charge in their nuclei and a negative charge in the electron shell space surrounding the nuclei.

Loss of electrons in atoms leads to the formation of an ion, which carries a charge and thus can both be easily manipulated in an electromagnetic field and easily detected. Such ions can be used for biological imaging both in the context of mass spectrometry imaging and helium ion microscopy (Figure 2.2). Heavy element ions, such as gadolinium or lanthanide play an indirect role in bioimaging as these ion beams can be used for sample preparation rather than imaging, i.e., to mill away unwanted material of a sample to expose the region of interest for subsequent imaging.

Bosons

With respect to bosons, the Standard Model of Particle Physics recognizes gluons as the carrier of the strong force inside the atomic nucleus, W- and Z-bosons as the carrier of the weak force inside the atomic nucleus, and photons as the carrier of the electromagnetic force, which resides outside the nucleus. Of all bosons only the photon is relevant for imaging (Figure 2.2), as it mediates all interactions between electrically charged particles, with the electromagnetic force changing as the inverse of distance with no limit.

While the photon does not possess a resting mass, it has energy and momentum due to its high velocity (i.e., traveling at the speed of light). Photons possess both particle-like and wave-like properties, a phenomenon referred to as the wave-particle duality. When detected by an instrument they register as particles. However, we utilize its wave-like properties when assessing the probability of detecting a photon in a particular space or when discussing diffraction and interference experiments. The energy of a photon is proportional to the photon's spatial frequency (also known as wave number), ranging from high-energy, very short wavelength (high frequency) ionizing radiation such as gamma-rays and X-rays, via the ultraviolet, visible, and infrared range to the lower frequency (longer wavelength) and thus lower-energy microwaves and radio waves. The most relevant parts of the electromagnetic spectrum are X-rays in the 0.01–5 nm wavelength range for X-ray crystallography and X-ray tomography/micro-CT, visible light in the 200–800 nm range for optical microscopy with its many flavors, near-infrared and infrared in the 900–2,500 nm range, as well as radio waves ranging from 0.33 m (900 MHz) to 300 m (1 MHz) for Nuclear Magnetic Resonance (NMR) Spectroscopy and Magnetic Resonance Imaging (MRI). It should be pointed out however that NMR and MRI only use radio waves indirectly for imaging, as will be discussed

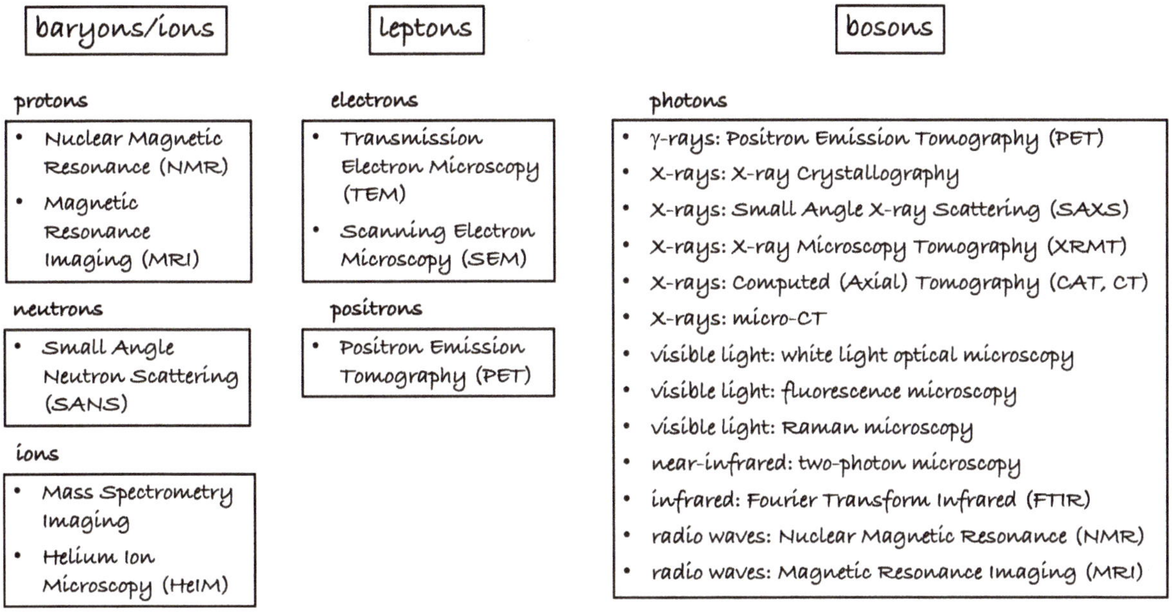

Figure 2.2 Role of baryons, ions, leptons, and bosons for different imaging modalities. With respect to baryons, protons are used not so much for direct imaging itself but in the context of nuclear magnetic resonance (NMR and MRI), neutrons play a small role in the context of SANS, and ions play a central role in mass spectrometry imaging and helium ion microscopy. Regarding leptons, electrons play a major role in bioimaging in the context of transmission and scanning electron microscopy, whereas positrons are used in medical imaging in the context of positron emission tomography (PET), although the emitted positrons are not detected directly, instead a pair of gamma-rays forms when positrons annihilate with electrons. Photons are the only bosons relevant for imaging and range in frequency from gamma rays (as detected in PET) over X-rays (used in X-ray crystallography, SAXS, XRMT, CAT/CT), visible light (white light optical microscopy, fluorescence microscopy, Raman microscopy), near-IR/IR (two-photon microscopy, FTIR) as well as radio waves (NMR/MRI).

in more detail in the respective chapters. Gamma-ray detection is used in Positron Emission Tomography in the context of medical imaging, when positrons that are created in the process of radioactive nuclear decay quickly annihilate electrons, with two gamma-ray photons being emitted.

Given the long history of experimenting with light, it is not surprising that the visual range of the electromagnetic spectrum is used for many specialized techniques, all of which are based on an atom- or molecule-associated transition of electrons to different energy levels.

Photons travel at the speed of light which in vacuum corresponds to ~$3 * 10^8$ m/s but is slower in material like glass. The change in speed of light in the material is reflected in the refractive index, which determines how much the light beam entering the material is bent. This property of glass has been used early on to craft lenses that can converge and thus focus light or disperse light, depending on the shape of the lens. The bending of the light beam is dependent on the wavelength, a phenomenon that is exploited in glass prisms where an incoming "white light" beam is split into a continuous spectrum, thus showing the different color components "white light" is composed of. The spectral properties of photons, i.e., the specific energy levels of the associated photons, are utilized in many imaging applications.

2.1.2 Atomic Structure

Atoms are the building blocks of ordinary matter, such as solids, liquids, or gases and form the chemical elements. Atoms consist of a nucleus and electron cloud. Atoms are typically in size ~100 pm (1 Å; 10^{-10} m), ranging from ~30 pm (0.3 Å) to 300 pm (3 Å), with the nucleus being in size of the order 10^{-15} m (1 fm) to 10^{-14} m (10 fm), and thus the nucleus is ~10,000–100,000 times smaller than the atom. The remainder of the atom is taken up by the electron cloud. Nearly 100% of the mass of an atom resides in the nucleus. To use an analogy, if the atom was the size of a large sports arena/stadium, the size of the nucleus would be the size of a mosquito in its center (Figure 2.3).

Electrons should not be thought of as negatively charged balls circulating the nucleus, despite the depiction commonly found. Classical physics is not useful to describe the events in this size range, instead, quantum physics with its probabilistic approach to physical phenomena such as the distribution of electrons in an atom is a more successful approach.

Atomic Structure: Nucleus

The nucleus typically consists of positively charged protons and electrically neutral neutrons, with hydrogen being

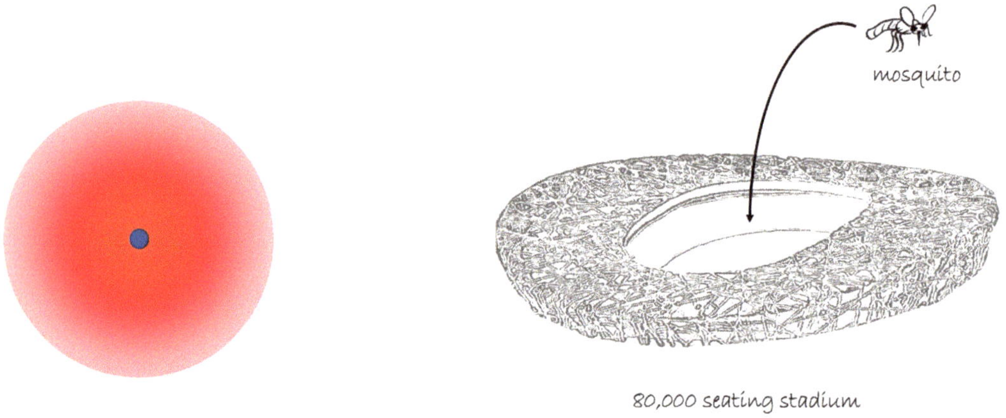

Figure 2.3 Structure of an atom with nucleus and electron cloud. Left: Typical depiction of an atom, with the relative size of a nucleus being depicted 1/10–1/20 of the size of an atom. Right: In reality, the size of an atomic nucleus is about 100,000 times smaller than the size of the atom. As an analogy, if one imagines a sports stadium with an ~80,000 seating capacity, the nucleus would be the size of a mosquito at its very center.

the exception as its nucleus only possesses a single proton. The number of protons (and thus the number of electrons) defines the type of chemical element the atom represents, and thus the characteristics of an element (Figure 2.4). Neutrons can be viewed as a glue that adds stability to the nucleus and prevents the element from disintegration. Protons and neutrons (also known collectively as nucleons) in the nucleus experience the nuclear force, also known as the strong (nuclear) force, which is a short-range force that leads to the attraction of nucleons and thus overcomes the repulsion by the electromagnetic force.

The same chemical element can exist in more than one isotope, depending on the number of neutrons being present in the nucleus. The chemical properties of the different isotypes of a single element are identical, as they are mediated by the electron cloud rather than the atom's nuclei. Electron cloud properties for each isotope of an element are identical for different epitopes, hence they cannot be distinguished by their chemical behavior. However, their nuclear stability often varies, with some isotypes being stable whereas others may enter radioactive decay.

For the lower mass elements, an equivalent number of protons and neutrons lead to stable nuclei, whereas higher mass elements often need a surplus of neutrons to balance out the large number of protons in the nucleus. Instable nuclei lead to radioactive decay, and thus to the formation of lower mass elements in addition to alpha-, beta-, and/or gamma-radiation, which refers to helium-nuclei, electrons/positrons, or high-energy electromagnetic photons, respectively. Also, different isotopes may interact differently with baryons such as neutrons (a property that is used in small-angle neutron scattering) or possess different spin properties (which is used in NMR spectroscopy).

Both protons and neutrons can be described as having spin, not in the Newton mechanical sense as a spinning motion, but in a quantum mechanical sense as a particle

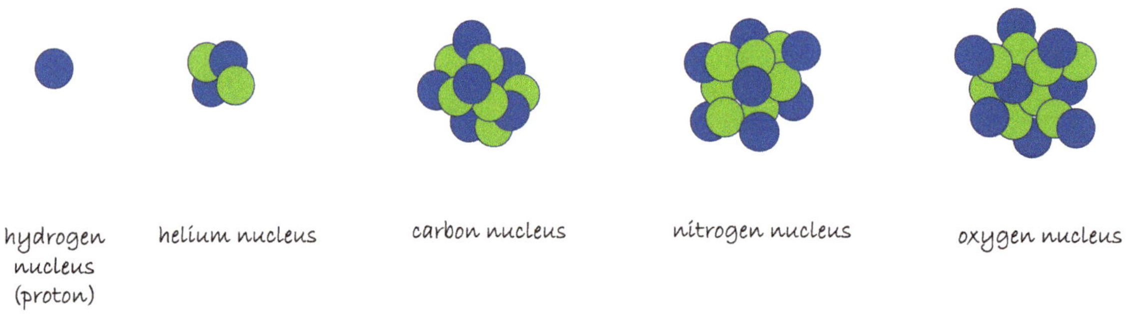

Figure 2.4 Atomic nuclei – Organization and element identity. Protons and neutrons form atomic nuclei, with the number of protons defining the identity of atom (chemical element) and different numbers of neutrons for a single number of protons lead to isotopes, which differ in atomic mass (weight). Isotopes of the same chemical element display identical chemical reactivity, but may differ in their stability of the nucleus, with some isotopes undergoing radioactive decay. Also, isotopes may behave differently upon nuclear magnetic resonance imaging or the scattering of neutrons.

property (with spin being typically defined as up or down). The net (total) spin of a nucleus can be zero, an integer or a half integer. If the number of both protons and neutrons are even, the net resulting spin of the nucleus is zero, as two protons and two neutrons each pair up, and cancel out each other's spin, not unlike two electrons forming a pair in their respective orbitals. Odd mass number nuclei have half-integer spins, such as ½ for ^{1}H, and ^{3}H, ^{13}C, 3/2 for ^{7}Li, or 5/2 for ^{17}O. Examples for integer spins are 1 for ^{2}H and ^{14}N or 3 for ^{10}B.

Nuclei with a non-zero spin can adopt a parallel or antiparallel spin orientation, and both states are typically occupied equally in the absence of an external magnetic field, as their respective energy is equivalent. However, upon experiencing an external magnetic field, the two states become energetically slightly different, hence the occupancy of the two states is no longer equal. Under certain conditions, such as in the presence of brief radio frequency pulses, spins can switch between these parallel and antiparallel orientations, which is the foundation of nuclear magnetic resonance (NMR).

Atomic Structure: Electron Cloud

In addition to the nucleus, atoms also contain an electron cloud, with negatively electrically charged electrons occupying different energy levels, also known as shells, which can be thought of as spherical spaces with their respective characteristic radii.

Initially, the Bohr model described electrons as circulating the nucleus like planets orbit the sun, with only certain orbits that could be occupied. Conceptionally it is still useful as a model in the sense that it explains electrons jumping between such "planetary orbits" when either emitting or absorbing photons (Figure 2.5).

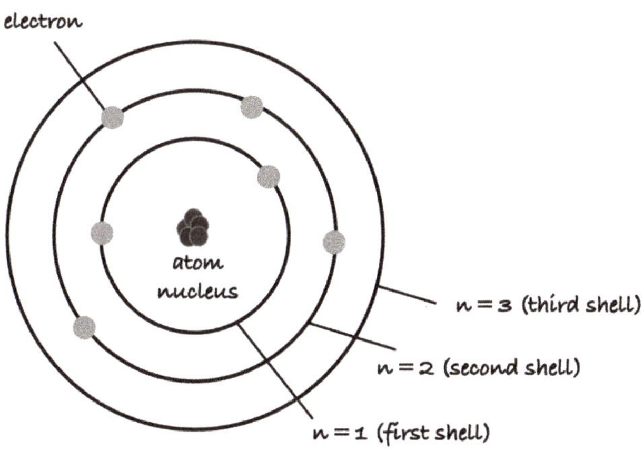

Figure 2.5 Bohr's atom model with electrons circulating the nucleus on discrete orbits. The Bohr atom model assumes stable circular orbits (shells) of discrete radius on which electrons reside. Upon absorption or emission of photons of defined wavelength/energy, electrons can "jump" between such orbits/shells.

However, a more refined model was developed that overcame the obvious problem that electrons circulating the nucleus could not maintain stable orbits as they would constantly lose energy.

Instead of depicting electrons as defined point charges on a defined circular path around the nucleus, they are now considered in a quantum mechanical way as having a certain probability to exist in certain spaces around the nucleus, called orbitals. In this new model, electrons still can jump to a new orbital by either absorbing or emitting photons. The refined model is also based on the de Broglie hypothesis that all particles at the (sub-) atomic level also behave like waves, and these orbitals can be thought of as standing waves inside an atom. This electron cloud atom model is significantly different from the Bohr model as shells are further subdivided into orbitals. Orbitals can be thought of as specific zones where the electrons reside with high probability. There are s-, p-, d-, f-, and g-orbitals which differ with respect to their shape.

In accordance with Schrödinger's mathematical description of the atom, electrons are considered as 3D standing waves, meaning waves that does not move with respect to the nucleus. Each possible state of an electron in an atom can then be described by four quantum numbers: the principal quantum number (electron shell number), the angular momentum quantum number (orbital number), the magnetic quantum number (defining orbital orientation in space) as well as the spin quantum number. Note that the spin of an electron is not a rotational momentum in the classical Newtonian physics sense, but a quantum mechanics property, and for an electron is either ½ or −½ (often also referred to as up or down).

Also note that such orbital shape considerations are an approximation only, as they based on the description a system with only one electron, a so-called hydrogen-like atom, which apart of the hydrogen atom is not a realistic system, yet the overall concept is believed to stand even for more complex atoms than hydrogen (Figure 2.6).

Shells are numbered 1, 2, 3, 4, 5, 6, and 7. For historical reasons the first five shells in X-ray crystallography are referred to as K, L, M, N, and O. Orbitals are named as s-, p-, d-, and f-orbitals (based on early spectroscopy that described spectral lines of alkali metals as **s**harp, **p**rincipal, **d**iffuse and **f**undamental, respectively, with s-orbitals accommodating 2 electrons, p-orbitals 6 electrons, d-orbitals 10 electrons, and f-orbitals 14 electrons. The nomenclature used for orbitals is to name the shell and the orbital, with an exponent depicting the number of electrons in respective subshells, e.g., $2s^2$ means that two electrons occupy a s-type orbital in the second shell, likewise $2p^4$-orbitals means that four electrons fill a p-type orbital in the second shell.

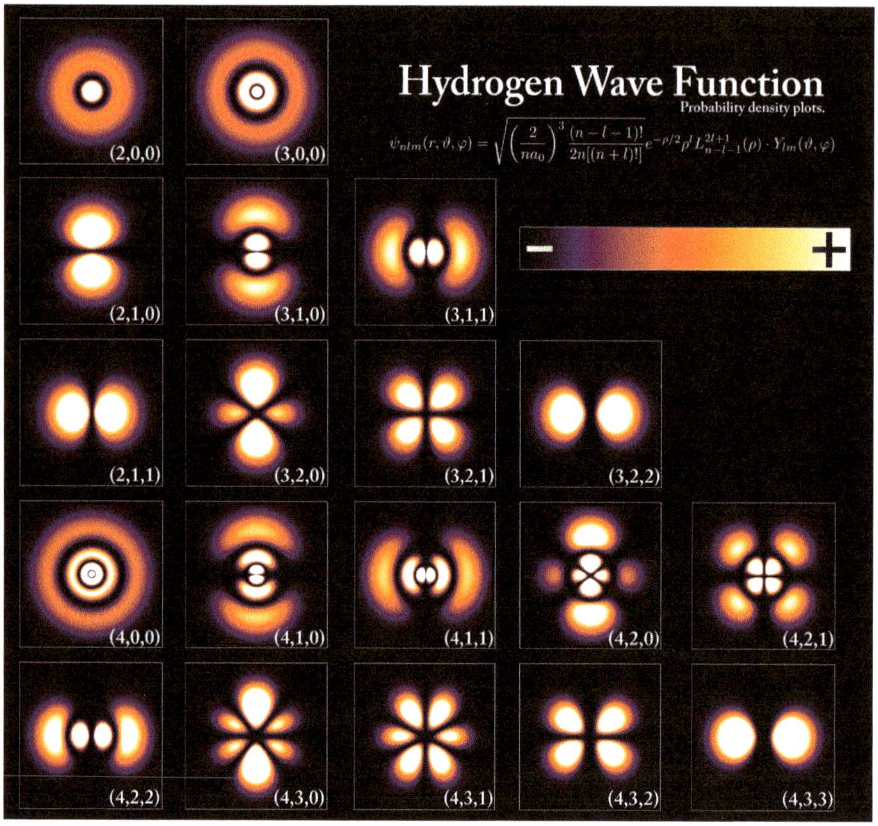

Figure 2.6 Electron cloud model/quantum mechanical model of the hydrogen atom. The commonly accepted atom model is based on quantum mechanics and assumes that electrons are matter waves, thus each electron can be considered a standing wave inside the atom. Electrons are no longer assumed to occupy an exact trajectory around the nucleus, and the exact position of an electron (in terms of being a particle) cannot be known. Instead, electrons reside with high probability in certain defined clouds, also known as shells and orbitals. The shape of the orbitals represents a solution for Schrödinger's equation describing electrons in the central electrical field of the nucleus. Four so-called quantum numbers are used for the description of an electron, namely the principal quantum number, the angular momentum quantum number, the magnetic quantum number, and the spin quantum number.
The principal quantum number (1–7) describes an energy level of an electron (and thus its average distance of that shell from the nucleus) in which the electron resides). It is equivalent to a shell in the classical Bohr model. The angular momentum quantum number (from 0 to 4) describes the shape of the orbitals (which are often referred to as s, p, d, f, and g-orbitals). The magnetic quantum number (−1, 0, +1) describes the orientation of the orbitals in space. The spin quantum number can have a value of −1/2 or +1/2. Two electrons occupying the same orbital must differ in their spin, which is also known as the Pauli exclusion principle. Shown here are cross-sections through the 3D-shapes of the orbitals (probability density plots) as calculated for a hydrogen atom. Bright areas indicate a high probability for an electron in the respective orbital. Note that beyond the second period with its s- and p-orbitals the shapes of d-, f-, and g-orbitals become rather complex. *Source:* PoorLeno / Wikimedia Commons / Public domain.

For the first (= the most inner) electron shell, there exists only one orbital, the so-called 1s-orbital, which can hold up to two electrons, for the second electron shell (which is on average further away from the nucleus than the first shell), in addition to the 2s-orbital there exist three 2p-orbitals, each of which can hold up to two electrons, bringing the total number of electrons the second shell can accommodate to 8. The third shell can accommodate a total of 18 electrons with 2 electrons residing in the 3s-orbital, 6 electrons in the 3p-orbitals, and 10 electrons in the d orbitals. From the 4th shell onward, there are additional f-orbitals that can accommodate up to 14 electrons (Figure 2.7).

For elements that have more than three shells, the energy of each of the shells and orbitals can overlap, resulting in lower energy orbitals from higher shells. For example, the 4s orbital has a lower energy and thus is filled before the 3d orbital. The order of how shells and orbitals are filled is as follows: 1s, 2s, 2p, 3s, 3p, 4s, 3d, 4p, 5s, 4d, 5p, 6s, 4f, 5d, 6p, 7s, 6d, 7p, 8s, 5g, 6f, 8p. Note that the chemical behavior of atoms corresponds to the outermost orbital that is (partially) filled with electrons. For a majority of biologically relevant elements, it is sufficient to focus on s- and p-orbitals and thus we neglect a discussion on d-, f-, and g-orbitals (Figure 2.8). Each orbital can only hold up to two electrons, with each electron of this resulting electron pair

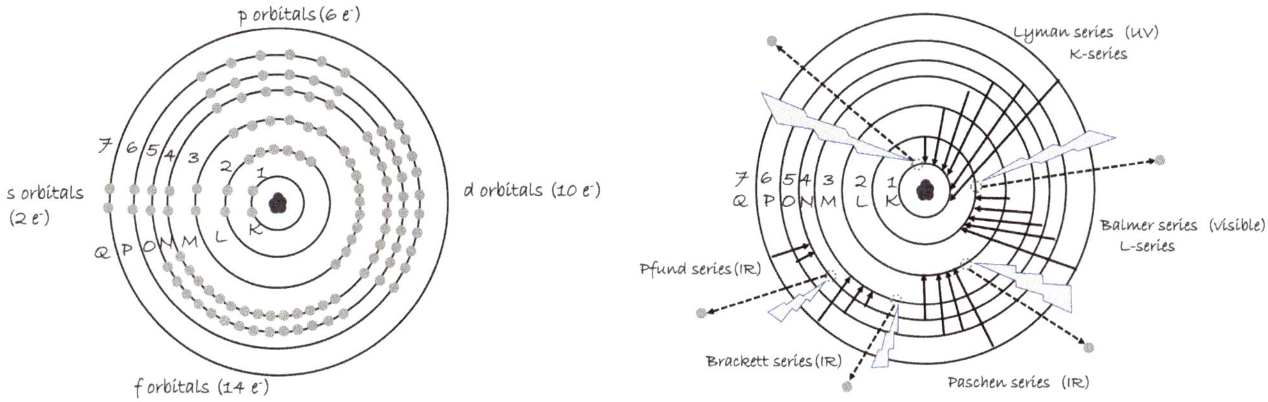

Figure 2.7 Maximal electron occupancy of shells in atoms and electron transitions from outer to inner shells. Left: The first shell can accommodate two electrons residing in the 1s orbital. The second shell can accommodate eight electrons, with two residing in the 2s orbital and six residing in the 2p-orbitals. The third shell can accommodate 18 electrons, with 2 residing in the 3s orbital, 6 residing in the 3p-orbitals and 10 residing in the 3d orbitals. From the 4th shell onward there exist f-orbitals, which can accommodate 14 electrons. Right: When electrons in inner shells are ejected due to high energy particle or high energy radiation, electrons from the outer shells transition to the inner shell, where they emit an element-specific and thus characteristic radiation in the UV range (Lyman-/K-series), visible light range (Balmer-/L-series) or IR range (Paschen-, Brackett-, or Pfund-series).

Figure 2.8 Atomic orbitals typical for biologically relevant elements such as carbon, nitrogen and oxygen, containing 1s, 2s and 2p orbitals.

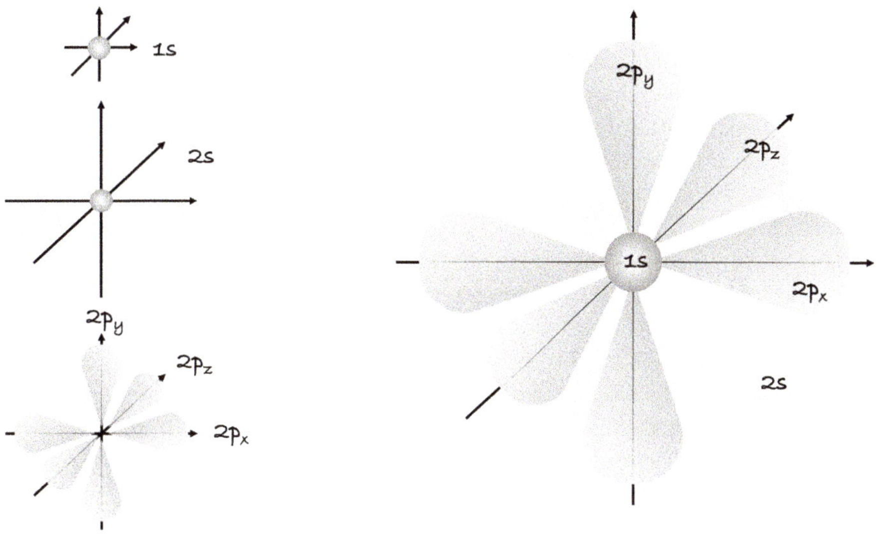

possessing a different spin. Figure 2.9 shows the orbital model and electron configuration for hydrogen, helium, carbon, nitrogen and oxygen atoms.

If high-energy radiation or high-energy particles knock out an electron from the inner shell, a vacancy in an inner shell is created that is filled with an electron from an outer shell that transitions from the outer shell into the lower-energy state of the inner shell. In the process of filling of the inner shell, a photon of characteristic energy and thus wavelength is emitted. For historical reasons such electron transitions are known as Lyman series (K-series) with photons being emitted in the UV light range, Balmer series (L-series) with photons being emitted in the visible light range, as well as Paschen-, Brackett-, and Pfund-series, with photons for these being emitted in the IR range (Figure 2.7).

The outermost electron shell of an atom is called the valence shell, and the electrons residing in this shell are referred to as valence electrons. The preferred state of an atom is to have either its valence shell empty or fully filled. Thus, alkali metals and alkaline-earth metals tend lose an electron, whereas halogens tend to gain electrons. They tend to become positively or negatively charged ions, respectively, which due to the electrostatic force attraction form an ion pair (ionic bond).

Noble gases, as their name implies, neither want to lose nor gain electrons and are therefore chemically inert (meaning that they tend not to react with other elements).

Elements like carbon on the other hand would need to lose four electrons to empty their valence shell, which would render them highly positively charged, or gain four

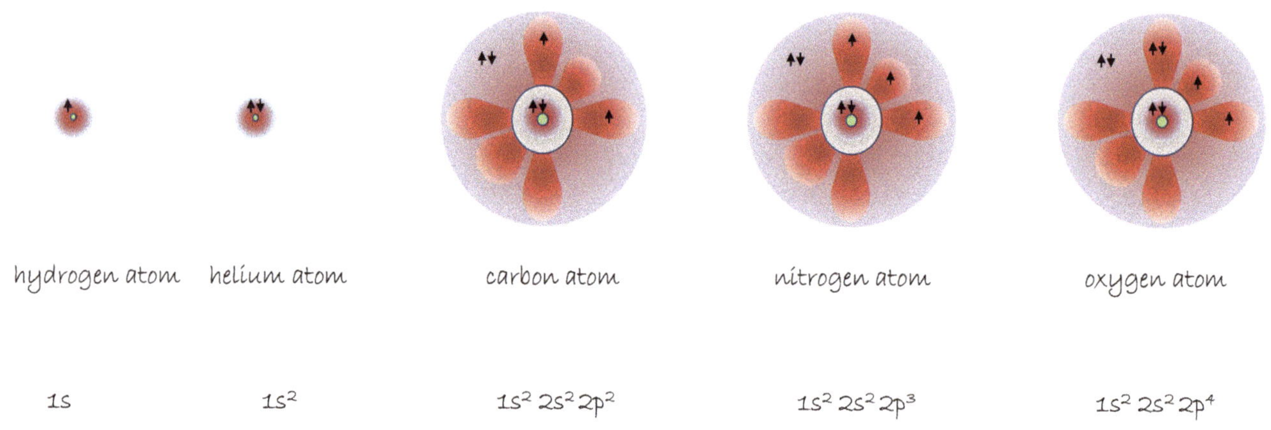

Figure 2.9 Electron configurations for several selected elements. The hydrogen atom is the simplest of all elements with only one electron, which resides in the 1s orbital. In the case of helium, two electrons differing only in spin occupy the 1s orbital. The carbon atom has two electrons in the 1s orbital, two electrons in the 2s orbital, and two electrons that occupy two of the three 2p orbitals. The nitrogen and oxygen atoms fill the 1s, 2s with two electrons each. Nitrogen has an additional electron for each of the three 2p orbitals, whereas oxygen fills one of the three 2p orbitals with two electrons and the other two with one electron.

electrons to fill their valence shell, which would render them highly negatively charged, neither of which is very likely to occur. Carbon therefore adopts a different strategy to fill its valence shell, namely by sharing its electrons with its partnering atoms and therefore forming covalent bonds. This leads to the formation of a group of atoms, known as molecules.

As will be discussed further in Section 2.1.6, each element is characterized by its electronegativity, a measure of an atom nucleus' ability to attract electron when sharing electrons in a covalent bond. When elements are organized into the periodic table of elements, electronegativity increases from the left to the right of the table and decreases from the top to the bottom. The difference in electronegativity of two atoms, linked by a covalent bond, leads to a higher probability of the two shared electrons to localize closer to the nucleus of the more electronegative atom. Such a bond is also called polar.

Hydrogen bonds exist between two different molecules, including but not restricted to water, where an electronegative partner such as oxygen or nitrogen in a molecule (being negatively polarized) forms a loose connection with a covalently bound hydrogen, that is typically in a polar covalent bond, and thus the hydrogen atom is positively polarized. Such hydrogen bonds are not as strong as covalent bonds but play an important role in the properties of water as a solvent and by stabilizing macromolecules (e.g., the tertiary structure of proteins).

In its electrically neutral state, the number of electrons in an atom matches the number of protons. Loss of electrons leads to ions, a process also known as ionization. Being ionized through either loss or additional uptake of an electron is the most abundant state for many elements, especially for alkali metals or halogens.

2.1.3 Periodic Table of Elements

The elements in the periodic table of elements are organized according to the principle of valency, with elements on the left-hand side tending to give off electrons to become cations, whereas elements near the right-hand side tending to accept electrons to become anions (Figure 2.10).

Emptying a partially occupied shell or filling shells to a maximum number of electrons are energetically favorable states, which defines the reactivity of elements. Alkali metals are likely to empty their most outer s-orbital and thus to lose electrons, whereas halogens like to receive electrons to fill their p-orbitals. Noble gases – at the very right-hand side of the periodic table – have their valence shell filled and thus are chemically inert (hence the name "noble gases").

While giving up or taking up one or two electrons is comparatively easy, elements such as carbon that either need to take up or lose four electrons to empty or fill their valence shell find it hard to do so: As the atoms is becoming ionized, the increasing electric charge makes the loss or uptake of additional electrons more difficult. Hence, rather than losing or receiving an electron, they fill up their valency by sharing the electrons with another atom to form a covalent chemical bond.

The magnetic moments of paired electrons cancel each other out, only when there is an odd number of electrons, and thus unpaired electrons, atoms display an overall magnetic moment. When orbitals of neighboring atoms overlap, spins can align with one another to form a lower

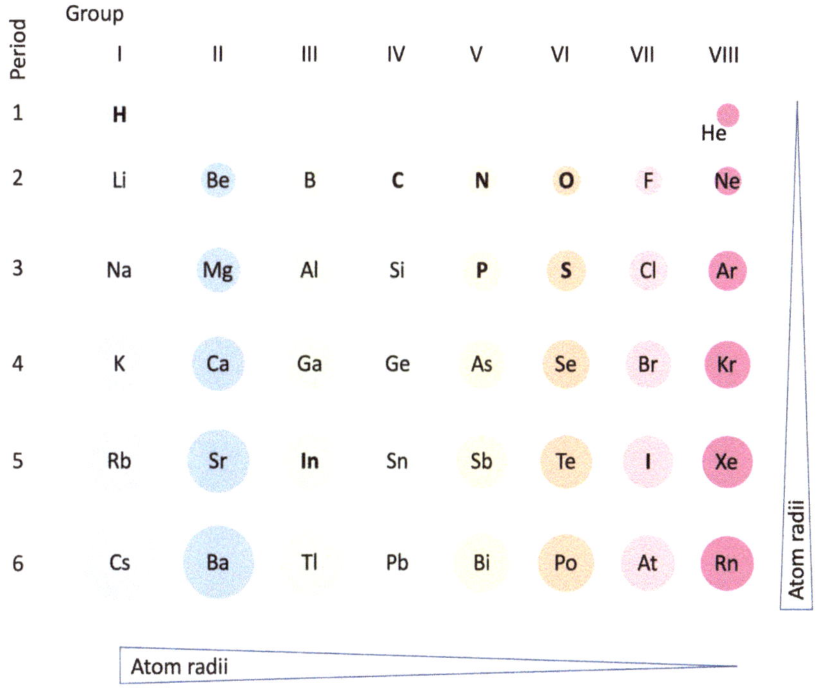

Figure 2.10 Periodic table of elements (excluding transition elements and rare earth elements). Elements are organized according to the principle of valency. Elements in group I–III tend to give off electrons to empty their valency shell, whereas elements in group VI and VII tend to take up electrons to fill their valency shell. Within one group elements with a higher period number are larger in terms of atom radius than elements with a lower period number. Within one period the atom radii decrease from the left to the right.

energy state, which can produce a measurable field, as is the case for ferromagnetic elements such as iron, cobalt, and nickel. In the case of paramagnetic elements, the magnetic moments of the atoms are in random orientation but can line up in the presence of an external magnetic field.

2.1.4 Transitions of Electrons

For an atom, each orbital represents a unique energy level of the electrons. The transition of an electron to a different orbital (with a higher or lower energy state) results in either the emission of a photon (with the electron moving from a higher energy orbital to a lower energy orbital) or requires the absorption of a photon to reach a higher energy orbital. For each element, these energies are precisely defined and are the reason for discrete emission or absorption lines in an electromagnetic spectrum. The electrons in an atom can only adopt certain states defined by their shell number, their orbital number, and the spin. Thus, they occupy certain spaces in an atom, with each such space having a certain energy associated with it. To remove an electron from the atom, a certain amount of energy, usually stated in units of electron volts (eV), is needed, depending on what shell and orbital the electron was taken from. An electron bound to an atom in its lowest energy state is described to be in its ground state. If it is found at any higher energy state, the electron is referred to as being in an excited state.

Absorption of a photon with a suitable energy leads to the transitioning of the electron from its ground state to an excited state. Return to its ground state from one of the excited states results in the emission of a photon with an energy (and thus a wavelength) that reflects the difference in energy level between the excited state from which it transitioned to the ground state. Absorption of photons and emission of photons can be seen as dark or bright lines absorption or emission spectra, respectively (Figure 2.11).

An electron in an excited state can also transition to a lower energy state upon interaction with a photon whose energy matches the energy difference between the excited and a lower energy state. This is called stimulated emission and leads to synchronized photons (of matching phases), which is the foundation of modern laser technology as well as of stimulated emission depletion microscopy.

2.1.5 Molecular Orbitals

Molecular orbitals are analogous to atomic orbitals and describe the space where the electrons between two bond-forming atoms are likely to reside. In the case of the carbon atom electrons will be shared between atoms. Instead of having the 2s orbital being filled with two electrons and, two of the three 2p-orbitals having one electron and one 2p-orbital being devoid of electrons, the carbon atoms can hybridize its 2s- and all three 2p-orbitals into four equivalent sp^3-orbitals. These sp^3-orbitals allow carbon to bind to four other atoms, such as for example hydrogen to form the molecule methane. The four orbitals arrange into a tetrahedral shape with an angle between each orbital of 109.5°.

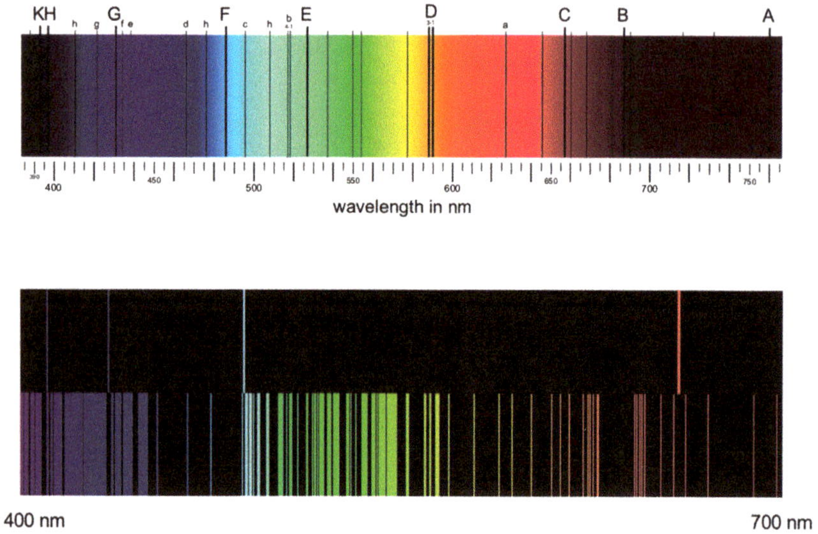

Figure 2.11 Atomic absorption and emission spectra. Top: Solar spectrum with Fraunhofer lines as an example of an absorption spectrum. Bottom: Emission spectrum of a hydrogen atom, showing only two lines, and an iron atom, showing many lines.

When other carbon atoms are the binding partners, long chain molecules can be formed, which is the foundation of organic chemistry. In addition to sp^3-hybridization, there is also the possibility for sp^2-hybridization and sp-hybridization. In sp^2-hybridization, one 2s-orbital and two of the three 2p-orbitals are combined into three sp^2-orbitals that form a plane with a 120° angle between the three sp^2-orbitals. The remaining 2p orbital is orthogonal to this plane. In the case of the sp-hybridization, one 2s-orbital and one 2p-orbital are combined into two sp-orbitals that are arranged linearly with an angle of 180° between the two sp-orbitals. The remaining two 2p-orbitals stand orthogonal to the axis defined by the two sp-orbitals (Figure 2.12).

2.1.6 Forces and Bonds Between Neighboring Atoms

Covalent Bonding

In a covalent bond, a pair of electrons is shared between neighboring atoms in a molecule. Typically, the formation of covalent bonds allows each of the atoms in the bond to attain a full valence shell and thus to achieve a stable electronic configuration. Covalent are particularly of interest

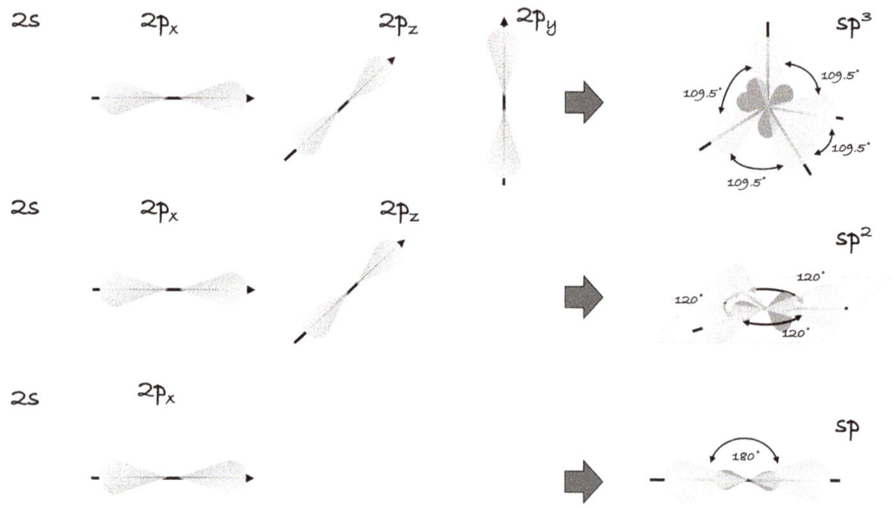

Figure 2.12 Molecular orbitals of carbon: sp^3-, sp^2-, sp-hybridization. In the case of sp^3-hybridization, one 2s-orbital combines with three 2p-orbitals into four equivalent sp^3-orbitals that are organized into a tetrahedron, with an angle of 109.5°; In sp^2-hybridization one 2s-orbital and two 2p-orbitals are hybridized, resulting in three sp^2-orbitals that are organized in a plane, with an angle of 120° between of them as well as one 2p-orbital; For sp-hybridization one 2s and one 2p orbitals are hybridized, with an angle between the two sp-orbitals being 180°. In this scenario, two additional 2p-orbitals are available for molecular bond generation.

in organic chemistry and thus in most of biochemistry, whereas ionic bonding being mostly found in inorganic chemistry (although charge–charge interactions can also play a role in biochemistry).

The bonds between atomic orbitals are termed by the Greek letters of the orbitals involved, hence a bond, forming between two sp^3-, sp^2-, or sp-orbitals, is a sigma-bond (σ-bond), whereas a bond between two p-orbitals is a pi-bond (π-bond). Double bonds contain one sigma-bond and one pi-bond, whereas triple bonds contain one sigma-bond and two pi-bonds (Figure 2.13). Pi-bonds are weaker than sigma bonds because the electrons in a pi-bond only overlap laterally, thus covalent sigma bonds are more stable. If double and single bonds alternate, one speaks of a conjugated pi-system, which is also called aromatic if the resulting structure is ring-like (Figure 2.14).

In conjugated pi-systems electrons are delocalized, which is of relevance in the context of fluorescence. Also, some molecules are charged (e.g., in a pH-dependent manner) and such charge can be stabilized via conjugated pi-electron systems. Some bonds such as hydrogen–oxygen or hydrogen–nitrogen bonds are polarized with the electrons having a higher probability to be found near the oxygen or nitrogen atom rather than near the carbon or the hydrogen atom, which leads to molecular dipoles (Figure 2.15).

Ion–Dipole and Dipole–Dipole Bonding

Ion–dipole interactions are stronger whereas dipole–dipole interactions are typically weaker than hydrogen bonding. As the name implies, forces occur either between ions and dipoles or between two dipoles, respectively.

Hydrogen Bonding

Hydrogen bonds are a form of dipole–dipole bond and occur between a hydrogen atom (being covalently linked to either nitrogen or oxygen) and another nitrogen or oxygen atom with a free electron pair (Figure 2.15). The nitrogen or oxygen are partially negatively charged (polarized), meaning that the electrons of the covalent bond with hydrogen have a higher probability to be found near the nitrogen or oxygen atom.

As the hydrogen atom is positively polarized, it seeks the presence of another electron pair, e.g., from a nitrogen or oxygen atom of a neighboring molecule. Hydrogen bonds are relatively strong, but weaker than covalent or ionic bonds. Hydrogen bonding is not only relevant for the physical properties of water (including its boiling point), but also play a significant role in the secondary, tertiary and quaternary structure of proteins, nucleic acids and other polymers.

Ionic Bonds

Ionic bonds are also referred to as salt bridges. They are the non-covalent interaction of atoms due to electrostatic forces between cations and anions. Ionic interactions are the strongest of all interactions between atoms or molecules. In a sense, ionic bonds are not really bonds as no electrons are shared between the anions and cations (Figure 2.15).

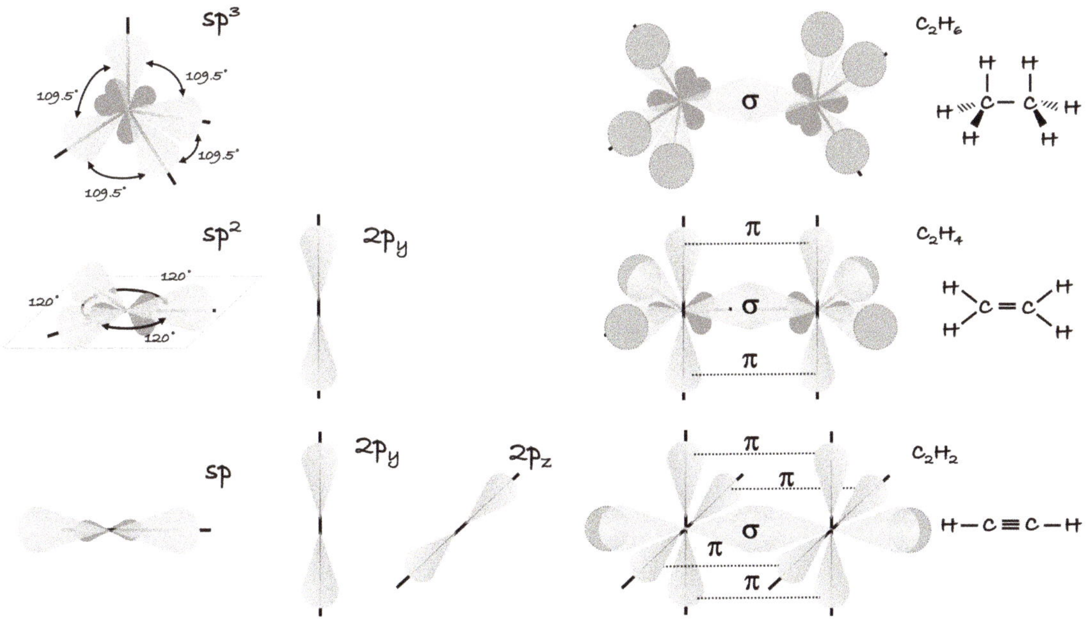

Figure 2.13 Covalent bonds – Sigma and pi-bonds. Covalent sigma-bonds are formed between s, sp^3-, sp^2-, or sp-hybrid orbitals, whereas pi-bonds are formed between adjacent p-orbitals. The combination of one sigma-bond and one pi-bond, or one sigma-bond and two pi-bonds are called double-bonds or triple-bonds, respectively.

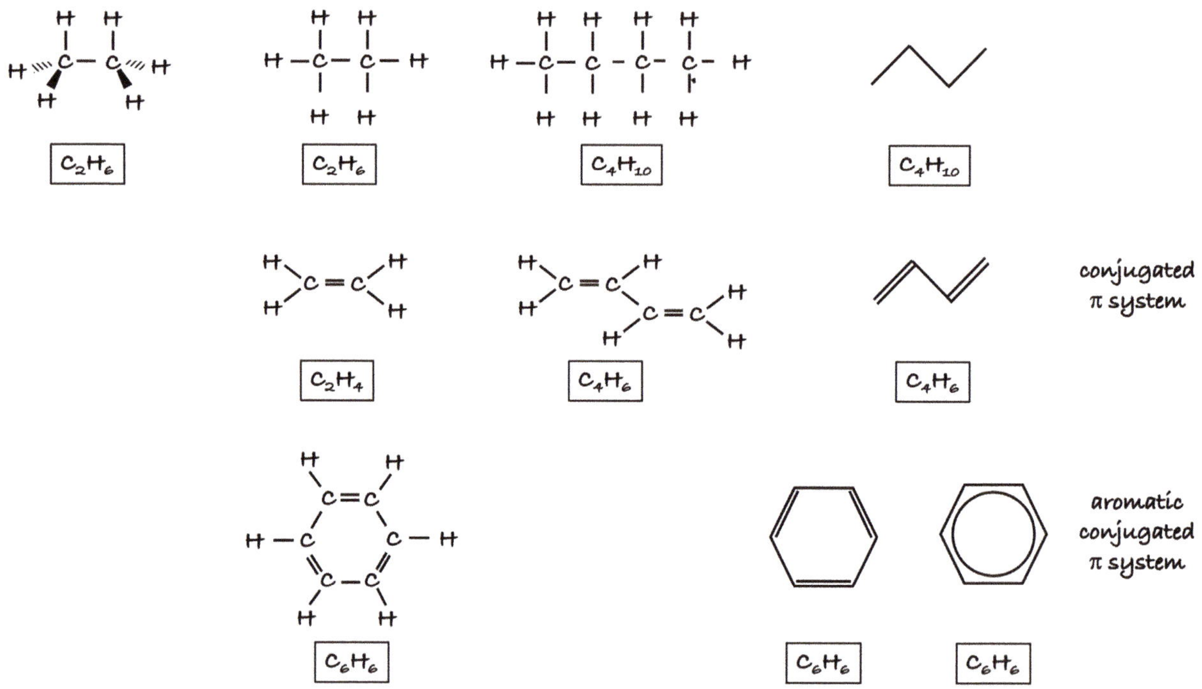

Figure 2.14 Molecular bonds in organic chemistry and conjugated pi-systems. There are different ways how the primary chemical structure can be shown: The chemical structure formula can depict the atoms as letters with bonds as lines between these letters. This may include an indication of the sterical configuration (see top left). Alternatively, the chemical structure formula depicts atoms as letters (e.g., C, H) on a flat two-dimensional plane without indication of the sterical configuration, with the type of chemical bond (e.g., single bond, double bond) in between the atoms being depicted as single or double lines (see middle section). An alternative is an abstracted version where carbon and hydrogen atoms are no longer explicitly depicted as letters, but instead carbon atoms implicit as hinges/corners of a set of lines. Hydrogen atoms are also implicit, and they are assumed to fill in all "free" valences. Conjugated pi-systems are characterized by alternating single and double-bonds. If such conjugated pi-systems exist as a ring-structure one speaks of aromatic conjugated pi-systems. The alternating double and single bonds are often replaced by a circle inside the polygon indicating that the electrons are distributed over the entire ring structure of the aromatic molecule.

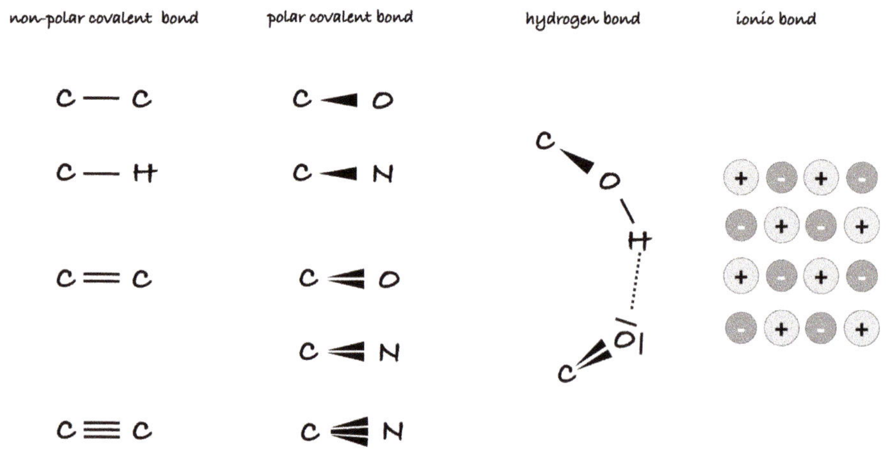

Figure 2.15 Non-polar, polar, hydrogen-, and ionic bonds. Carbon–carbon and carbon–hydrogen bonds are non-polar covalent bonds, with electrons being equally shared by the neighboring atom nuclei, whereas covalent bonds between carbon or hydrogen atoms and oxygen or nitrogen atoms are polarized, with the electrons residing closer to the electronegative oxygen or nitrogen atoms than to carbon or hydrogen atoms. Hydrogen-bonds form between the hydrogen atom of a hydroxyl- or an amine-group and the oxygen of a carbonyl group. Of course, the classical hydrogen bond exists between water molecules. Electrostatic forces are the foundation of ionic bonds between cations and anions.

Van-der-Waals Forces

Van-der-Waals forces are often used as a summary term, and include the Keesom-, Debye-, and London-dispersion forces. They are weak forces of attraction between uncharged molecules, due to correlations in the fluctuating polarizations (transient shift in electron density) of nearby particles. These intermolecular forces are short-range, thus only nearest neighbors need to be considered.

Hydrophobic Effect

The hydrophobic ("water-fearing") effect is a term used to describe the tendency of nonpolar molecules to aggregate in an aqueous solution. Separation of non-polar molecules from water and the resulting aggregate formation minimizes contact between water molecules and nonpolar molecules, while maximizing hydrogen bonding between water molecules. It is often argued that the hydrophobic effect is an entropic effect, with nonpolar molecules disrupting hydrogen bonding between the liquid water.

2.2 Electromagnetic Spectrum

The electromagnetic spectrum refers to the continuous range of frequencies of electromagnetic radiation, with the electromagnetic force being carried by photons. Each photon is characterized by its energy, corresponding to the frequency of its wave function and thus by its wavelength, which can vary from a fraction of the size of the atomic nucleus to hundreds of meters. Short-wavelength (high-frequency) photons (such as gamma-rays and X-rays) possess high energy, whereas long-wavelength (low-frequency) photons (such as microwaves and radio waves) are low in energy. The continuous spectrum historically has been divided into separate bands. Each of these bands is different in terms of photon characteristics, mode of photon generation, interaction with matter and thus its respective application in bioimaging (Figure 2.16).

The longest known and by far the most studied band is the visible light band, dating back to the ancient Greeks, who knew that light traveled in straight lines and were aware of reflection and refraction of light. By the 17th century, there were conflicting theories with respect to the nature of light, as some experiments suggested light acted as particles whereas others suggested light acted as waves. This discrepancy was later reconciled in the wave-particle duality of light, which states that photons, depending on the experiment they are subjected to, behave either as particles or as waves.

Infrared light was discovered in 1800 by William Herschel, when using a thermometer he measured the temperature of different light colors of light, split by a glass prism. He found that the region beyond red (i.e., the infrared region), which is not visible to the naked eye, was the hottest of all regions examined.

Working on the other end of the visible light band, Johann Ritter noticed in 1801 that light rays, behaving similarly to visible violet light but being beyond the visible spectrum, were able to cause chemical reactions. This radiation was later named ultraviolet radiation.

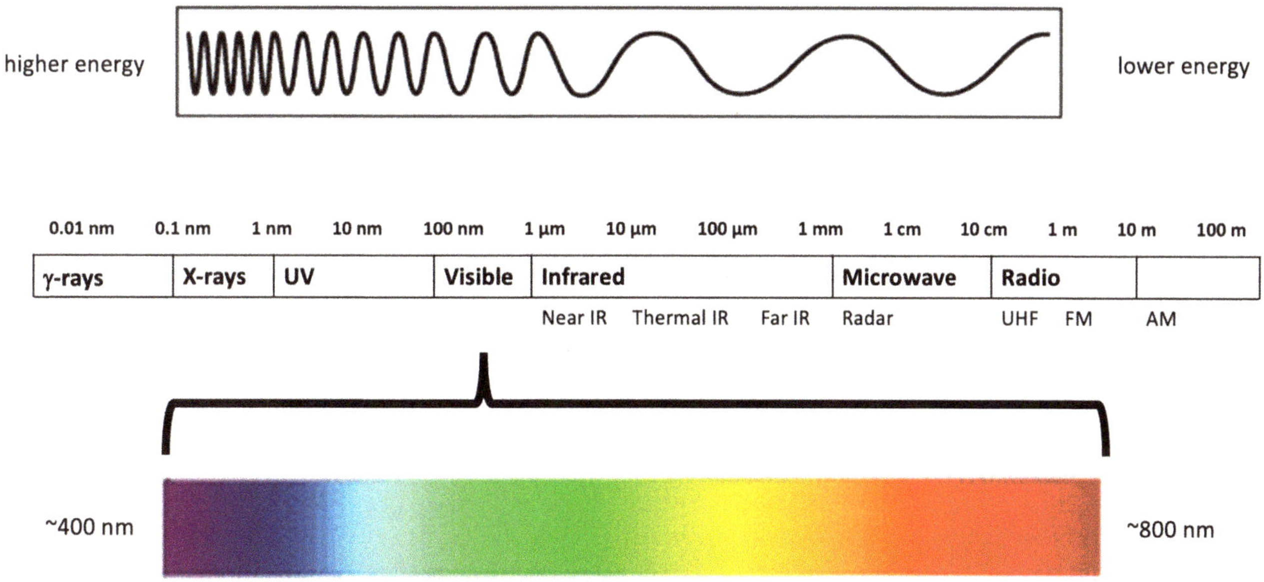

Figure 2.16 Electromagnetic spectrum. The electromagnetic spectrum ranges from gamma-rays (short wavelength/high frequency/high energy) to radio waves (long wavelength/low frequency/low energy). Photons in the visible range from violet/blue to red are at the center of optical microscopy.

After Michael Faraday realized in 1845 that light responded to a magnetic field, and James Maxwell in the 1860s developed a mathematical description of electromagnetism, it became clear that light itself was just one type of electromagnetic radiation, and that there would be radiation beyond the infrared, which could be created by oscillating charges in an electrical circuit. In 1886, Heinrich Hertz built such an apparatus to first generate radio waves and later microwaves and showed that radio waves, like light, could be reflected and refracted by dielectric media, which paved the way for modern telecommunication.

X-rays were discovered in 1895 by Wilhelm Röntgen, who noticed a new type of radiation emitted by an evacuated tube subjected to a high voltage, and called it X-rays. These rays can penetrate parts of the human body. They are reflected or absorbed by denser matter such as bones, a discovery that ultimately led to the use of X-ray for radiography.

The last missing part of the electromagnetic spectrum was discovered in 1900 by Paul Villard, who studied radioactive emission of radium. He examined what he first thought to be radiation being like the known alpha and beta particles, but he noticed that this new radiation was able to penetrate matter even more. This new form of radiation was named gamma rays in 1903 by Ernest Rutherford. In 1910 William Henry Bragg showed that gamma rays did not consist of particles but were a form of electromagnetic radiation. In 1914 Ernest Rutherford and Edward Andrade measured the wavelengths of gamma rays and showed that gamma rays were like X-rays but displayed even shorter wavelength (higher frequencies).

It should be clear by now that the different names for each band of the continuous electromagnetic spectrum are largely a consequence of the historical discovery of each band. The difference in name of each band reflects how photons in these different bands interact with matter in different ways, courtesy of the different energies they carry. This will be discussed in more detail in Section 2.3 of this chapter that deals with the interaction of radiation with matter. Briefly, gamma rays, X-rays and hard ultraviolet light are classified as ionizing radiation since they are capable of knocking electrons off atoms, creating reactive ion species that can damage chemical and thus biological material. Radio waves on the other end of the electromagnetic spectrum are relatively low in energy and are considered a non-invasive way to investigate biological systems. Microwave radiation leads to molecular rotation, near infrared light causes molecular vibration, whereas photons from the visible light band are linked to electron transitions in molecules.

There are no sharp boundaries between the bands of the electromagnetic spectrum, instead the spectrum is quantitatively continuous, yet it has proven practical to treat each band of the spectrum separately. Photons in the boundary zones show characteristics associated with each of its neighboring band. Both particle and electromagnetic radiation are used for imaging of biological samples (see Figure 2.17).

2.2.1 Gamma Rays

Photons in the gamma ray band are the most energetic with a very high penetration ability. The distinction between hard X-rays and gamma rays is founded in part on how the radiation is generated, with radiation originating from decay of atomic nuclei being termed gamma-rays, whereas X-rays are emitted during transition of highly energetic inner shell atomic electrons. Gamma rays are produced by a number of radioisotopes, and play a diagnostic role in nuclear medicine, such as in Positron Emission Tomography (PET) imaging, or as a therapeutic in radiation cancer therapy.

2.2.2 X-Rays

X-ray is the band of the electromagnetic spectrum between gamma-rays and hard ultraviolet light, and like its direct neighboring band regions, X-ray radiation ionizes atoms and molecules by ejecting electrons from the atoms. X-ray photons can also interact with matter by Compton scattering, a form of inelastic scattering interaction of the photon with a charged particle like an electron, where the photon initially deposits its energy into the electron before the recoiling electron emits another X-ray photon of slightly lower energy. Hard X-rays can penetrate many materials without significant absorption, a phenomenon that is used as a diagnostic tool in medicine (radiography).

2.2.3 Ultraviolet Radiation

Ultraviolet (UV) radiation is the band between soft X-ray and visible light bands. Like gamma-rays and X-rays, hard UV light can ionize atoms. The boundary of ionization is not sharply defined in the UV band, as different atoms and different molecules are ionized at different energies. However, even though longer-wavelength UV radiation does not possess ionizing capabilities, it still can directly damage biochemical molecules and cause mutations in the DNA molecules.

2.2.4 Visible Light

The visible light band is the band between ultraviolet (UV) radiation and infrared (IR) light bands. As the name implies, visible light is the part of the electromagnetic spectrum (typically ~380 to ~760 nm) that can be detected by the

type of radiation	wavelength	energy (eV)	major field of application for bioimaging
leptons			
electron	~1 nm	~1	
electron	~0.04 nm	~10^4	electron microscopy (EM)
electron	~0.004 nm	~10^5	electron microscopy (EM)
positron	~1 nm	~1	positron emission tomography (PET)
baryons			
proton	~0.03 nm	~1	
proton	~0.0003 nm	~10^4	
proton	~0.0001 nm	~10^5	
neutron (thermal)	~0.2 nm	~10^{-2}	small angle neutron scattering (SANS)
neutron (fast)	~0.00003 nm	~10^5–10^6	
hadrons			
helium-ion	~0.02 nm	~1	
helium-ion	~0.0002 nm	~10^4	helium ion microscopy (HeIM)
helium-ion	~0.00004 nm	~10^5	
bosons (photons)			
gamma-rays	0.003–0.03 nm	~10^4–10^9	positron emission tomography (PET)
X-rays	0.03–10 nm	~10^2–10^4	X-ray crystallography Small Angle X-ray Scattering (SAXS) X-ray microscopy (XRM) computed tomography (CT, CAT)
ultraviolet	10–400 nm	~3.1–10^2	
visible	400–750 nm	~1.7 –3.1	optical light microscopy (LM) fluorescence microscopy (FLM) Raman micro(spectro)scopy bioluminescence
near infrared	750–1.3 μm	~1.2 –1.7	near-infrared (near-IR) microscopy
infrared	1.3–100 μm	~10^{-2}–1.2	infrared (IR) microscopy
microwave	100 μm to 10 cm	~10^{-5}–10^{-2}	
radio wave	10 cm to 300 m	~10^{-9}–10^{-5}	nuclear magnetic resonance (NMR) spectroscopy magnetic resonance imaging (MRI)

Figure 2.17 Use of particle radiation and photons in bioimaging. One distinguishes particle radiation including electron, positrons, proton, neutrons, and atomic ions from electromagnetic radiation with photons ranging in wavelength from gamma-rays to radio waves.

human eye. Visible light is absorbed and emitted when electrons move from one energy level to another in atoms and molecules. This part of the spectrum has been explored for imaging for a long time, and all forms of optical microscopy are using this band of the electromagnetic spectrum. Light with a wavelength just above 760 nm is often referred to near-IR.

2.2.5 Infrared Radiation

The infrared (IR) band is the band between the visible light and the microwave bands. IR is the part of the electromagnetic spectrum between 750 nm and 1000 μm/1 mm and is typically divided into three parts: near IR 750 nm to 2,500 nm/2.5 μm, mid-IR 2.5–10 μm, and far-IR (10 μm to 1,000 μm/1 mm). Near-IR is similar to visible light and can be detected by photographic film or solid-state image detectors. Near-IR is also relevant in terms of two-photon fluorescent light microscopy. Mid-IR radiation is what we would consider as heat emitted from a hot object (also known as a black-body radiator) or human skin. Since mid-IR is absorbed by molecular vibrations around their equilibrium position, the mid-IR range is relevant for identification of molecules and used in IR microscopy, as many molecules have their own characteristic spectral fingerprint of absorption. The far-IR is closer in its physical behavior to microwaves, and often this region is also referred to as terahertz radiation or as sub-millimeter radiation. It is absorbed by so-called rotational modes of molecules in their gaseous phase or by motions of molecules in their liquid phase, and does not play a significant role in bioimaging.

2.2.6 Microwave Radiation

The microwave radiation band is the band of the electromagnetic spectrum between the infrared and radio wave bands, ranging from 1 mm to 10 cm. They are absorbed by polar molecules (such as water) through vibrational and rotational modes. Microwaves unlike IR penetrates deep into materials, where they cause heating of the material such as water. Microwaves are not used for imaging of biological samples, but can be useful in sample preparation as short exposure to low-power microwave radiation can speed up the diffusion process for penetration of tissues by chemical fixatives or heavy metal stains.

2.2.7 Radio Wave Radiation

The radio wave radiation band is at the low-energy/long-wavelength end of the electromagnetic spectrum ranging from 10 cm to hundreds of meters. Radio waves are widely useful in telecommunication. In terms of biological imaging, radio frequencies are used by nuclear magnetic resonance (NMR) spectroscopy and magnetic resonance imaging (MRI), as the radio waves can probe the intrinsic spin properties of atomic nuclei, and thus influence transitions between nuclear energy levels via resonance phenomena.

2.3 Interaction of Radiation with Matter

When electromagnetic radiation interacts with matter, photons can transfer their energy to electrons residing in atoms and molecules or to atoms' nuclei. The wave-particle duality says that both particles (such as electrons, atoms, or molecules) and photons have particle-like and wave-like properties. In 1924, Louis-Victor de Broglie formulated a hypothesis that all matter exhibit wave-like properties, including a wavelength and momentum, for which he was awarded the Nobel Prize in Physics in 1929. His hypothesis was substantiated by subsequent experiments by George Paget Thomson and Clinton Joseph Davisson, for which they were awarded the 1937 Nobel Prize in Physics.

The interaction of photons/particles with matter depends on the energy they carry (such as frequency/wavelength or momentum) (Figure 2.18).

2.3.1 High-Energy Photons

Absorption of high energy gamma rays can lead to an instability of the nucleus, which disintegrates in a radioactive decay and emits electron, positrons, neutrons, protons, or alpha particles (helium nuclei). Also, high-energy X-ray photons (with an energy greater than 1 MeV) can form a pair of an electron and a positron near a nucleus. However, photodisintegration and pair production do not play any significant role for imaging of biological samples and will not be discussed further.

When photons with a high-enough energy, such as gamma rays, X-rays, and hard UV rays, interact with an electron, they can transfer their energy to the electron, which in turn can be ejected from its host atom, leaving behind a positively charged atom or molecule, in a process called photoionization. A certain amount of energy (also known as the binding energy) is needed to eject the electron, the remainder of the energy photon contributes to the kinetic energy of the ejected electron.

The process where an electron is ejected from a metal surface (or any other material surface) due to the bombardment with photons is called the photoelectric effect. It is important to notice that a low intensity (few photons) of short-wavelength (blue) photons leads to ionization of the metal, whereas even a high intensity of longer-wavelength (red) photons fail to do so. Hence, the incoming photon must possess a threshold energy to eject electrons from the surface of certain metals. Higher intensity of photon irradiation (with appropriate frequency) simply increases the number of electrons being ejected but does not affect their energy.

Building on Max Planck's hypothesis that the energy carried by electromagnetic waves could only be released in packets of energy, Albert Einstein theorized in 1905 that the energy in each quantum of light was proportional to its frequency. The proportionality constant was later called Planck's constant. Einstein's theory could explain experimental data collected for many years by several physicists and was a key step in the development of quantum mechanics.

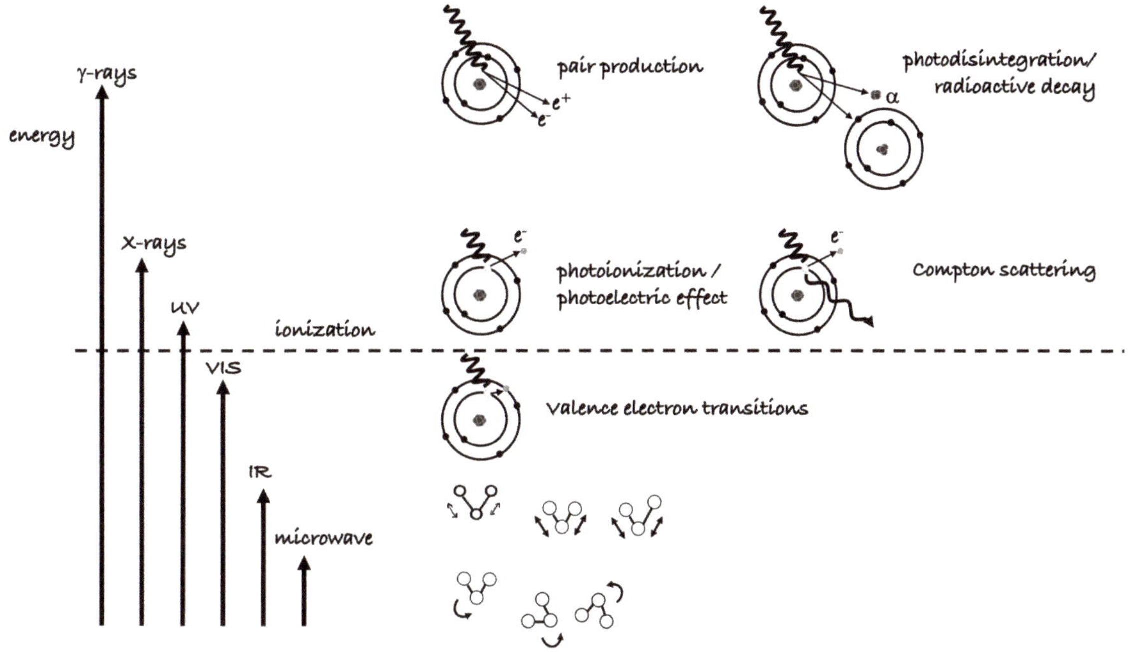

Figure 2.18 Interaction of electromagnetic radiation with matter. Gamma-ray bombardment can lead to electron–positron pair production in the vicinity of an atom's nucleus or to radioactive decay (photodisintegration). X-ray bombardment can lead to photoionization (photoelectric effect) and to Compton scattering. Visible light interacting with matter results in valence electron transitions, whereas IR and microwave radiation lead to changes in the vibrational and rotational state of molecules.

Hence, it was the energy (and hence the frequency/wavelength) of the photon that determined its ability to eject the electrons. Einstein's theory was further experimentally supported in 1914 by Robert Millikan. The study of the photoelectric effect was an important milestone in physics, as it was strong evidence for the dual wave-particle nature of light. For their theoretical and experimental work on the photoelectric effect, Albert Einstein was awarded the Physics Nobel Prize in 1921 "for his services to Theoretical Physics, and especially for his discovery of the law of the photoelectric effect" and Robert Millikan in 1923, for "his work on the elementary charge of electricity and on the photoelectric effect."

The photoelectric effect also plays an important role in photomultiplier detector technology for biological imaging.

Yet another mode of interaction of high-energy X-rays with matter is Compton scattering, a form of inelastic scattering, where the incoming photon deposits its energy into an electron, which in turn emits a photon, although at a slightly lower energy/longer wavelength. The remainder of the energy goes to the recoil of the electron.

2.3.2 High-Energy Particles

Free electrons are created when particles of sufficient energy (e.g., electrons or ions) hit the surface of a metal (or other material) in a vacuum tube (secondary emission). The emission of secondary electrons is important in the function of photomultiplier tubes and image intensifier tubes, and thus in the field of detector technology, but also plays a major role also for scanning electron/ion microscopy imaging.

"Bremsstrahlung" (X-ray radiation) is produced when charged particles are deflected or when an electron is being decelerated by an atomic nucleus. Such events result in the emission of photons that reflect the energy difference of incoming and decelerated particle. This process is the basis of X-ray generation in laboratory sources, like the rotating anodes, which is widely used for X-ray crystallography. In a broader sense, "Bremsstrahlung" is also produced when high energy (high velocity) particles (e.g., accelerated electrons) are forced by a magnetic field to alter their trajectory, resulting in a broad spectrum of high-intensity radiation, like that found at cyclotrons and synchrotrons.

2.3.3 Middle-Energy Photons

The inner photoelectric effect (also referred to as internal photoelectric effect) refers to a process where lower-energy photons (e.g., in the energy range of visible light) hit a suitable semiconductor material, which leads to the excitation of an electron from the valence band to the conduction band, and to the internal generation of an electron/hole pair, increasing the conductivity of the semiconductor.

This process is of importance in semiconductor-based detector technology, such as CMOS or CCD technology, which will be discussed in detail in Section 5.6.5.

Absorption

Absorption is the process by which matter (typically electrons being part of atoms or molecules) take up electromagnetic radiation, and are elevated to a higher energy level, from which they either return to a lower energy level either by emitting photons (as is the case in fluorescence) or by transforming their energy into internal energy (such as thermal energy, i.e., heat).

Attenuation (in the context of imaging) is the gradual loss of flux intensity of light propagating through a medium, viewed from a macroscopic perspective.

Absorption of photons occurs in a molecule (i.e., a chromophore) often by a conjugated pi-bond system, with alternating single and double bonds or aromatic ring systems. Absorption of a photon in the visible light range, leads to the perception of color, with the portion of light that was not absorbed being reflected or scattered.

Fluorescence

Fluorescence is the emission of longer-wavelength (lower-energy) photons (typically in the visible light range) by a molecule after it has absorbed photons of shorter wavelength (higher energy). Fluorescing molecules (fluorophores) stop emitting photons immediately (within nanoseconds) after the fluorophores are no longer irradiated. In the case of phosphorescence, light continues to be emitted for some time (up to minutes or hours) after irradiation stops. The underlying mechanism for phosphorescence are crystal defects, as they trap and store the energy for a longer period. The process of phosphorescence is of some significance in bioimaging in the context of detector technology with the development and application of phosphor imaging plates.

Fluorescence will be discussed in more detail in Section 3.15. For fluorescence to occur, electrons inside atoms, molecules or other nanostructures first must absorb a photon, resulting in an excited state. That state may have multiple levels of energy, including vibrational energy. A fluorophore in such an excited state will relax to the lowest vibrational level of the excited state by transferring energy to the solvent (in form of heat) before it emits a photon of lower energy (longer wavelength) to return back to its ground state. This emission of light is known as fluorescence, and competes with other ways of energy transfer, including triplet state formation, transfer to another molecule (known as Förster resonance energy transfer or short Förster transfer), quenching (e.g., by molecular oxygen O_2), or internal conversion. The efficiency of fluorescence is given by the quantum yield, i.e., the ratio of emitted to absorbed photons, which is ≤ 1.

Apart from the above-mentioned organic molecules and inorganic nanostructures, in the 1980s (after their first discovery in 1962 in the jellyfish *Aequorea victoria*) genetically encoded fluorescent proteins emerged in the field of biology, typically in the form of a fusion protein, where a fluorescent protein is linked to the target protein of interest. The 2008 Nobel Prize in Chemistry was awarded to Osamu Shimomura, Martin Chalfie, and Roger Y. Tsien "for the discovery and development of the green fluorescent protein, GFP." GFP has been joined since by a large variety of fluorescent proteins with different colors and properties, including photo-switchable probes, which have helped to revolutionize diffraction-limited fluorescence light microscopic imaging and thus to develop modern "superresolution" optical imaging.

Bioluminescence

In bioluminescence, which is another biological process where light is being emitted, with the energy for the emission of light stemming from chemical processes rather than the absorption of a photon. There are also cases where both processes, bioluminescence and fluorescence go hand in hand, e.g., with the bioluminescence creating the light source for subsequent fluorescence.

Raman Scattering

Raman scattering is the inelastic scattering of photons by matter, due to the transmission of part of the energy of the photon to the photon-interacting molecule's vibrational state (Stokes Raman scattering), followed by the emission of a red-shifted (longer wavelength) photon.

2.3.4 Low-Energy Photons

Infrared imaging is based on the absorption of infrared photons, whose energy of near-IR or mid-IR, is transmitted to molecules, which respectively undergo a transition from a vibrational ground energy state of molecular bonds, resulting in stretching, bending, twisting. Infrared radiation absorbance is lower than for visible light but higher than for microwave radiation.

Absorption of microwaves in non-metals leads to excitation of quantum states of molecular rotation and to a torque of molecules that possess an electric dipole moment (e.g., water). Absorption of microwaves by metals leads to the generation of electrical currents, which in turn leads to rapid heating of the metal.

While radio waves are not directly absorbed by biomolecules, they can play an important role in bioimaging, e.g., when atomic nuclei of the molecules, aligning with a strong external magnetic field, can undergo magnetic resonance upon perturbation by a short pulse sequence. This is the underlying principle in nuclear magnetic resonance spectroscopy and magnetic resonance imaging. It is useful to discuss the interaction of the particles or photons first in macroscopic terms before we consider the actual interactions that occur at the atomic and molecular levels. A radiation beam interacting with matter either penetrates the medium, is absorbed by the medium, is reflected or refracted at the medium's boundary, is scattered by an objected or undergoes diffraction (Figure 2.19). Considering incoming wavefronts encountering a medium boundary is another macroscopic way to describe transmission, absorption, reflection and refraction (Figure 2.20).

Penetration/Absorption – A Macroscopic Perspective

Particle radiation consists of a stream of moving charged or neutral particles, including alpha particles (helium nuclei), beta particles (electrons, positrons), neutrons and ions of other chemical elements. Like electromagnetic radiation (photons), particle radiation shows wave-particle duality, meaning that in the interaction with matter, they show aspects of both corpuscle (particle) and wave-like behavior.

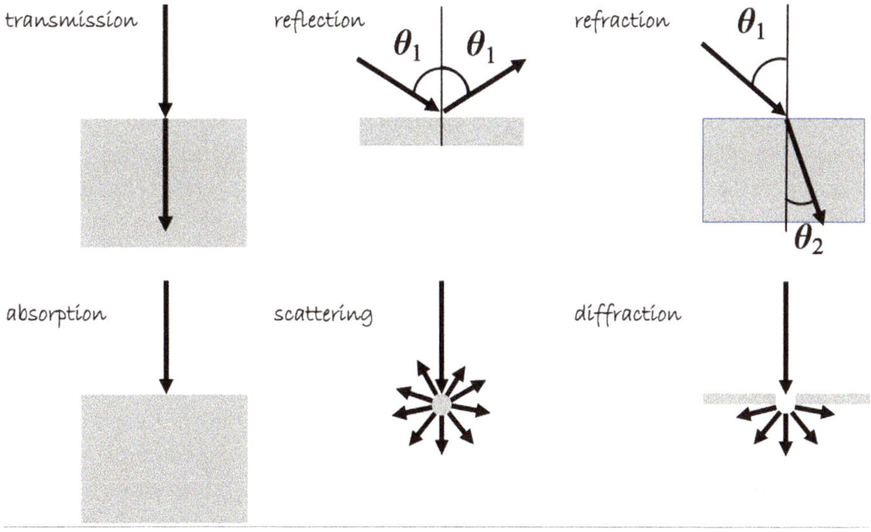

Figure 2.19 Macroscopic description of radiation interacting with matter. Using a macroscopic approach, a radiation beam can interact with matter in different ways: It is either transmitted, absorbed, reflected, refracted, scattered, or diffracted.

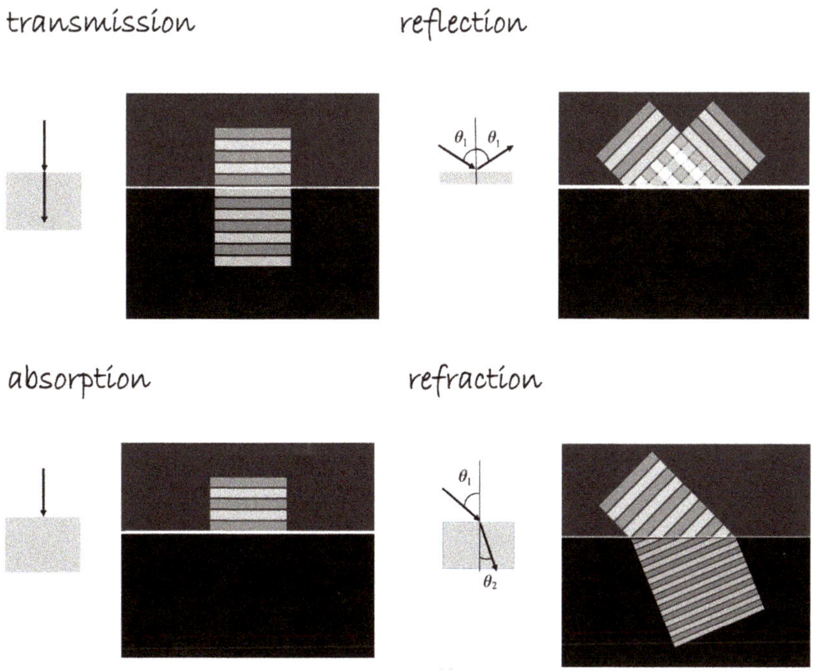

Figure 2.20 Behavior of a radiation wave front at a medium boundary. An incoming wave front is either transmitted at the medium boundary, absorbed at the medium boundary, reflected, or refracted at the medium boundary, with refraction altering the wavelength of the wave front.

According to the Lambert–Beer law, the intensity of the electromagnetic wave falls off exponentially when traveling through matter. The penetration depth is the distance in a material at which the incoming radiation is weakened to 1/e (~37%) of its original value. Absorption is the flip side of penetration and describes how the photon's energy is taken up by matter (typically by electrons in the atoms). For example, visible light traveling through matter may be absorbed and the energy dissipates and is given off as thermal energy. The absorbance of matter describes how much of the incoming light is transmitted/absorbed, reflected, or refracted.

One medically important example of absorbance is X-ray imaging (radiography), where different tissues (such as the calcium-rich bones) absorb more X-rays than tissue with high water content (or consisting predominantly of other light elements). Different materials absorb a certain radiation type differently, and certain parts of the electromagnetic spectrum are absorbed by a material more strongly than others, e.g., UV light is absorbed in sunglasses, whereas the visible and/or infrared light penetrates undisturbed.

Regarding particle radiation, alpha particles are the least penetrating and can be stopped by a piece of thin paper. Beta particles are absorbed by a few millimeters of aluminum or other low atomic weight materials such as plastic. Neutrons are highly penetrating as they need to be absorbed by atomic nuclei. Regarding electromagnetic radiation, gamma-rays and X-rays are the most penetrating and must be shielded by atoms with heavy nuclei, such as several centimeters of lead (Figure 2.21). UV light on the other hand, while being ionizing and thus damaging, can be easily shielded, e.g., by thin layers of sunscreen or fabric.

Absorption/Emission – A Quantum Mechanics Perspective

One of the key concepts to understand absorption and emission of photons by molecules is grounded in quantum mechanics and thus in the understanding that energy levels in atoms and molecules are quantized, meaning that changes of state by absorption or emission of photons reflect precise energies (wavelengths) of the absorbed/emitted photons.

Fluorescence can also be thought of as a form of inelastic scattering, where a molecule absorbs a photon to one of the excited states before it relaxes back to one of the ground states, emitting a photon of lower energy (longer wavelength) in the process.

Scattering

Scattering describes a physical process where a moving particle (e.g., an ion or an electron) or electromagnetic radiation (photons) does not follow a straight trajectory due to the interaction with a scattering center (scatterer). This is probably the most frequent interaction of particles or electromagnetic waves with matter (Figure 2.22).

There are different ways to think of scattering, some originating from a time, when quantum mechanics and atomic particle physics had not yet been developed. Instead, the phenomenon was described in more macroscopic terms, such as a scattering cross section, which is a measure of the probability of scattering to occur, usually given as the fraction of the irradiance power per area, a free mean path, which is a description of an average distance over which a moving particle substantially changes its direction or energy, e.g., as a result of collision(s) with other particles, or attenuation coefficient, which is a

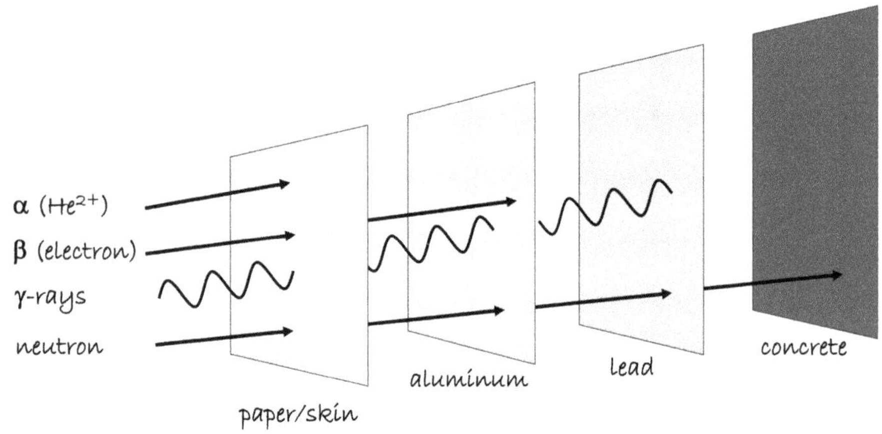

Figure 2.21 Penetration/absorption of alpha-particles (helium nuclei), beta-particles (electrons), gamma-rays, and neutrons. Alpha-particle (helium nuclei) radiation is most easily stopped by a thin piece of paper or by our skin. Beta-radiation (electrons) penetrates paper and skin but will be stopped by aluminum shielding. Gamma-rays will penetrate paper, skin, and aluminum, but will be stopped by lead shielding, whereas neutrons even penetrate lead shielding and will only be absorbed by concrete.

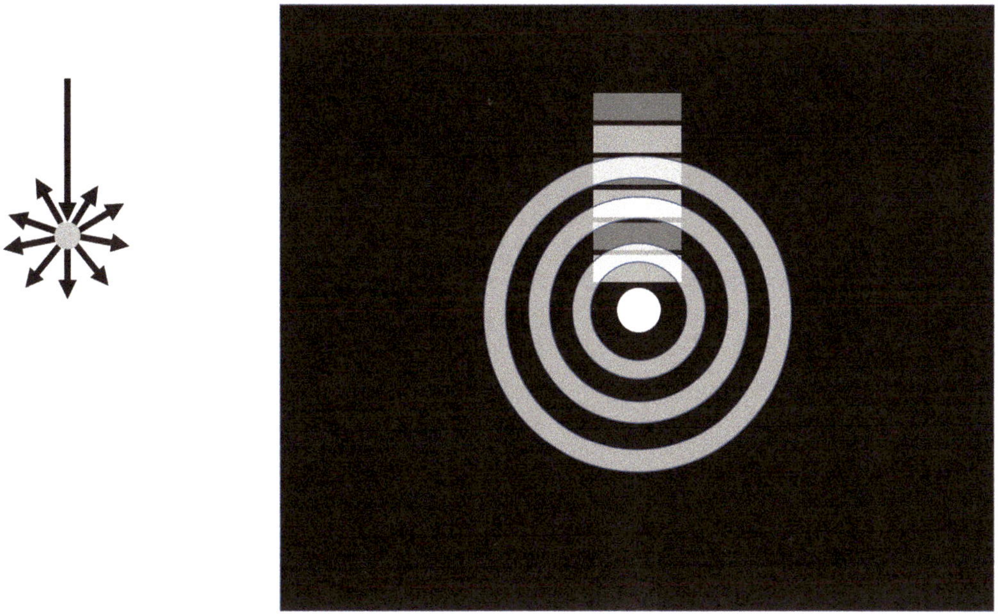

Figure 2.22 Scattering. In scattering, incoming particle or photon radiation encounters a scattering center (scatterer) with the incoming wave front being scattered in all directions.

characteristic of the ability of a beam to penetrate a certain volume of material, with a large coefficient suggesting a lot of attenuation, and a small coefficient suggesting little loss of beam intensity. The historically older term extinction coefficient is still in use in chemistry.

Along its path, moving particles or photons may scatter only once (single scattering) or many times (multiple scattering). While a single scattering event is stochastic and its result (e.g., its direction) cannot be easily predicted, multiple scattering events are often linked with one another, and thus considering a large number of scattering events due to the averaging out of the random contribution of individual scatterers, it is easier to model the result of multiple scattering, e.g., by diffusion theory. However, the assumption no longer holds true if the scattering events are not linked or only a few scattering events have happened.

A somewhat special way of scattering happens when alpha particles (helium nuclei) hit gold atoms (nuclei), with alpha particles being elastically scattered (meaning the entire kinetic energy of the helium particles is preserved, just the angle of the trajectory changes, not unlike billiard balls hitting each other on a billiard/pool table. This is known as Rutherford scattering. In a more general scattering theory, one considers particles or waves interacting with a scattering center.

Historically, elastically scattered electromagnetic waves have been described as Rayleigh scattering, Mie scattering or geometric scattering, depending on whether the particle size is small, comparable to the radiation wavelength, or large, respectively, with respect to the electromagnetic wavelength.

Inelastic scattering includes Raman Scattering and Compton scattering. In Raman scattering, photons are inelastically scattered, which means that part of the energy of the photons leads to increased vibrational and/or rotational energy of the chemical bonds, and photons of a lower energy (longer wavelength) are being emitted as a result. Multiple photon absorption can also lead to the coherent emission of anti-Stokes photons, which have a higher energy than the original photons, which is an important concept in Raman spectroscopy/microscopy. For the discovery of the so-called Raman effect in 1928, Sir Chandrasekhara Venkata Raman was awarded the Nobel Prize in Physics in 1930. Compton scattering (also known as the Compton effect, for which Arthur Compton received a Nobel Prize in Physics in 1927) is the inelastic scattering of high-energy electromagnetic radiation, such as X-rays or gamma-ray photons, by a charged particle (typically an electron), resulting in a lower-energy photon being re-emitted (although higher energy photons can occur, which is referred to as inverse Compton scattering). However, it should be noted that many electrons are scattered elastically with no shift in wavelength. Elastic scattering for high-energy electromagnetic radiation is also known as Thomson scattering and can be modeled as elastic scattering of electromagnetic radiation by a free charged particle (an electron) (Figure 2.23). As the charged particle absorbs the energy of the photon it will accelerate the particle, then emits a polarized photon in a direction perpendicular to the direction of its motion.

Our human experience of the interaction of an electromagnetic wave of the visible light range with matter can be described by either the phenomenon of absorption or scattering. White, matte surfaces usually indicate high levels of scattering, with glossy appearance does not. Spectral absorption of light in certain color ranges determines the color of most objects, however the apparent color of an object can also be the result of scattering, such as the blue daylight sky and the red-colored sunsets, both being the result of Raleigh scattering.

For Raleigh scattering to occur, the scattering center must be much smaller (10% or smaller) in diameter than the wavelength of the scattered wave. Shorter wavelengths are much more effectively scattered (by the power of 4) than longer wavelengths.

If the scattering centers are comparable in size to the wavelength of the scattered wave, Mie scattering (named after the physicist Gustav Mie) is used to describe the interaction. In Mie scattering the precise shape of the scattering center becomes more important. For objects significantly larger than the wavelength of the scattered wave, geometric scattering approaches (the laws of geometric optics) are sufficient to describe the outcome of the interaction.

Among these three forms of scattering, Raleigh scattering is the most significant for bioimaging. If the electromagnetic radiation is scattered by a moving scattering center, it undergoes a Doppler shift, a systematic change in wavelength (and thus change in energy), characteristic of the velocity of the scattering centers.

Diffraction

Although scattering and diffraction of wave phenomena are sometimes used interchangeably, there is a difference between the two terms. When a single wave encountering a scatterer (an obstacle) it changes its direction, we call it scattering, whereas in the case of diffracting, the overall direction of propagation is retained, which does not mean that some waves do not change direction, it just means that on average the direction of propagation stays the same. So, one could say that diffraction describes the forward spreading of waves, and the resulting diffraction patterns are the result of individual scattering events. A scatterer or an opening (such as an aperture or a slit), comparable in size to the wavelength of the waves, becomes a new source of a spherical wave, which (according to the Huygens–Fresnel principle) then can combine with other spherical waves into a wavefront at a distance from the scatterers/aperture (also known as the far-field zone) (Figure 2.24). Note that the angular distribution is not uniform, there is a maximum in the direction of propagation but also adjacent regions of low intensity followed by higher-order maxima.

In the presence of multiple scatterers or apertures, the propagating wavefront is also not uniform, but will contain regions of constructive interference and destructive interference of the waves, resulting in "bright" (high amplitude) and "dark" (low amplitude) regions. These regions of high or low amplitude are the result of the superposition of

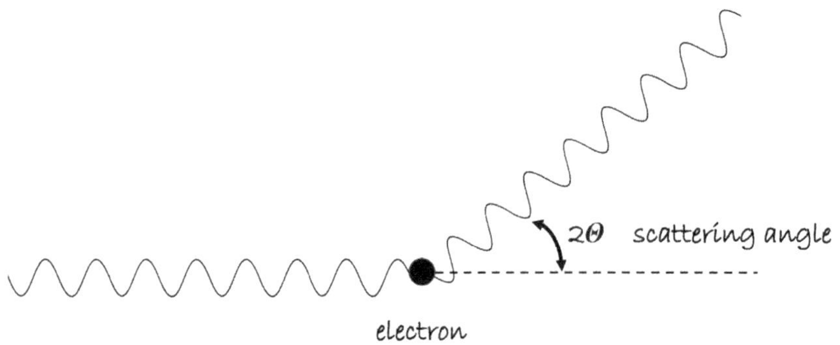

Figure 2.23 Scattering of X-ray by single electron. In this highly simplified depiction of a scattering event of an X-ray wave by an electron, the incoming X-ray interacts with an electron either elastically (no change in wavelength/energy) or inelastically, which leads to an X-ray wave that is changed with respect to trajectory/direction and polarization, and that has undergone a phase shift upon scattering. While this is depiction is not entirely precise, it is often used in the context of discussion of Bragg diffraction in X-ray crystallography.

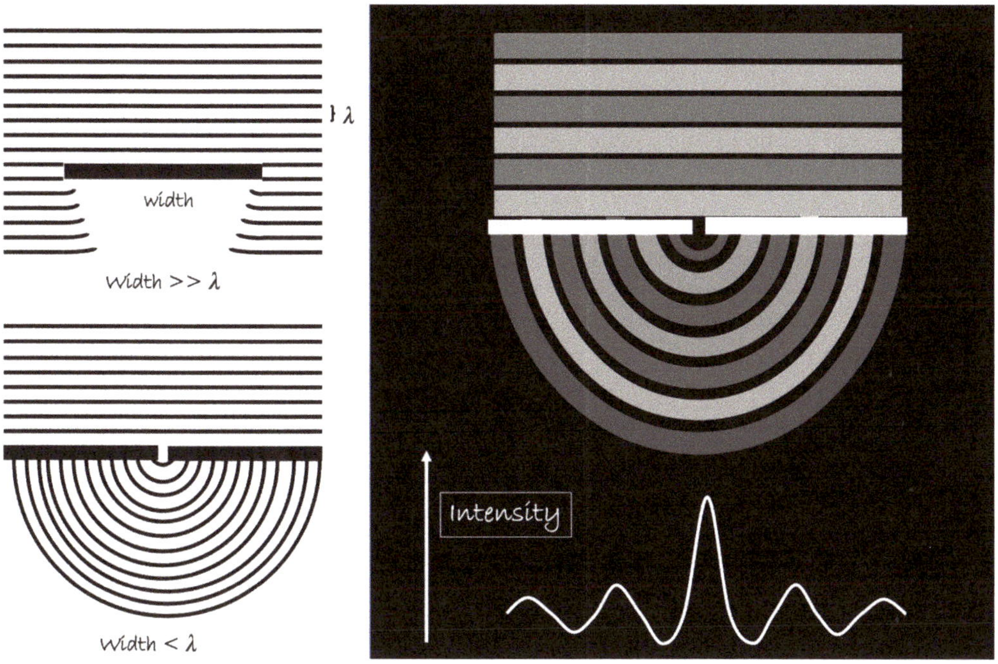

Figure 2.24 Diffraction: Single obstacle and single slit. Waves, encountering an obstacle (or opening/aperture) much larger than their wavelength, are bent around the corner of the object. However, if the obstacle or aperture is of similar size compared to the wavelength, it effectively becomes the source of a secondary propagating wave. If one records the wave amplitude in a plane behind the aperture, one notices a distribution with a maximum at the center, as well as higher order side maxima with smaller amplitude, with minima in between.

multiple individual waves, that arrive with a different phase. This results in a reinforcement or cancelation of the amplitudes.

Due to the wave-particle duality, particles also display wave-like properties (and vice versa waves show particle-like property like momentum), but only very small particles, such electrons, neutrons, atoms, ions, and small molecules have a wavelength that can be observed, larger particle have a wavelength that is far too small to be of practical value for bioimaging.

3

Basics of Optics

3.1 Properties of Light

Optics is a discipline in physics that examines the propagation of visible light and its behavior when encountering matter. For historical reasons visible light has been singled out, but since it only represents a small band in the electromagnetic spectrum, many of the concepts developed in the context of visible light also apply to the remainder of the electromagnetic spectrum, including X-rays, UV rays, as well as IR light, microwave radiation and radio waves.

Light (and thus all electromagnetic radiation) can be described as an electromagnetic field that oscillates in space as a sine-wave function. It has an electric field component (a plane with the propagation direction being one axis) as well as a magnetic field component that constitutes another plane with the propagation axis being one axis, with strength of the magnetic field component being perpendicular to the electric field axis component (Figure 3.1).

Like all wave functions it is defined by an amplitude, a frequency (and thus a wavelength), a phase-offset (with respect to a regular sine wave), as well as a plane of polarization of the electric field and magnetic field components both of which are normal to the axis of propagation. The product of the frequency and wavelength is the speed of light, which is a constant in vacuum but varies in all other media, where the speed is lower. This forms the basis of refraction, where the index of refraction (refractive index) is the ratio between the speed of light in vacuum over the speed of light in the medium.

Light paths are usually represented either by waves (usually in two dimensions), simple rays (usually in form of an arrow or just lines), or as wavefronts with a single line or vector that defines the direction of the light propagation, and perpendicular lines that periodically intersect the line or vector; the perpendicular lines represent the crests (maxima) of the waves and the spacing indicates the wavelength.

3.2 Classical Optics

Classical optics is an oversimplification of the underlying often complex physical processes, however its simplicity and its ability to explain many optical phenomena makes its discussion worthwhile.

In its simplest form, geometric optics uses the simple concept that light rays travel from the light source in a straight line until they encounter an interface between different media, where reflection and refraction laws apply. Their path satisfies Fermat's principle that the path taken between two points by the light ray is the path that can be traversed in the least time. The fact that the speed of light varies in different media lies at the core of refraction and dispersion.

Physical optics borrows concepts from classical wave mechanics to describe phenomena such as positive and negative interference, diffraction and polarization, which cannot be explained by ray optics alone. If the light source moves toward or away from the observer, its spectrum becomes blue-shifted or red-shifted, respectively, which is known as the Doppler effect.

The realization that light displayed both wave-like and particle-light properties, as exemplified by the pattern obtained in diffraction experiments and the photoelectric effect, respectively, required a new theory of light, which is based on quantum mechanics.

Atom and molecule model theory lies at the center of our understanding fluorescence, phosphorescence, infrared and Raman microscopy with changes in electron valency, vibrational and/or rotational molecule modes. Quantum mechanics with its implications on the atom and molecule model theory are needed to truly understand the photoelectric effect, as well as the underlying mechanisms of fluorescence, phosphorescence, vibrational and rotational state imaging, as well as stimulated emission, including laser technology.

Introduction to Biological Imaging, First Edition. Manfred Auer.

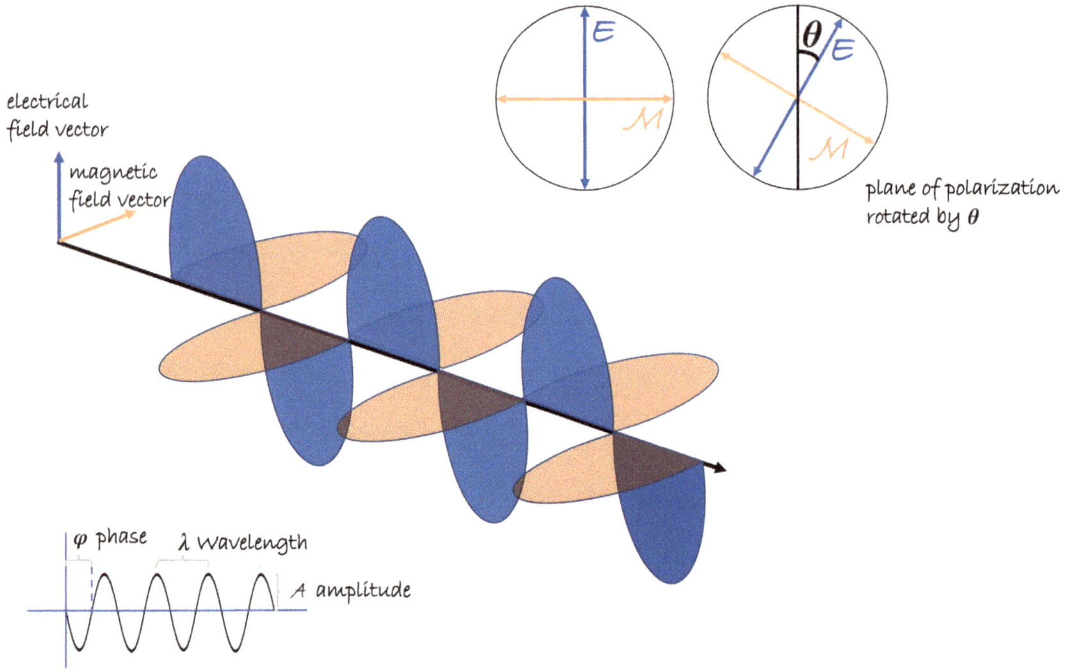

Figure 3.1 Properties of an electromagnetic wave. Electromagnetic waves are defined by a direction of propagation. Along this direction there is an oscillating electrical field plane, with a wave characterized by its amplitude, wavelength, as well as the phase shift (as compared to a sine wave with zero degree phase shift at the origin). The magnetic field vector is perpendicular to the electrical field plane. The orientation of the axis of the electrical field plane (and thus the orthogonal magnetic field plane) is known as polarization of the electromagnetic wave.

3.3 Interaction of Light with Matter

In our discussion of the interaction of light with matter/objects, we will start with the simplest concept of light rays that encounter a boundary/surface, which led to the empiric laws of reflection and refraction. We will then examine the wavelength-dependent changes in refractive index in transparent materials, which underlies the phenomenon of dispersion.

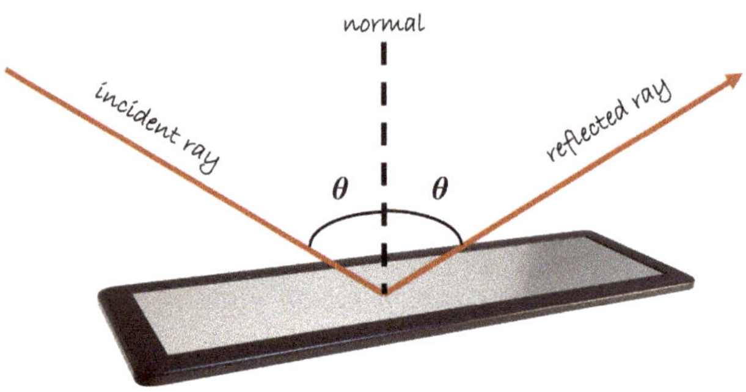

Figure 3.2 Reflection. When light rays encounter a mirror surface the angle of the incident ray is the same as the angle of the reflected ray. The image appears as same size and upright but left–right inverted.

3.3.1 Reflection

According to geometric optics a light ray hitting the boundary between two transparent materials is divided into a reflected and a refracted ray. The reflected ray is reflected from the surface at the same angle as the incident ray. For a single flat mirror (as curved mirrors alter the magnification of an object), the image is the same size, upright, and left–right inverted (Figure 3.2).

3.3.2 Refraction

When light enters glass from air only about 96% of the light penetrates, whereas 4% of the light is reflected from the glass surface, with a minimal fraction of the light being absorbed (Figure 3.3). The refracted beam continues at an angle that according to Snell's law depends on the refraction indices of each of the two materials (which in turn are related to the speed of light in the respective medium). If the light ray travels from a material with high refraction index (e.g., water, glass) to a material with low refraction index (e.g., air), depending on the angle, the light can be reflected. This is called total internal reflection, a phenomenon that is relevant not only for fiber optics illumination but also for an imaging technique known as Total Internal

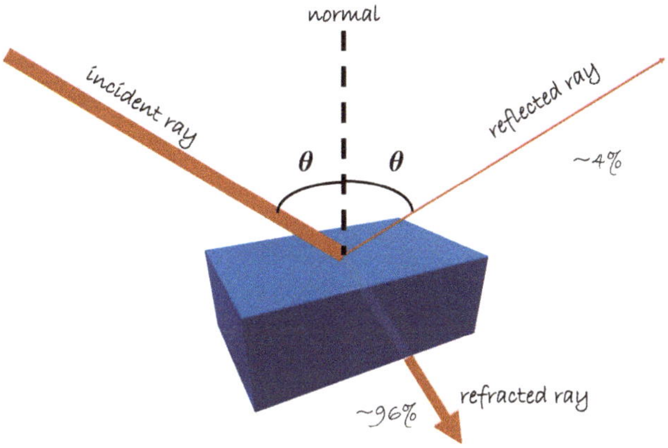

Figure 3.3 Refraction. Light at the boundary of two different media is either reflected or refracted, with the refracted beam continuing at an angle that depends on the refraction indices of the two media (Snell's law). The underlying cause of refraction is the change of the speed of light at the media's boundary.

Reflection Fluorescence (TIRF) microscopy. TIRF allows very thin cellular regions to be studied, thereby eliminating much background from the rest of the sample.

Refraction and reflection are basically the same concept: if in Snell's law both refraction indices are equal (as would be the case for reflection), their angles have to be also equal, which is basically what the law of reflection states.

3.3.3 Dispersion

Dispersion is caused by a decrease in the index of refraction for radiation at increasing wavelength, which is common for most transparent materials. The term normal dispersion refers to this process taking place in bands of the electromagnetic spectrum that are not absorbed by the dielectric material, whereas significant absorption can lead to an increase of the index of refraction, in which case we call it anomalous dispersion. Refractive indices depend on the wavelength of the light, which is the basis of obtaining a color spectrum of white light by a prism (Figure 3.4).

3.4 Lenses

Refraction is also the basis for understanding the properties of lenses. Lenses are simply devices that either converge or diverge light rays because of refraction.

Lenses that converge are called convex lenses, whereas lenses that diverge light rays are called concave lenses. Lenses are typically characterized by their focal length, with converging lenses having a positive focal length and diverging lenses having a negative focal length. The smaller the focal length the stronger is its converging or diverging

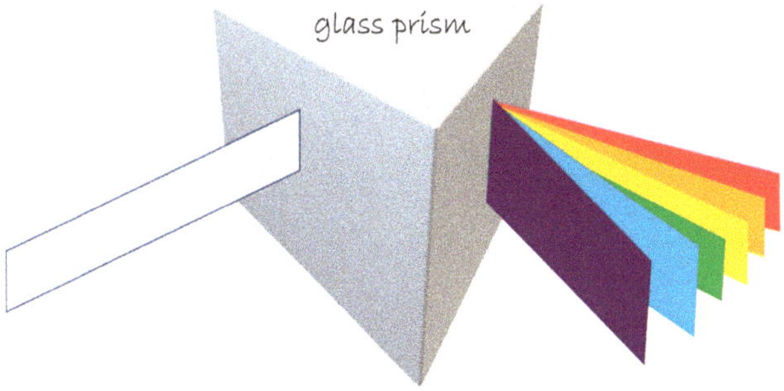

Figure 3.4 Dispersion. White light (which is a mixture of light of different colors), entering a transparent material such as glass, is spatially split into its different components, resulting in a spectrum. This phenomenon is called dispersion and is based on differences in the index of refraction for different wavelengths.

effect. If parallel rays encounter a convex lens, they will be focused onto a spot on the far side of the lens, defined by the focal length of the lens. There are different kind of lenses such as positive meniscus, plano-convex, biconvex (double convex), negative meniscus, plano-concave and biconcave (double concave) lenses (Figure 3.5).

There are three guidelines that allow ray tracing in geometric optics of lenses:

(1) Parallel rays entering a lens converge at its focal plane; (2) Rays originating from the back-focal plane entering a lens exit as parallel rays; (3) Rays that pass through the center of the lens will not be refracted and thus exit the lens unaffected in straight line (Figure 3.6).

Light is considered collimated if the light from a point source is converted into a beam of parallel light rays.

The magnification M is given as the ratio of the distance of the image from the lens to the distance of the object from the lens (Figure 3.7).

3.5 Numerical Aperture

Lenses in optics are characterized by the numerical aperture (NA), which reflects the ability to collect light (acceptance cone) and to resolve features of a specimen. The wider the range of angles the lens can gather light from, the higher its resolving power. The numerical aperture (NA) value is calculated as: NA = n (sin μ), with n being the refractive index of the medium between the cover slip (specimen) and the objective lens and μ being the maximal angle of light cone and the center of the lens. The highest refractive index n is 1.0 for air and 1.51 for immersion oil, with n for water being 1.33 and n for glycerin being 1.47. Given the angular range limit of ~60–70°, the NA for imaging in air is typically less than 0.95 for a 60× (magnification) lens. NA values above 1.0 require the use of water or

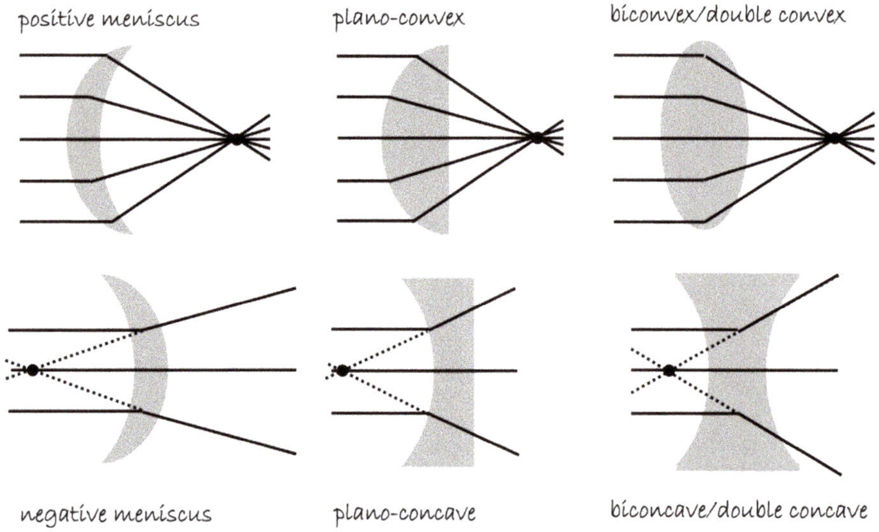

Figure 3.5 Lenses. Lenses with a positive focal length (converging lenses) are either positive meniscus, planoconvex, or biconvex/double convex lenses. Lenses with a negative focal length (diverging lenses) are either negative meniscus, planoconcave, or biconcave/double concave lenses.

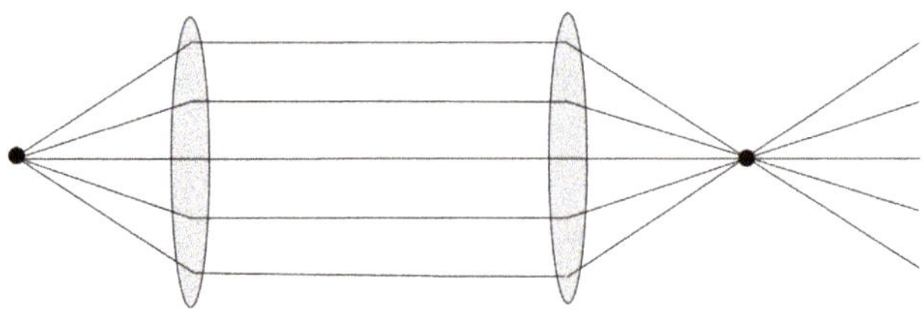

Figure 3.6 Ray tracing/geometric optics. There are a three rules that guide ray tracing in geometrical optics. Rays originating from the back-focal plane and entering a lens will exit the lens as parallel rays. Parallel rays entering a lens will converge at the lenses focal plane. Furthermore, rays that pass through the center of a lens will be unaffected by the lens and will continue as a straight line.

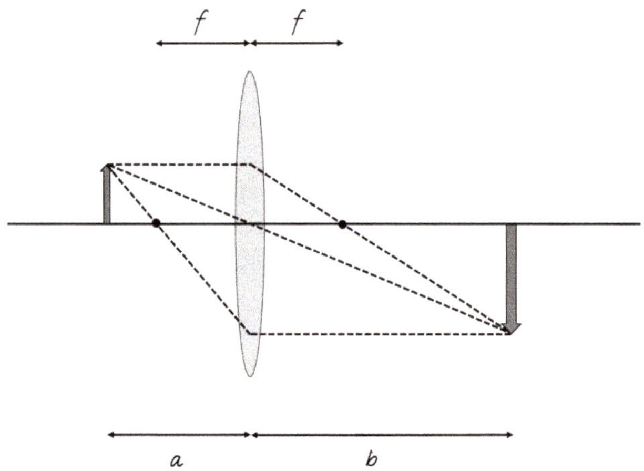

Figure 3.7 Lens magnification. The magnification of an object is given by the ratio of the distance of the image from the lens (*b*) to the distance of the object from the lens (*a*).

immersion oil, with lens NA values of 1.0–1.35 being most common. Aberration-corrected lenses typically have a higher numerical aperture compared to lower quality lenses.

For narrow light cones (e.g., at 7°) the NA is reduced to 0.12, but one enjoys a large working distance between the lens and the specimen although at only low magnification (e.g., at 4× magnification). The working distance (how close an objective lens must be to the specimen) can be an important experimental consideration and may limit what kind of objective lens can be chosen for imaging. Lenses with magnification powers of 60–100× typically are designed for use in conjunction with immersion oil (Figure 3.8).

The lower the numerical aperture the lower the resolving power of the lens. 4× lenses with a NA of 0.1–0.2 can resolve objects spaced 2.75 to 1.375 μm apart, 10× lenses with an NA of 0.25–0.45 can resolve objects spaced 1.1 μm to 610 nm apart, whereas 100× lenses with an NA of 1.25–1.4 achieve a resolution of 220–200 nm. The total resolving power of a microscope depends not only on the NA of the objective lens but also on the NA of the condenser lens.

3.6 Scattering

To understand scattering and its many related consequences, ray tracing as a concept is not sufficient, thus we will need to include the concepts of wave mechanics.

Scattering is the process when a wave front encounters an object. The object (scatterer) then become the source of another wave. In essence, the underlying mechanism for all phenomena in optics are based on scattering, including

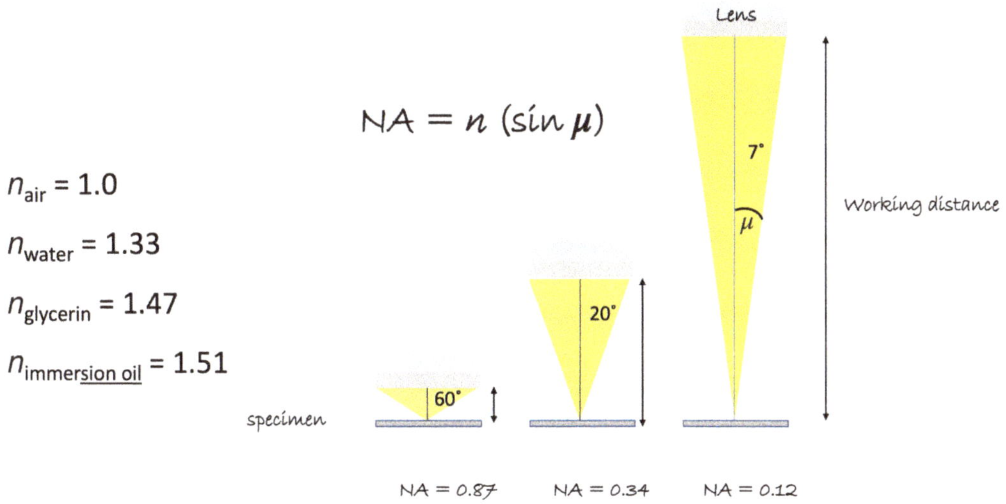

Figure 3.8 Numerical aperture. The numerical aperture (NA) reflects a lens' ability to collect light and resolve features of a specimen. The higher the NA, the wider is the range of angles that the lens can gather light from and the higher is the resolving power of a lens. Refractive indices range from 1.0 in air to 1.51 for immersion oil. Highest quality lenses have an NA of ~1.4. Note that the higher the NA the shorter is the working distance, which means the closer the lens needs to be to the object.

reflection, refraction, diffraction, dispersion and polarization as well as fluorescence and phosphorescence. So, in that sense, scattering is the most fundamental of all processes.

In the case of elastic scattering the scattered wave front has the same energy is as the incident wave front, where in the case of inelastic scattering energy is transferred to the scattering object, and thus the scattered wave front has a lower energy.

In Rutherford scattering, the collision of alpha-particles with atomic nuclei is also a form of scattering and can be thought of as being similar to billiard/pool balls hitting one another. Bragg scattering is the scattering of X-rays by an array of atoms and can be elastic or inelastic in nature.

3.7 Interference

Interference is an optical phenomenon that cannot easily be explained by light traveling as rays, instead one needs to acknowledge the wave-like properties of electromagnetic and particle radiation.

The concepts of constructive and destructive interference are shown when two waves interfering with one another to create a new wave that will have different amplitude and possible different wavelength. Constructive interference occurs when wave crests of both waves overlay on top of one another, whereas destructive interference occurs when the waves are phase-shifted, e.g., when wave crests of one wave overlay with wave troughs of the other wave. If the two wave have different amplitudes, the resulting wave becomes weaker, if the amplitudes happen to be the same, they completely cancel each other out. A more complicated picture emerges when different waves have both different amplitudes and frequencies (Figure 3.9).

As waves originate from a point source, they diverge as spherical waves with the intensity of the light being proportional to the square of its electrical field amplitude, hence doubling the amplitude leads to a fourfold increase in light intensity. Individual spherical waves are also referred to as wavelets. Wavelets originating from several point sources will combine into a wavefront. When such a wavefront encounters a double slit, new wavelets will originate from each slit (scattering object) and will be in phase. Depending on position on a screen behind the double slit, there will be regions where the two wavelets will constructively interfere and thus strengthen each other, whereas in regions in between wavelets interfere destructively and thus wipe each other out, depending on the relative position of wave crests and wave troughs for each of the waves. If the waves have the same wavelength and are in phase, interference is constructive and the resulting amplitude will be at a maximum, whereas in destructive interference, phases will be out of phase and thus wave crests of one wave will align with wave troughs of the other wave and they will cancel out each other's amplitude (Figure 3.10).

3.8 Diffraction

Diffraction, which literally means "breaking into pieces," can be thought of as a systematic pattern of wave interference caused by scattering elements that are arranged periodically (gratings). This is analogous to a multi-slit

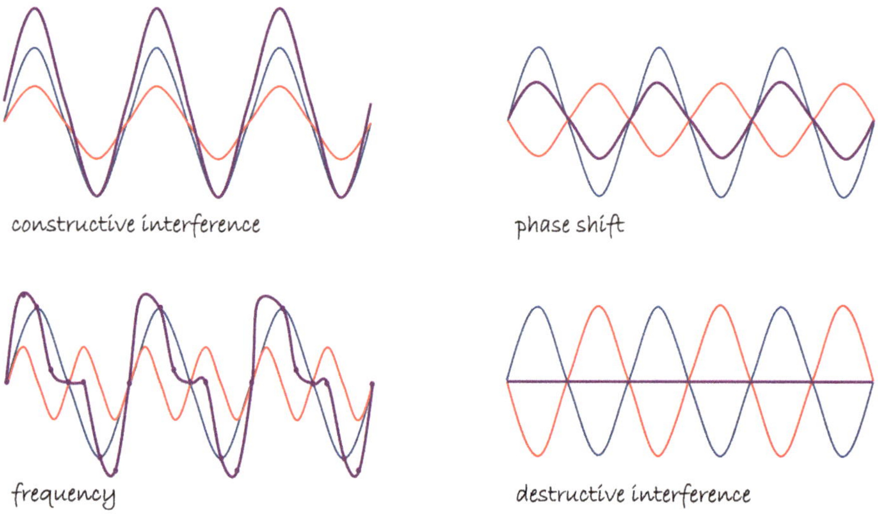

Figure 3.9 Constructive and destructive interference. Two waves with the same frequency and phase will interfere constructively, whereas two waves with same frequency that are phase shifted will interfere destructively. If waves of different frequencies interfere with one another, there will be regions of the resulting wave where the interference was constructive and other regions where the interference was destructive. Note: The two waves are shown in red and blue, with purple being the result of their interference.

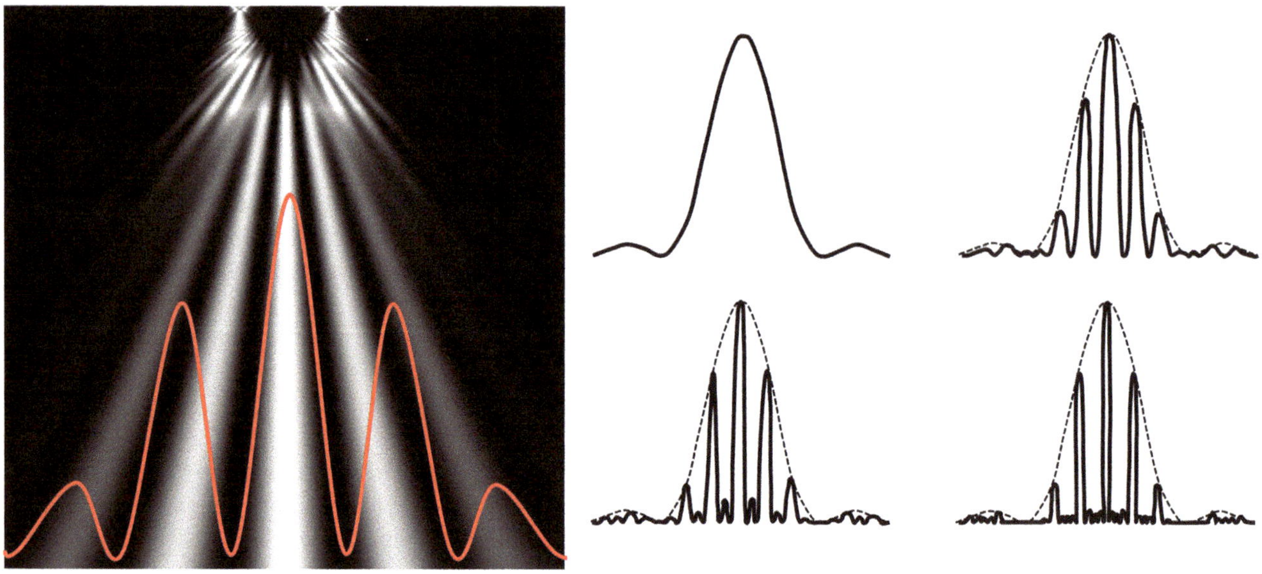

Figure 3.10 Single-slit, double-slit, and multi-slit wave interference. Left: Result of a double-slit experiment with the one-dimensional intensity distribution shown in red. Right: Single-slit diffraction experiments lead to a maximum peak at the center and a shoulder peak. In double-slit diffraction experiments, the central peak sharpens, and additional shoulder peaks become apparent. The more slits are used the sharper the peaks of the resulting diffraction pattern become. Note that peak height distribution follows the envelope (dashed line) of the single-slit experiment curve.

interference experiment, with the light being split up into a regular pattern of discrete spots. Diffraction can be explained if one assumes light to be wave-like rather than corpuscle-like. Diffraction plays a major role in bioimaging, and Bragg diffraction is the foundation of X-ray crystallography for high resolution structure determination of biological macromolecules (Figure 3.11).

In Bragg diffraction, each atom in a macromolecule resides at a particular position in the unit cell and serves as a scattering center. Constructive interference from these scattering centers will occur under certain angles that can be determined by imagining planes connecting these scattering centers in each unit cell of the crystal, from which X-rays are reflected. Crystal planes in different orientations

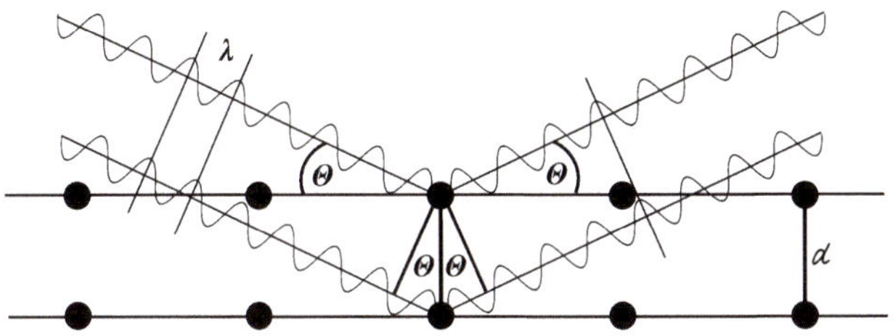

Figure 3.11 Bragg diffraction. In a crystal, atoms are organized into a periodic 3D array. They serve as scattering centers for incoming X-ray wavelets. The scattered X-ray wavelets from different scattering centers interfere constructively only in certain directions, leading to discrete diffraction spots (similarly to a multi-slit diffraction pattern). In the space in between the diffraction spots, the wavelets cancel each other out. Historically, discrete diffraction spots were interpreted as reflections of X-rays from parallel crystal lattice planes whose (d) spacing leads to a path difference of the X-rays to allow constructive interference (Bragg reflection).

lead to discrete diffraction spots in space with a specific relationship between the distance of each plane in the crystal and the angle at which the X-ray encounters the imagined crystal plane.

The two different ways of thinking about Bragg diffraction are not mutually exclusive, as the underlying idea of constructive interference of X-rays that are scattered by each atom residing in a crystalline (and thus periodically repeating) unit cell is common in both approaches. The X-rays can only interfere constructively in certain spots in 3D whereas in between they cancel each other out. In essence, X-ray passing through a 3D crystal is analogous to light passing through gratings, both result in a discrete pattern of diffraction spots.

3.9 Airy Disk

Diffraction not just happens when light encounters periodic objects like gratings, but even when passing through a single aperture onto a screen. The resulting far-field wavefront is not uniform. Instead of a single point, the screen will show a distinct pattern, also known as Airy pattern of concentric rings with a bright central spot (also known as the Airy disk) whose intensity dims radially toward the first minimum, only to reach a second maximum, a second minimum, a third maximum and so on (Figure 3.12).

Each maximum is dimmer than the previous. Eighty four percent of the light is in the Airy disk, 16% in the surrounding maxima. The diameter of the Airy disk depends on the size of the chosen aperture. The formation of an Airy disk instead of a single point by an aperture is what ultimately limits the resolving power of an imaging system. If in an image there are two point-sources, each of them will produce an Airy disk. If the two point-sources are spaced apart both can be detected, and the center of each Airy disk becomes the location of the corresponding point source. If the two point-sources become closer in space, the two Airy disks will start to overlap. According to the Rayleigh criterion, one considers the two point-sources as resolved, if they are separated by the radius of the Airy disk, which means that the first minimum of the Airy disk from the one point source falls onto the maximum of the second Airy disk (see also Section 3.11).

3.10 Point-Spread Function

The point-spread function (PSF) can be thought of as the shape that a point source will adopt once it passes through the imaging system or in other words in what way a point source will be blurred by the imaging system. Mathematically speaking is the resulting image of the point source a convolution of the object with the PSF. Deconvolution is the process by which the image of the original object (e.g., the point source) can be restored. This can be accomplished by mathematically taking the PSF into consideration when calculating the image. An Airy disk can be thought of as the PSF of an aberration-free imaging device with an aperture. The PSF of an imaging system can be modeled, but there will be uncertainties about its exact shape, so one should be always careful when

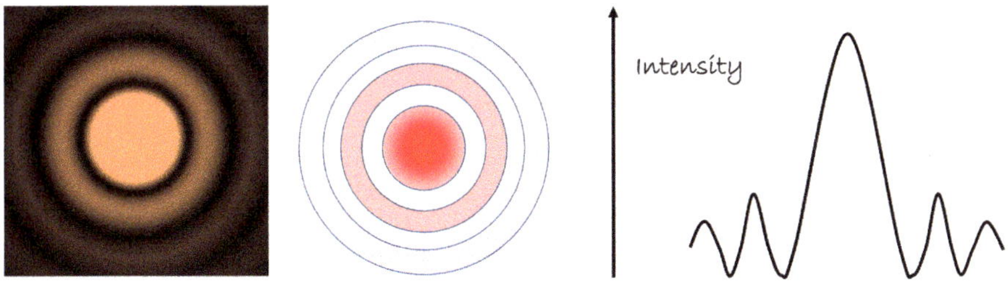

Figure 3.12 Airy disk. Light passing through an aperture (e.g., in a microscope) and being detected on a screen leads to an Airy pattern of concentric rings, with a central peak (Airy disk) containing 84% of the intensity, with the remaining 16% of the intensity being distributed over the surrounding maxima.

attempting deconvolution, as incorrect assumptions about the PSF can lead to an incorrect image of the object. In a typical high-end microscope with an appropriate high-end objective lens, the PSF – the distance from the center of the Airy disk to its first minimum ring – is about 200–250 nm (225 nm) wide in *x*, *y*, and about threefold worse in *z*. Shorter wavelengths used for imaging result in a comparatively smaller PSF than for longer wavelengths. The PSF (with its lateral and axial component) is a key measure when comparing different types of fluorescence light microscopy (Figure 3.13).

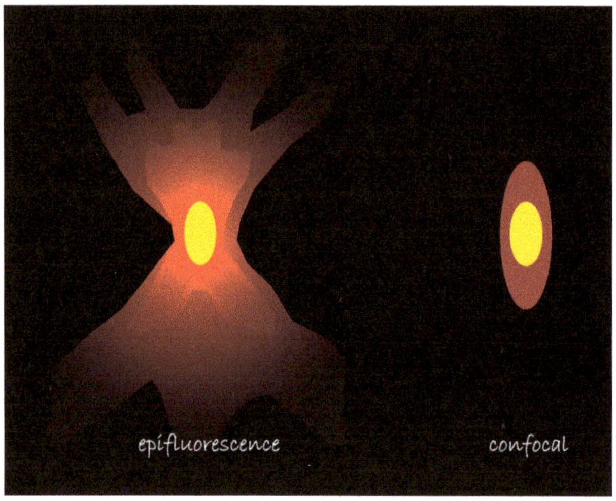

Figure 3.13 Point-spread function. The point-spread function indicates how light from a point source is spread out in 3D, with *XY* cross-section typically being round (the equivalent to an Airy disk), whereas *XZ* or *YZ* cross-sections having an elliptical shape. In other words, the point source is more spread out along the light path compared to the direction perpendicular to the light path. For confocal microscopy, the PSF has the shape of an ellipsoid. In the case of epifluorescence, the PSF in *XZ* or *YZ* planes resembles more an hourglass, as the irradiation by the illuminating beam and the emission of fluorescence also occurs outside the focal region.

3.11 Resolution

The term resolution is often used loosely. Angular resolution refers to a microscope's ability to distinguish object details that are spaced at a small angular distance, and angular resolution is closely related to the term spatial resolution, which refers to the measurement of the smallest distance of two points in a specimen that can still be perceived as being separate from one another.

In optical (visible light) microscopy, for a typical 4× lens at an NA value of 0.2, the resolution that can be achieved is ~1.4 μm, whereas 40× lenses with an NA of 0.95 can resolve features as closely spaced as 0.29 μm (or 290 nm) and 100× lenses with an NA of 1.4 are capable of resolving two points that are ~0.2 μm (~200 nm) apart. However, the resolution also depends on the wavelength at which image data is recorded: For an NA of 0.95, the resolution at 360 nm, 400 nm, and 700 nm are 190 nm, 210 nm, and 370 nm, respectively (approximately one half of the image data wavelength).

Naturally, the resolution that can be achieved by shorter wavelengths of the electromagnetic spectrum or high energy particles (such as electrons) is higher (meaning shorter distance details can be detected), whereas longer wavelength electromagnetic spectrum radiation such as IR or microwave, have inherently lower resolution. The resolution of imaging techniques employing X-rays or high-energy particles such as electrons is in the nanometer or subnanometer (Angstrom, 1 Å = 0.1 nm) range, whereas IR radiation is in the micrometer (μm) range.

When it comes to resolution or the resolving power of an imaging device (such as a microscope), often the Raleigh criterion is used, which states that two objects are considered resolved if the distance of center of two Airy disks is equal or larger than the radius of the Airy disk, or in other words, when the center of the Airy disk of the first object is falls into the first minimum of the Airy disk of the second object (Figure 3.14). Smaller Airy disks are characteristic of

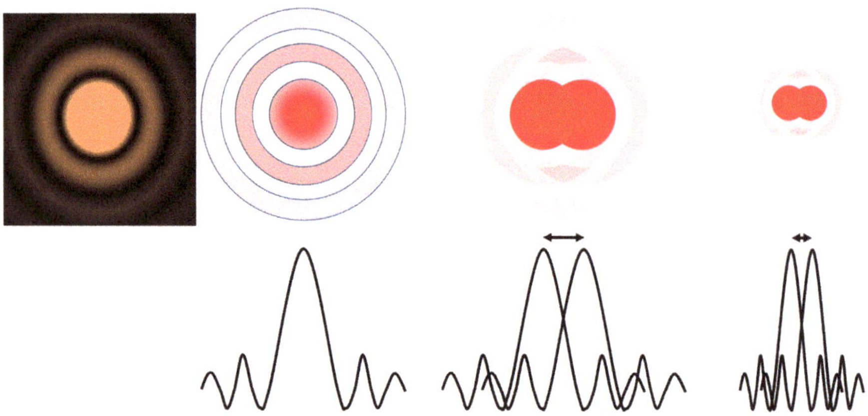

Figure 3.14 Raleigh criterion in resolution. The Raleigh criterion states that two objects are considered resolved when the center of one Airy disk falls into the first minimum of the Airy pattern of the other Airy disk. Note that sharper/smaller Airy disks can resolve closer-spaced point sources.

aberration-corrected fluorite and apochromat lenses and allow higher resolution images. The maximum value of diffraction limited resolution in optical imaging is often given as ~225 nm laterally and ~860 nm axially, or ~0.4 to ~0.5 of the wavelength used for imaging.

While the resolution criteria of a microscopic system may be an appropriate way to judge instrument performance, one also needs to realize that it is not the only criterium by which to judge data quality, proper illumination, and specimen contrast, as well as a number of sufficient photons for image formation are important components to record high-information content images.

3.12 Aberrations

Lenses rarely are perfect and suffer from a variety of distortions/aberrations. An aberration is a characteristic of an optical system (such as a lens), which results in the blurring of an image. The blurring occurs when light is not perfectly focused onto a single spot but rather spread out over some region of space. Such imperfections of an optical microscope can be corrected for by instrument makers using additional lenses.

Aberrations can be understood in the context of geometrical optics by ray tracing analysis. There are two types of aberrations: monochromatic aberrations and chromatic aberrations. Monochromatic aberrations depend on lens (or mirror) geometry and can occur both with reflected and refracted light rays. Chromatic aberrations are caused by wavelength-dependent variations of the lens' refractive index (dispersion). Hence in case of chromatic aberration, light of different color (wavelength) is focused onto different points. As the name implies chromatic aberration does not occur for monochromatic (single wavelength) light (Figure 3.15).

Among the monochromatic aberrations are defocus, spherical aberration, and astigmatism. Defocus is usually not considered a lens aberration since it can easily be corrected by moving the lens or the image plane into focus. Spherical aberration occurs in lenses (or curved mirrors), which contains spherical surfaces. In such systems, rays that pass through the center of the lens will be focused differently than rays that pass toward the edge. This deviation from an idealized lens is the case for real lenses even if they are perfectly manufactured. Astigmatism on the other hand means that rays propagating in two orthogonal planes along the optical axis are focused at two different distances. This results in an elliptical Airy pattern, with the distances of the maxima and minima being different when examining the pattern in orthogonal directions.

Adaptive optics are rather new in biological imaging but common in the field of astronomy to compensate for the effects of atmospheric distortion. In adaptive optics, deformable mirrors or liquid crystal arrays can correct wavefront distortions that are measured by, e.g., a wave front sensor. In astronomy, a laser beam is sent into the night sky as a "guide star" to account for atmospheric disturbances. Rare-earth nanoprobes can provide a similar "guide star" in biological sample.

3.13 Polarization

Electromagnetic waves oscillate in a plane with the electrical and magnetic field vectors being perpendicular to one another. If all wave packages have a field vector (and thus also magnetic vectors) that align in orientation, we call this form of light polarized. Polarization can occur in a single direction, in which case we call it linear polarization, or the oscillation direction rotates as the wave travels, in which case we call it circular (or elliptical) polarization. For circularly polarized light, waves either rotate to the right (clockwise) or to the left (counterclockwise).

Certain dichroic devices block light in all directions, except for one direction where the material is transparent, in which case the transmitted light becomes polarized in the direction where the material is transparent. Note that in polarizers not all light will be transmitted, which means that the overall intensity of the light beam will go down significantly.

Molecules with centers of chirality, can alter the direction of polarized light, which can be used as a diagnostic tool (in

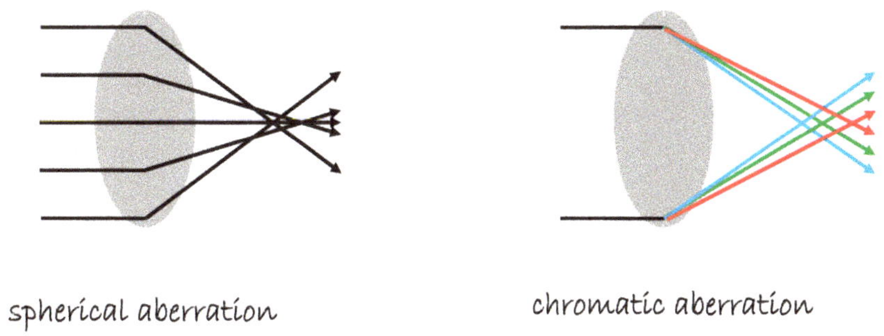

Figure 3.15 Spherical and chromatic aberration. In the case of spherical aberrations light rays near the center of the lens are focused onto a different focal point compared to light rays that pass near the edge of the lens. Chromatic aberration is the result of wavelength-dependent variation of a lens' refractive index. Light of different colors (different frequencies) are focused onto different focal points.

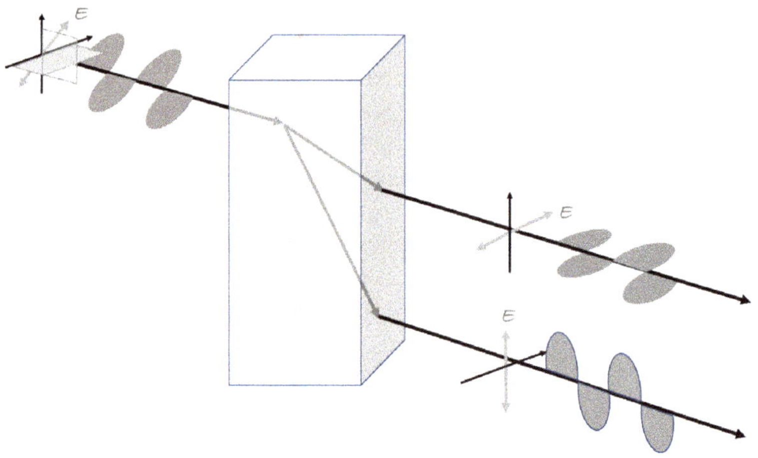

Figure 3.16 Birefringence. Calcite crystals show birefringence, a phenomenon of double refraction, where an incident light beam is split by polarization into two rays that in the crystal take different paths. Birefringence plays an important role in differential interference contrast (DIC) microscopy.

combination with other tools for molecular identification) for the presence of a chiral molecule (e.g., D, and L-sugar molecules).

Birefringence as found in calcite is a phenomenon of double refraction due to differences in polarization (Figure 3.16). Mitotic spindles show weak birefringence, which is used for contrast formation. Birefringence plays an important role in differential interference contrast (DIC) microscopy.

3.14 Photoelectric Effect

An understanding of the photoelectric effect requires the acknowledgment that in atom and molecule model theory electron energy levels are quantized and require photons of sufficient energy to knock an electron off an atom, any additional energy beyond freeing the electron from the atom adds to the kinetic energy and thus the velocity of the freed electron. In an appropriate setup, such freed electrons can be captured and counted, and thus measured as an electrical current.

In the inner photoelectric effect, the electrons do not leave the atoms altogether, but absorption of the photons leads to separation of charges, namely a negatively charged electron and positively charged "hole." The separation of charges can then be detected (Figure 3.17).

3.15 Valence Electron Transitions

Short-wavelength visible light possess the right amount of energy to cause a transition of electrons from a ground-state to one of several excited states, with the energy

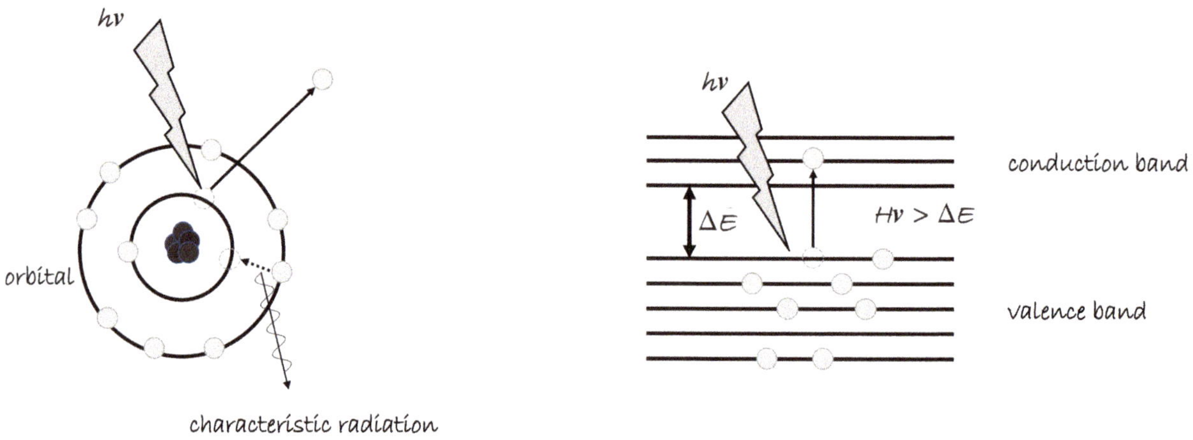

Figure 3.17 Photoelectric effect and inner photoelectric effect. Photons with sufficient energy can eject an electron from an atom, leading to a free electron with a kinetic energy that can be detected. In the inner photoelectric effect, the electrons are not ejected from the atom, instead the absorption of a photon of appropriate energy leads to the elevation of the electron from the valence band to the conduction band. This also leads to an electron-hole pair.

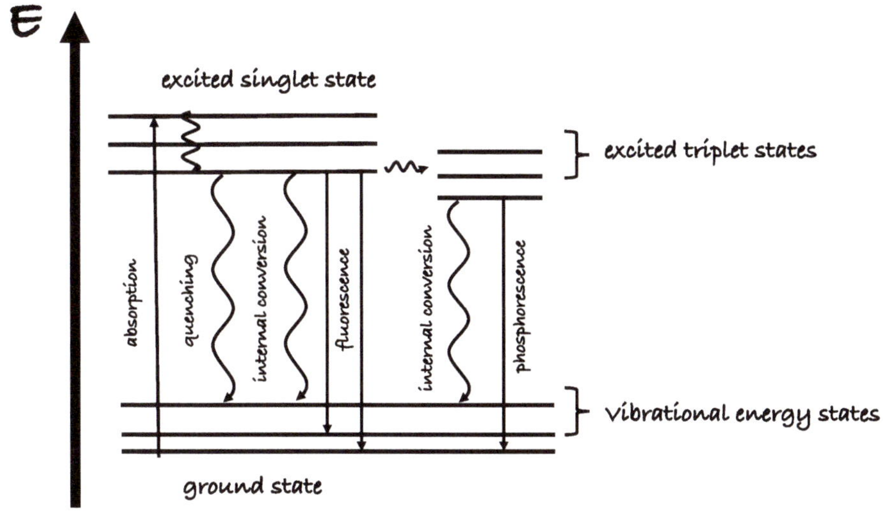

Figure 3.18 Jablonski diagram. The Jablonski diagram depicts the various ways how photons can be absorbed and emitted by a fluorophore. Photons that possess the right amount of energy (the correct wavelength) are absorbed by molecules, which leads to the transition of an electron from a ground state to one of excited singlet states. Note that both valence electron ground state as well as valence electron excited states have multiple levels due to different vibrational energy states of the molecule. Electrons will first relax to the lowest level of the excited state before they relax back to the ground state, which results in the emission of a photon of slightly lower energy (and thus longer wavelength) than the photon that originally absorbed. This is known as fluorescence. Competing processes are quenching and internal version, where the system relaxes to the ground state without the emission of a photon. Also, some systems can adopt an excited triplet state that is more stable (minutes to hours) than a singlet state (nanoseconds), and hence emission of a photon can occur at a later time. In this case we speak of phosphorescence.

difference from the ground state to any of the excited states being much larger than the energy differences of the various excited levels. Absorption of photons elevates electrons to a higher energy excited level. The electron then relaxes from a higher vibrational level of the excited state to a lower vibrational level of the excited state before relaxing back to a ground state, emitting a longer-wavelength photon in the process. This process is the same for both fluorescence and phosphorescence, the difference between these two processes is that in fluorescence absorption and emission occur within nanoseconds, whereas in phosphorescence emission can occur up to minutes or hours later.

A Jablonski diagram lists the various ways photons can be absorbed and emitted by a fluorophore (Figure 3.18).

3.16 Vibrational and Rotational Transitions

Transitions of molecular states do not only occur at the level of valence electrons but also at the level of vibrational and rotational energy. Energy differences between vibrational states are much lower (and even lower for different rotational states) than for valence electron states, hence it takes much lower energy (hence even longer-wavelength) photons for such vibrational ground-state to excited-state transitions to occur. Hence, these transitions occur at the infrared light range of the electromagnetic spectrum (Figure 3.19).

3.17 Stimulated Emission

As discussed above, absorption of a photon with a specific frequency by a molecule typically leads to the elevation of an electron from a ground state to an excited state, from where is relaxes back to the ground state in a process called spontaneous emission. Spontaneous emission lies at the heart of fluorescence imaging (and also thermal emission, which does not play a significant role in bioimaging).

However, if the system is already predominantly in an excited state (which is known as population inversion), the interaction of an atom in the molecule with a photon of appropriate energy can lead to a induced (stimulated) drop from an excited state to a ground state. Two photons are emitted in the process with both emitted photons having the same energy (frequency), polarization, as well as direction of trajectory (Figure 3.20).

This parity in polarization and trajectory is what distinguishes spontaneous and stimulated emission. Stimulated emission is also a light intensity amplification process, as one incoming photon leads to two photons. The rate of

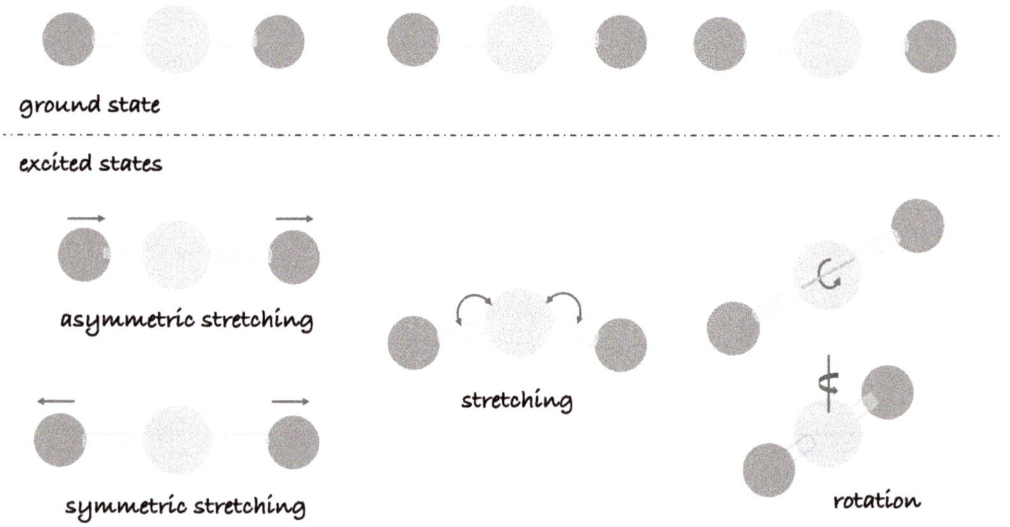

Figure 3.19 Vibrational and rotational states. Molecules can exist in vibrational and rotational ground states, as well as excited states. Vibrational energy lies in the symmetric or asymmetric stretching of bond lengths and in changes of bond angles. Rotational energy lies in rotation of the entire molecule as well as rotation around the axis of individual bonds.

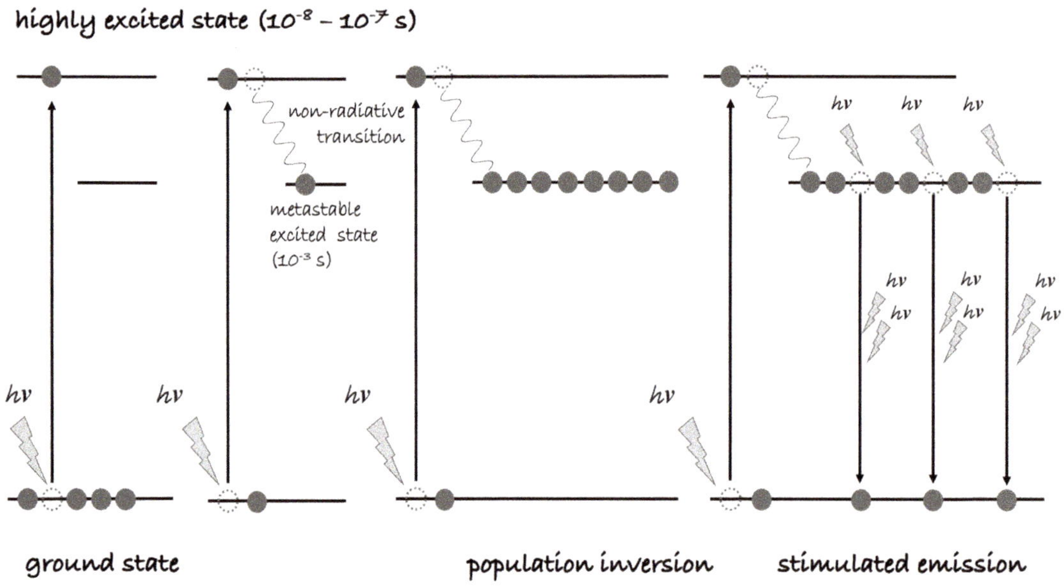

Figure 3.20 Stimulated emission. For stimulated emission to occur the system must be predominantly in a metastable excited state (which is known as population inversion), typically courtesy of a pump laser that continuously excites electrons that then transition in a non-radiative manner to this metastable excited state. Once population inversion has been achieved, absorption of a photon can lead to the simultaneous emission of two photons with the same frequency, polarization, and direction of trajectory. Stimulated emission is a light amplification process and underlies laser technology.

emission is proportional to the number of atoms in an excited state and to the density of the incident photons. In addition to stimulated emission there is also absorption, which elevates electrons from the ground state to an excited state.

Naturally, the energy to get and keep the system in a predominantly excited state comes from a pump laser. Light amplification by means of a so-called gain medium along with an optical resonator is the foundation of laser technology.

4

Basics of Fourier "Math"

Fourier transforms lie at the heart of many aspects of biological imaging, be it in the context of diffraction in X-ray and electron crystallography, image formation in an optical microscope, the conversion of the free-induction decay signal into an NMR-resonance spectrum, frequency modulation in radiotechnology, and the conversion of interferogram signal into an FT-IR spectrum.

In essence, a Fourier transform allows the transition between different kinds of datasets or domains, e.g., transitioning between a time domain and a frequency domain, or between real space scattering object positions (density map as a function of x, y, z-coordinates) and Fourier space structure factor domain, with the amplitude, phase, and frequency components for each of the diffraction spots (h, k, l-indices). In other words, real space and Fourier space are two different representations of the same data.

Fourier transformation is based on sinusoidal functions in part because sinusoids are a convenient set of functions that are easy to deal with as a base, with each sinusoidal function being characterized by a corresponding frequency, amplitude and phase shift. Fourier series allow the description of any periodic function by the sum of sinusoids (sine-functions), if appropriate parameters (amplitude and phase) can be determined for each of the sinusoids at a certain frequency that is included in the process.

First, let us consider the effect of changing the amplitude of sine wave as well as changing the frequency of the sign wave (Figure 4.1) and the role of amplitude and frequency changes upon superposition of waves (Figure 4.2).

A phase shift of $\pi/2$ (90°) turns a sine wave into a cosine wave, whereas a 180° phase shift (π), results in another sine wave, where wave crests have become wave troughs. Superposition of waves depend on both amplitudes and phase-shift, where at certain points waves may reinforce one another or destroy one another (Figures 4.3 and 4.4).

Adding several sinusoids with different amplitudes and frequencies allows the approximation of a rectangular step function by sinusoids. As a matter of fact, the shape of any function (such as a 3D dimensional density distribution) can be recreated by adding up many sinusoid (sine and cosine) functions.

Note that the approximate shape of the rectangular step function is defined by the low frequency sinusoid, whereas higher-frequency sinusoids are needed to better approximate the fine details of the rectangular step function, in other words: low-frequency data thus provides an overall shape and higher frequency data reveals the details (Figure 4.5).

In X-ray crystallography, to take one (prominent) example, the structure factor $F_{(hkl)}$ is a vector with an amplitude and phase for each of the discrete spot positions, each with its unique h, k, and l index. $F_{(hkl)}$ is the result of the superposition of the scattering factors from each scattering center in the unit cell of the crystal that diffracts X-rays. Discrete spots of regular spacing in a diffraction pattern are the result of the periodic arrangement of molecules within each unit cell. The diffraction pattern is then a convolution of the structure factor of the unit cell with the crystal lattice. Non-periodic arrangements and/or even a single unit cell (e.g., single molecule) will also have a structure factor, but the resulting Fourier space distribution will be continuous and not discrete, and it will be highly susceptible to noise. A periodic arrangement is one way to strengthen the signal by concentrating the signal into discrete locations (diffraction spots). The entire structure of the unit cells (i.e., its scattering centers) contribute to each of the diffraction spot, and therefore all information about the scattering centers in the unit cell is distributed over the entire diffraction pattern, and thus the entire diffraction pattern needs to be decoded appropriately to reconstruct the

Introduction to Biological Imaging, First Edition. Manfred Auer.

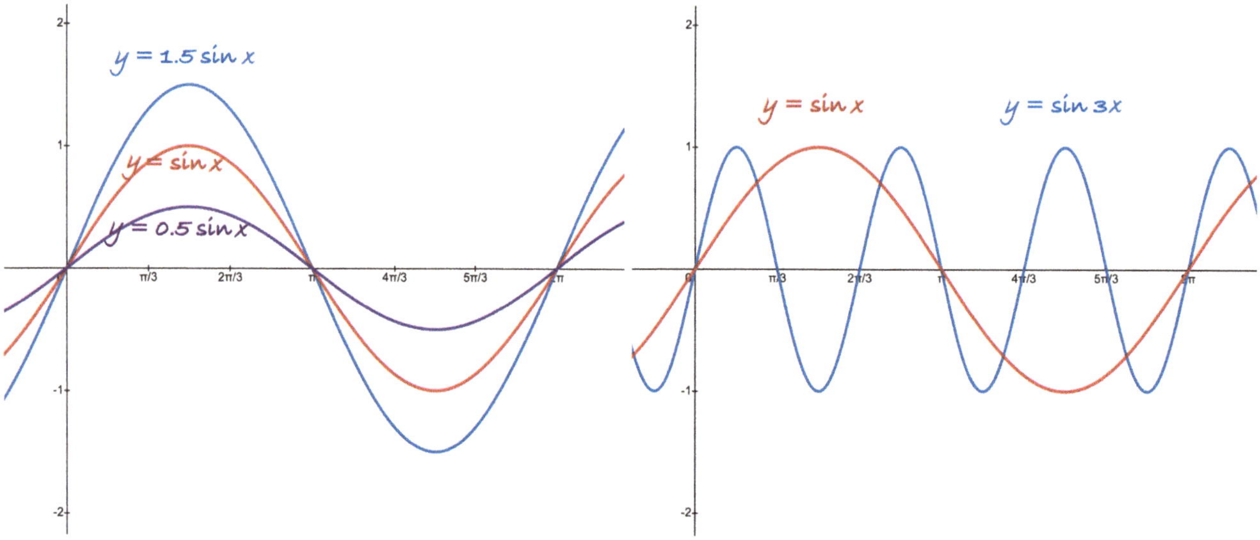

Figure 4.1 Waves: Amplitude and frequency. Sine waves are characterized by their amplitude, frequency, and phase. Left: Three sine waves with the same frequency, an amplitude of 0.5 (purple wave), of 1.0 (red wave), and 1.5 (blue wave), and a phase shift of zero. Right: Two sine waves, with the blue wave having a frequency of three times the frequency of the red wave.

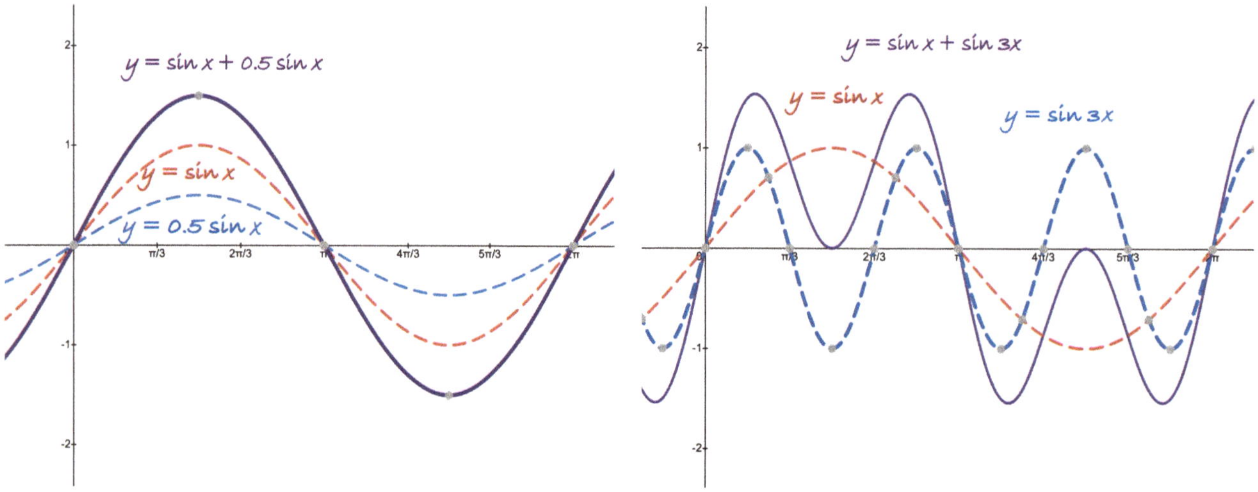

Figure 4.2 Superposition of waves: Role of amplitude and frequency. Superposition of two waves (red and blue dotted lines) leads to the addition of the *Y*-axis value at every *X*-value position (purple continuous line). Note that some numbers may be negative and hence the sum of a negative number is effectively a subtraction of the negative value from the positive number. When all waves have the same frequency and phase shift, the superposition will result in a wave with a higher amplitude but the same frequency and phase shift. The superposition of two waves with different frequency but same amplitude and phase shift results in a more complicated curve, where at some positions the resulting superposition will lead to constructive or to destructive interference.

electron density (the position of all the scattering centers) in the unit cell.

To say that the structure factor $F_{(hkl)}$ is a vector is to say that $F_{(hkl)}$ can be written as a complex number. As a complex number it constitutes a Cartesian plane with a so-called real (*x*-axis) and imaginary axis (*y*-axis). As a vector in this Cartesian plane, $F_{(hkl)}$ has a vector length, also referred to as its amplitude and a phase (ϕ) which is the angle the vector includes with the real axis (i.e., the *x*-axis).

Euler's formula describes the vector as an amplitude $|F_{(hkl)}|$ times $e^{i\phi}$, which can be thought of as a vector sum of the vector cos (ϕ) along the real axis and the vector sin (ϕ) on the imaginary axis. We can write $e^{i*\phi} = \cos(\phi) + i\sin(\phi)$ with ϕ being the phase shift of the wave (Figure 4.6).

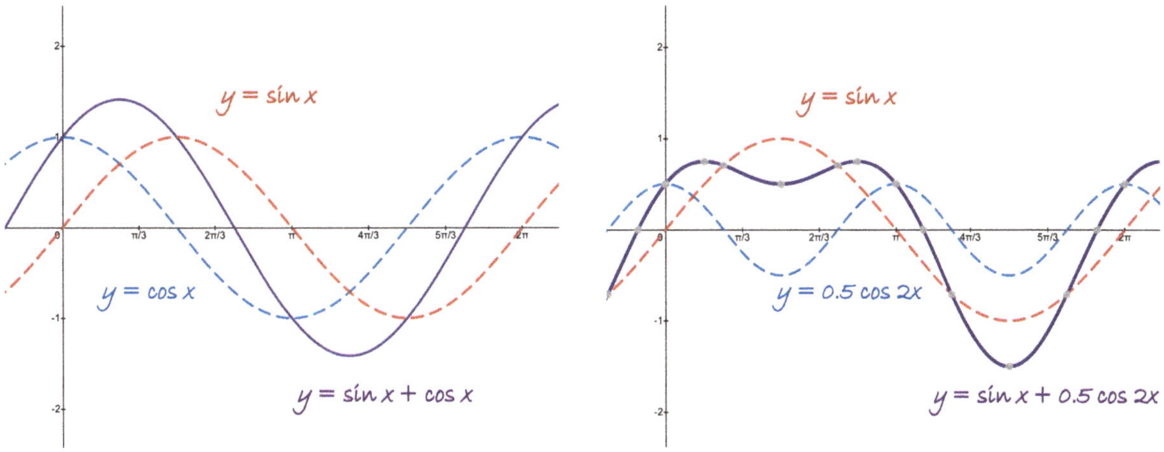

Figure 4.3 Superposition of waves: Role of phase shift, amplitude, and frequency. Left: Phase shift of $\pi/2$ (90°) turns a sine wave into cosine wave. Superposition of the two waves lead to a third wave (purple) with a higher amplitude but the same frequency. A phase shift of π or 180° between the two waves would lead to a completely destructive interference with all Y values being zero (not shown). Right: Superposition of two waves with different amplitudes, frequency, and phase shifts results in a more complicated function (purple) with some constructive and some destructive interference.

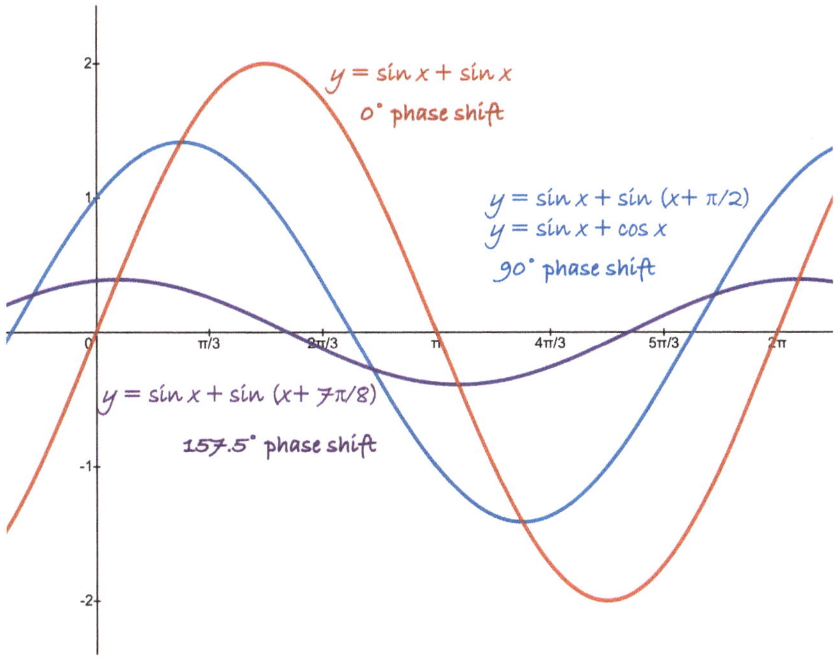

Figure 4.4 Constructive and destructive interference depends on the phase shift between the two waves. Three different waves are shown that are the results of the sum of two waves. The three waves differ from one another in the phase shift that the second wave has compared to the first wave. The red wave (0° phase shift between the two waves) is an example of constructive interference, whereas the purple wave (with a $7\pi/8$; 157.5° phase shift) is an example of destructive interference. The blue wave is somewhere in between with positive and negative interference.

We can then write the formula for the structure facture $F(hkl)$ for a particular hkl-index position in the diffraction 3D-lattice, by summing up all n scattering factors (atoms) at each x, y, z coordinate of the unit cell.

$$F(hkl) = \sum_{j=1}^{n} f_j e^{2\pi i[hx+ky+lz]}$$

In other words, if we know the position of each atom in the unit cell and its scattering factor (which depends on the atomic number of the atom and thus its elemental identity), we can calculate what the diffraction pattern in reciprocal (diffraction) space will look like, and thus determine the structure factor with its amplitude and phase for each reflection (diffraction spot).

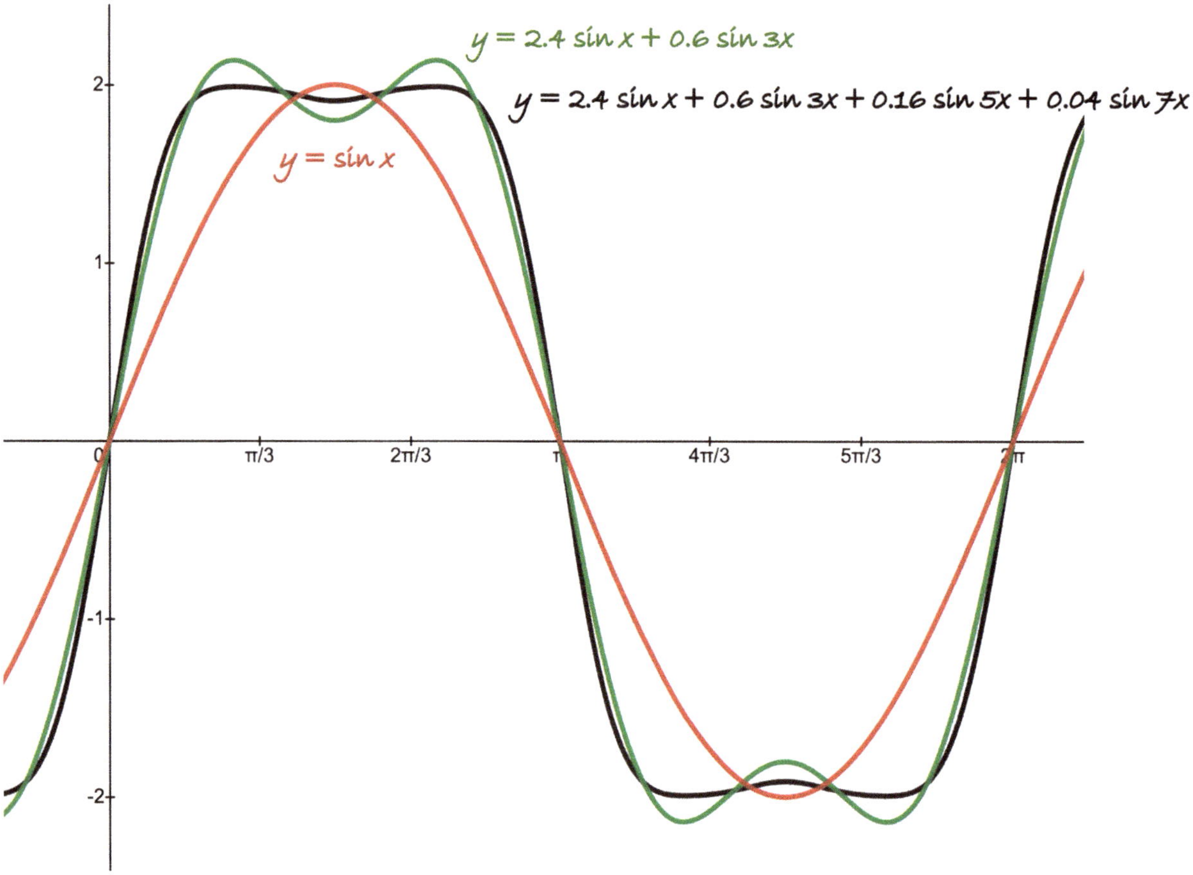

Figure 4.5 Approximation of a step function by adding sinusoid wave functions. Adding many sinusoid (sine and cosine) wave functions with different amplitudes, frequencies and phase shifts allows the approximation any function, e.g., a step function. Note that lower frequency waves define the rough outline, whereas higher frequency (higher resolution) terms allow a closer approximation of the function that is to be modeled.

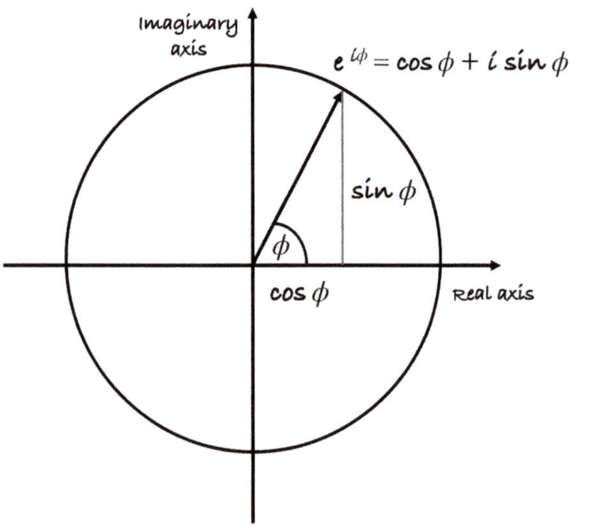

Figure 4.6 Description of a vector as a complex number. A vector can be described in a Cartesian plane as complex number with a real axis (*X*-axis) and an imaginary axis (*Y*-axis). The vector has a length (also referred to as an amplitude) and a phase ϕ. Euler's formula describes the vector as the vector sum of cos ϕ on the real axis and sin ϕ on the imaginary axis.

Likewise, if we can determine the structure factor at each *hkl*-indexed diffraction spot, and know its amplitude and its phase, we can for any specific *x*, *y*, *z* coordinate in the unit cell determine the scattering power, which we refer to as the electron density at the position *x*, *y*, *z*.

$$\rho(xyz) = \frac{1}{V}\sum_{hkl\,-\infty}^{+\infty} |F(hkl)| \cdot e^{-2\pi i[hx+ky+lz-\phi(hkl)]}$$

Repeating this calculation for every *x*, *y*, *z* combination (for every point in the unit cell) results in a 3D electron density map, which is a distribution of atoms in the unit cell. The resulting model of atoms placed in the *x*, *y*, *z* coordinate space of the unit cell is called an atomic model or the atomic structure of the (macro)molecule. Note that Euler's formula applies, and thus that the above formulas can be written as a combination of sinusoids to replace the exponential expression.

It should be obvious now that determining a diffraction pattern with an amplitude and phase for each reflection from an image is straight forward, and simply requires the mathematic exercise of multiplications and sums of terms with known arguments. Likewise, the inverse Fourier transform is straight forward if amplitude and phase are known for each position in reciprocal (diffraction) space. The same principle applies also to non-crystalline macromolecules, where the Fourier transform is continuous instead of discrete.

Fourier transforms can also be used to distinguish high frequency (high resolution) from low frequency (low resolution) contributions, and thus can be used for noise filtering (which tends to be more of a high frequency phenomenon). In real space pixel to pixel variations constitute a high frequency signal, whereas in the case of a sizeable object the intensity of neighboring pixels is related to one another.

The situation becomes more complicated when the phase information is lost, as is the case in an experimental X-ray diffraction experiment. Here only the intensity (as the scaled square of the amplitude) of a diffraction spot can be measured, and the phase information is lost upon the impact of the photons on the detector. This is known in X-ray crystallography as the phase problem, and thus the very essence of structure determination in X-ray crystallography lies in restoring reliable phase information for each of the *hkl*-indexed reflections.

In a Fourier transform of an image, the low-resolution information is near the center of the Fourier transform, whereas the higher-resolution information resides near the periphery with a maximal value at the edge of the Fourier transform that relates to the sampling step size (in accordance with the Nyquist–Shannon theorem). Hence, by circular masking one can ignore the higher frequency contributions, in which case we speak of low pass filtering.

Lenses in an optical system in essence carry out a Fourier transform, which leads to a diffraction pattern/image in the back focal plane that with the use of another lens is reversed back to an actual image of the object, with both amplitudes and phases being known.

Fourier–Bessel series is a special case of Fourier series, and particularly helpful when cylindrical or spherical coordinates are used. Fourier–Bessel methods have been used for 3D reconstruction of specimen with helical symmetry, such as actin filaments, microtubule tubes or 2D crystals of the acetylcholine receptor or the Calcium ATPase. Fourier–Bessel methods remain in use even though single particle-based approaches in the form of iterative helical real space reconstruction (IHRSR) methods have recently replaced Fourier–Bessel methods in helical reconstruction.

Bessel functions were first defined by Daniel Bernoulli and then generalized Friedrich Bessel. Bessel functions are known as cylindrical harmonics and are used in the solution of partial differential equations in cylindrical (/spherical) coordinate systems. The Fourier transform of a projection image of a helical object is equivalent to a central section through the 3D Fourier transform with its layer planes, which results in a 2D power spectrum with layer lines that can be described with Fourier-Bessel series (Figure 4.7).

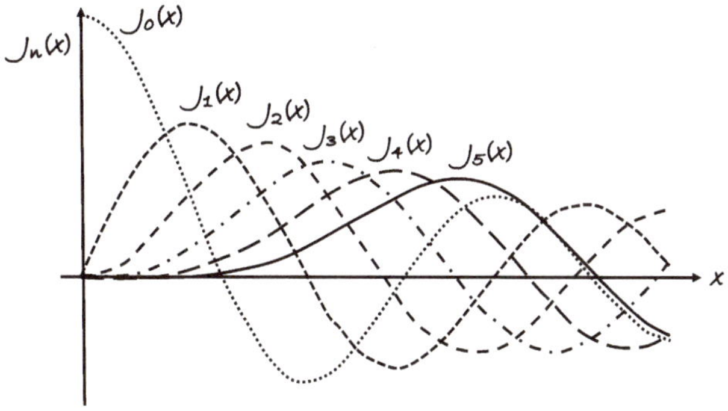

Figure 4.7 Fourier–Bessel series. Fourier–Bessel series are a special case of Fourier series. They are particularly useful in systems that use cylindrical or spherical coordinates, such as filaments or tubular structures with helical symmetry.

5

Basics of Imaging and Image Formation

5.1 Goals of Imaging

When considering bioimaging, we need to define the goal of imaging, such as the determination of precise shapes of macromolecules (Chapter 7), the architectural interplay of macromolecular inventory (Chapter 8), the spatiotemporal localization of selected macromolecules (Chapter 9), or the composition of the molecular (and possibly macromolecular) inventory (Chapter 10) (Figure 5.1).

For a structural biologist the goal is to determine the exact shape, ideally at atomic resolution of a well-defined macromolecule or ensemble of macromolecules. At high resolution, where the position of individual atoms can be established, one can determine the mechanism of an enzymatic reaction, drug–target interactions, or the molecular interactions between macromolecules, such as viruses docking to their cellular receptors. Historically, structural biologists tended to focus either on X-ray crystallography or NMR spectroscopy, but due to the "resolution in revolution" cryo-EM in the last decade, single particle analysis has become the dominant discipline in structural biology in recent years.

Many cell biologists are more interested in the localization and the dynamic behavior of proteins rather than their precise 3D structure. Detailed macromolecular interactions with other (macro-)molecules at atomic detail are of secondary interest. They are in the category: "nice to have, but not essential." Fluorescence light microscopy has become the work horse for cell biology imaging, since it is ideally suited for real-time live-cell imaging, which is often the key for cell biological understanding.

Neurobiologists interested in "connectomics" aim to determine the 3D organization of interacting neurons in the brain, and therefore aren't interested at all in macromolecules. Light microscopy can cover a larger field of view/volume at moderate resolution, whereas electron microscopy (particularly large volume 3D scanning electron microscopy) reveals higher resolution details, but typically is restricted to a much smaller volume. Note however that in fluorescence light microscopy one only images what is labeled, whereas in electron microscopy all structures are visible.

Systems biologists are much more interested in the protein, lipid, and metabolite composition as a function of cellular state or as a response to a cellular perturbation.

Developmental biologists are interested in the patterning of cells to form tissues or organs and their breakdown due to genetic mutations. One of the key aspects of developmental biology imaging is to minimize light exposure during imaging to allow long-term assessment of tissue and organ development, hence light sheet imaging is a key technique.

Naturally, there are hybrid disciplines that borrow concepts from its flanking discipline, such as structural cell biologists, who are interested in the 3D architectural organization of macromolecules, including their shape but also their spatial distribution with respect to organelles and other cellular landmarks, as well as the shape (geometric/volumetric properties) of supramolecular complexes (such as the cytoskeleton) as well as of organelles.

Increasingly, there is an interest in correlative imaging, which aims to identify a particular region of interest by using reporter molecules and fluorescence light microscopy. That region of interest is subsequently studied at higher resolution by electron microscopy.

As it should have become clear by now, there is no goal that is "per se" worthier than any other, as all the different approaches are valuable in their own right, and each goal will require a certain set of imaging techniques, with each imaging technique having its own sample preparation requirements, source of radiation, imaging optics as well as detection system.

Introduction to Biological Imaging, First Edition. Manfred Auer.

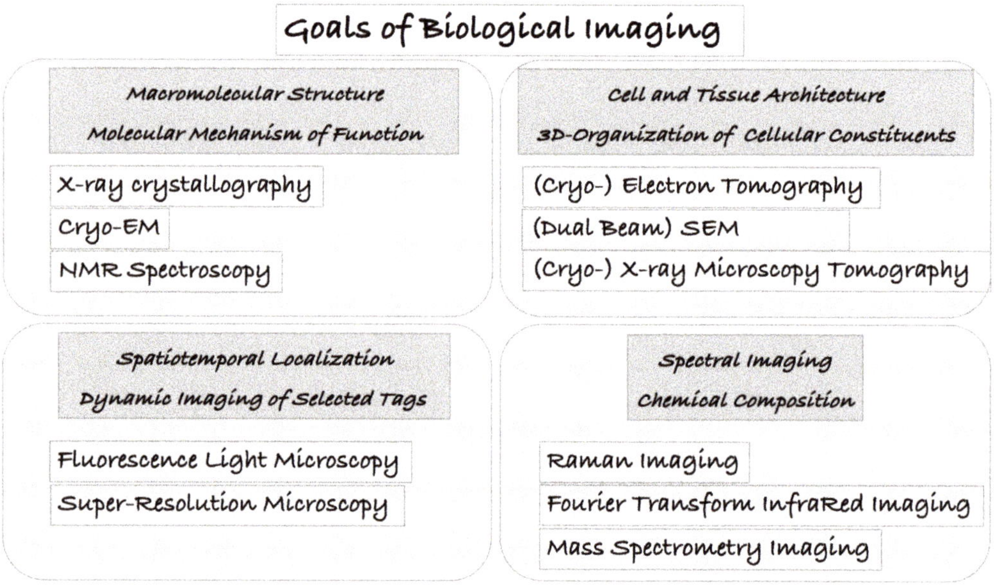

Figure 5.1 Goals of bioimaging. There are different goals in biological imaging: Methods for macromolecular structure determination, such as X-ray crystallography, Cryo-EM, and NMR spectroscopy, aim for atomic-level, high-resolution that will reveal molecular mechanisms of function. Determination of cell and tissue architecture, relies on (Cryo-) Electron Tomography, large volume/ dual beam Scanning Electron Microscopy and X-ray Microscopy Tomography. Here the goal is to determine the 3D organization of cellular constituents. In the case of spatiotemporal localization a few selected tags provide dynamic information using diffraction-limited and superresolution fluorescent light microscopy. Spectral imaging in the form of Raman imaging or FTIR imaging and chemical imaging such as mass spectrometry imaging can reveal the chemical molecular and/or macromolecular composition of a sample.

5.2 Source of Radiation

Each imaging technique requires its own type of equipment, some of which are benchtop-sized (most visible light imaging techniques fall into this category), some require their own room or building, such as for transmission electron microscopy, X-ray crystallography or NMR spectroscopy. Others yet are in size in between, where multiple instruments can be fit into one room, with each instrument having the footprint of a large dining table. Particle accelerators relevant for bioimaging, such as synchrotrons, fall into a completely different category, as synchrotrons occupy a space equivalent of a football field, some even the size of several football fields, with individual measuring stations for a specific radiation type being much smaller, typically the size of a single room. Nearly the entire range of the electromagnetic spectrum is used for imaging of biological samples (Figure 5.2). Gamma-rays are the result of a positron-electron annihilation, with radionuclides being the source of positron emission. X-rays are produced either by using rotating anodes or in synchrotrons. UV, visible and near infrared light is produced by arc lamps, light emitting diodes (LED) or lasers. Mid-infrared radiation is generated by a Globar®, microwaves by magnetrons and radio waves by radio transmitters in combination with an antenna.

Synchrotrons produce electromagnetic radiation from hard X-rays to infrared waves, and frequently the entire spectrum of electromagnetic radiation is used for high-energy flux imaging. Synchrotrons use varying electric and magnetic fields to accelerate charged particles (typically electrons) and force them onto a circular trajectory, which leads to the tangential emission of electromagnetic radiation. These radiation beams are then used in different workstations (often referred to as hutches) for imaging experiments. Cyclotrons were the precursors of the modern synchrotrons, where charged particles (e.g., protons) are accelerated in a spiral trajectory from the center in a constant magnetic field. Cyclotrons are nowadays still used for creating radioisotopes for nuclear medicine.

5.2.1 Gamma-Rays

Gamma rays are not really used in bioimaging as a radiation source, although gamma-rays are ultimately detected in Positron Emission Tomography (PET). However, the radiation source for PET is a radioactive tracer substance that is administered to the patient, typically intravenously, and that undergoes radioactive beta decay, creating positrons in the process, which annihilate with an electron to produce a pair of gamma rays, which is then detected.

Source of Radiation

electromagnetic radiation		
gamma-rays	electron–positron annihilation	positron emission tomography
X-rays	rotating anode, synchrotron	X-ray crystallography, SAXS, X-ray microscopy tomography, CT
UV/Vis/near-IR	arc lamp, LED, laser	bright light, fluorescence, and Raman microscopy
infrared	Globar (SiC), synchrotron	FTIR microscopy
microwave	magnetron	
radio wave	radio transmitter with antenna	NMR spectroscopy, MRI imaging

Figure 5.2 Source of electromagnetic radiation and application in bioimaging. Nearly the entire electromagnetic spectrum is used for bioimaging purposes, ranging from gamma rays to radio waves except for microwaves.

5.2.2 X-Rays

The classic way to produce X-rays is to bombard a target metal anode with electrons, which leads to the production of X-rays. Since this process generates significant amount of heat, such anodes are usually rotating for the purpose of cooling. Rotating anodes have been the workhorse for X-ray crystallography until access to the much brighter synchrotron radiation facilities became widely available. Nowadays, most structures being determined by X-ray crystallography use synchrotron radiation. Synchrotrons in the context of bioimaging are particle accelerators, where electrons are accelerated to high velocity and forced onto a circular trajectory, which results in tangential electromagnetic radiation. Undulators are highly specialized periodic arrays of dipole-magnets who force electrons to undergo oscillations and thus radiate energy. Undulators produce a much higher-intensity X-ray beam, which is both coherent and collimated, and thus ideally suited for X-ray crystallography experiments. Undulators are not specific to X-rays and can also be designed to yield other types of collimated high-intensity electromagnetic radiation.

5.2.3 UV-Rays/Visible Light Rays/Near-IR Light Rays

Arc Lamps

Arc-lamps have been used for many decades as they are a high-powered light source. There are a variety of arc lamps, such as the Xenon gas discharge lamps, where electricity passing through ionized xenon gas leads to a white (broad spectrum) bright light, not unlike sunlight. However, such lamps are very hot (up to 10,000 °C), and thus often need to be (water-)cooled, with an average lifetime of only ~500 hours. This type of light is still being used today in movie theaters. In mercury-vapor lamp, vaporized mercury is the filling gas. Such lamps are fairly energy efficient with a much longer lifetime of ~24,000 hours, creating high-intensity white light, however they require a warm-up time of several minute for full light output, as the mercury needs to vaporize.

Such lamps are frequently used in sports arenas. They face strong competition from metal halide lamps, which are made of an amalgam of mercury with sodium iodide.

For high-end spectroscopy, where a continuous UV spectrum is needed, with little output in the visible and IR range, deuterium lamps are the illumination source of choice. Deuterium lamps are more expensive than hydrogen lamps, but they are superior as they have a longer life span and better emission in the far UV range with continuous emission between ~180 and ~370 nm. However, they need ~20 seconds of warm-up time, and have a lifetime of about 2,000–5,000 hours.

Light Emitting Diode (LED)

Light-emitting diodes are a semiconductor-based light source, which emit light when an electric current flows. In some way, one can think of LED as the reverse effect of the inner photoelectric effect, which underlies semiconductor light detector technology. For LEDs, white light can be obtained by using a mixture of semiconductors of different frequency (such as red, green, and blue LEDs) or by coating the LED with a layer of light emitting phosphor. There are LED for UV light, visible light as well as the IR light range.

LED have low power consumption, long lifetime, physical robustness, small size, and fast switching. Some LEDs emit in the blue and UV range, with some diodes emitting down to 240 nm. The 2014 Nobel Prize in Physics was awarded to Isamu Akasaki, Hiroshi Amano, and Shuji Nakamura for the invention of efficient blue light emitting diodes which enabled bright and energy-saving white light sources.

Laser

As the word laser (short for "light amplification by stimulated emission of radiation") implies, a laser is a device that emits a high amount of light, based on the concept of stimulated emission. Historically, the foundation of laser technology was laid in the 1950s by Alfred Kastler, who won the Nobel Prize for Physics in 1966 for proposing an optical pumping mechanism. Charles H. Townes, Nikolay Basov, and Aleksandr Prokhorov shared the 1964 Nobel Prize in Physics for their fundamental work in the field of quantum electronics, which has led to the construction of oscillators and amplifiers based on the (microwave amplification by stimulated emission of radiation) maser–laser principle. The first functioning laser was built in 1960.

What makes a laser so different from other sources of light (such as thermal sources) is that the emitted light is spatially coherent, allowing the laser light to be collimated to a small spot that stays narrow, even over great distances. Laser can also be spectrally coherent with the spectral emission window being very narrow. Light waves produced by a laser are also temporally coherent, which means that even over great distances, the wave stays in phase, or to word it differently: laser have a long coherent length. Lasers can be operating continuously or be pulsed, which means that ultrashort pulses (as short as femtosecond duration) can be produced.

Historically, lasers followed the invention of masers, which stands for "microwave amplification by stimulated emission of radiation," and the concept is exactly the same. This already implies that lasers can be built for all the different regions of the electromagnetic spectrum, from gamma-ray lasers to infrared lasers (with the word maser being reserved for microwave or radio wave radiation).

At the center of a laser is a so-called gain medium, a material that allows light amplification through stimulated emission. This gain medium requires energy in form of light at a different wavelength, a flash lamp or an electric current (a process that is also known as pumping) in order to populate the excited state until there are more electrons in the excited state than in the ground state, at which point one reaches population inversion. Once the system is in such a state, there are more electrons that relax back from the excited state to the ground state than electrons absorbing the photons to reach an excited state, which leads to the amplification of light (a gain in photons). In addition, the gain medium reside inside what is called a resonant optical cavity, where light travels back and forth between a pair of mirrors. Each time the light beam is gaining strength, meaning there is an increase in the number of polarized coherent photons, before a portion of the light beam can escape through one of the mirrors, which is partially transparent.

The gain in photons is explained by the quantum mechanics phenomenon known as stimulated emission, where an electron already at an excited state interacts with a photon of appropriate energy (wavelength) and relaxes back to its ground state, and in the process giving off two photons of the same energy (wavelength), which also show the same polarization and path of propagation (direction). It should be noted that the temporal coherence of laser light, is the result of the resonant optical cavity setup and is not a direct consequence of stimulated emission.

Stimulated emission stands in contrast to spontaneous emission, where electrons in the ground state are elevated to an excited state by absorption of photons, and spontaneously relax back to the ground state, which case photons are emitted which have the same wavelength (energy) but are random in terms of direction and polarization.

The gain medium can be a gas, liquid, solid, or even plasma, but requires defined properties with respect to purity, size, concentration, or sometimes even shape. For a laser to be effective, the amplification in the gain medium must be larger than the losses of the resonator set-up. Also, each time a photon is gained, electrons in the excited state are lost and electrons in the ground state accumulate, hence reducing the gain of the medium until a gain medium saturation is reached.

There are a variety of different lasers, some operate as gas discharge lasers, such as the commonly used helium neon laser, emitting at 633 nm, or so-called excimer lasers, a specialized sort of gas lasers (e.g., ArF, KrCl, KrF, XeCl, XeF) that emit in the UV range.

In addition to gas discharge lasers, there are also solid-state lasers, some of which operate in the visible light range or the near-IR range. Titanium-doped sapphire lasers are used as highly tunable infrared lasers for spectroscopic applications and can be used as a mode-locked laser with high peak-power ultrashort pulses.

Semiconductor lasers are diodes, which are electrically pumped, with the recombination of electrons and holes (the reverse of the inner photoelectric effect) induced by the applied current leading to optical gain, and the crystal itself acting like an optical resonator. Such diodes can emit wavelengths from near UV to mid-IR.

Dye lasers employ an organic dye as the gain medium, with a wide spectrum of dyes (and mixture of dyes) being available, these lasers can be tuned to a variety of frequencies.

Free-electron lasers operate in a way different from the classical atomic or molecular valence states and instead use accelerated electron beams for the generation of high-power coherent radiation range in frequencies from the X-ray range, over UV, visible light, and IR range to the microwave range.

For continuous wave (CW) lasers, there must be an equilibrium found between pump power gain and the combination of gain medium saturation and optical cavity/resonator losses. Some lasers cannot be run as CW lasers, but give off their energy as repetitive laser pulses, which can be very short (nanosecond to femtosecond range) and very high-powered. So-called mode-lock lasers can produce perfectly periodic pulses with perfect phase-coherence. Pulsed pumping is another way to create a pulsed laser beam.

In general, due to the many complications UV light presents for biological samples, including radiation damage, limited choices for microscope optics and that fact that there aren't that many interesting biological questions in that UV-light window of the electromagnetic spectrum, UV imaging is rarely used.

5.2.4 IR Radiation

Near-IR radiation with wavelengths ranging from 1 to 2.5 µm is emitted by tungsten-halogen lamps. Also as discussed above, IR lasers are available, particularly for the near-IR region of the spectrum. For the mid-IR range of the electromagnetic spectrum, the most commonly used source is a so-called Globar® (sometimes referred to as a "glow bar"), which consists of a silicon carbide (SiC) rod that is heated electrically to between 1,000 and 1,650 °C. Its emission spectrum is close to the ideal case of a black body (Planck) radiator. For the far-IR at wavelengths greater than 50 µm, mercury discharge lamps are an alternative thermal source, however, far-IR radiation is not relevant for biological imaging. The most powerful and spectrally tunable source of IR radiation is synchrotron radiation.

5.2.5 Microwave Radiation

Microwaves have a wavelength ranging from millimeter to meter. Microwaves do not play much of a role in bioimaging, as there is little relevant information about biological systems in that wavelength/size range. Microwaves do play a role in certain sample preparation protocols that rely on the diffusion of chemicals into tissues and organs. In such cases, low intensity microwave irradiation can speed up the diffusion of such chemicals, but care must be taken not to "cook" the sample, as microwaves induce polar molecules such as water to rotate and thus produce heat, a process that is also known as dielectric heating.

Microwaves are produced in a magnetron, which is a high-power vacuum tube, where electrons, produced at a heated cathode, move to the anode. If such a system is placed into an appropriate magnetic field, the electrons are forced on circular trajectories between cathode and anode, emitting microwave radiation, in a process very similar to cyclotrons. However, in its simplest form, production of microwave radiation is not very efficient, hence current day devices rely on a resonant cavity magnetron, which is not based on external circuits or fields, but on the oscillation of electrons based on the shape of the anode. The cavity magnetron looks similar to the cylinder of a revolver handgun, into which a central hole has been drilled that carries a wire serving the function of the cathode. Each circular cavity of the revolver drum has a narrow opening to the center cavity of the magnetron, which acts as capacitor, while the circular cavities form an inducer. Electrons travel along the surface of the circular cavities, and when placed into a magnetic field, they move on arched trajectories toward the anode. Oscillating currents form a flow around the cavities, which results in microwave frequency radiation being produced inside this cavity magnetron. This microwave radiation is being detected and then transmitted to the outside via a loop-shaped wire, called a tap. The size of the cavities determines the resonant frequency, and thus the microwave frequency being produced.

5.2.6 Radio Wave Radiation

Radio waves have a wavelength ranging from meters to kilometers and are thus not directly useful for bioimaging. However, they are central to nuclear magnetic resonance (NMR) spectroscopy and the related magnetic resonance imaging. Radio waves are generated and detected by radio transmitters and receivers, using antennas. Radio wave transmitters are simply devices producing an alternative current at radiofrequency, which is then coupled to an antenna that emits radio waves.

5.2.7 Particle Radiation

Particles such as electrons, positrons, neutrons, and ions can also be used to probe biological samples. It is helpful to remind ourselves that both particles and photons possess both particle-like as well as wave-like properties, and thus possess a wavelength and momentum energy, which will be important to consider when the radiation interacts with matter. The energy of a particle beam depends on how much the particle has been accelerated. While accelerated

Source of Radiation

particle radiation		
electrons	thermionic emission electron gun field emission electron gun	Transmission and Scanning Electron Microscopy
positrons	radioactive decay	Positron Emission Tomography
ion beam	field emission electron gun in presence of helium gas	Helium Ion Microscopy
neutrons	research reactor, spallation source	Small Angle Neutron Scattering

Figure 5.3 Source of particle radiation and application in bioimaging. Accelerated particles not only possess particle-like properties such as momentum but also wave-like properties such as wavelength. Among the particles, electrons feature most prominently for bioimaging, but ion beams are becoming more prominent not only for sample preparation (milling of the sample) but also for imaging (e.g., helium ion microscopy).

protons could in principle be used for imaging, there is hardly any application in biological imaging that uses a proton beam. Likewise, the use of neutrons in imaging is not very wide-spread, with Small Angle Neutron Scattering being a niche technique. Widely used are electrons in transmission electron microscopy (TEM) or scanning electron microscopy (SEM). SEM is often used in conjunction with an ion beam that trims the samples. This approach is known as Focused Ion Beam Scanning Electron Microscopy (FIBSEM) or Dual Beam SEM. However, ion beams can also be used directly for imaging. Helium ion microscopes show promise to outperform scanning electron microscopes in terms of achievable resolution, focal depth and blurring, which is due to specimen charging (Figure 5.3).

5.2.8 Particle Radiation: Electrons

Electrons are being extracted from an electrode either by thermionic emission or by field emission. Thermionic emission (also referred to as the Edison effect) is the process by which free electrons are produced at a hot cathode residing in a vacuum tube. The cathode material is either a metal such as tungsten (W) or a transition metal borides (or carbides) such as lanthanum boride (LaB_6). The thermal energy provided can overcome the work function of the material, i.e., the minimal amount of energy for an electron to leave the surface (which is typically in the order of a few electron volts). According to band theory in solid-state physics, electrons in a large, periodic lattice of atoms or molecules can adopt a range of energy levels (electronic bands) and are free to move from atom to atom. In this sea of electrons, the velocities of individual electrons adopt a statistical distribution, with some electrons having enough energy to exit the surface of the material (and thus to overcome the work function). Increase in thermionic currents depend exponentially on the temperature of the wire. Oxide coatings on metal filaments decrease the work function. Owen Willans Richardson was awarded the 1928 Nobel Prize in Physics for his work on thermionic emission.

The second mechanism for extraction of electrons from a material surface is known as field electron emission or simply as field emission (FE). For field emission to occur, a high electrostatic field is applied to a sharp (oxide-coated) metal tip, which results in the quantum-mechanical tunneling and thus release from the surface of the electron.

In electron guns used in electron microscopes, electrons are produced either by thermionic emission (e.g., by tungsten or lanthanum hexaboride) or by field emission. Such free electrons are accelerated from the cathode to an anode, through a cylinder with repulsive electrical field to collimate the electron beam. A central hole in the anode allows the narrow electron beam to pass through.

Field emission guns (FEG) are preferred for high resolution electron microscopes as the electron beam is smaller, much brighter, and more coherent, both in terms of spatial and temporal coherence. Electrons originate from a smaller volume and with a better-defined kinetic energy, as there are no thermal differences in energies of the electrons that need to be considered. FEG can be operated at room temperature, but heating is often preferred as it prevents build up of contamination at the tip.

Electron guns are not only used for electron microscopy, but can also be used for ionization purposes, like in mass spectrometry or to remove electrons to create ion beams in helium (scanning) ion microscopy (HeIM). For HeIM, tips consisting of a three-atom triangle are used for the ionization of the helium gas in the vacuum to produce a very narrow helium ion beam. Furthermore, electron guns can also be used to create microwave frequencies and most importantly in linear accelerators, where a high energy electron beam to hits a target to produce X-rays.

5.2.9 Particle Radiation: Positrons

Positrons are emitted as part of the radioactive beta decay and requires the generation of radioactive nuclei that undergo radioactive beta decay. Positrons emitted by the radioactive nuclei annihilate with electrons, leading to a pair of gamma-rays emitted in opposite directions that can be detected. Positrons play a prominent role in Positron Emission Tomography (PET), a medical imaging technique, but otherwise have no role in bioimaging.

5.2.10 Particle Radiation: Alpha-Radiation/ Helium Nuclei

Alpha particles are positively charged helium nuclei, consisting of two protons and two neutrons thus possessing two positive charges. They are the result of radioactive alpha decay and thus exist naturally. However, in this form, they are not used for biological imaging. Instead, helium ions are produced by ionization of helium gas.

5.2.11 Particle Radiation: Ion Beams

Helium ion beams can be obtained from helium gas by heating the apex of a metal (e.g., tungsten) tip in a vacuum. As a result, helium gas atoms are ionized to form helium ions with a single positive charge. Helium ions are accelerated and collimated into a narrow beam. Atomically sharp tips can be produced, consisting of three atoms arranged in a triangle, which are highly effective in creating helium ion beams.

Apart from helium ion beams there are other sources of charged particles/ion beams (such as argon), which are usually obtained in a similar way to helium ions (e.g., in duoplasmatrons), but many of these ion beams are often not used for imaging purposes, instead they are used for sample preparation, e.g., the ablation/milling of a sample in focused ion beam scanning electron microscopy and/or excavation of thin lamella, e.g., for cryo-electron tomography.

5.2.12 Particle Radiation: Neutrons

Free neutrons can be emitted as a result of nuclear fission of highly enriched (typically 20%) uranium in a research reactor (also known as non-power reactors) or by nuclear fusion, e.g., when alpha particles collide with a beryllium nucleus resulting in a carbon nucleus. Neutron moderators such as graphite, ordinary water (light water) and heavy water slow down fast neutrons allowing an effective fission chain reaction. Another source of neutron radiation are high energy particle accelerators (spallation neutron sources), where protons are accelerated to high energies before hitting a target, prompting the emission of neutrons.

5.2.13 Particle Radiation: Protons

Protons are not used in routine biomedical imaging applications, although their use has been proposed in the 1960s as proton computed tomography (pCT). While absorption of a proton by a tissue (its relative stopping power) can be determined, it is less clear how to interpret the loss of the signal in biologically/biochemically relevant terms.

5.3 Beam Collimation

A beam is considered collimated when the electromagnetic rays run parallel to one another, thus spreading minimally (limited only by diffraction) along its path. Another way to state it is to say that collimated electromagnetic radiation is focused on a point in infinity, which also means that perfectly collimated radiation can be thought of plane waves (even though we started with spherical wavelets).

The concept of collimation also applies to particle beams and implies that the trajectories of the particles is parallel to one another and thus that beam divergence is minimal over the scale of the experimental setup.

Some radiation sources are inherently collimated such as synchrotrons or lasers. For other radiation sources, which can be thought of as point sources, a variety of mechanisms can be used for beam collimation. Whereas visible is relatively straight-forward to collimate, e.g., using mirrors and lenses, other types of radiation are much more difficult to collimate, such as X-rays. For X-rays, focusing can be achieved either by total internal reflection at very small angles (grazing incidence reflection) or multilayer coatings, or by the principles of diffraction and interference at zone plates. Zone plates for X-rays fulfill the function of lenses for optical imaging but are highly chromatic and thus must be adjusted to a small wavelength range. Hence zone plates are best suited for monochromatic X-ray radiation. Gold- or iridium-based mirrors to reflect X-rays do exist but are not widely in use.

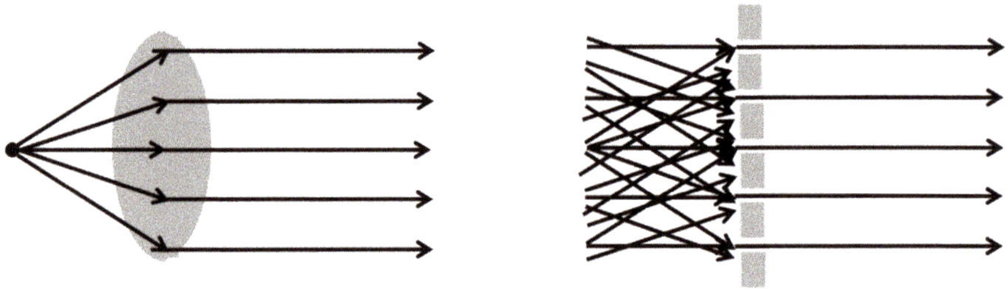

Figure 5.4 Beam collimation. Radiation can be either collimated by lenses or pinholes/apertures. Light can easily be focused through optical lenses, and electrically charged particles such as electrons or ions can be focused/collimated by electromagnetic lenses. Other forms of collimation/focusing can be grazing incidence reflection or by diffraction.

For electrons, which are negatively charged, electrostatic fields can be used to focus the beam. Pinholes/apertures (or related forms of radiation shielding) are another way to simply stop any beams that are not parallel, but pinholes will reduce the amount of radiation available for imaging (Figure 5.4).

5.4 Lenses

Refraction is the basis for understanding the properties of optical lenses. Lenses are simply devices that either converge or diverge light rays because of refraction. Lenses that converge are called convex lenses, whereas lenses that diverge light rays are called concave lenses.

Lenses are typically characterized by their focal length, with converging lenses having a positive focal length and diverging lenses having a negative focal length. The smaller the focal length the stronger is its converging or diverging effect. If parallel rays encounter a lens, they will be focused onto a spot on the far side of the lens, defined by the focal length of the lens. There are different kind of lenses such as biconvex, plano convex, positive meniscus, negative meniscus, plane concave and biconcave lenses.

There are three guidelines that allow ray tracing in geometric optics of lenses:

Parallel rays entering a lens converge at its focal plane. Rays originating from the back-focal plane entering a lens exit as parallel rays. Rays passing through the center of the lens are not refracted and thus exit the lens unaffected in a straight line (Figure 5.5).

The magnification M (h_i/h_o) is given by the ratio of the distance of the image from the lens (d_i) and the distance of the object from the lens (d_o). The lens equation states that $1/f = 1/d_o + 1/d_i$, with f being the focal length of the lens (Figure 5.6).

Lenses are rarely perfect and suffer from a variety of distortions/aberrations, with monochromatic aberration reflecting the geometric lens imperfection of a lens to direct rays to a single point, and chromatic aberration reflecting differences in refraction indexes for different wavelengths (thus colors) of the light.

Depth of focus describes the tolerance of placing a recording device in relation to the lens. It is sometimes also referred to as depth of field, and although the two have a slightly different meaning, both describe how far from the focal plane an object or the recording device can be placed outside the focal plane and still be seen at acceptable sharpness. The smaller the aperture the larger the depth of field and the depth of focus (note also: less light is collected by a smaller aperture).

The concept of lenses is most intuitive in the case of optical light microscopy, where differences in refractive index combined with lens geometry can lead to a convergence or

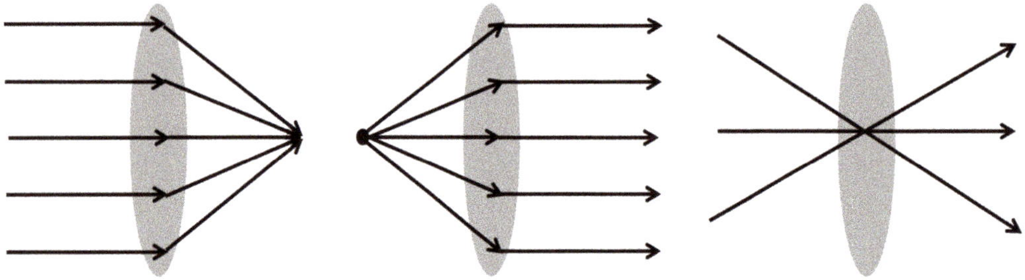

Figure 5.5 Ray tracing in geometric optics of lenses. There are three guiding rules for ray tracing in geometric optics: (1) Parallel rays entering a lens converge at its focal plane (point); (2) Rays originating from the back-focal plane entering a lens exit as parallel rays; (3) Rays passing through the center of a lens continue as straight lines.

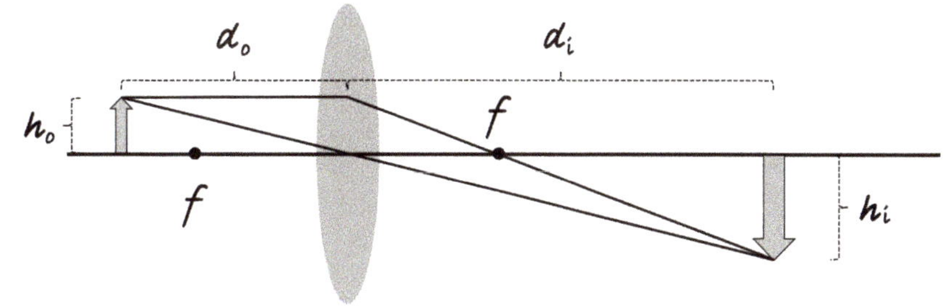

Figure 5.6 Lens magnification. The magnification M (h_i/h_o) is given by the ratio of the distance of the image from the lens (d_i) and the distance of the object from the lens (d_o). The lens equation states that $1/f = 1/d_o + 1/d_i$, with f being the focal length of the lens.

divergence of light rays. However, other forms of radiation can also be focused albeit by different mechanisms. Accelerated charged particles such as electrons and ions can be focused by electromagnetic lenses. Although the path of electrons in electromagnetic lenses is often depicted as straight, in reality the electromagnetic field of the magnetic pole piece (which is surrounded by a solenoid of wires through which an electrical current flows) forces the high velocity particles onto a spiral path. One big advantage of electromagnetic lenses is the wide range of magnification accomplished by a single lens, whereas in optical microscopy the lenses have a constant magnifying power, and changes in magnification require an exchange of the objective lens. However, electromagnetic lenses show a higher degree of aberrations (which can be corrected for), and are also often plagued by hysteresis, particularly when rapidly switching between high and low magnification modes.

Some forms of radiation such as X-rays cannot be focused by traditional lenses. Instead, zone plates, which are based on diffraction, are used for focusing the X-ray beam. In zone plates the concentric rings of radiation-transparent and radiation-absorbing (Fresnel zones) lead to constructive interference. The ring-width becoming increasingly smaller toward the edge, which eventually presents a manufacturing challenge. The width of the outermost zone defines the maximal resolution of the zone plate.

5.5 Lens-Free Imaging/Near Field Imaging

The vast majority of optical imaging is lens-based, and therefore diffraction-limited. One way to overcome the diffraction limit of far-field lens-based optical imaging is to bring laser light into close proximity to the sample, e.g., with the help of a scanning probe microscope, similar to what is done for atomic force microscopy (AFM). The tip of the probe emits an evanescent field that is concentrated in proximity but dies off exponentially. Hence only fluorophores being in direct contact with the probe tip will get excited and emit photons (Figure 5.7). Near-field scanning optical microscopy (NSOM) has been shown to reach a lateral resolution of 6 nm and a vertical resolution of 2–5 nm.

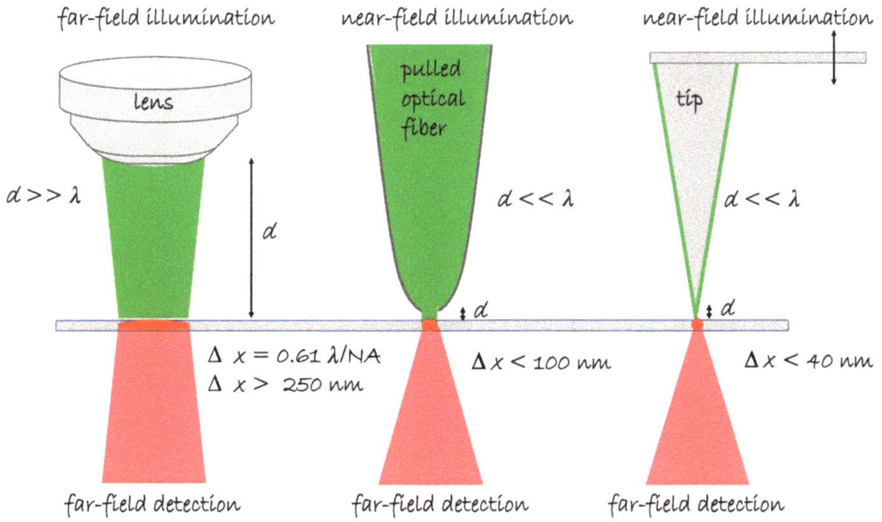

Figure 5.7 Far-field and near-field illumination. Left: Far-field illumination in combination with far-field detection leads to diffraction-limited images. One way to overcome the diffraction limit is to only illuminate a very small volume by near-field illumination using either a pulled optical fiber (middle) or a scanning probe microscope tip (right). While detection is far field (and hence diffraction-limited), it seems safe to assume that only fluorophores close to the optical fiber or scanning probe tip were excited and hence the diffraction-limited signal can only come from a very tiny volume, which in turn leads to high resolution images.

Several experimental challenges need to be overcome, particularly when imaging samples in water, but the development of NSOM has been recognized by the 2014 Nobel Prize in Chemistry awarded to William E. Moerner, along with the other two diffraction/Abbé limit-breaking far-field techniques, which are based on either sequential precise localization of individual molecules or point-spread function engineering. Combining NSOM with spectral imaging seems a particularly promising approach for chemical imaging.

5.6 Signal Detection and Detectors

A detector is a device that interacts with or captures a photon of the electromagnetic spectrum or a particle, and reports the encounter to an observer, ideally with as little time delay and error as possible. While some detectors can report each encounter in real time (with a small delay), thus allowing for a real-time count of the interacting photon or particle, others accumulate and thus integrate the signal, and need to be read out after the detecting process has ended. Some detectors are also able to measure the energy of the incoming radiation.

Detector technology is a wide and active field of research, and thus it can only be discussed here in broad terms.

Among the characteristics of a detector is its ability to count individual encounters or integrate the signal before read-out. Detection efficiency and sensitivity, noise, its dynamic range, linearity and uniformity of response, as well as its geometric, spatial, temporal and spectral properties, its size and detection area, angular and energy resolution, and possible distortions, as well as trivial considerations such as robustness, size, weight as well as cost and ease to retrofit existing equipment need to be considered (Figure 5.8).

Furthermore, besides the physical phenomena of interaction of the radiation with the detector, there are other ways to categorize detectors. We can discriminate between detectors that measure the flux of photons (point detectors) or particles in a particular state, whereas other detector types provide information about the spatial distribution of the photons/particles (spatial image detectors). Point detectors can only provide spatial information if the detector and the object move respect to one another (e.g., to detect the angular distribution of radiation or to raster across a flat object). Data collection with a point detector has the disadvantage to be tedious and time consuming, still it is still frequently used in bioimaging.

5.6.1 What Are the Different Types of Radiation That Need to Be Detected?

Radiation means the transmission of energy occurs through space (in a vacuum or filled by a material medium) by either subatomic particles or electromagnetic waves. The distinction between particles and waves is not always that strict, as elementary particles display wave-like properties, and in turn electromagnetic waves under certain conditions behave like a particle.

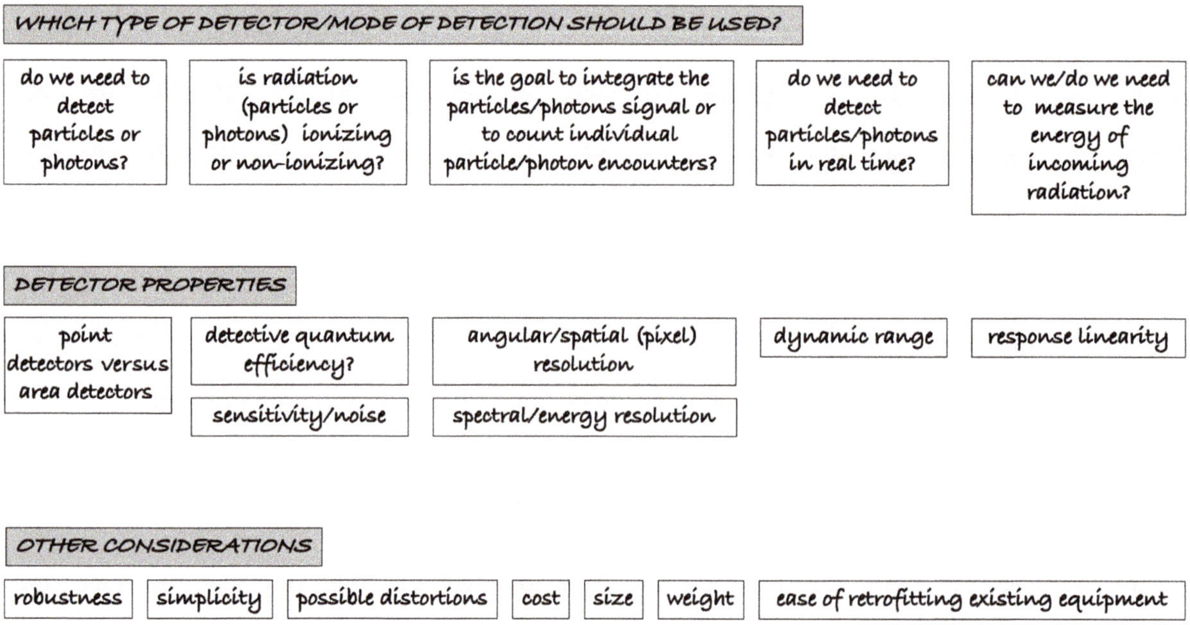

Figure 5.8 Detectors – Choice of detectors. A variety of factors need to be considered when choosing a detector for the imaging task at hand, including the type of radiation to be detected, detector properties as well as more practical considerations. Choosing the right kind of detector is crucial for a successful bioimaging experiment.

In terms of particle radiation, the most significant types for bioimaging are electrons, and to a much smaller degree also helium ions, and neutrons. Note that particles are not resting but are accelerated and thus possess high kinetic energy as they are emitted.

When we speak of wave radiation, we speak of electromagnetic radiation with ranges (in declining order of energy) from gamma-rays and X-rays, over ultraviolet (UV), visible and infrared (IR) light to microwaves and radio waves.

Radiation is also often categorized as either ionizing or non-ionizing, depending on the energy of the particles or the waves, with energies above 10 eV being able to ionize atoms or molecules, and/or chemical bonds, and thus harm living organisms (Figure 5.9).

All particle radiation can be considered as ionizing (except for thermic neutrons that penetrate many materials as the interaction with many materials is rather low). For electromagnetic radiation, ionizing potential depends on the energy and thus the frequency of the wave radiation, with gamma-rays, X-rays, and hard UV light possessing enough energy to eject one or several electrons, thus ionizing atoms and molecules. On the other hand, visible light, IR, microwaves, and radio waves are non-ionizing, even though in biological material soft-UV can also lead to disruption of chemical bonds in molecules. High intensities of visible lights can lead to conjugated-double bond/aromatic systems-mediated radical singlet oxygen formation, and thus to phototoxicity, which is known to harm living organisms. Also, upon irradiation, the hereditary macromolecules of all living beings can mutate and thus harm the cell and organism. Furthermore, high intensity IR and microwave radiation causes bond vibrations and thus while they are not ionizing, they can heat up the sample.

5.6.2 Detection of Particle Radiation

Due to the momentum of the particles in particle radiation electrons are ejected from the atoms of the sample, which then can be detected (Figure 5.10).

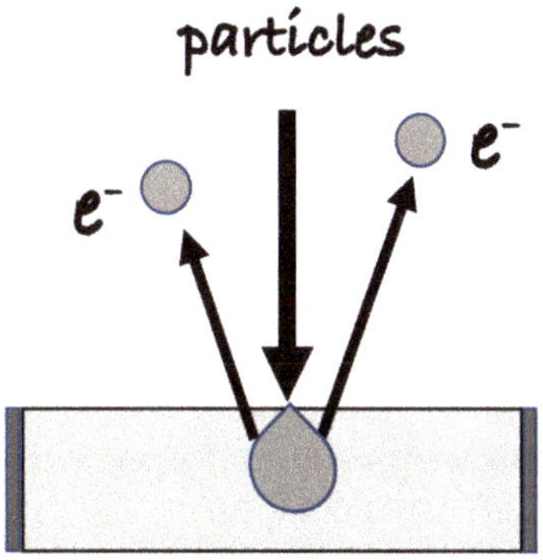

Figure 5.10 Electron microscopy and helium ion microscopy. In scanning electron microscopy (SEM) and helium ion microscopy, the sample is bombarded by electrons or helium ions, which leads to the emission of secondary electrons. Apart from secondary electron emission, electrons can also be backscattered from the surface of the sample.

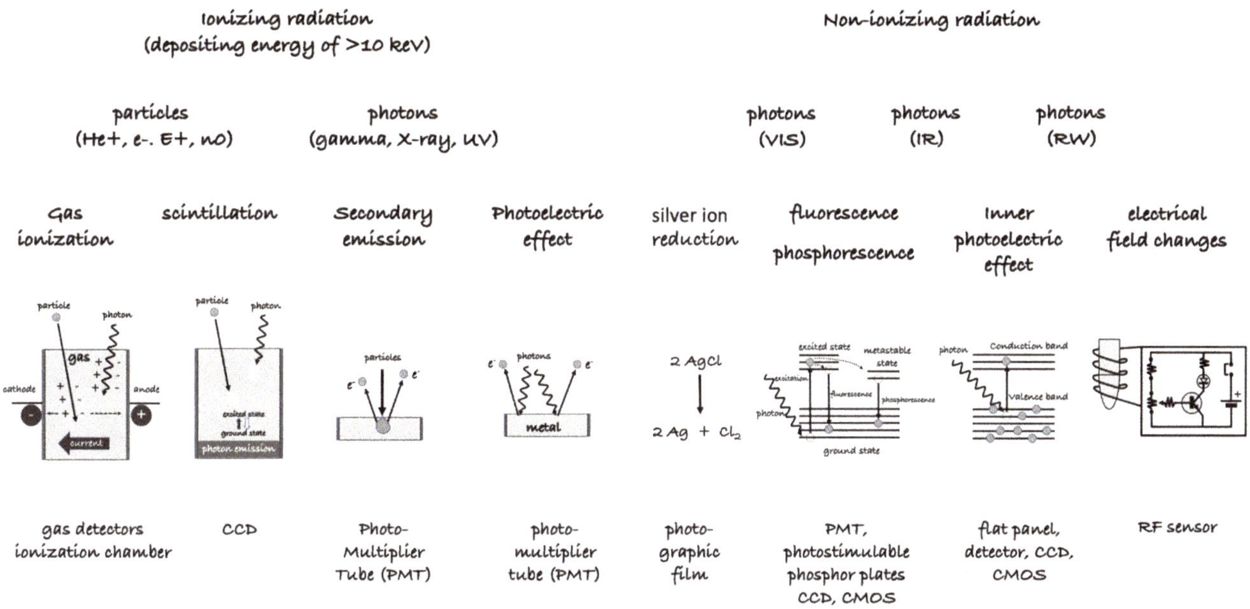

Figure 5.9 Types of radiation and detection principles. There are a variety of detectors, suitable to detect different types of particle radiations or photons, including ionizing and non-ionizing radiation. The mode of detection varies greatly, ranging from gas ionization, scintillation, secondary emission, photoelectric effect, silver ion reduction, fluorescence, phosphorescence, inner electric effect to electrical field changes.

Alpha Radiation (Helium Nuclei)

Alpha particles consist of two protons and two neutrons and basically are helium nuclei typically emitted at high speed. Given their size, mass, and charge, they interact strongly with matter and will only travel a few centimeters in air or a few millimeters in light weight solid material. Detection of alpha particle is best done in gas chambers where they leave a trace of gas ionization. They are not suited for detection by scintillation. However, alpha radiation does not play a role in biological imaging.

Helium Ions

The more frequent use of helium in biological imaging are helium ions. In the high vacuum and high electric field of a field emission gun helium molecules are ionized and are accelerated as He^{+}-ions with a single positive charge.

Beta-Radiation

Beta-radiation is produced by radioactive decay of an atomic nucleus and consists of high-energy, high-speed **electrons** (beta-minus decay) or **positrons** (beta-positive decay). Positrons are the antimatter of electrons, and thus upon encountering an electron, the positron will annihilate the electron, resulting in two high energy gamma-ray photons that are emitted (and thus can be detected) in exact opposite directions. Positrons are used in positron-emission tomography (PET), which is an important imaging technique in medical imaging, typically using radioisotopes as the source for positrons.

Electrons

Electrons for biological imaging do not stem from radioactive beta-minus decay but arise from the acceleration of electrons generated by thermionic or cold emission in electron guns. Electrons are widely used in bioimaging, such as in transmission electron microscopy and scanning electron microscopy, because they allow imaging at high resolution. Since electrons interact much more strongly with matter than for example X-rays, samples probed by electrons must be studied in a vacuum, which in turn puts strict restrictions on sample preparation.

Neutron Radiation

Neutrons are emitted in induced nuclear fission events, such as found in nuclear reactors. As thermal (non-resting) neutrons, they can be absorbed by atomic nuclei, which leads to unstable nuclei, which then in turn emit particles or gamma-ray electromagnetic radiation (neutron activation). Hence, neutrons are indirectly ionizing. Some atoms can absorb neutrons without becoming unstable, like hydrogen and oxygen, which simply turn into stable, heavier isotypes. High-energy (high-speed) neutrons on the other hand can ionize atoms directly, e.g., by ejecting their nuclei, or emission of high-energy protons from atomic nuclei. Effective shielding for high-energy neutrons can be thick layers of water and/or concrete. The ionizing potential of particle radiation can be exploited for detection, e.g., in gas detectors with ^{3}He as an inert gas or in scintillation materials (Figure 5.11).

5.6.3 Detection of Ionizing Electromagnetic Radiation

Depending on the energy (frequency) of the photons, electromagnetic radiation can be ionizing or non-ionizing. High-energy photons can be detected by gas ionization, by scintillation, by the photoelectric effect, or by the inner photoelectric effect (Figure 5.12).

Gamma Radiation

Gamma rays are most typically created as a by-product of a nuclear reaction, but unlike alpha and beta radiation

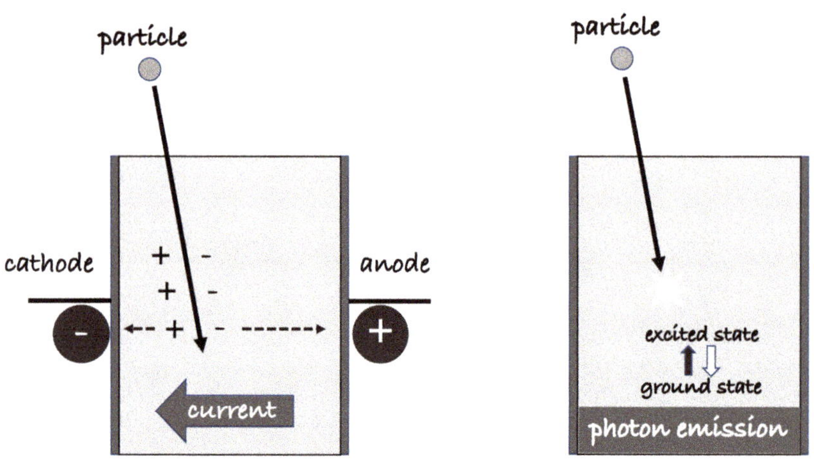

Figure 5.11 Particle radiation detection by gas ionization or scintillation. Particle radiation can be detected by gas ionization, with an ion pair forming after interaction with the neutron, resulting in an ion current. Alternatively, they can be detected by scintillation, where the interaction with the neutron leads to the emission of photons that can be readily detected.

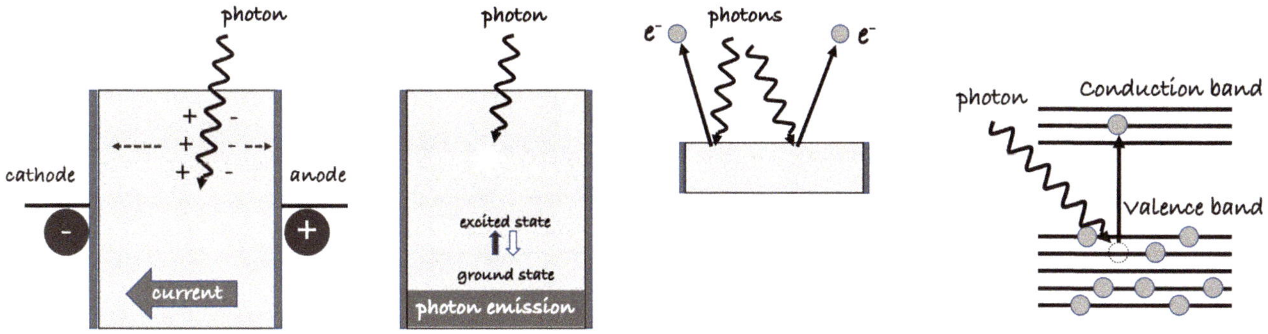

Figure 5.12 Detection of electromagnetic radiation. Depending on their energy photons can be detected by gas ionization, by scintillation, by the photoelectric effect, or by the inner photoelectric effect.

(which are subatomic particles), gamma-rays consist of mass-less, charge-less photons, characterized by a very short wavelength, less than 1 pm (10^{-12} m) and high frequency (10^{20}–10^{24} Hz), and thus gamma-ray photons possess a high amount of energy. Gamma-rays are best shielded by heavy metal material, such as lead or by large volumes of lighter materials. Detection of gamma-ray photons is best done by one of these processes: ionization, photoelectric effect, Compton scattering or pair production, the latter of which dominates at higher energies. The energy is fully deposited in the case of the photoelectric effect and pair production, whereas it is only partially deposited during Compton scattering.

X-Ray Radiation

X-ray radiation is composed of high-energy photons, characterized by wavelengths ranging from ~10 nm to ~1 pm (10^{-8}–10^{-12} m) and a frequency of ~10^{16} to ~10^{20} Hz. X-rays are considered high energy and typically cause damage upon interaction with matter through ionization. Larger atoms are more likely to absorb the impact of an X-ray photon without ionization, and may inelastically re-emit, and thus scatter the X-ray photon in a process called Compton scattering. Detection of X-rays occurs through gas ionization, the photoelectric effect in metal surfaces, scintillation, phosphorescence, fluorescence, or electron/hole pair formation in semiconductors.

Ultraviolet Radiation

Ultraviolet (UV) radiation consists of photons with a wavelength ranging from ~400 nm to ~10 nm ($4 * 10^{-7}$ to 10^{-8} m) and a frequency of ~10^{16} to ~10^{17} Hz. Shorter-wavelength (higher energy) UV photons possess sufficient energy for direct ionization of atoms and molecules, whereas longer-wavelength UV photons can be detected by devices that are based on the inner photoelectric effect. Semiconductor-based detectors can be used either with or without the need for a scintillator layer, which transduces UV light into visible light and in this process also acts as a protective layer.

5.6.4 Detection of Non-Ionizing Electromagnetic Radiation

Visible light and infrared light are part of the non-ionizing portion of the electromagnetic spectrums since these photons do not possess the energy to ionize atoms or molecules. Instead, they change the electronic valence, vibrational or rotational state of molecules and atoms. Excitation of molecules by the absorption of a photon is the foundation of fluorescence and phosphorescence. There are several ways to detect non-ionizing photons including by exploiting the photoelectric effect, where electrons are ejected from the surface of a metal, or the inner photoelectric effect, where electrons from the valence band are elevated to the conduction band in semiconductors (Figure 5.13).

Visible Light Radiation

Visible light radiation consists of photons with a wavelength ranging from ~800 to ~400 nm (~$8 * 10^{-7}$ to ~$4 * 10^{-7}$ m) and a frequency of ~10^{15} Hz. While photons do not possess sufficient energy for ionization of atoms and molecules, they change the electronic valence configuration of many molecules and atoms. Such photons can also be detected by the inner photoelectric effect in semiconductors that creates a pair of electrons and (electron) holes, a process that can be readily measured as an electric current.

Infrared Light Radiation

Near infrared (near IR) light radiation consists of photons with a wavelength ranging from ~2.5 μm (= 2,500 nm) to ~800 nm (~$2 * 10^{-6}$ to ~$8 * 10^{-7}$ m) and a frequency of ~10^{14} Hz. Infrared (IR) light radiation consists of photons

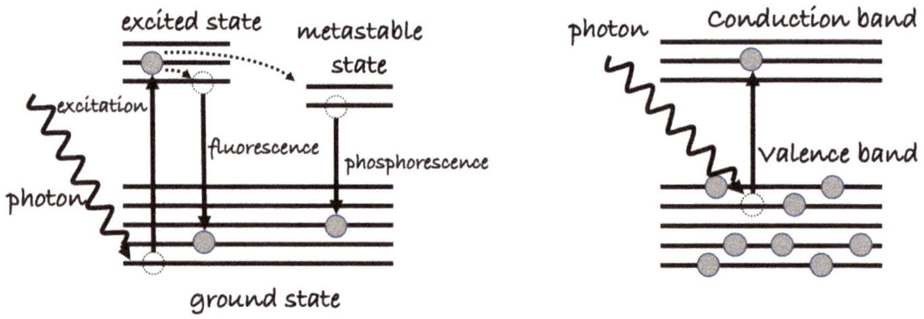

Figure 5.13 Detection of fluorescence photon signal by the inner photoelectric effect. Interactions of photons in the visible light range with molecules alter their electron valence configurations, which forms the basis of fluorescence and phosphorescence. Photons in the infrared range alter the vibrational and rotational states of molecules. Photons can be detected by a variety of different approaches, including the inner photoelectric effect, where electrons from the valence band are elevated to the conduction band.

with a wavelength ranging from ~25 to ~2.5 μm (~2 * 10^{-5} to ~2 * 10^{-7} m) and a frequency of ~10^{13} to ~10^{14} Hz. There are two main IR detector types, which are based on either pyroelectric or photonic detection (via the thermoelectric effect). Pyroelectric detectors contain temperature-sensitive materials such as deuterated triglycine sulfate (DTGS) or lithium tantalate ($LiTaO_3$) that operate at room temperature and show adequate sensitivity for many routine applications. DTGS as well as indium gallium arsenide photodiodes are typical choices for experiments in the near-IR range. Due to higher sensitivity and faster response rate, liquid nitrogen-cooled mercury cadmium telluride (MCT) detectors are the detector of choice for mid-IR radiation. Liquid helium-cooled silicon or germanium bolometer (via temperature-dependent changes of electrical resistance) are the method of choice for the far-IR range.

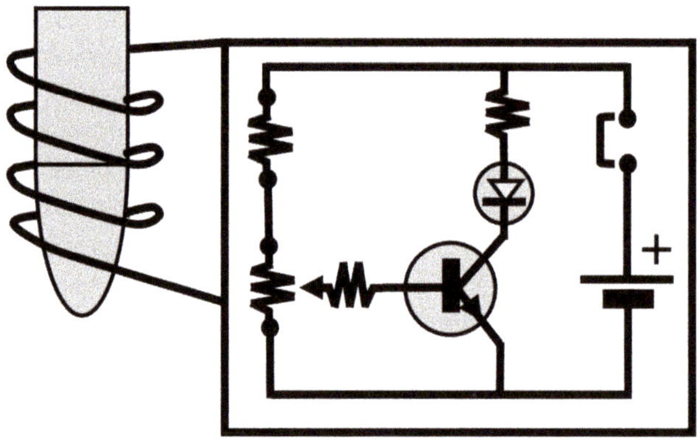

Figure 5.14 Detection of radio waves by a radio frequency (RF) detector electrical circuit set-up. Radio waves and their precise frequencies can be detected by an appropriate antenna – receiver electrical circuit set-up, as is used for NMR spectroscopy and MRI imaging.

Microwave Radiation

Microwave light radiation consists of photons with a wavelength ranging from ~1 mm to ~25 μm (~10^{-3} to ~2.5 * 10^{-5} m) and a frequency of ~3 * 10^{11} to ~10^{13} Hz. While they can be detected using an antenna and receiver setup like radio waves, microwaves do not play much of a role in bioimaging.

Radiowave Radiation

Radio wave radiation consists of photons with a wavelength larger than ~1 mm (~10^{-3} m) and a frequency less than 3 * 10^{11} Hz. Likewise, radio waves are picked up by an appropriate antenna (some form of a wire) and receiver setup (Figure 5.14). Radio waves are relevant in nuclear magnetic resonance of molecules/atoms' nuclei, residing in a strong external magnetic field. The two important examples are NMR spectroscopy for macromolecular structure determination, as well as for functional MRI imaging/medical MRI imaging.

5.6.5 Principles of Signal Detection

The precise mechanism of detection depends on the type of radiation and their respective energies, and it falls into one of these categories:

1) Gas ionization: Photons/particles enter a gas-filled chamber and ionize the gas, allowing for a current to flow between the anode and the cathode.
2) Photoelectric effect: Photons lead to ionization of a surface (e.g., of a metal) and the ejection of electrons.
3) Luminescence, Phosphorescence, Scintillators, Storage Phosphors: High-energy photons transfer their energy to either a scintillator or a storage phosphor material, which in turn emits photons in the visible range spontaneously or by photostimulation, respectively, which is then detected by a photodetector.
4) Fluorescence: Photons excite an electron in a molecule to a higher energy level (excited state), from which it returns almost immediately to the ground state,

emitting a longer-wavelength photon, which is detected by a photodetector.

5) Generation of carriers/electron–hole pairs by means of the inner photoelectric effect: Photons elevate electrons in semiconductors from the valence band to the conduction band, producing two mobile carriers, namely a negatively charged electron and a positively charged hole.
6) Photon-induced reduction of silver halides produces silver grains that through a development process (increase of size of silver grains) and fixation process (removal of non-reduced silver halides) create a physical image. For computational image processing and analysis, a physical image needs to be digitized.
7) Chemical Effect: The presence of a chemical and its binding to the sensor leads to a concentration-dependent change of measurable physical signal (rarely used in bioimaging).

Gas Detectors

Gas detectors provide a direct account of how many detection events have happened and belong to the category of photon counting devices. High-energy photons enter an inert gas and ionize gas atoms by ejection of an electron. Since there is a voltage gradient across the gas volume, the electrically charged entities (electrons and gas ions) move in different directions and along the way, like an avalanche, this leads to many more charged particles, so one high-energy photon may result in a million electrons. The best-known example of such a gas detector is the Geiger–Müller counter, which due to its high electric field, gives a strong signal. Gas detectors in their simplest form are single pixel detectors but can be used to measure a spatial distribution by using multiple crossed wires in form of a wire chamber.

Photomultiplier Tube Detectors

Photomultiplier tubes (PMT) are vacuum tubes that are very sensitive to light in the UV, visible light and near-IR range of the electromagnetic spectrum. They can amplify the signal from the incoming light by eight orders of magnitudes ($10^8\times$). In low light conditions individual photons can be detected. PMT are characterized by high gain, low noise, and high frequency response. PMT play a role in low light level spectroscopy, confocal microscopy, Raman spectroscopy, fluorescence spectroscopy, some high-end image scanners (e.g., drum scanners).

Photomultiplier tubes consist of a photocathode, several dynodes, and an anode (Figure 5.15). At the cathode, a photon hits the photocathode material and ejects an electron via a mechanism known as the photoelectric effect. The ejected electron is accelerated to the first dynode, held at a more positive potential, where it provokes the ejection of several electrons (through a process call secondary emission), which are then accelerated to the next dynodes. The total count of electrons multiplies at each subsequent dynode, before the total number of electrons hit the anode, where the total signal is read out as an electrical current. Different photocathode materials are sensitive to different photon energies, so that a broad spectrum of photons can be detected. Semiconductor devices, silicon photomultipliers and avalanche photodiodes are alternatives to classical photomultipliers.

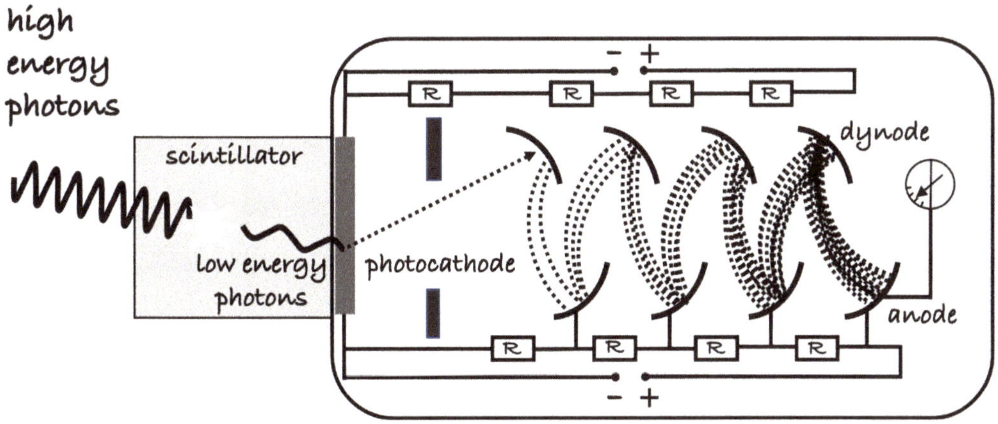

Figure 5.15 Photomultiplier tubes (PMT). Photomultiplier tubes (PMT) are sensitive to photons ranging in wavelength from UV over VIS to IR. Photons hitting the photocathode eject an electron (photoelectric effect) that in the vacuum of the PMT is accelerated to the first dynode where multiple electrons are ejected (secondary emission), all of which are being accelerated to the next dynode. At each step, more and more electrons are being ejected, which are finally hitting the anode, where the signal is read out as an electrical current.

Film

Film represents probably the oldest technology for the detection of photons. According to the Gurney–Mott model of latent image formation, incoming photons interact with small silver halide particles, that are suspended in a gelatin film emulsion (Figure 5.16). The photons with an appropriate energy will elevate electrons from the valence band to the conduction band. These electrons move through the silver halide particle until they encounter and get trapped at a crystal defect site where they will reduce highly mobile interstitial silver ions. Between 6 and 30 photons need to be absorbed to form stable silver clusters of 3–5 atoms (grains). The sum of all stable silver clusters leads to a latent image. At this point the exposed film is exposed to a photographic developer (e.g., using hydroquinone as a chemical reducing agent). During this process, all exposed grains are converted to opaque silver which then forms the visible image, with areas of high illumination result in being darkest. In the following fixation process, the remaining silver halide grains are removed so that the film emulsion can be exposed to light without altering the image. Film played a major role in data collection for a long time, but has several disadvantages, which ultimately led to its replacement by digital detectors. Among the disadvantages of film is its low dynamic range, its poor energy discrimination, the fact that the dose needed is typically higher than for digital detectors and cannot be corrected in real time, and that for subsequent image processing subsequent digitalization is required. To achieve high resolution either a point detector or 1D-line scanner is needed, which makes the process of digitalization very tedious.

Photostimulable Phosphors

In the 1980s, imaging plate systems were pioneered by Fuji, who utilized the phenomenon of photostimulated luminescence to create a Europium-doped phosphor-powder device. It uses the oxidation of Eu^{2+} to Eu^{3+} by a high-energy photon, which leads to a stable state, until the stimulation by a red laser results in a detectable light signal that is proportional to the original high-energy photon flux (Figure 5.17). Among the advantages over film are the significantly better dynamic range, the low price of plastic imaging plate and the fact that image plates unlike film is re-usable. However, energy discrimination is poor, and the readout of each image by the red laser is rather slow and can take several minutes.

Semiconductor Detectors

Developed since the 1970s, semiconductor detectors entered medical imaging in the early 2000s. Detection of radiation by semiconductor material is based on the photon-induced generation of electron/hole pairs (also known as the inner photoelectric effect). High-energy photons create electron–hole pairs in semiconductor crystals, with one high-energy photon being able to evoke a current of several thousand electrons, which can be easily read out. In general, the energy required to produce electron/hole pairs in semiconductors is much lower than to

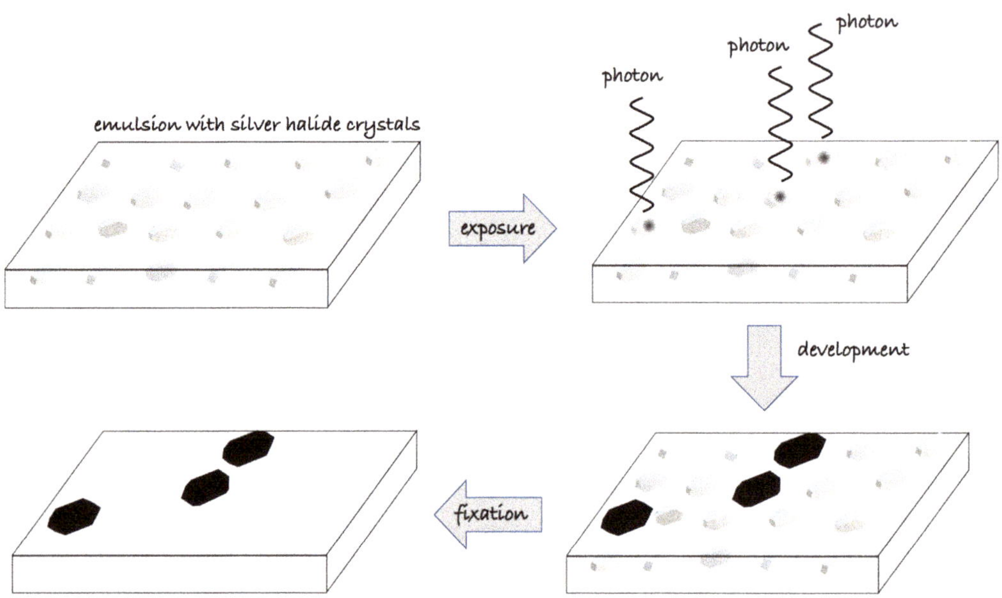

Figure 5.16 Photographic film processing. When a silver halide crystal emulsion is exposed to light, photons knock out free electrons that get trapped in crystal defects. Silver ions are attracted to such charged crystal defects, forming clusters of transparent silver atoms (grains). In the development process, these grains are converted to opaque silver forming the visible image. The fixation process that follows the development process removes the remaining silver halide grains.

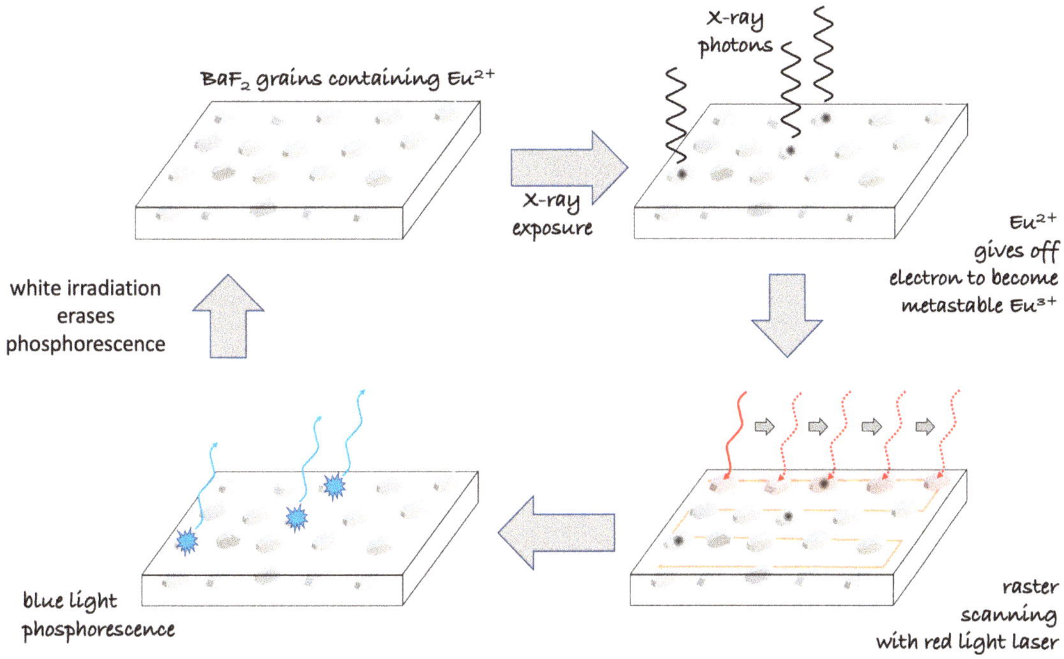

Figure 5.17 Photostimulable phosphor plates. High energy photons oxidize a Europium-doped phosphor-powder. Upon stimulation by red laser light, photons are emitted that can be detected, with the signal being proportional to the original high-energy photon flux.

produce ions in a gas detector. The exact material used depends on the energy of the photons to be detected. X-rays may be directly detected by cadmium–zinc–telluride or indirectly by using a scintillator material (such as cesium iodide or gadolinium dioxide sulfide), which converts X-ray photons into visible light photons.

Flat Panel Detectors Flat Panel Detectors (FPD) are an example for direct detection of X-rays, based on amorphous selenium as the X-ray sensitive material that can convert X-ray photons directly into an electrical charge. Flat panel detectors are widely used today in medical and dental applications.

Charge-Coupled Devices (CCD) Solid state semiconductor detectors can be operated in a direct photon-counting mode or in a photon-integrating mode. There are different kinds of photosensitive semiconductor-based detector designs, such as photodiodes, photoconductors, charge-coupled-devices (CCD).

For each of these devices, electron/hole pairs are being generated and then further processed by some integrated circuit, such as an array of thin film transistors (TFT), complementary metal oxide semiconductor (CMOS) or shift register approach in a CCD. For each of these detectors readout noise and dark currents (currents created in the absence of photons) must be determined and accounted for through calibration. CCD have held a prominent role in detector technology, with the 2009 Nobel Prize in Physics being awarded to Wiliam S. Boyle and George E. Smith "for their invention of an imaging semiconductor circuit – the CCD sensor."

Charge-Coupled Devices (CCD) are widely used in bioimaging, and consist of a photoactive region, i.e., a photosensitive layer (made of silicon), as well as metal-oxide-semiconductor (MOS)-based transmission region, which acts like a shift register (Figure 5.18). This integrated circuit contains an array of linked (coupled) semiconductor-based capacitors (also referred to as wells). Each of these wells can accumulate electrical charges proportional to the number of photons detected. The maximum capacity for each well is ~10^5 electrons. Too long an exposure may lead to an overflowing of each well to its neighboring "bins," resulting in a phenomenon called blooming.

Under the control of an external circuit each capacitor transfers its charge to its neighbor (hence the term shift register), with the last capacitor in the array transferring its charge to an amplifier that converts the charge into a voltage. As a result, all pixels are read out as a sequence of voltages, which are stored in memory.

The best way to operate a CCD is to divide into two separate phases: an exposure phase and a readout phase. As the name implies, upon exposure to light, electron charges are created and stored. In the readout phase, where the CCD is no longer exposed to light, the charges for each cell are

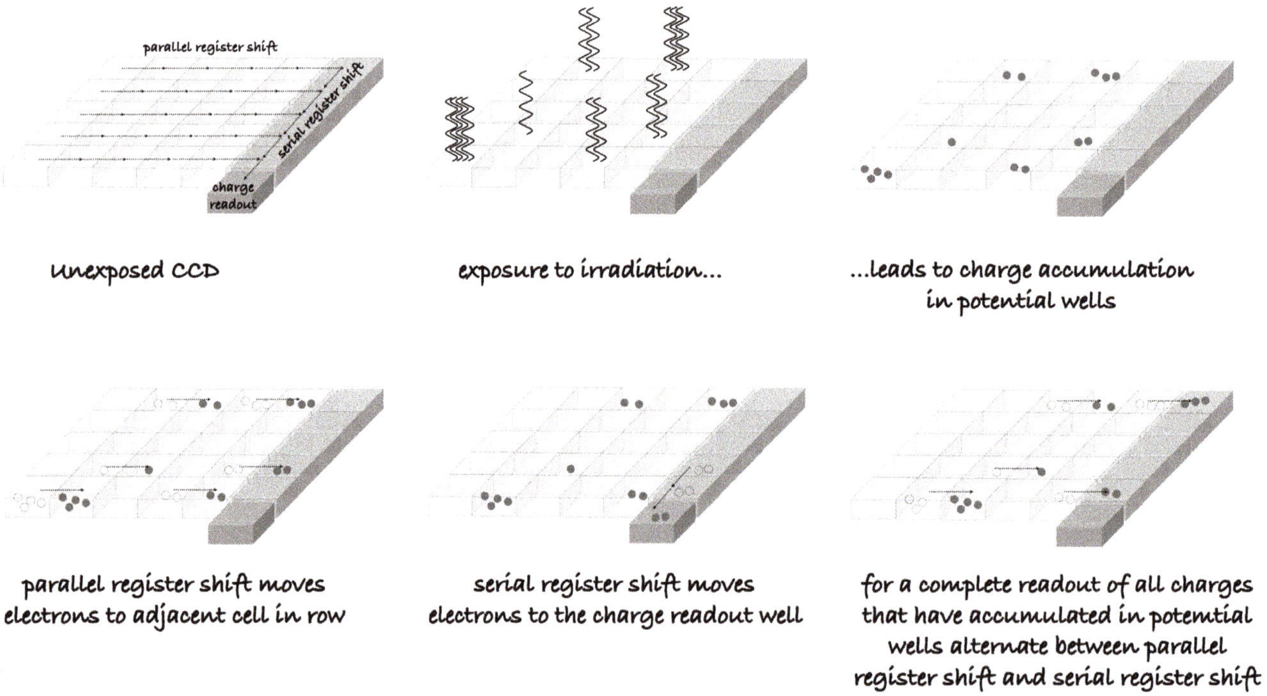

Figure 5.18 Charge-Coupled Device. Charge-Coupled Devices (CCD) contain a photosensitive silicon layer in combination with a metal-oxide-semiconductor (MOS)-based shift register. Each pixel acts like a capacitor, capable of accumulating electrical charges. Photons hitting each pixel of the CCD leads to an accumulation of electrical charges in each well (capacitor). After exposure, the integrated circuit shifts the charges to the neighboring pixel, not unlike a bucket-brigade, and through a parallel and serial register shift until each charge is eventually read out.

shifted to its neighboring cell, all the way down to the last cell of the entire area of the CCD. Naturally the readout of the CCD is somewhat slow, which means that the CCD cannot be re-used for detection until this readout process is finished.

A faster way to accomplish the readout is to shift the entire charge distribution of the exposed CCD onto a shielded empty CCD array, before the somewhat slow readout of each well can be accomplished. This is the principle behind frame transfer CCD, allowing the light-sensitive part of the CCD to be re-used much faster for subsequent signal detection. Frame transfer CCD are more expensive, as the cell area is double and control electronics is more complex.

For so-called intensified CCD (ICCD), an image intensifier (consisting of a photocathode, a microchannel plate, and a phosphor screen) is mounted in front of the CCD. Hence photons hitting the photocathode leads to electrons, which are multiplied before hitting the phosphor screen. This then presents a much brighter signal to the CCD via a fiber optic or a lens system.

An alternative to the expensive ICCD is the so-called electron multiplying CCD (EMCCD), the signal is amplified at the step of charge transfer between the last CCD cell and the output amplifier through the process of impact ionization, in a way like avalanche diodes. To keep the noise low, EMCCD need to be kept at low temperature, which adds cost and can cause condensation problems in the detection setup. Sensitivity of ICCD and EMCCD are comparable, but EMCCD show a slightly better performance under low-light conditions.

Complementary Metal Oxide Semiconductor (CMOS) An alternative semiconductor-based concept for photon detection is the complementary metal-oxide semiconductor (CMOS), which is a metal-oxide semiconductor field effect transistor (Figure 5.19). CMOS technology is also widely used for constructing integrated circuit chips, including microprocessors. Another advantage of CMOS sensors for imaging is that they have very little noise, and they are characterized by a favorable detective quantum efficiency (DQE), which measures the level of the signal retained by a camera at a particular spatial frequency. Over the last decade CMOS have become the dominant technology, largely replacing CCD image sensors, and have led to a resolution revolution in single particle cryo-electron microscopy, which has replaced X-ray crystallography as the number one technology for macromolecular structure determination.

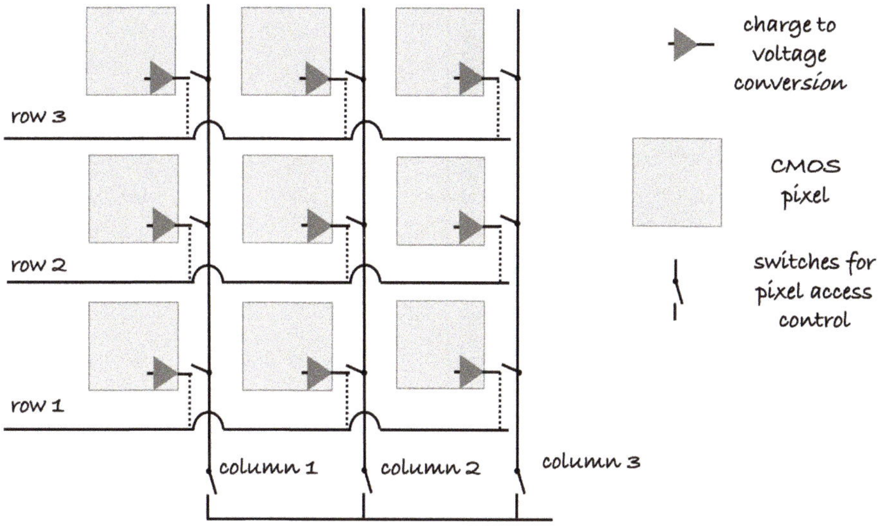

Figure 5.19 Complementary metal-oxide semiconductor. Complementary metal-oxide semiconductor (CMOS) technology is widely used for microprocessors. CMOS detectors show little noise and high detective quantum efficiency (DQE). CMOS has largely replaced CCD technology.

5.7 Modulation-, Contrast-, and Optical-Transfer Function

The modulation transfer function (MTF) describes a microscope's performance to transfer contrast from the specimen to the intermediate image plane as a function of resolution (frequency) (Figure 5.20). This concept stems from electrical engineering, where the degree of modulation of an output signal is plotted as a function of the signal frequency.

The MTF is just a mathematical way (and therefore a useful concept) to describe the optical properties of microscopes, such point spread function and Airy disks.

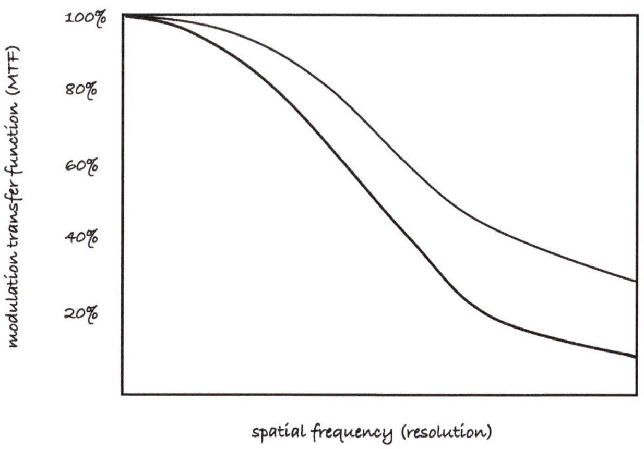

Figure 5.20 Modulation transfer function. The modulation transfer function (MTF) is a measure of an instrument's performance of relative signal output as a function of signal frequency. In electron microscopy the related term contrast transfer function (CTF) is frequently used where relative contrast is blotted as a function of spatial frequency (resolution).

If the original signal used for assessing microscope performance is a step function/high contrast square wave (e.g., when imaging a periodic grating target), then one speaks of a contrast transfer function (CTF), hence MTF and CTF are very similar concepts.

The optical transfer function (OTF) is the ratio of image contrast to specimen contrast as a function of spatial frequency, while considering possible phase shifts between the real image and the ideal image position. The OTF is a complex variable with the MTF as its amplitude. Its imaginary component is the phase transfer function. The MTF (CTF) is very closely related to the point spread function (PSF) and the Airy disk shape. Optical aberrations (including defocus) and numerical aperture variations affect the MTF (CTF) and thus also the shape of the Airy disk/PSF. The MTF is usually decreased at higher spatial frequencies, which is to say higher resolution signals are typically weaker than low-resolution components, where the contrast transfer can be close to 100%. Near the Abbe limit the contrast transferred is too low, which is another way of saying that optical imaging is diffraction-limited.

Imaging at defocus (or other kinds of aberrations) will also affect the MTF/CTF, so that the MTF/CTF will oscillate between positive and negative values (Figure 5.21), which means that in the regions of negative values of the MTF/CTF, contrast is inverted (and thus phase shifts need to be corrected during image reconstruction). The regions between positive and negative values show little to no contrast. These regions can be thought of as spatial frequency blind spots (or gaps of resolution). CTF is particularly important in transmission electron microscopy where image data is typically collected at a small defocus. Changing the defocus changes the zero positions of the

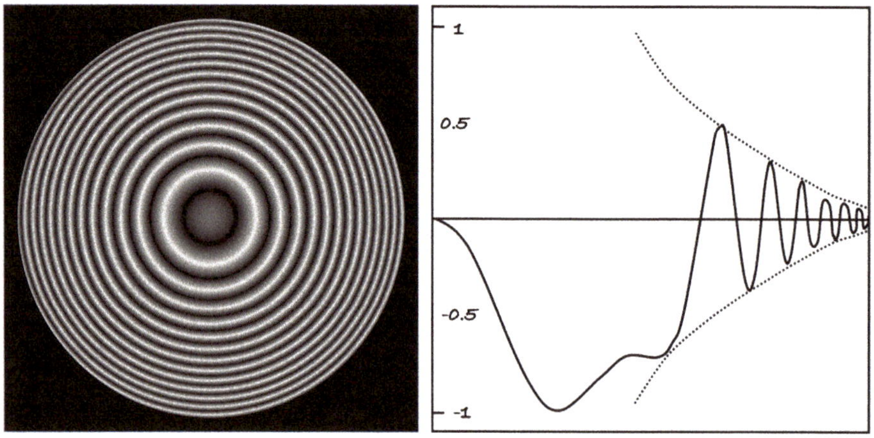

Figure 5.21 Contrast transfer function (CTF) in electron microscopy. In transmission electron microscopy of unstained samples, images are typically recorded with a certain amount of defocus (underfocus) to generate contrast. Defocus affects the Contrast Transfer Function (CTF), which oscillates between positive and negative values (contrast inversion). For each defocus there will be resolution ranges in which the microscope does not transfer any contrast, hence such regions are blind spots with no information about the sample being transferred. Note that there is an overall envelope function that dampens the amplitudes. Contrast inversion requires adjustment of the phases. Furthermore, the higher the resolution the more frequently the function oscillates. Determining the CTF and correcting the amplitudes and phases accordingly is key to structure determination by cryo-electron microscopy.

MTF/CTF. Hence, to record data at all frequencies, one needs to record images at different defocus settings.

Imaging at a larger defocus leads to an increase in the number of oscillations of the MTF/CTF, hence more spatial resolution regions where the contrast is inverted. In electron microscopy Thon rings constitute the pattern in the Fourier transform of an image of an amorphous carbon film, recorded at a defocus, and show the CTF of the electron microscope. In the dark regions the CTF is near zero. Studying Thon rings as a function of defocus and other aberrations (including astigmatism) is an excellent way to visually observe the contrast transfer function, and Thon rings can be used in electron microscopy to calculate the defocus value for each image and thus to correct the phases for image reconstruction. The MTF/CTF is a characteristic property of an (electron) optical system. Without CTF correction there would be no high-resolution TEM structure determination.

5.8 Field of View, Coverage

The area of a sample that can be imaged by a microscope camera is called a field of view and is a combination of lens properties and camera sensor size. While it may seem trivial, it should be explicitly pointed out that the field of view/coverage of the sample, resolution, and data collection time/data storage space are connected. As much as one is tempted to want to image an area/volume as large as possible at a resolution as high as possible, one should keep in mind that such an attempt will result in long data collection times and a gigantic amount of image information that presumably needs to be analyzed in detail, further increasing the time needed to deduce useful biological information from the imaging data.

On the other hand, focusing the imaging on a region of interest too small may lead to missing out on important contextual information or providing insufficient statistical coverage. There is furthermore the danger to select regions for imaging that match expectation of the experimenter, thus biasing the conclusions. It is always advisable to take lower-resolution overview images (possibly at different magnifications) either before or after taking the high-resolution dataset, in order to be able to place the higher-resolution dataset into a larger cell and tissue context (Figure 5.22).

In general, it is advisable to be conscious of the overall dimensions in the images taken at different magnification, and when evaluating the images to always include scale bars, as they are very helpful to evaluate the information in the images. Since images are often said to be "more convincing than a thousand words," image information should be collected and analyzed without bias (like any other data in science), and not be treated as mere "eye candy" or support for a foregone conclusion. Imaging the whole range of phenomena rather that always imaging only one appearance may lead to the discovery of rare or unexpected phenomena and possibly to change in the underlying hypothesis and thus may lead closer to a correct conclusion (Figures 5.23 and 5.24).

The issue of imaging at multiple scales (possibly with multiple imaging techniques) will be discussed again in Chapter 12.

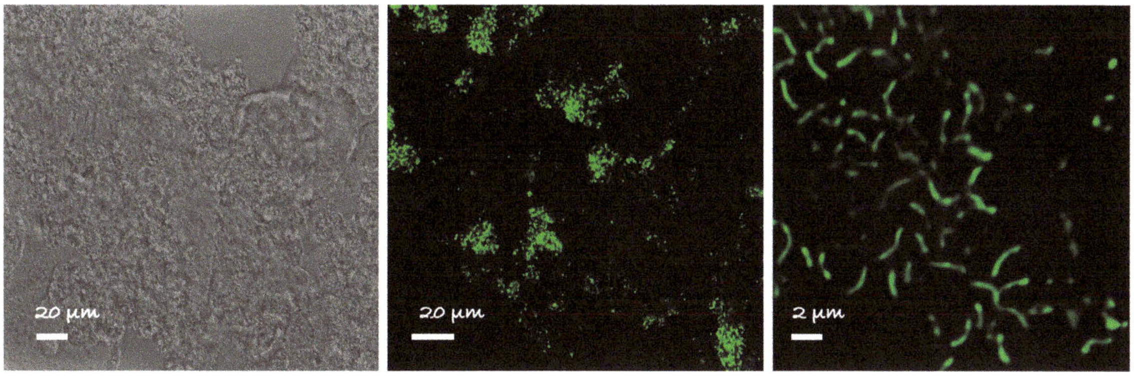

Figure 5.22 Field of view/coverage – Large scale heterogeneity and difficulty in selecting a representative region. As high-resolution microscopy can only cover a small region, it is important to take images at different scales and magnification to assess heterogeneity in a specimen. Left: Phase contrast image of a thin *Desulfovibrio vulgaris* biofilm that has been genetically engineered to express glutamine synthase as a SNAP-tag fusion protein. Middle: Fluorescent light image of BG505-labeled biofilm. Note that there are islands of glutamine synthase fusion protein expression, with equally or even larger biofilm regions with little or no glutamine synthase fusion protein expression. Right: Higher-magnification images reveal glutamine synthase fusion protein localization in individual bacteria in the biofilm.

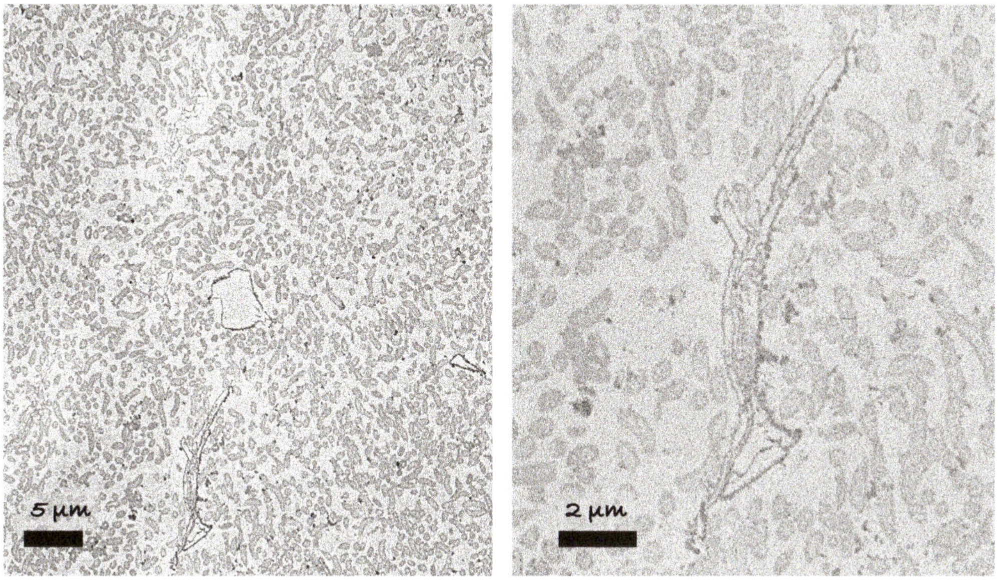

Figure 5.23 Field of view/coverage – Detection of rare events. In a 45 µm × 45 µm × 100 µm volume of a biofilm of the anaerobe bacterium *Desulfovibrio vulgaris*, one can find extracellular metal deposits that appear to be membrane-based. Such deposits are relatively rare but once they are found they can be very prominent, extending as sheets for many tens of micrometers. Hence it is important to select the right region at lower magnification for higher-resolution imaging.

5.9 Spot-Scan Versus Flood-Beam Imaging

The decision to image a single point of the sample or a large area of the sample (flood beam) often depends on the type of detector available for signal collection. Point-detection requires point-illumination, whereas area detectors allowing larger areas to be illuminated simultaneously. In the case of point-illumination/point-detection a beam will sweep over the sample in a raster-like pattern (Figure 5.25).

A typical example of single-point imaging is laser-scanning fluorescence light microscopy, whereas light sheet fluorescence imaging is an example for flood beam illumination. Another example is electron microscopy where samples are either imaged in a spot scan or flood beam mode. Scanning electron microscopy, and many spectroscopic techniques that require each pixel of data collected to be spectrally analyzed, are imaged by spot scan illumination and detection, whereas transmission electron microscopy typically uses flood beam illumination.

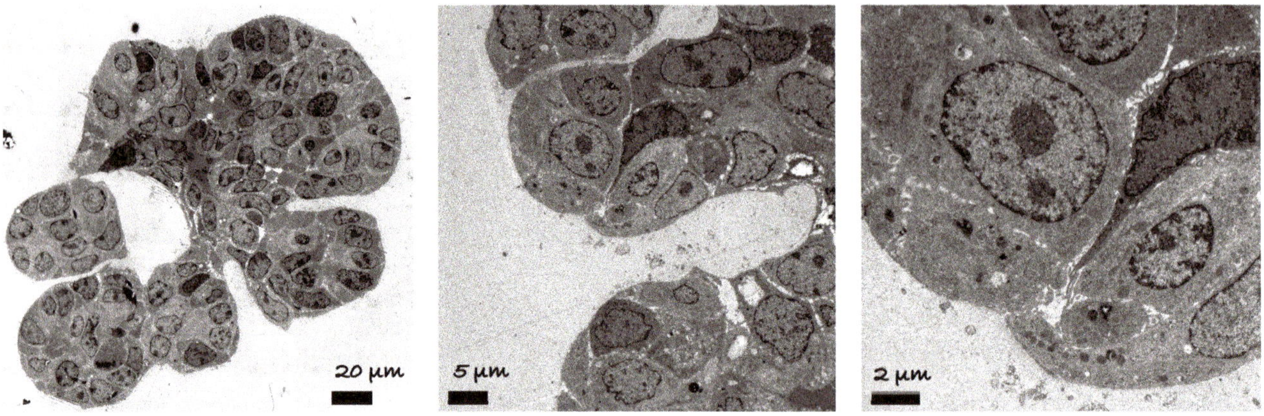

Figure 5.24 Field of view/coverage – Cell-to-cell heterogeneity and new cell populations. Typically, TEM images of cells are recorded as with a 2k by 2k pixel field of coverage, corresponding to 2 µm × 2 µm at 1 nm pixels size or 10 µm × 10 µm at 5 nm pixels size, which is about the size a typical individual cell. Small tissues or organoid, such as the mouse mammary gland undergoing branching morphogenesis, which is shown here, consist of hundreds of cells. Trading resolution for a larger field of view cannot be a solution, instead the collection of larger data sets such a 10 × 10 montage of individual 2k by 2k images at high resolution is a promising path. Left: Montage of high-resolution images of a field of view of ~200 µm by ~200 µm. Note that cells are highly heterogeneous with respect to shape and image contrast. Middle and right: Close inspection of cellular ultrastructure reveals that there are cells present with thin membrane protrusions indicative of migratory cells. The presence of migratory cells within a tissue were subsequently independently confirmed by time lapse fluorescence microscopy.

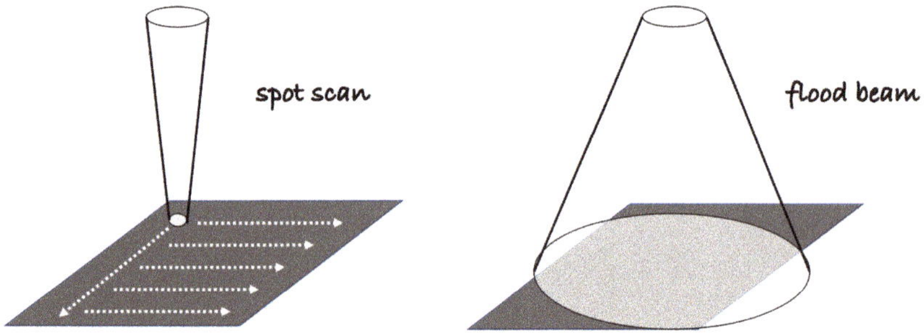

Figure 5.25 Spot scan versus flood beam illumination. In spot scan illumination mode, a narrow beam is raster-scanned across the sample, and the signal is recorded for each image point. In flood beam illumination the entire field of view is illuminated simultaneously, and an image of the entire region is recorded, typically by an area detector such as a CCD or a CMOS detector.

Among the downsides of single-point illumination/detection is the long data acquisition time required for raster image formation, which often limits the area that can be imaged altogether. One solution to this problem is to use an array of multiple beams that simultaneously scan the sample. Flood beam imaging is much faster but the size of the area that can be imaged is limited by the detector size. Larger areas can be obtained by collection of multiple images that can be stitched together as a montage into a larger image. Typically, for a montage images of neighboring regions have a 10% overlap, which significantly helps the montaging process.

5.10 Radiation Damage

As discussed in the section on the interaction of radiation with biological samples, many types of radiation cause damage to the sample. Radiation damage is prominent and easy to understand for ionizing radiation, such as X-ray, electron, or ion beams, where covalent bonds are broken, resulting in radicals (unpaired electrons) that are highly reactive and can lead to additional bond breakage. As a result, macromolecules disintegrate and fragment into pieces, which obviously alters their 3D structure (Figure 5.26). Non-ionizing radiation (such as visible light) can also be damaging to biological sample, particularly in high doses, due to fluorophore bleaching and phototoxicity due to singlet-oxygen-mediated metabolic damage to living cells.

One of the key objectives in biological imaging is to utilize the overall photon budget available to maximize the imaging signal and to minimize background (e.g., out-of-focus contributions). This point will be discussed in more detail in Chapter 9 on optical/fluorescence microscopy.

5.11 Spectroscopic Imaging

Spectroscopic imaging is a pixel-by-pixel study how electromagnetic radiation interacts with matter as a function of the radiation wavelength/frequency. The concept

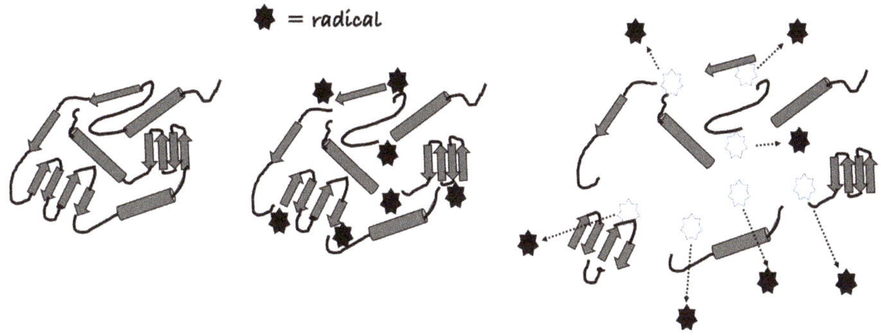

Figure 5.26 Radiation damage. Ionizing radiation can damage biological macromolecules through covalent bond breakage and resulting radical formation, which can lead to fragmentation of the macromolecule.

can also be extended to matter waves, such as electrons, where the kinetic energy of the electrons needs to be considered. Spectroscopy is most intuitively understood for the visible light range, where the absorption or emission of photons at discrete frequencies corresponds to different lines in the absorption or emission spectrum.

Absorption of a photon results in the decrease or total loss of intensity at a particular spectral line and is the key in understanding atomic absorption spectroscopy or X-ray spectroscopy to determine the elemental composition. Changes in the molecular electronic states results in the emission of visible light at a particular frequency and thus at a particular color, a concept that is prominent in fluorescence light microscopy, which is one of the major techniques in bioimaging. Changes in molecular vibrational and molecular rotational states underlie both Raman spectroscopy and infrared spectroscopy. Furthermore, changes in the nuclear spin states that are exposed to a strong external magnetic field and its resonance behavior are probed in nuclear magnetic resonance (NMR) spectroscopy.

In all these different techniques, the intensity of the signal is sampled as a function of frequency (wavelength) of the electromagnetic radiation. In the most basic implementation of spectroscopic imaging, a monochromator, blocking all but a small window of the electromagnetic spectrum, sweeps through a range of frequencies (wavelengths). In such a dispersive spectrometer, the full spectrum is recorded by detecting a specific signal for each wavelength/frequency.

Fourier-Transform (FT) Spectroscopy

While dispersive spectrometers are perfectly adequate for data collection, they are increasingly replaced by Fourier-Transform (FT) spectroscopy approaches. As can be illustrated by the example of FTIR spectrometers, FT spectroscopy offer a variety of advantages, including higher signal-to-noise ratio (~100-fold) of the spectrum with a high accuracy of the wave number and wide scan range, a short scan time and high spectral resolution (by a factor of 10,000). The difference to dispersive IR spectrometers is in essence that FTIR spectrometer contain a Michelson interferometer with a beam splitter and two perpendicular mirrors, one of which is stationary, and the other one is movable. The FTIR spectrometer allows many wavelengths of light to irradiate the sample and record the total beam intensity as a function of time and thus mirror position. A second data point is recorded at a different movable mirror position, where the measured intensity corresponds to a second set of wavelengths/frequencies.

This process is repeated many times, with the signal of the superposition of the two beams being measured as a function of time (and thus movable mirror position and thus differences in beam path length) and ultimately lead to an interferogram. For each mirror configuration, due to wave interference, certain frequencies/wavelengths pass through whereas others are not.

Such interferograms (as the raw data is sometimes called) can be turned into an IR absorption spectrum via a Fourier transform (Figure 5.27), as was discussed in Chapter 4. Fourier Transform spectroscopy can be used for both absorption and emission spectroscopy. Pulsed Fourier transform techniques are widely using in biological imaging, e.g., radio frequency pulses in a strong ambient magnetic environment lie at the heart of nuclear magnetic resonance (NMR) spectroscopy.

5.12 Multidimensional and Multi-channel Imaging

Strictly speaking, any form of biological imaging is already multidimensional, as an image usually has already two independent dimensions, namely x and y, and for volumes the dimensionality is three. Typically, in biological imaging the term multidimensional imaging is reserved for dataset that exceed three dimensions. Spectral imaging is an example of multidimensional imaging, where each pixel in an image is more than a single gray-value, but contains spectral information, hence a gray value for every frequency scanned. It thus opens other dimensions than just spatial information (Figure 5.28).

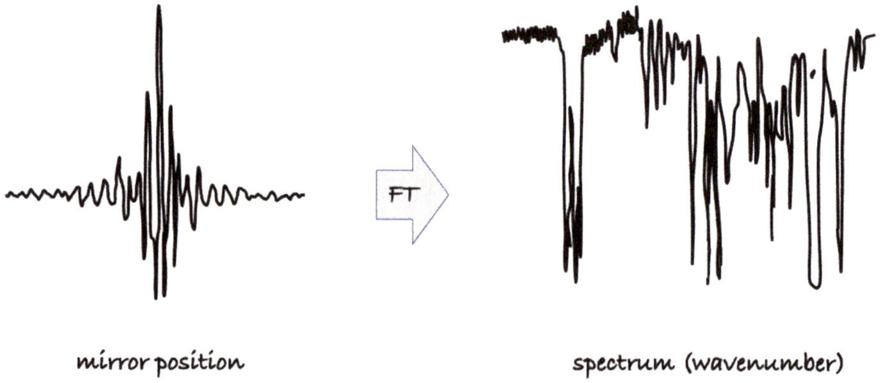

Figure 5.27 FTIR spectroscopic imaging. In FTIR imaging one uses a Michelson interferometer design, where the beam is split between a stationary mirror and a perpendicularly oriented movable mirror. The data is recorded as a function of relative mirror position, which upon Fourier transform will yield a wavenumber spectrum.

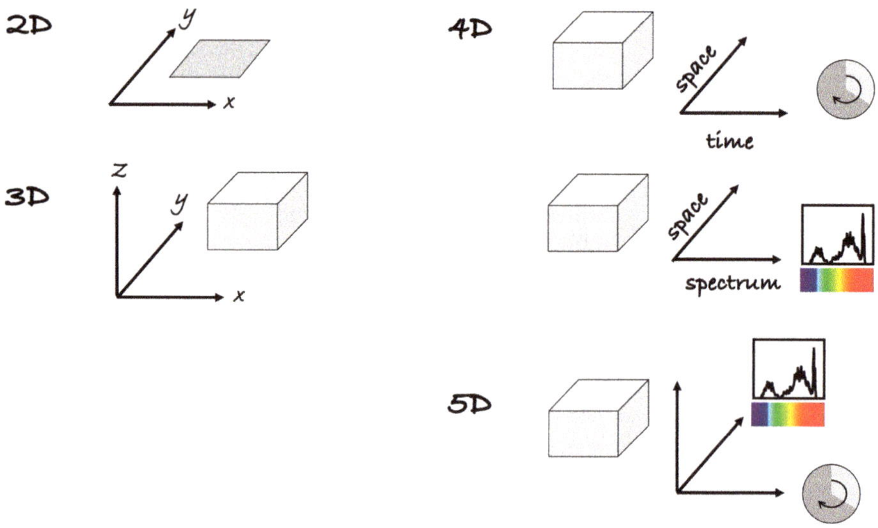

Figure 5.28 Multidimensional imaging. A typical 2D image is a gray value as a function of *X* and *Y* coordinates (two spatial dimensions; pixel). Adding a third spatial dimension (*Z*) results in a 3D volume with an observed gray value for each *XYZ* coordinate (voxel). A fourth dimension can be added such as time or spectral information, adding both leads to five-dimensional data. Such high-dimensional datasets are difficult to display and comprehend as raw data, and thus some form of analysis and segmentation/annotation is needed such as the identification of certain (macro-)molecular components.

For this reason, one speaks of multidimensional data. Other example of adding another dimension is temporal imaging, when a sample is monitored over time, an approach that is typically referred to as video-rate (if in real time at more than 20–30 frames per second) or time lapse (where an image is taken every few seconds, minutes, or hours). A temporal dimension can be added to two-dimensional images, in which case the time domain turns a 2D data set into a 3D data set and can be visualized as such. Adding time to a spatially three-dimensional data set (3D volume) turns the data set four-dimensional, and if spectral information is added, yet another dimension is added. In this case we would be dealing with a five-dimensional data set. Typically, colors are recorded, e.g. through the use of respective color filters, in three channels (blue, green and red). We can think of color imaging as three-channel imaging. The combination of the values for these three different channels at least in principle yields millions different colors. However, there are applications such as in Raman imaging or hyperspectral imaging, where data collection occurs in finer increments, and an entire intensity spectrum is recorded as a function of wavenumber/frequency.

Anything bigger than a three-dimensional data set is difficult to visualize and comprehend for the human brain.

For this reason, one may want to collapse other dimensions (e.g., focusing on a single plane of a 3D volume) to be able to display additional dimensions. Even 3D information, particularly if the data space is rather densely populated and the features are complex, can be difficult to visualize, and often requires simplification, e.g., by extraction of certain features of interest from its complex surrounding, and or by replacing of the feature with simplified and idealized models of the feature. This dilemma will be further discussed in Chapter 6 in the section on bioimage informatics.

Yet another complication for spectral information is that the actual spectrum (signal intensity as a function of frequency) is not particularly meaningful. Certain combinations of peaks in a spectrum may be indicative of the presence of certain molecules, and hence, may be interpreted that way. Instead, translating the spectrum into a map showing the presence (and possibly the abundance) of certain (macro-)molecules might be more intuitive and meaningful.

However, it is rarely the case that one pixel corresponds to only one (macro-)molecule signal, hence multiple (macro-)molecules will likely contribute to each pixel, making the analysis and the display of that information even more challenging. Since for many (hyper-)spectral datasets, the actual contribution from a (macro-)molecules cannot be independently established and thus is not known with certainty, classification of images in terms of self-similarity of the spectral distribution can be a way to analyze such (hyper-)spectral datasets. Such self-similarity may allow an investigator to come to a biologically relevant conclusion, even if the exact (macro-)molecular composition cannot be determined.

Color imaging is yet another type of imaging. It is not multidimensional imaging where the data is dependent on a variety of independent data, it better fits in the category of multi-channel imaging, where different detectors measure different signals (e.g., wavelengths and thus colors), all of which depend on the same spatial X,Y-dimensions typical for a 2D image (Figure 5.29). Multi-channel and multidimensional are not mutually exclusive, a dataset may be both multi-channel and multidimensional.

Regarding optical imaging, there is a limit how many independent channels can be recorded by fluorescence imaging due to the finite filter and detector bandwidths, and thus possible overlaps in absorption and emission spectra of the fluorophores.

5.13 Sample Preparation Requirements

5.13.1 Macromolecular 3D Structure

Among the "unsung heroes" in biological imaging is sample preparation, as adequate sample preparation ensures faithful sample preservation. This is obvious for macromolecular imaging, where molecules must be isolated and

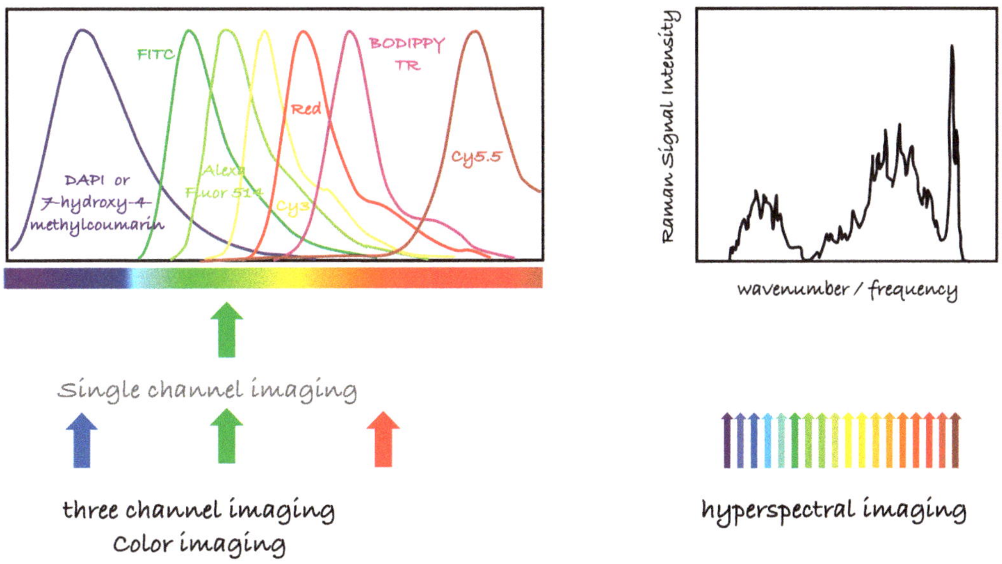

Figure 5.29 Multichannel imaging versus multi-dimensional imaging. Color imaging is an example of multichannel imaging where multiple (typically three) color regions are selected for data recording and thus image generation. The color image, with its many colors, is the result of the mixture of the colors used for each individual color. Hyperspectral imaging (such as Raman imaging) show signal intensity as a function of entire spectral wavelength/frequency range, which puts this kind of data into the category of multidimensional imaging.

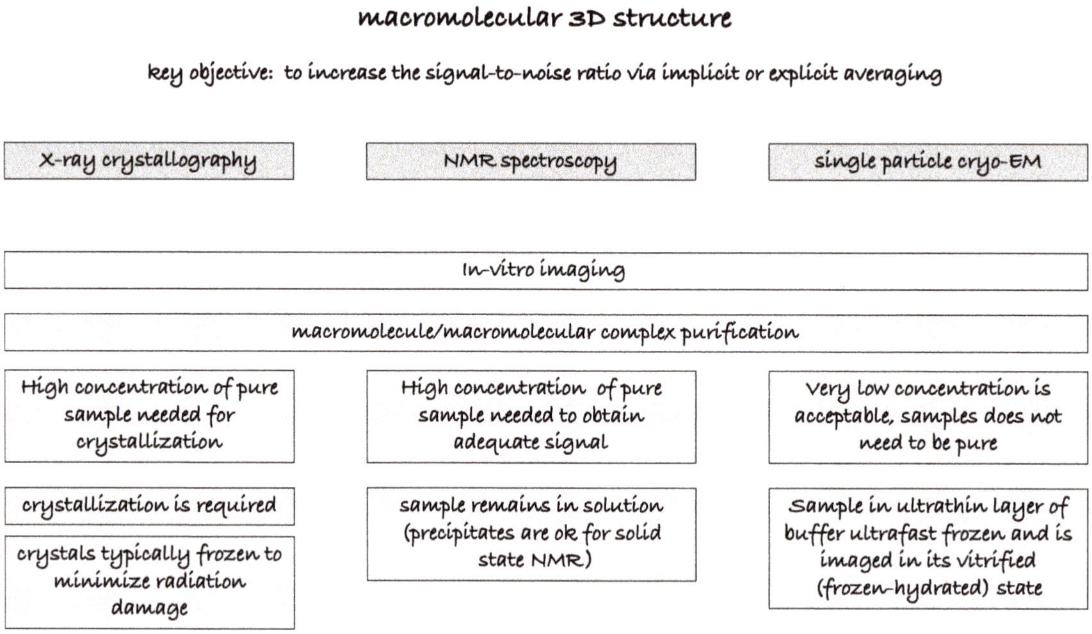

Figure 5.30 Sample preparation for macromolecular imaging. The key objective in macromolecular 3D structure imaging is to increase the signal-to-noise ratio either by implicit or explicit averaging. Typically, the sample must be purified to homogeneity with respect to macromolecular identity and/or conformational state, although recent day cryo-electron microscopy may be able to get away with a highly enriched sample and may not require high purity.

purified in a biologically relevant state (Figure 5.30). Too many impurities or different conformational states may be detrimental to the macromolecular crystallization process in X-ray crystallography, cause problems in picking the right particles for single particle cryo-EM or render NMR spectra uninterpretable. In the case of NMR, and to some degree also of X-ray crystallography, macromolecules must tolerate high concentrations, and/or be stable under non-physiological pH or ionic environment.

5.13.2 Subcellular, Cellular, and Tissue 3D Architecture

For cellular imaging with the goal of determining subcellular, cellular and tissue 3D organization and architecture, sample preparation ranges from little (as is the case for soft X-ray microscopy tomography) to extensive (as is the case of electron microscopy) (Figure 5.31).

Early histology work relied on extensive sample preparation (e.g., Golgi's stain with its heavy metals) to provide contrast in tissue sections for optical imaging. This pioneering work on heavy metal stains became the foundation for staining cells and tissues for electron microscopic imaging.

Electron microscopy (EM) is notorious for its extensive sample preparation protocols which aim for faithful preservation of the samples. Since the interaction of electrons with matter is very strong, samples must be imaged in the (high) vacuum of the electron microscopy and typically be very thin (unless surface-scanning EM is utilized for imaging). These sample preparation requirements are not compatible with live cell imaging. Cryogenic preparation techniques such as high-pressure freezing (millisecond freezing and thus immobilization of all dynamic cellular processes), followed by freeze-substitution (the exchange of frozen cellular water against organic solvents at low temperature) have minimized sample preparation artifacts that plagued earlier cellular EM imaging. This process is often followed by heavy metal staining, resin infiltration and polymerization as well as the cutting of ultrathin resin-embedded tissue sections.

Alternatively, cryo-sections or cryo-lamella can be produced, and the sample can be imaged by cryo-electron microscopy, in an unstained, frozen-hydrated state, which is thought to faithfully represent the 3D macromolecular, supramolecular, and cellular structure. Such cryo-imaging approaches can be very challenging, with sample preparation being the most critical aspect in the process. Sample requirements for cryo X-ray tomography of unstained, frozen-hydrated samples and X-ray tomography of stained samples are similar to the sample requirements for cryo-electron microscopy, with a sample thickness limit of about 15 μm (roughly the diameter of a eukaryotic cell). Thicker samples can be imaged by X-ray tomography of heavy metal-stained samples, including tissues and organs, as well as entire small animals such as zebrafish larvae.

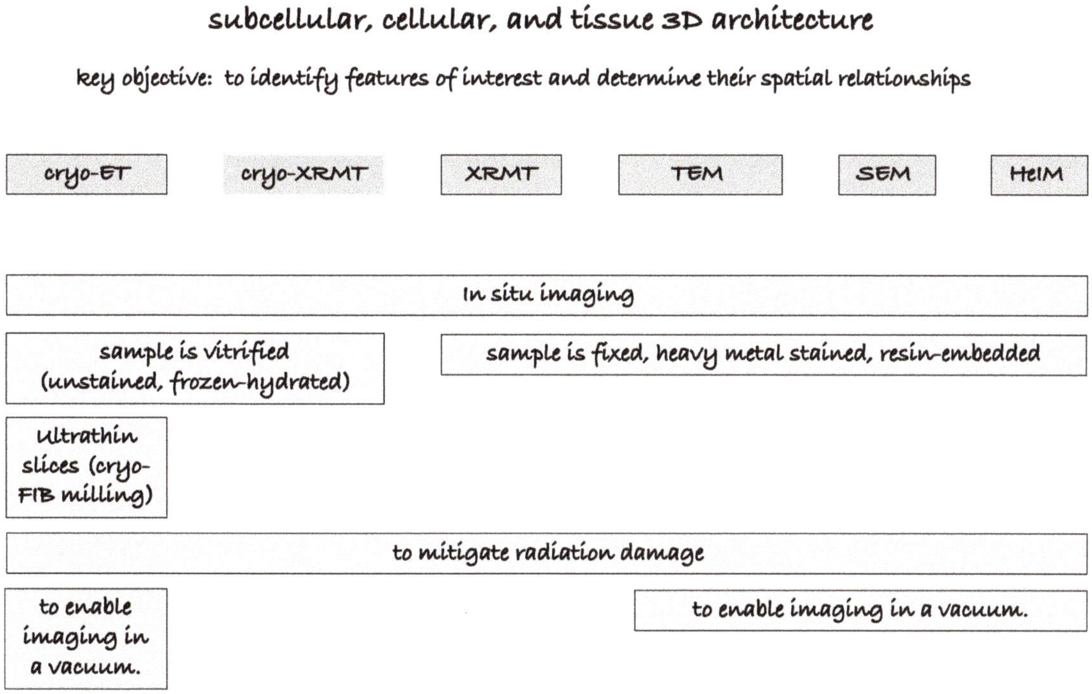

Figure 5.31 Sample preparation for 3D architecture determination. Sample preparation requirements for each of the techniques are different with cryo-electron tomography (cryo-ET) and cryo-soft X-ray microscopy tomography (cryo-XRMT) require the sample to be ultra-rapidly frozen so they can be imaged in an unstained, frozen-hydrated state. For cryo-ET, sample should be less than 0.5–1 µm in thickness (the size of a prokaryotic cell), whereas for cryo-XRMT sample thickness limit is ~15 µm (the size of a eukaryotic cell). Thicker samples require heavy-metal staining for contrast generation. Sample either need to be critical point dried to and heavy metal coated as is the case for conventional scanning electron microscopy (SEM) and helium ion microscopy (HeIM) or dehydrated, resin-infiltrated, resin-embedded is the case for either block-face SEM imaging or for ultra-thin sectioning and subsequent transmission electron microscopy (TEM) imaging. Hard X-ray microscopy tomography (XRMT) requires heavy-metal staining but works with either fully hydrated or resin-embedded samples.

5.13.3 Dynamic Localization of Macromolecules in Cells and Tissues

In the context of cellular imaging, optical microscopy with the goal of dynamic localization of macromolecules in cells and tissues requires the least sample preparation, but often requires specific labeling (Figure 5.32).

The introduction of specific labels can have its own demands on sample preparation, as is the case for immunolabeling, with the targeting of a reporter molecule via affinity of antigen-specific antibodies.

Also, for some fluorescent imaging approaches the presence of singlet oxygen scavenger molecules is required to reduce phototoxicity. Also, not all optical imaging techniques are suited for live-cell imaging, so for some applications, the cells and/or tissues are chemically fixed with paraformaldehyde.

For imaging of thick samples, tissues are often chemically treated (a process also known as clearing) to reduce absorption and scattering of light. Even thicker tissue samples are not suitable for optical microscopy imaging and thus require physical sectioning prior to imaging, which requires freezing of the sample or chemical fixation, dehydration and embedding into a resin that can be hardened. Yet in other applications, e.g., in neurobiological imaging, fluorescent stains that partition into cell membranes are either added to the water or injected into selected cells, e.g., to reveal the extensive network of dendrites and the axon.

Correlative imaging approaches, such as correlative fluorescence and electron microscopy (CLEM) may put additional strain on sample preparation. What is ideal for one technique may turn out to be detrimental for another imaging technique. Care must be taken at each step of sample preparation to avoid the trash-in/trash-out trap, as there is little point to image a sample, whose preservation is compromised and where its structural organization was significantly altered during the sample preparation process.

5.13.4 Chemical Inventory of Cells and Tissues

For cellular imaging with the goal of determining the chemical inventory of cells and tissues, sample preparation is typically minimal. The methods are often label-free and

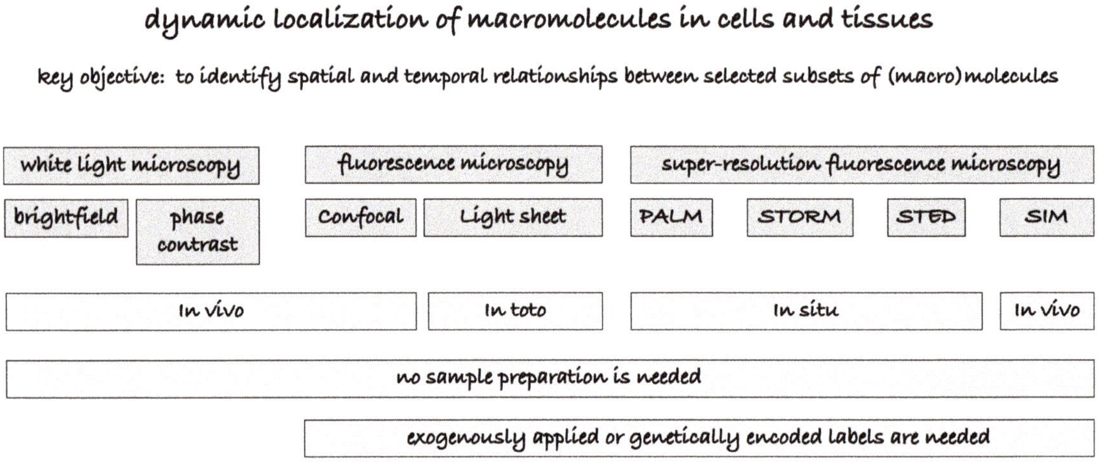

Figure 5.32 Sample preparation for localization of macromolecules. In general, optical microscopy requires little to no sample preparation, in many cases, samples can be imaged in vivo. However, for fluorescence microscopy applications, the fluorophore label either needs to be specifically targeted to the macromolecule or be genetically encoded as an intrinsic or extrinsic fluorescent fusion protein. Thick tissues often need to be chemically treated to minimize scattering of light (also known as clearing).

free of stains. Fourier Transform InfraRed (FTIR) imaging and Raman imaging do not require any sample preparation and are compatible with in-vivo imaging. For mass spectrometry, imaging nano-DESI ionization does not require any sample preparation, whereas MALDI-ionization may require the sample to be embedded in a matrix. The only method that requires significant sample preparation is X-ray microanalysis, since the sample is imaged in a vacuum, the sample needs to be either dried, frozen, or embedded in a resin (Figure 5.33).

Also, certain optical techniques such as Raman imaging rely on the suppression of autofluorescence signals and may thus require chemical treatment prior to imaging.

5.13.5 Medical Imaging of Tissues and Organs

For medical imaging (imaging of tissues and organs) there is no sample preparation needed in the classical sense of the word, as imaging happens in a living organism. However, people undergoing medical imaging procedures

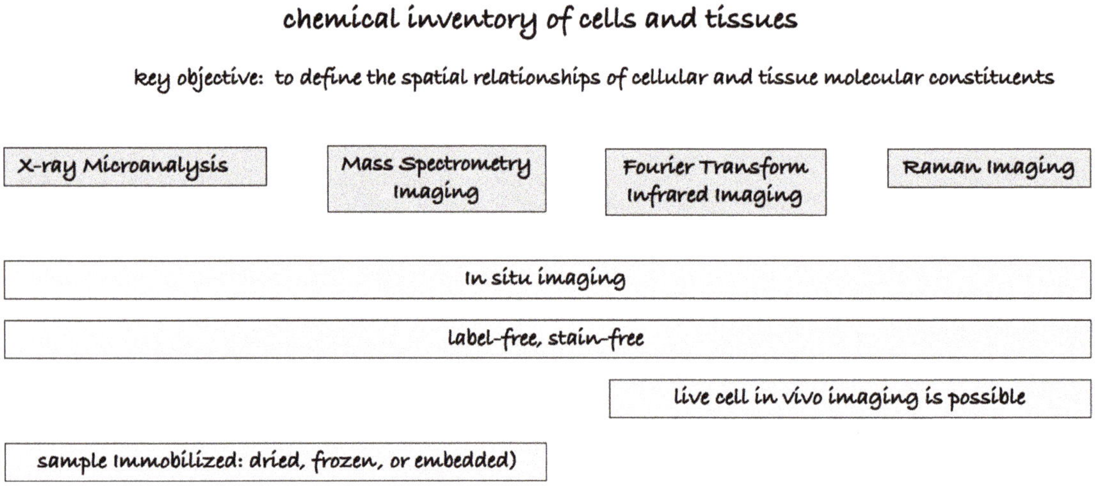

Figure 5.33 Sample preparation for determining the chemical inventory of cells and tissues. Most techniques require minimal sample preparation, as the technique are typically label-free and do not require staining for contrast generation. For X-ray microanalysis, one needs to image the sample in a vacuum, which means that the samples either need to be dried, frozen, or resin embedded. While X-ray microanalysis and mass spectrometry are destructive techniques that will damage the biological sample, other approaches such as Fourier Transform InfraRed (FTIR) imaging and Raman imaging are compatible with in-vivo imaging.

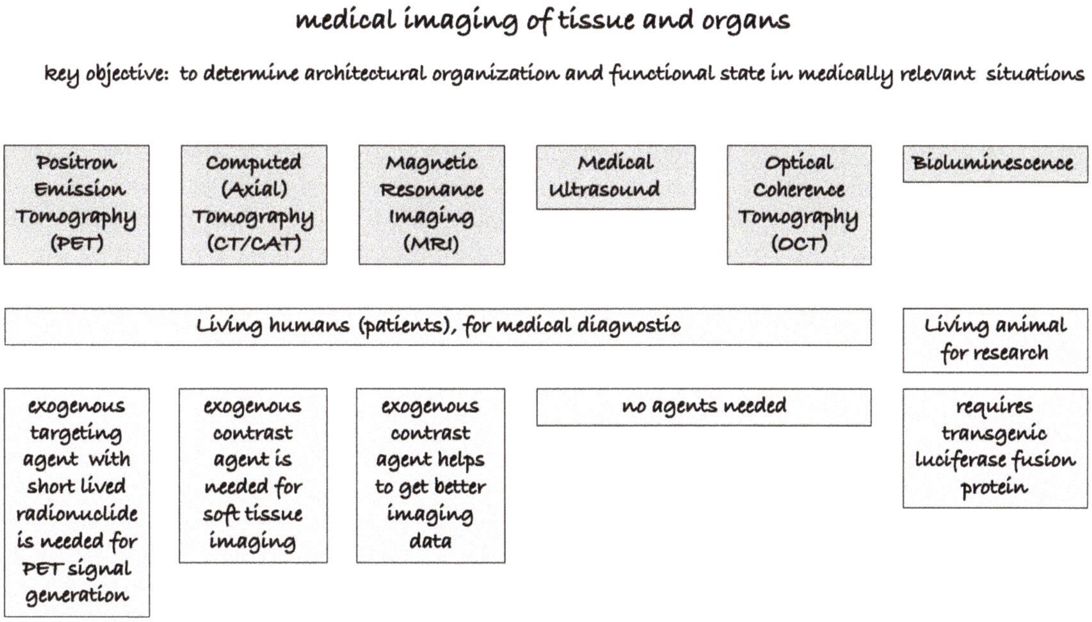

Figure 5.34 Sample preparation for medical imaging of tissues and organs. Many of the medical imaging techniques do not require a specific sample preparation of the tissue or organ to be imaged, however, a person may need to take up reagents that improve contrast. Positron Emission Tomography (PET) relies on a radionuclide to emit positron radiation, which annihilates with an electron in its immediate surrounding to emit two gamma-rays in opposite directions, which then can be detected. So, while the tissue/organ does not require sample preparation per se, the source of radiation needs to find its intended target tissue/organ. Computed (Axial) Tomography (CT/CAT) does not need contrast reagents as long as the tissue to be imaged is dense, such is the case for bones. However, if soft tissue needs to be imaged an appropriate contrasting reagent needs to be administered. Similarly, Magnetic Resonance Imaging (MRI) does not require sample preparation per se, but gadolinium is frequently used as a contrasting agent to shorten the relaxation time of tissue water protons, which in turn yields contrast. Contrasting agents are typically administered through the blood stream or are taken orally. In terms of sample preparation ultrasound and optical coherence tomography are the simplest as no prior preparation is needed. Bioluminescence is not carried out in humans as genetic engineering of the organism is needed to express the luciferase protein, which catalyzes the oxidation of luciferin, which in turn creates light that can be detected.

may need to take up chemicals that will lead to enhanced contrast (Figure 5.34).

In the case of Positron Emission Tomography (PET), radionuclides must be administered prior to imaging, as the radioactive substances will emit positrons (due to radioactive decay), which in their immediate environment will annihilate with electrons to produce two gamma-ray photons with opposite trajectories. The detection of such a pair of gamma-ray photons is the basis of PET imaging.

In Computed (Axial) Tomography (CT/CAT) imaging, contrasting agents are not needed when imaging dense tissues such as bones with its high density and high amount of calcium, but is needed when imaging soft tissues. In these cases, iodinated reagents or barium salts serve as contrasting agents, but kidney function must be closely monitored as such reagents can be nephrotoxic.

Magnetic Resonance Imaging (MRI) relies on differences in T1 relaxation time of water protons in different tissues. Contrasting agents like gadolinium shorten the time for T1 relaxation and thus provide a higher proton signal wherever the contrasting reagent is present. Contrasting reagents are typically administered through the blood stream or ingested orally, although take up through the rectum is also possible.

Ultrasound and Optical Coherence Tomography do not require any contrast enhancement or sample preparation of any sort. Bioluminescence is used in pre-clinical research, but cannot be employed for human beings, as the luciferase protein needs to be genetically introduced. Luciferase catalyzes the oxidation of luciferin to oxyluciferin. In the process light is being produced, which can be detected as bioluminescence.

5.14 Labels and Labeling

Biological systems are characterized by their (macro-) molecular composition and localization as well as the higher structural organization these macromolecules form (subcellular, cell, and tissue architecture). Equally important is an understanding of their dynamic behavior (macromolecular localization). Localization of individual macromolecular components requires labeling techniques that render these components and only these components visible. By focusing on one to several labels one can simplify the analysis as many other aspects of these complex systems can simply be ignored. Label-free systems may not require specific labeling but due to the complexity of the signal, analysis can be very complicated.

With respect to labels, fluorophores represent the largest group of labels, but others such as radiotracers for PET imaging also fall into the category of labels, which means that they have a specific biological target that will be selectively imaged through the label. In the case of fluorophores, there are three classes: 1. synthetic dyes, 2. Quantum dots, 3. genetically encoded fluorescent proteins (Figure 5.35).

Organic chemistry synthetic dyes often have favorable imaging properties, however they require extrinsic specific targeting to the macromolecule of interest. Small (few nm-sized) semiconductor-material based probes (such as Quantum dots) have the advantage of being very bright and bleaching-resistant, but also need to be targeted to the macromolecule of interest. Genetically encoded fluorescent proteins that are genetically fused with the target protein do not require targeting as each fluorescent signal stems from the target molecule. However, only intrinsically fluorescent proteins do not require any chemical labeling as the label is fully genetic encoded. Extrinsically fluorescent proteins consist of a genetically encoded tag (typically in form of a fusion protein) that will selectively bind a label that still needs to be extrinsically provided. The big difference to synthetic organic chemistry dyes is the way the dye finds its target. For extrinsically fluorescent proteins the target is genetically encoded and has a high affinity for the label, whereas without a genetically encoded tag the dye must be delivered to its target by some other affinity probe.

Hence, introducing labels to a biological sample relies on the affinity of a probe for the target molecule or genetic encoding via intrinsically or extrinsically fluorescent fusion proteins.

Immunolabeling is one example how labels (fluorescent or otherwise) can be targeted specifically to (macro-)molecules, where one exploits the affinity (and hopefully specificity) of an antibody to the (macro-)molecule of interest. There are other examples where there is a natural affinity of a small molecule to bind to macromolecules, such as phalloidin having a high affinity for filamentous actin, or DAPI which binds to DNA. Such small molecules, if conjugated with a suitable synthetic fluorophore, can be very powerful for specific targeting and subsequent fluorescence imaging.

Genetic encoding of fluorescent proteins is a powerful approach to deliver a fluorescent label to a macromolecule of interest. Initially based on discovery of the jellyfish green

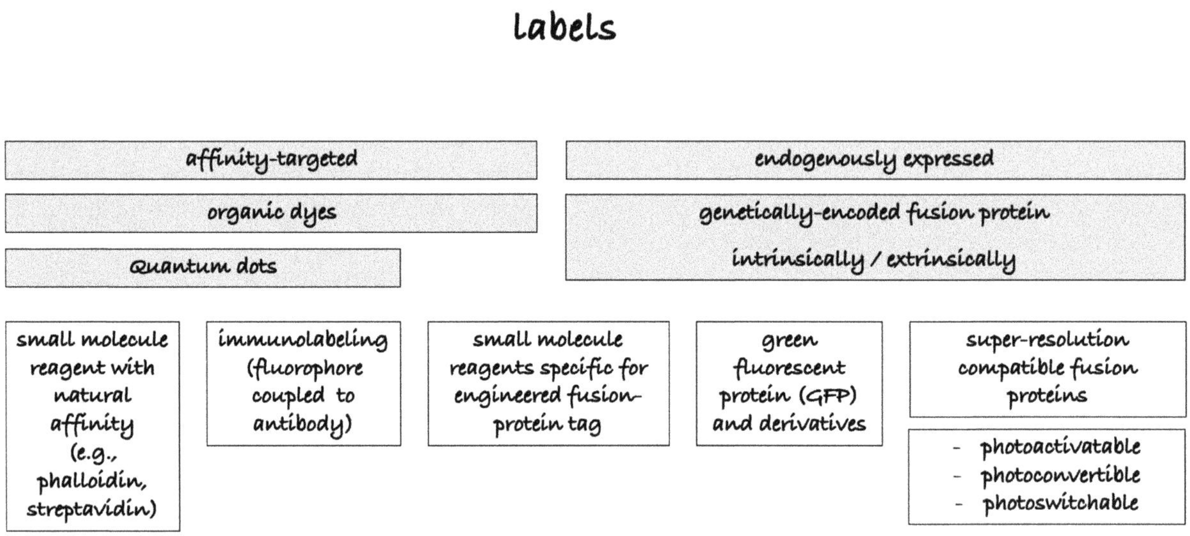

Figure 5.35 Affinity-targeted labels and endogenously expressed fusion proteins for localization of (macro-)molecules. Labels are delivered to their target (macro-)molecule either through some form of affinity probe that will deliver the label or through the expression of a fusion protein where a fluorescent protein is genetically fused to the proteins of interest. Intrinsically fluorescent proteins do not require any further labeling. Extrinsically fluorescent proteins are genetically engineered/fused to the macromolecules of interest but are not intrinsically fluorescent. They are tags that bind a fluorescent label with high selectivity and with high affinity. Affinity probes are either antibody based or exploit a natural affinity of a small molecule for certain macromolecules such as phalloidin for filamentous actin. With respect to intrinsically fluorescent proteins, the classic example is green protein fluorescent proteins (GFP) and its many spectral derivatives. Furthermore, some of these fluorescent proteins have additional properties such being photoactivatable, photoconvertible or photoswitchable, which makes them ideal labels for superresolution light microscopy.

fluorescent protein (GFP) the probe repertoire was expanded to include different segments of the visible light spectrum and thus to allow fluorescence imaging in different colors. Genetic encoding and thus expression of fluorescent proteins as a fusion protein has revolutionized cell biology, a fact that has been recognized by the 2008 Nobel Prize in Chemistry.

Affinity-based probes often require a biological sample to be fixed as cells need to be penetrated for the affinity probe to find its target, whereas genetically encoded fluorescent protein fusion proteins are usually compatible with live cell imaging, which is key for cell biological imaging. Since the early days of GFP, a whole arsenal of fluorescent protein probes has been developed, some of which now are photoactivatable, photoconvertible, or photoswitchable, which in turn allows superresolution fluorescence imaging that can localize macromolecules with a precision beyond the diffraction limit of optical light microscopy imaging.

Extrinsically fluorescent proteins which bind a synthetic fluorophore with high affinity, represent a hybrid between affinity-based and genetically encoded tags. Tags are often moderate-size oligopeptides or small proteins that are genetically engineered as fusion proteins to the target protein. Some tags even bind covalently a small molecule that is conjugated to a synthetic fluorophore with favorable fluorescence imaging properties. Such tags/labels allow pulse-chase experiment, e.g., to measure protein turnover. This approach allows nearly background-free imaging like it is the case for fluorescent protein imaging, as non-specific signals from unbound fluorophores can be readily washed away. SNAP-tag, HALO-tags, CLIP-tags and tetracysteine tags are examples of this approach.

5.15 Label-Free Imaging

While labeling has become increasingly easier for many biological model systems, not every species that may be of interest is genetically accessible. A prominent example is human tissue that is obviously of interest to understand disease mechanisms, yet for good ethic reasons human cells cannot be genetically manipulated.

Label-free imaging can present an alternative to the use of labels. Another reason to consider label-free imaging is the fact that labeling only allows the experimenter to visualize what has been labeled, all other aspects that may show interesting patterns of spatiotemporal change remain invisible. To stay with optical light microscopy techniques, there are several techniques that are label-free, including brightfield imaging, phase contrast microscopy and differential interference contrast (DIC) microscopy, the latter two of which are superior to standard brightfield imaging in terms of contrast and subcellular details. In phase contrast imaging, cells appear dark on a light background, and in DIC imaging mode, they appear with a pseudo-3D shadow. One big advantage is that cells are being analyzed in their native unperturbed way, free of any change in behavior that may arise due to phototoxicity (as can be the case for long-term fluorescence imaging of cells and tissues). The experiments are straight forward, as no genetic modification of cells or exogenous fluorophore labeling of cells is necessary, and no complex laser or optics are needed to obtain results. Hence, unlike fluorescence imaging, label-free imaging approaches can be non-invasive, fast, and cheap, as cellular dynamics and cell morphology can be studied over long periods of time and phototoxicity usually is not an issue.

While bright light imaging is typically carried out at lower resolution than is typical for localization microscopy, the study of morphology and behavior as a function of experimental intervention (genetic mutation, response to drugs or to changes in environmental culturing conditions, e.g., to changes in the extracellular matrix properties) can be very revealing. Cell division, proliferation, motility as well as differentiation/senescence and cell death can be recognized even at lower resolution by the above-mentioned optical techniques. Individual cells can be identified and tracked over time, which can monitor migratory behavior of cells and determine distance and speed of migration. Cell morphology can even be quantified, such as the total area of the cellular footprint, changes at the tissue periphery including protrusions, a cells aspect ratio or changes in orientation and organization.

Raman imaging is another important label-free optical imaging technique, that like Fourier Transform InfraRed (FTIR) imaging can reveal molecular composition, or at least address the question of homogeneity of distribution of molecular components through a self-similarity analysis of the compositional distribution. Raman signaling has been successful in a few cases, as has FTIR imaging, but the computational analysis of Raman and FTIR imaging data remains a challenge.

One could argue that electron microscopy (EM) and X-ray microscopy tomography (XRMT) are label-free imaging techniques in the sense that one can examine biological systems at a range from very low to very high resolution without the need for a specific label. The lack of a label means that everything is visible in EM and XRMT, but it also means that features of interest can be selected from the entire data set only after data collection, in a process known as segmentation (feature extraction).

5.16 2D Versus 3D Imaging

Individual images typically are two-dimensional. Stacks of images build up a 3D volume (and in a computer 3D volumes are often stored as stacks of 2D images). There are good reasons to collect 3D datasets, particularly, if the 2D images are taken from a sample that is too thick to allow unambiguous interpretation as a 2D projection. In such cases important structural details are positioned on top of one another and thus cannot easily be discriminated (Figure 5.36).

Usually, it is much easier to collect 2D image datasets than 3D volume datasets. Also, visualization and analysis of 3D volumes typically is more complicated and involves more steps. Therefore, when deciding whether to record 2D or 3D data, one should first ask one-self what additional information will be obtained by recording a few 3D volume image data sets rather than a much larger number of 2D images, and whether the *Z*-direction is important to answer a biological question, both in terms of localization and cellular architecture. While 3D data may seem to be more "elegant" and appear more sophisticated, often it may not provide important information, and due to the more complicated analysis of 3D volumes, one may not be able to get as many independent measurements, hence one may end up with a lower statistical coverage.

Depending on the imaging techniques employed, there are multiple ways to collect 3D datasets. For example, in the case of laser scanning fluorescence microscopy, each 2D image is taken by raster-scanning the laser beam across the sample as the sample is moved along the *Z*-axis through the focal plane. This results in a stack of 2D-images that can be readily combined into a 3D volume. However, there will be some contributions of out-of-focus fluorescence light above and below the sample that will degrade image resolution in the *Z*-direction. Out-of-focus illumination and thus unnecessary fluorophore excitation also can lead to photodamage to the sample, even when such out-of-focus photons do not contribute to the recorded image. In the light sheet imaging mode, only one thin slice of the sample will be illuminated at any given time, with the image being recorded by an area detector (e.g., a CCD or CMOS camera). The advantage is that the light sheet illumination only excites fluorophores whose light is being recorded. Two-photon microscopy with its near-perfect sphere-like point-spread function is another way to collect 2D stacks, with neighboring pixels along the *Z*-axis being independent. For some light sheet applications, one rotates the sample through the light sheet, in which case the 3D volume is reconstructed as a function of the rotation angle and its corresponding image (as will be discussed below).

Optical techniques that employ a shift of the focal point (or the sample) along the *Z*-axis are referred to as optical sectioning microscopy, to distinguish older techniques that rely on physical sectioning to obtain thin enough sections that can be imaged as 2D images (Figure 5.37). Imaging of consecutive physical sections is still in use for serial section transmission electron microscopy (TEM) cellular imaging, however the cutting of many consecutive sections with reliable and consistent thickness without the loss of sections or compression/damage to sections can be experimentally demanding, particularly when picking up such ribbons of consecutive sections with transmission electron microscopy grids.

Array tomography SEM or automated tape-collecting ultramicrotome (ATUM) SEM employ automated approaches for cutting long ribbons of sections that attach to a

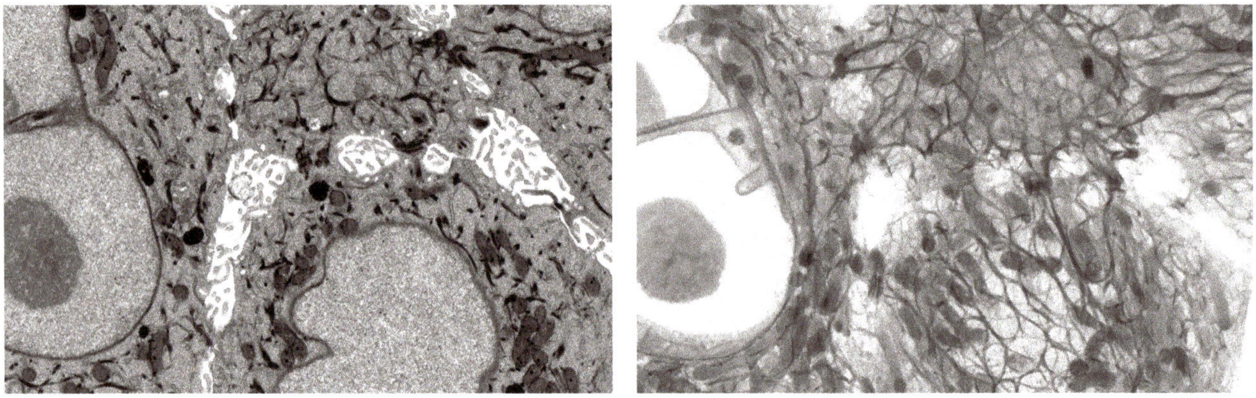

Figure 5.36 2D versus 3D imaging. 3D volume of mammary gland cells cultured in a 3D matrix forming an acinus. Left: Single 5 nm thin slice through 3D volume showing cell nuclei, mitochondria, and the cytoskeleton. Right: 3D organization of the cytoskeleton in a 1 μm thick slab. Note that projecting through the 3D volume of the slab gives an overall impression of cytoskeletal organization, which is not appreciated when inspecting individual slices. However, segmentation of individual strands of the cytoskeleton requires an analysis of 200 thin slices at 5 nm-thickness.

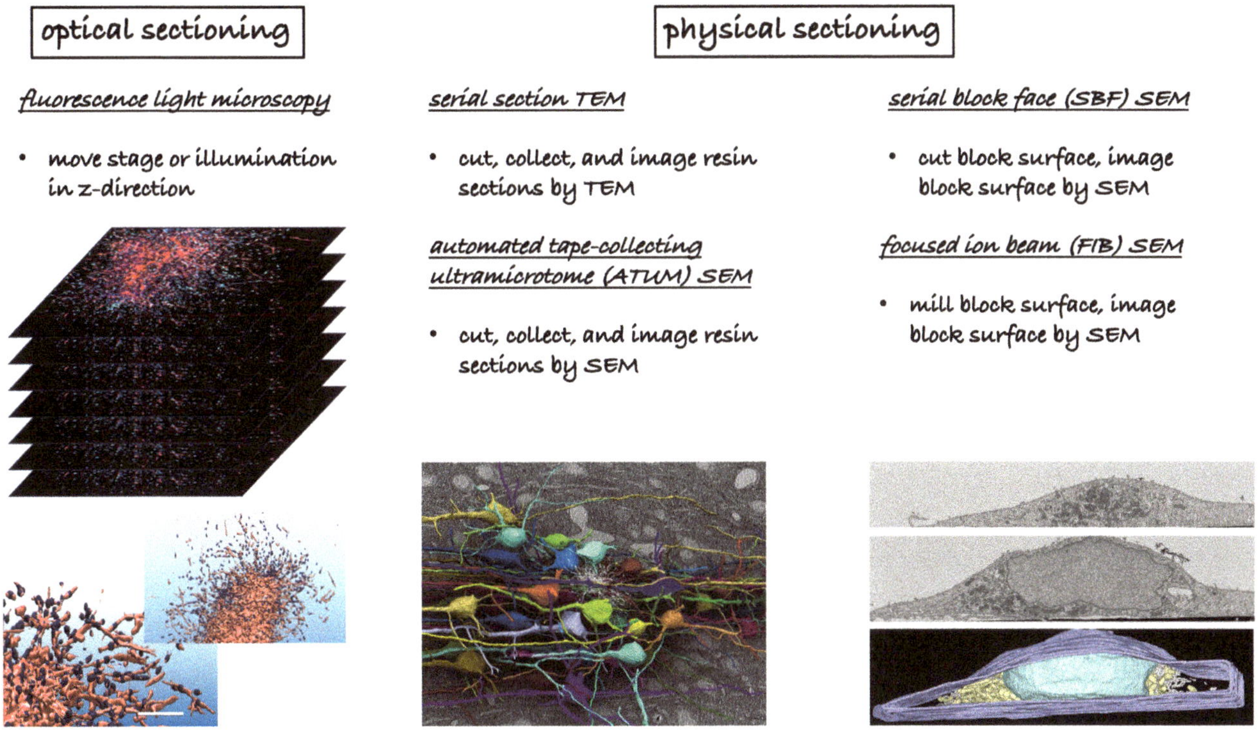

Figure 5.37 Optical sectioning and physical sectioning. Optically transparent samples can be imaged by optical sectioning, e.g., in fluorescence light microscopy, where either the illumination or the sample are being translated along the *Z* direction (along the beam). Physical sectioning involves cutting sections of the sample, which is embedded in a resin-block (or in a frozen sample block). Sections are then collected and studied by either transmission or scanning electron microscopy (TEM or SEM), resulting in the generation of a 3D volume from such serial sections. Note that the 3D volume will display anisotropic resolution as the physical section thickness is much larger than the lateral resolution. Block surface imaging is another form of physical sectioning where images are taken of the block surface. After imaging, the block surface is removed either by a diamond knife (serial block face SEM at anisotropic resolution) or by a focused ion beam (focused ion beam SEM at isotropic resolution).

continuously moving tape that is then mounted onto a silicon waver for scanning electron microscopy. Such approaches can yield image information for very large volumes, but given that the lower limit of section thickness (and thus the *Z*-axis step size) is much larger than the *X,Y* imaging resolution of the scanning electron microscope (SEM), there is a large discrepancy in *X,Y* versus *Z*-axis resolution, hence the 3D volume is anisotropic. Furthermore, at the very surface of the section, there could be artifacts due to the physical cutting of the resin with a diamond knife. However, this is usually not a problem (particularly if the section is imaged as a 2D projection image), and can be neglected. Physical sectioning of samples embedded in resin-blocks followed by 2D imaging of the serial sections by TEM is yet another example of stacks of 2D images that amount to a 3D volume. However, serial section TEM often battles with a variety of artifacts, which complicates 3D reconstruction, as upon physical sectioning and section collection two adjacent serial images may show differences in overall rotation angle and scale due to sectioning compression artifacts.

Yet another way to build up a 3D volume as a stack of 2D images is to obtain serial images of the very surface of a resin-embedded block of the sample (Figure 5.38) by either Serial Block Face SEM imaging or Focused Ion Beam SEM (FIBSEM). The difference between these two approaches is how the block face is refreshed for each imaging cycle. In the case of Serial Block Face SEM imaging (also known as volutome), a diamond knife cuts 30–50 nm sections from the block face, whereas in the case of Focused Ion Beam SEM (also known as Dual Beam SEM) an ion beam abrases the surface of the block at ~5 nm step size. Hence, FIBSEM can accomplish an isotropic *X, Y, Z* resolution of ~5 nm, whereas Block Face SEM imaging suffers from the same data anisotropy as serial section TEM or array tomography SEM.

(Cryo-) Electron tomography and (Cryo-) X-ray tomography use a similar principle for volume data collection and 3D reconstruction, which is different from the physical sectioning approach discussed above. Using specimen rotation and collection of tilt series 2D images, 3D volumes are reconstructed from aligned tilt series images by back-projection and related approaches (Figure 5.39). As both

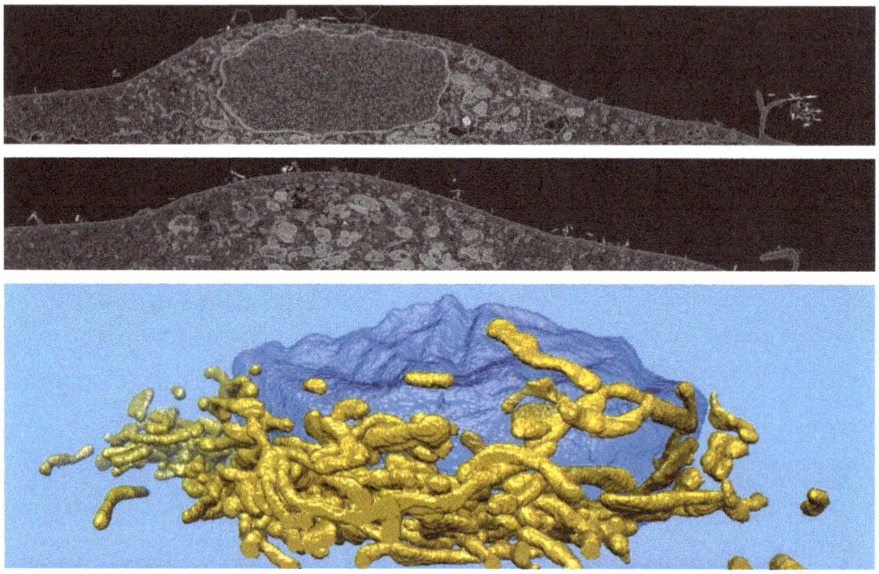

Figure 5.38 Example of 2D versus 3D imaging. Top and middle: Two non-adjacent ~5 nm slices of a 3D volume of a Petri-dish cultured eukaryotic cell; Bottom: 3D rendering of the 3D volume, with segmented cell nuclear membrane in blue and mitochondria in golden. From the segmented 3D volume, it becomes apparent that many mitochondria form a continuous 3D network, whereas in 2D slices mitochondria appear as disconnected.

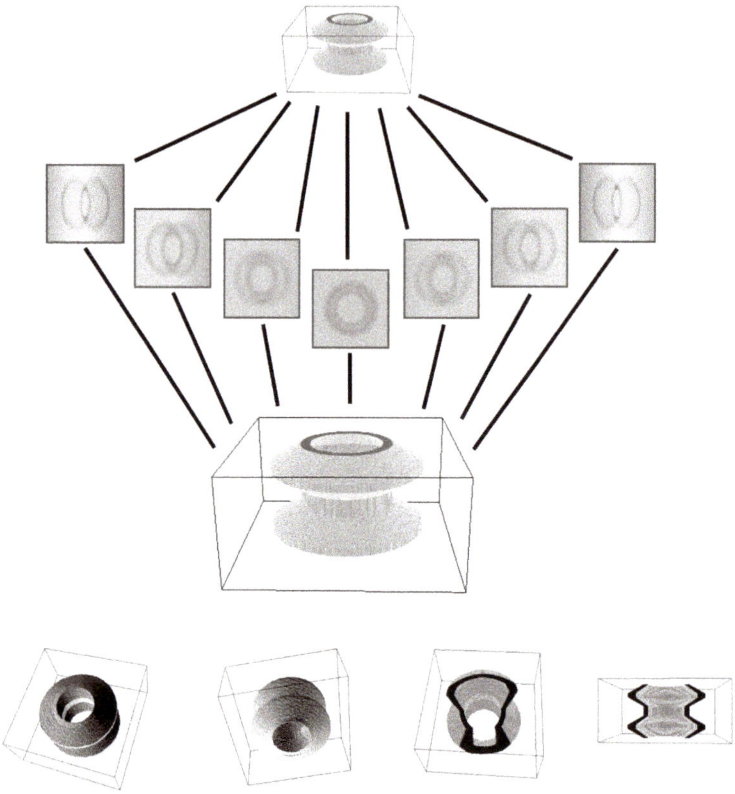

Figure 5.39 Tomographic 3D reconstructions by back projections. For imaging approaches where the radiation penetrates the sample and thus only 2D projection images can be obtained, back projection is a way to reconstruct a 3D volume from a series of these 2D projection images recorded at different tilt angles (tilt series). Note that for samples that cannot be rotated for a full 180° range, the resolution along the *Z*-axis (which is also the axis of penetration of the sample by the beam) is lower than the resolution perpendicular to the *Z*-axis.

imaging approaches rely on the transmission of electrons or X-rays, respectively, each 2D image is recorded as a projection image, with electrons or X-rays penetrating through the sample. To reconstruct a 3D volume from projection views, one needs to rotate the sample through the electron/X-ray beam. In X-ray tomography the sample can be rotated through a full 180° angle range, which leads to isotropic information, whereas in electron microscopy, the rotating angle is limited to about ±70° (~140° altogether), in part due to the support grid that blocks views at higher angles. Hence, there is a missing wedge of data where views of the sample cannot be recorded.

Furthermore, for sample geometries like a slab (resin-section or a frozen-hydrated lamella), the thickness of the sample increases at higher tilt angles. As a result, the resolution of the tomogram is not uniform, but decreases from the center toward the periphery of the tomogram.

Dual axis imaging (rotating the sample by 90° between the recording of the two tilt series) reduces the missing wedge of information to a missing pyramid of information, but it does not fully eliminate the resolution discrepancy between the XY-plane and the *Z*-direction of the resulting 3D tomographic volume. Reconstruction of the 3D volume is typically done by weighted (filtered) back projection (WBP) algorithms, which is a variation of the simple back projection approach, modified by a weighting function in Fourier space. More sophisticated approaches such as iterative reconstruction techniques can be used but they tend to be computationally rather expensive, but often the algebraic reconstruction technique (ART) yield better results than conventional WBP. As discussed, for electron tomography the *Z*-resolution typically is significantly worse (typically by a factor of three) than the resolution in *X*,*Y*, as the sample often cannot be tilted more than ±60 to ±70° (sometimes even only ±45°).

As only the very central region of the tomogram offers the highest resolution, care should be taken to ensure the volume of interest is at the very center of the tomogram, and the *X*, *Y* versus *Z*-direction data anisotropy should be taken into consideration in the 3D analysis.

5.17 Structural Versus Functional Imaging

Structural and functional imaging are two imaging approaches with very different goals. The structural imaging approach focuses on the 3D structure and thus 3D organization of cells, tissues, and organs. Functional imaging on the other hand focuses on the physiological activities of a tissue or organ. In positron emission tomography (PET) tracers are targeted toward certain receptor molecules or they accumulate in certain tissues or organs.

One prominent example is the glucose-derivative ^{18}F-fluorodesoxyglucose (FDG), which accumulates in cancerous tissues with a high glucose demand. FDG but also can be used to study glucose metabolism in heart and brain. Functional magnetic resonance imaging (fMRI) takes advantage of the difference in magnetic sensitivity to discriminate between oxyhemoglobin and deoxyhemoglobin and uses the signal difference of oxygen-rich and oxygen-depleted blood flow as a proxy for brain activity. The goal of functional imaging often is not so much spatial resolution but instead temporal resolution. As the signal by itself may be difficult to interpret, it is often being placed into a structural imaging context. For this very reason, functional imaging is often combined with structural imaging, as is the case for PET being combined with Computed Tomography (CT). The combination of two different imaging techniques will provide complementary information, leveraging their respective strengths.

5.18 Correlative Imaging

The example of PET–CT imaging (as discussed above) is just one of many, where the use of different imaging techniques provides leverage and helps illuminate a bigger picture, revealing different aspects of a biological system, e.g., cellular architecture and dynamics, cellular architecture and molecular composition, localization of macromolecules (including their dynamics) and cellular architecture. Using a combination of imaging techniques on the same sample is known as correlative imaging, as the goal is to correlate information from the same specimen region obtained from different platforms. One can also speak of a multi-platform or multimodal imaging. Often the two imaging modes also happen to be imaging at different scales, in which case we also need to consider multiscale imaging.

For example, optical imaging (e.g., epifluorescence microscopy) maybe used to determine the location of certain macromolecules in cells (attached to a sapphire disk or embedded in a thin extracellular matrix). Upon studying the dynamics of the system and the location of the labeled macromolecules by optical microscopy, the sample is then chemically fixed or ultra-rapidly frozen, with the fluorescence signal being converted into a heavy metal precipitate. This is called photoconversion and is based on fluorescence-driven singlet oxygen reaction that precipitates diaminobenzidine, which as a precipitate shows high affinity for the heavy metal compound osmium tetroxide.

Subsequent further processing for electron microscopy imaging then results in darkly stained areas where there was a fluorescence signal before. Upon sectioning and electron microscopy imaging one is then able to determine at high resolution the immediate ultrastructural context of the precipitates and see whether they are associated with certain organelles or supramolecular assemblies (cytoskeleton, adhesion complexes, vesicles, etc.). Since these two imaging techniques often operate at different scales, low-resolution electron microscopy images can provide an overview and serve as a bridge to correlate the two datasets.

Correlative imaging can be tricky to accomplish and works best for thin individual cells in cell culture, where cells are well spaced from one another, and an individual cell can be easily identified. It helps that cells in 2D culture often appear as flat, further reducing the number of sections that need to be studied.

It is much more difficult in 3D organoids or tissues where individual cells are closely packed in all three dimensions. There it is difficult to distinguish individual cells a priori from one another, particularly if resolution is limited and the scenery is crowded. In such instances, 3D datasets may need to be recorded both by optical microscopy and by electron microscopy. However, it is vastly underestimated how long it takes to find the exact same region of interest for high resolution imaging given the large mismatch in scale between the different techniques. Further complications arise from the possibility of non-specific heavy-metal signals that may arise from other sources during the photoconversion process.

While clearly a worthwhile goal, correlative imaging is technically very challenging and has specific sample geometry and imaging geometry requirements. Furthermore, often there are sometimes conflicts with respect to sample preparation requirements of different techniques, which may result in compromises with respect to sample preservation or contrast. Also given the difficulties associated with correlative imaging, datasets are often small and sparse, which makes it difficult to assess, how typical presented results really are.

6

Basics of Image Processing and Image Analysis

6.1 Overview

Image Processing

The roots of digital imaging processing date back to the 1960s, when the Bell Laboratories, the Jet Propulsion Laboratory, the Massachusetts Institute of Technology, the University of Maryland, and others were dealing with images from satellites, medical diagnostic, text/character recognition and photographs of the lunar surface by using computer algorithms to enhance image data quality.

Image processing includes image restoration (e.g., motion blur correction), image enhancement (e.g., contrast enhancement, edge detection, geometrical transformation such as rotation of the image), and compression. Early efforts have focused on 2D images.

In image processing, both the input and the output are images. Image processing typically does not include an analysis or interpretation about image content. There is significant overlap of image processing with the interdisciplinary field of computer vision, whose goal is to achieve a higher-level understanding of the scenery depicted in 2D or 3D images (or in videos).

Computer Vision

Computer vision seeks to emulate the process of the human visual system, from receiving the image data and basic processing of the image data to extracting and analyzing the useful and relevant portion of the information (segmentation) and deriving meaning from such visual data. Computer vision should not be confused with the field of computer graphics where 3D models are used to generate image data (e.g., to create animations), although some overlap of computer graphics and computer vision exists, e.g., in the form of augmented reality where image data and model data are combined into a new (enhanced) representation of the visual reality.

Among the many challenges that computer vision addresses are the more mundane tasks such as image registration and image morphing, panoramic image stitching and motion tracking as well as the more sophisticated challenges tasks such as classical texture-based, region-based or edge-based image segmentation/feature extraction (e.g., by *K*-means clustering, graph cuts, region growing and contour levels as well as other approaches), feature annotation, and feature (object) recognition. Image segmentation can mean to divide an image into a foreground and background, into multiple categories of self-similarities or to extract single or multiple features with specific characteristics.

Feature-based approaches have resurged with advances in Machine Learning (ML) and Deep Learning (DL) techniques that are based on classical or convolutional neural networks (CNN), respectively, which can "learn" feature characteristics without being given explicit instructions on what specific characteristics to pay attention to. Typically, in supervised DL, a large amount of ground truth data is provided that serve as examples of what constitutes a certain feature of interest and thus a desired solution for learning. The more varied the examples are for training, the more robust will the CNN success rate be for new examples that were not part of the training data set. In unsupervised learning, no specific ground truth is given, and the algorithm looks for similarities and differences between different image data sets.

Bioimage Informatics

Bioimage informatics is closely related to the fields of computational biology, computer science, computer vision, and bioinformatics. There is also significant overlap with data mining. The focus of bioimage informatics lies on the use of computational approaches to analyze bioimages, often at cell and tissue level resolution, and often recorded at

Introduction to Biological Imaging, First Edition. Manfred Auer.

large scale with high data content and/or at high throughput. The goal is to turn complicated and heterogeneous image data (along with its metadata) into useful biological knowledge. Automation of image processing and analysis is an important step to deal with the increasing number of large-scale datasets that are recorded by automated microscopes and to analyze such datasets without the bias of desired outcome. There are still a variety of aspects of bioimage informatics that require further development, including computer vision, image processing, data mining, and database science. Regarding visualization there are several open-source point-and-click visualization packages with intuitive graphical user interfaces (GUI) available, including ImageJ, Fiji, CellProfiler, Icy (and others). Figure 6.1 shows a workflow for an in-depth image analysis, including steps for image restoration and enhancement, visualization, feature of interest extraction and annotation, as well as quantitative analysis.

Data Mining

Data mining is part of computer science that aims to extract information from large data sets to discover patterns, and thus to gain knowledge about a system, by using advances in machine learning/deep learning (ML/DL), statistics, visualization, and database systems. In a more general sense, the term data mining refers to data analysis and analytics at a scale large enough that it can no longer be handled by an individual person. As for any analysis, the goal is to detect hidden patterns in large data sets, such as the clustering of certain data characteristics, relationships (associations, dependencies) between variable, as well as the detection of abnormalities, deviations, or changes, which could either be simply data errors or may point to interesting phenoms. The goal is to use a known data structure to classify new data into different categories, and to mathematically model the data, like fitting a curve that has the least error (e.g., by using regression analysis). The goal is to summarize the complex data by representing it in a more compact and simplified/abstracted way und using visualization for report generation.

In this process, datasets often need to be pre-processed to remove data of insufficient quality (where some data is missing or data that only contribute to noise). Data mining relies on efficient database management and ML for data analysis including cluster analysis, decision trees as well as neuronal networks.

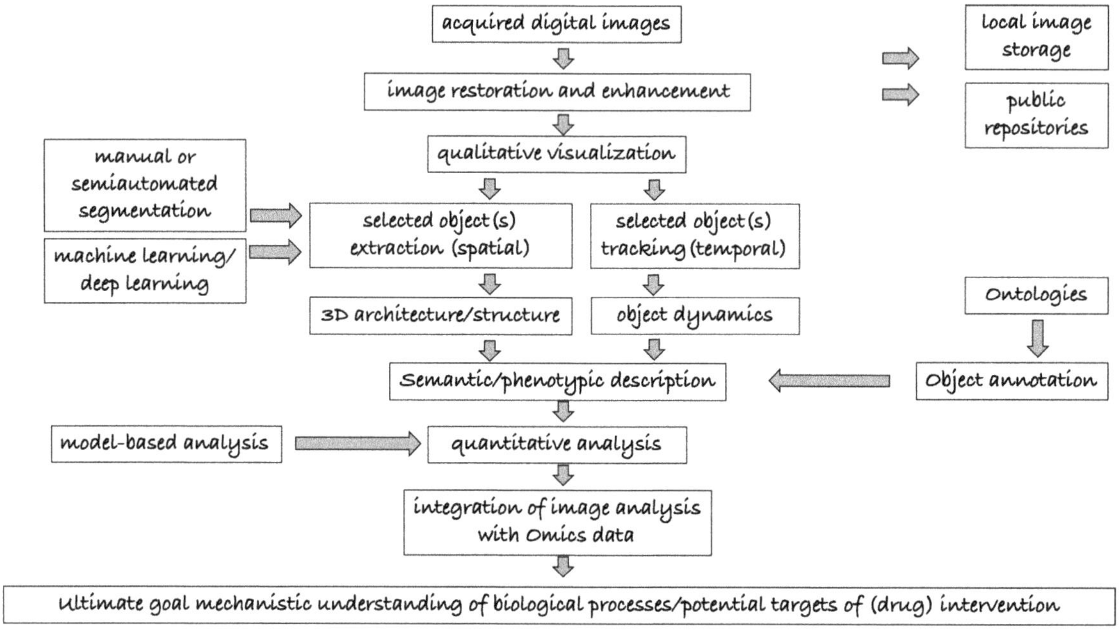

Figure 6.1 Image processing and analysis. Acquired digital images undergo image restoration and image enhancement (if necessary) before images are qualitatively visualized. Images can be stored locally for subsequent analysis, or deposited into public repositories, including all their meta-data. After an initial qualitative visualization, efforts should be made to select features of interest spatially and for video/time lapse data also to track such features temporally, either by manual or semiautomated segmentation approaches or by the use of machine learning/deep learning. Through these approaches, 3D architectures as well as object dynamics can be determined. Through defined vocabularies/ontologies and thus object annotation we will come to a semantic/phenotypic description of the scenery at hand. Using a model-based analysis and statistically rigorous quantitative analysis, as well as an integration of the analysis with omics-data, we may be able to reach the ultimate goal of a mechanistic understanding of biological processes and/or identify potential targets for drug intervention.

6.2 Characteristics of Digital Images

A digital image is a measurement of light (or other forms of radiation) signal intensity in two dimensions. It is usually depicted as a rectangular array of numbers (a matrix) with an *X*-coordinate and a *Y*-coordinate, with the maximum numbers depending on the bit depth of the image (Figure 6.2). 3D volumes consist of voxels (volume elements), and can be thought of as z-stacks of 2D images of pixels with their respective *x,y*-coordinates. Each voxel is defined by a *x,y,z*-coordinate and a density value (Figure 6.3).

At a bit depth of 1, each picture element (known as pixel) is either a 0 (black) or a 1 (white). At bit depth of 2 there would be 2^2 and thus 4 values, thus the pixels would either be black, dark gray, light gray or white. 8-bit images contain 256 values (1 black and 1 white and 254 gray values in between). 8-bit is also known as 1 byte.

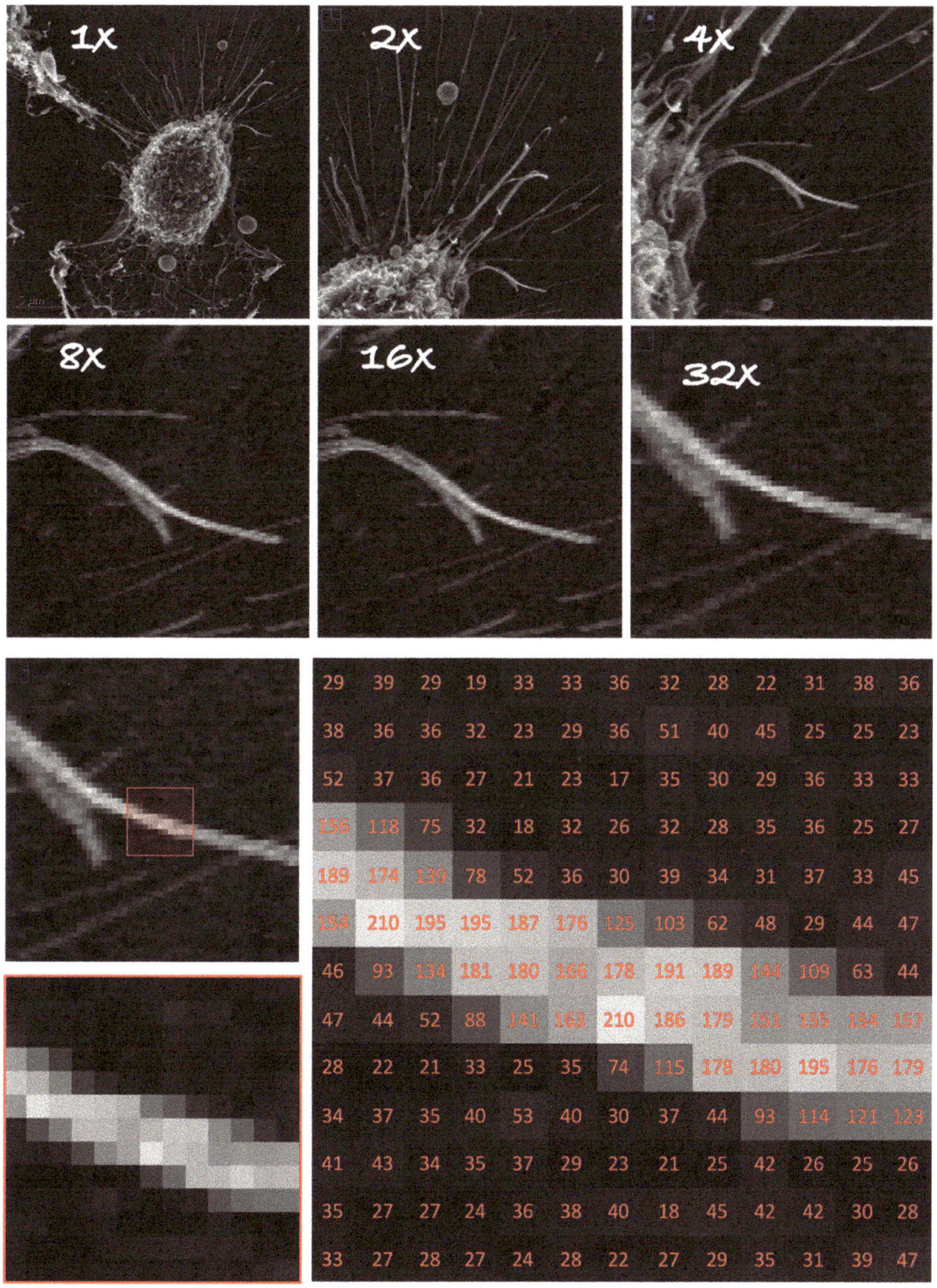

Figure 6.2 Digital image: An image is a rectangular array of pixels (picture element) with a *X,Y*-coordinate and a density value, e.g., ranging from 0 to 255 (for a 8-bit grayscale image).

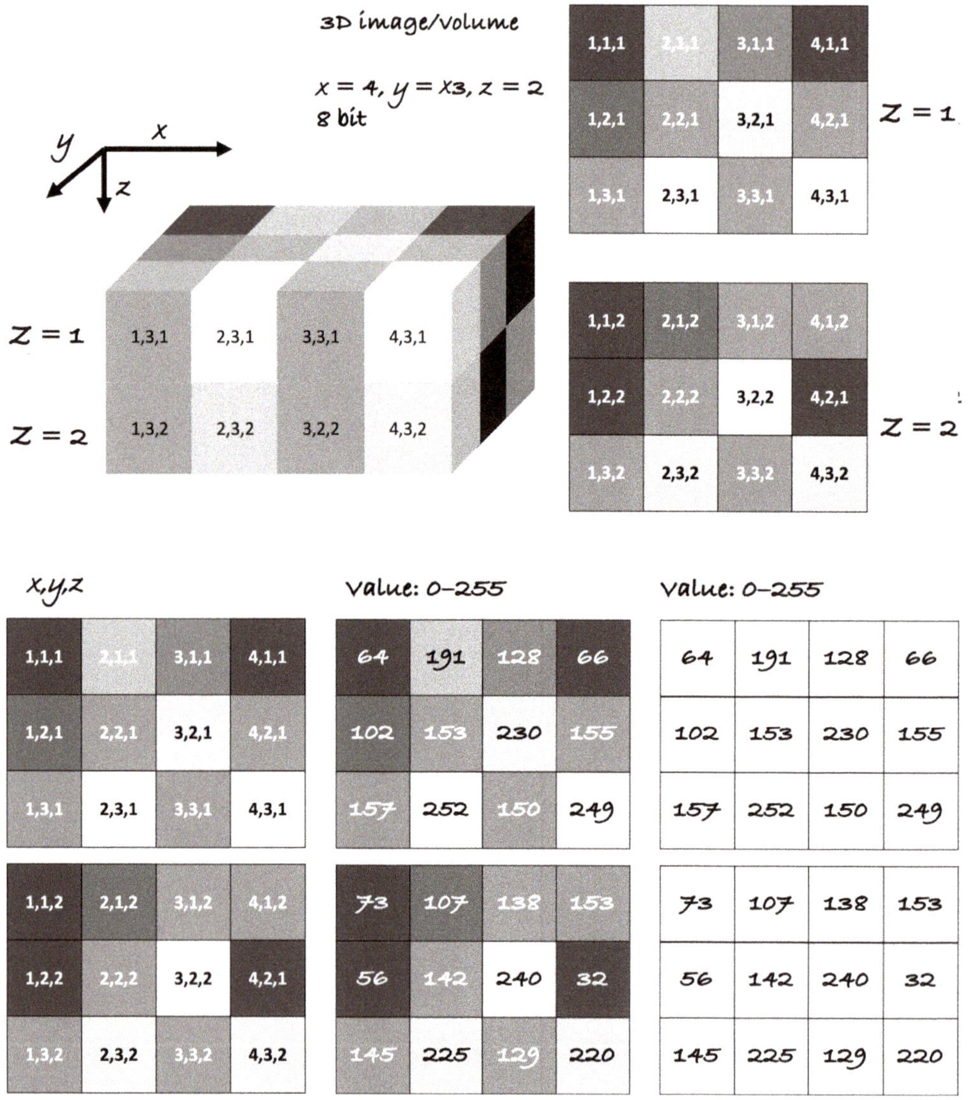

Figure 6.3 Characteristics of a 3D volume image. For three-dimensional data, the rectangular volume is defined by *X,Y,Z*-coordinates and an associated density value, in which case we speak of an individual point of the 3D volume as a voxel (volume element). Each voxel has a density value, which for 8-bit data ranges between 0 and 255.

All images with a bit depth up to 8-bit will have storage requirements of 1 byte, whereas images with a bit depth of larger than 8 bit such as 12 bits or 16 bits require 2 bytes of storage per pixel. 16-bit images offer 1 white, 1 black, and 65,534 gray values (Figure 6.4). A 2D image of 1,000 pixels by 1,000 pixels at an 8-bit dynamic range takes up 1 megabyte (MB) of storage space, at 16-bit dynamic range it takes up 2 MB. In addition, there is space needed for the header information, which is comparably small.

Header and Image Type

While an image may appear as a continuum of gray values, a digital 2D image is always a raster, divided into individual pixel (picture elements), with each pixel having its defined *X,Y* coordinate and a discrete intensity (density) value. For an 8-bit image with 256 intensity bins, this number ranges between 0 and 255. With respect to computer hard drive storage, the *X,Y* coordinate is not explicitly stored, but the file reserves for an 8-bit image 8 bits (=1 byte) for each pixel. Depending on the convention of the program used to write that file, the *X,Y* dimensions either start at 0,0 or as 1,1.

As the 2D image is stored as a one-dimensional string of numbers which could be 8-bit, 16-bit gray scale, but also 24-bit or 32-bit color image (without or with an alpha channel for transparency, respectively), there need to be clear instructions for any program trying to read the image file. Such instructions are stored in an image header that precedes the image density values (Figure 6.5).

The minimum information needed to read the image file correctly, is whether one pixel is 8-bit or 16-bit, and what

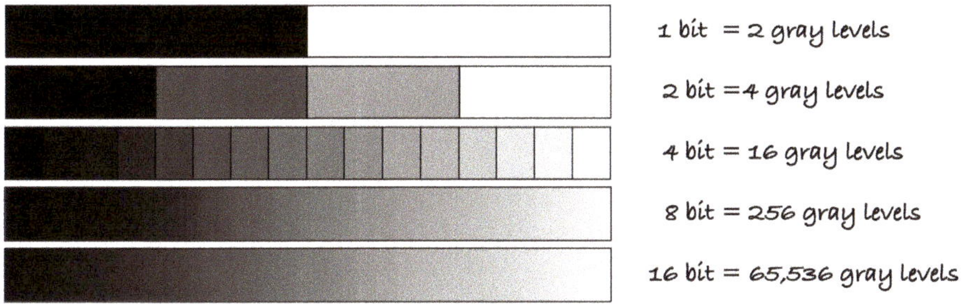

Figure 6.4 1-bit, 2-bit, 4-bit, 8-bit, 16-bit. 1-bit encoding means that the value can be either 0 or 1. At 2-bit there are four values that can be encoded. For a gray scale image at 2-bit, each pixel can be either black, dark gray, light gray, or white. At 4-bit there are 16 gray values, whereas at 8-bit there are 256 gray values, which are more shades of gray than the human eye can perceive. At 16-bit depth 65,536 different gray values can be encoded.

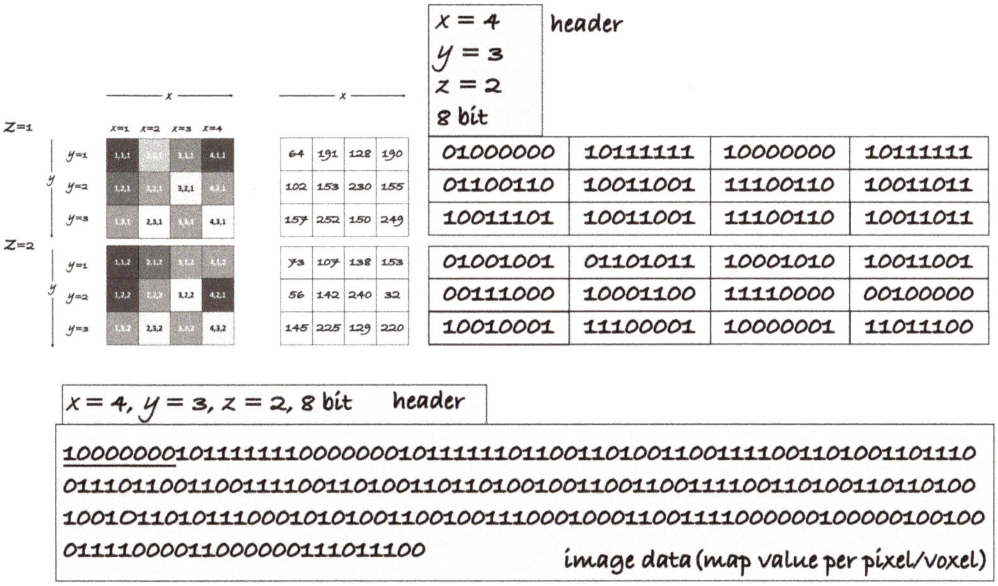

Figure 6.5 File structure including a header and a data block. An image typically consists of a header, which at the minimum contains information about the dimensions for the *X*-, *Y*-, and *Z*-coordinates, as well as number of bits that are allocated for each pixel/voxel. The data block is a continuous string of 0 and 1, which encodes a density value for each pixel/voxel.

the number of pixels in *X*, *Y* are. It is important to have a defined (standardized) header structure so that each program trying to open the image file knows what to expect and how to read and interpret the string of ones and zeros.

The image file extension tells the program, reading the image file, what type of header structure to expect. Among the additional information typically stored in an image header is which axis is considered the fast and the slow axis, whether the angles of the axes are 90° (which is true for most images recorded with an array detector/camera, but may not be true for diffraction experiments, where there could be non-orthogonal unit cells), and the size one pixel represents at the level of the specimen. Also, Fourier transforms can be displayed as images, but have an entirely different data structure (depicting complex numbers). An example for an image header is shown in Figure 6.6.

Fast, Medium, Slow Axes

When reading an image file, there is a fast, medium, and slow axis for accessing the content of a file. Pixels of the *X*-axis are stored consecutively, meaning the information for pixel 1 (0,0) and 2 (1,0) of the *X*-axis are next to one another, whereas the information of pixel one (0,0) and two (0,1) of the *Y*-axis are separated by all the other pixels of the *X*-axis before one reaches the second *Y*-axis pixel, in other words any program trying to access the information along the *Y*-axis must jump to the right position along the linear array.

Hence in 2D images the *X*-axis is referred to as the fast axis and the *Y*-axis is the slow axis for read-out. In the case of 3D data, the *X*-axis is the fast axis, the *Y*-axis is referred to as the medium axis, as the *Z*-axis is the slow axis (Figure 6.7).

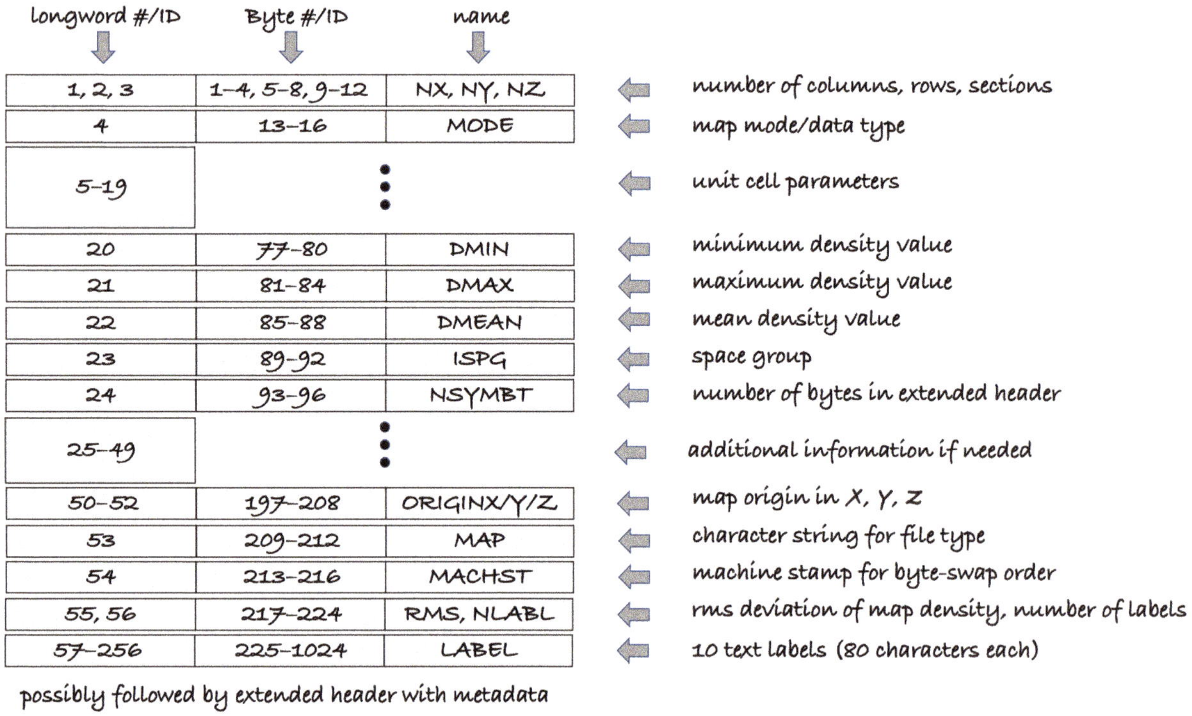

Figure 6.6 Example of an image header: MRC-format. This example of an image header provides information about the X-, Y-, and Z-dimensions of the image/map, the type of data (how many bits are allocated for each pixel and whether the data is grayscale or color), the dimension of the image, minimum, maximum and mean density values for the entire image, whether or not there in an extended header and how big such an extended header would be, the origin of the map (which is not necessarily at 0,0,0 e.g., if a smaller volume has been trimmed from a larger volume), whether the data needs to be byte-swapped or not, and other information.

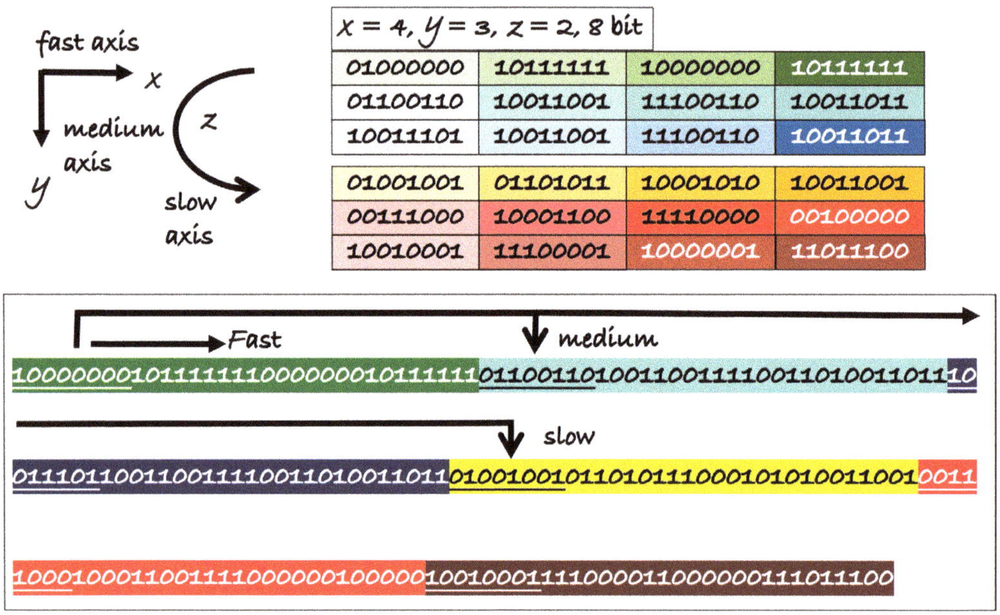

Figure 6.7 Image data block: Fast, medium, and slow axes. The fast axis in image file formats is the axis (direction) where all pixels are next to one another and can be read without needing to jump over data. For example, if one wants to read the values of the voxels in the first row of the image (in the X-direction, i.e., the green pixels), one can read the data string continuously. If one wants to read the values of the voxels only in the first column of the image (in the Y-direction), one will read the first voxel value, then jump over three voxels, before reading the second voxel, then jump again over three voxels before reading the third voxel (green to cyan to blue). This direction is called the medium axis, as there is a slower axis, namely the Z-axis. If one reads out the slow axis, one needs to jump in position from each image of the image stack to the next image in the stack (e.g., from light green to light yellow, or from cyan to red), and thus after reading the first voxel, one needs to jump over 11 voxel to come to the voxel with the same X,Y- but different Z-value.

Color Images

Color images are typically encoded (and thus stored) as 24-bit pixel data, with three independent channels (red, green, and blue) each containing 8-bit information (i.e., 256 shades for each of the red, green, or blue channels). The combination of 8-bit data in the red, green, and blue channels (RGB) results in over 16 million colors, a little more than humans can discriminate. This is also referred to as true color. Adding an alpha channel (which then results in a 32-bit image) allows transparency to be encoded in the image (Figure 6.8). Figure 6.9 shows a RGB color image, as well as pixel intensities in the red, green and blue channel.

Historically speaking, first color representations used 4 bits or 8 bits, e.g., on early Commodore 64, Macintosh, or Atari computers only certain colors were available using a color table (indexed color), later 12-bit color depth (3 channels at 4-bit color RGB depth) was used in Silicon Graphics workstations resulting in 4,096 colors. 15-bit or 16-bit color depth has been known as high color and has been used in some lower-end mobile phones.

There are different color spaces that are used to assign color to a pixel/voxel in an image, the most prominent of which is the RGB (red, green blue) and the CYMK (cyan, yellow, magenta, key/black) color spaces (Figure 6.10). The RGB system is an additive color model system and is thus well-suited for computer display. Red, green, and blue screen diodes emit light at an intensity ranging from 0 to 255. The emitted light is added up, with 0 for red, 0 for green, and 0 for blue adding up to black and 255 for red, 255 for green, and 255 for blue adding up to white.

To get a bright red color, one chooses a value of 255 for red, 0 for green and 0 for blue. If the number in the red

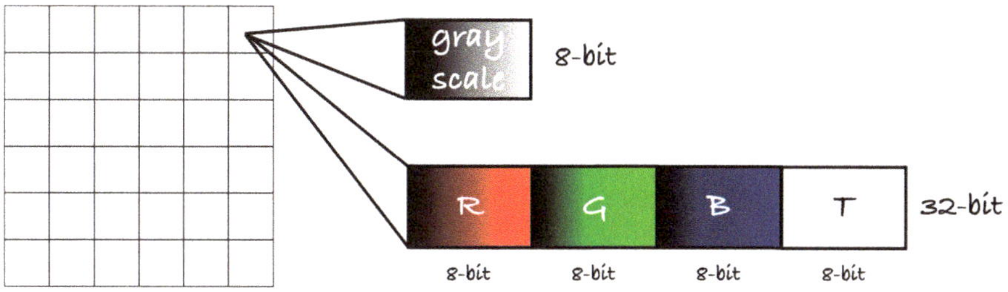

Figure 6.8 Grayscale and color raster images. Images are composed of a raster of pixels (or voxels for 3D data). Each pixel/voxel is either a gray scale image with 256 gray scales for 8-bit data or over 65,000 gray scales for 16-bit data. There are different ways color images can be encoded and stored, a prominent way is the RGB color format, which is based on the concept that computer screens can emit red, green, and blue light, and thus over 16 million colors can be created as a mixture of these three different light channels. In color images every pixel/voxel can be encoded as 24 bits, with 8 bit each being reserved for the red, green, and blue channel, respectively. If one also wants to encode transparency, one needs 32 bits per pixel/voxel.

Figure 6.9 RGB color images: Intensity of the red, green, and blue channels. A color image can be encoded as grayscale images in the red, green, and blue channels, respectively. Note that regions of red color feature prominently as white in the red channel but dark in the blue channels, whereas blue regions in the RGB original as expected are bright in the blue channel but dark in the red channel. White regions in the original RGB image feature prominently (bright) in all three channels.

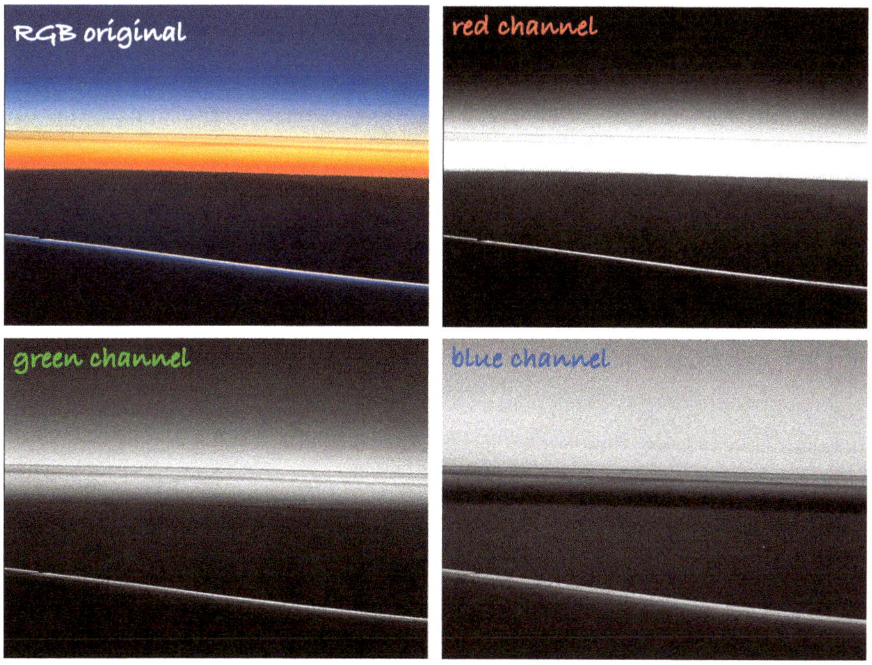

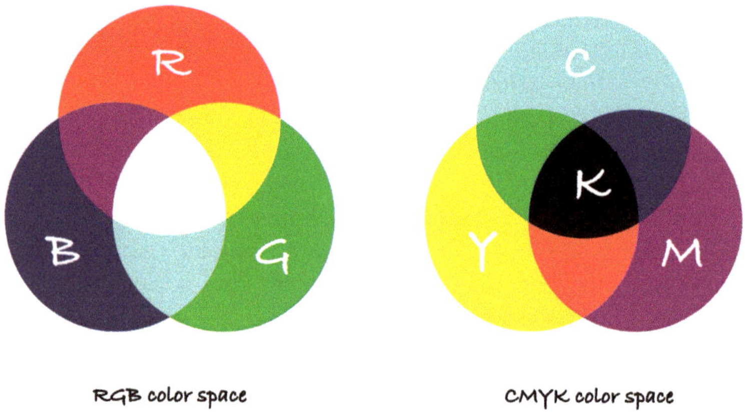

Figure 6.10 Color spaces: Additive (RGB) and subtractive (CMYK). Depending on the medium chosen (e.g., computer screen versus color print-out), there are additive or subtractive color spaces. RGB color format is a prominent example of an additive color space, whereas CMYK is a prominent example of a subtractive color space. In an additive color space, light is emitted, e.g., by diodes of different colors, and the light from the red, green, and blue channels is added up. Equal amounts of red, green, and blue light add up to white, equal amounts of red and blue (with no contribution from green) leads to magenta, whereas equal amounts of red and green (with no contribution from blue) leads to yellow, and equal amounts of green and blue (with no contribution from red) leads to cyan, as colors are added on top of one another. In a subtractive color space, a mixture of magenta and yellow yields red, whereas a mixture of magenta and cyan yields blue, and mixture of cyan and yellow yields green. A mixture of magenta, cyan, and yellow results in black. For printing purposes, the CMYK is a very important color space. To print a blue color, magenta and cyan ink are mixed in equal amount, likewise magenta and yellow yields red, and cyan and yellow yields green. Black on the other hand for printing purposes is usually not the result of mixing cyan (abbreviated as C), magenta (abbreviated as M), and yellow (abbreviated as Y) but is usually given its own color (abbreviated as K for key/black).

channel is lower than 255, the red color becomes darker. Equal amounts of red and green with 0 in the blue channel adds up to the various shades of yellow, equal numbers in all three channels (but below 255) results in gray tone.

Beside the additive RGB color space, there also exists a subtractive color model system, which is called CMYK, standing for cyan, magenta, yellow, and key (black). The CMYK is the dominant color space for printing colors on paper. Mixing magenta and yellow results in a red color, whereas a mixture of magenta and cyan yields a blue color, and mixture of cyan and yellow yields a green color.

While the combination of cyan, magenta, and yellow should be sufficient for obtaining black, black ink is used instead for black, in part to save color ink, and in part to ensure that black is truly black and not some very dark gray or brown. Halftoning is needed if one does not want the full saturation of primary colors and is accomplished by printing sparsely for each pixel only small number dots of ink onto the white paper space, hence leaving much of the white paper background empty.

Other color spaces are HSV/HSB or HSL, which defines the colors by either Hue, Saturation, Value/Hue, Saturation, Brightness or Hue, Saturation, Lightness, respectively (Figure 6.11). Yet another color space is the (Commission Internationale de L'Eclairage = International Commission on Illumination) CIE 1976 Lab color space, which is rarely used in science, but prominent in various industries (e.g., the LED light industry and in colorimetry). The CIE 1976 color space takes human perception of colors by the human eye's cone cells (i.e., their absorption spectra) into consideration.

File Formats

One of the most general (and portable) file formats is the TIFF (tagged image file format) which can exist in various forms, such as an 8-bit or 16-bit gray scale or 24-bit RGB (red, green, blue) color format. PNG (portable network graphic) is a widely portable image file format that supports grayscale and 32-bit color information (i.e., 16 million colors and a transparency alpha channel) and is an excellent alternative to the GIF format and JPEG formats, both of which have their shortcomings.

Apart from file formats that store images as a raster pixel by pixel, there are formats such as EPS and PDF that are better suited for graphics in vector space (Figure 6.12). Raster graphics files are either uncompressed or compressed with compression being either lossy or lossless.

Many microscope manufacturers have their own proprietary image data acquisition, displaying and analysis software with their respective own file formats, which are optimized for equipment and specialized analysis tasks. Such software packages often provide solutions for the quantitative analysis of multidimensional data, including metadata handling and data warehousing. One big downside

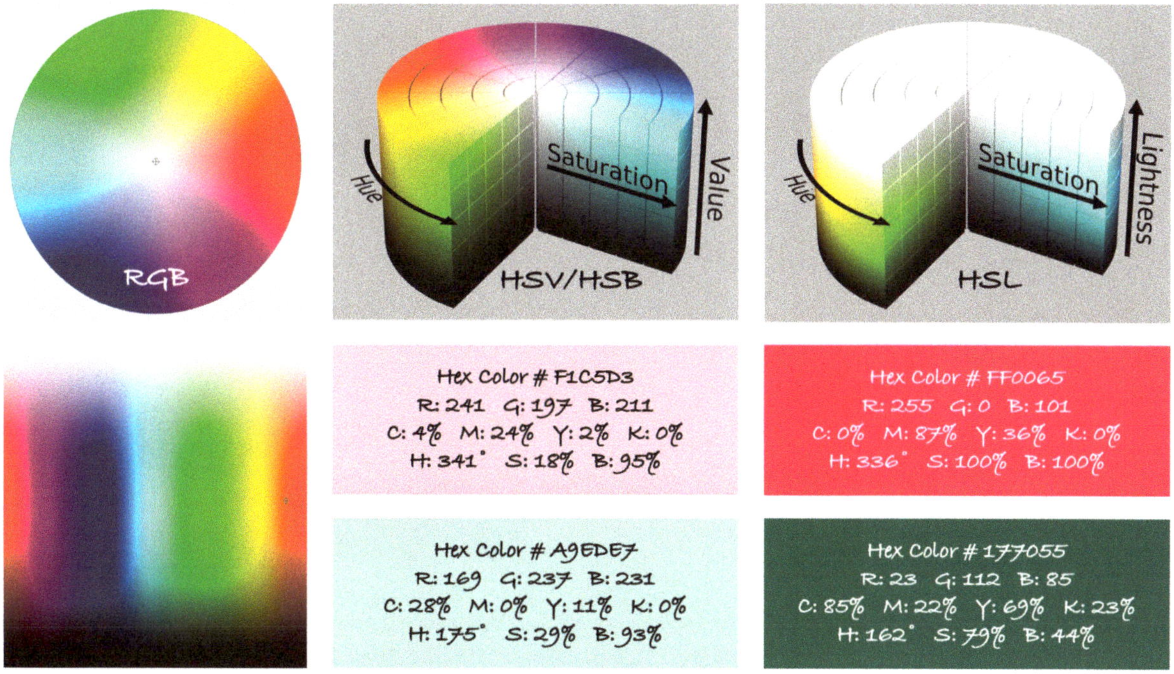
RGB
Hue
Saturation
Value
HSV/HSB
Hue
Saturation
Lightness
HSL
Hex Color # F1C5D3
R: 241 G: 197 B: 211
C: 4% M: 24% Y: 2% K: 0%
H: 341° S: 18% B: 95%
Hex Color # FF0065
R: 255 G: 0 B: 101
C: 0% M: 87% Y: 36% K: 0%
H: 336° S: 100% B: 100%
Hex Color # A9EDE7
R: 169 G: 237 B: 231
C: 28% M: 0% Y: 11% K: 0%
H: 175° S: 29% B: 93%
Hex Color # 177055
R: 23 G: 112 B: 85
C: 85% M: 22% Y: 69% K: 23%
H: 162° S: 79% B: 44%

Figure 6.11 Color spaces: RGB, HSV/HSB, HSL. Apart from the above-mentioned RGB and CMYK color spaces, there also exist alternative color spaces, such as HSV/HSB, which stands for hue, saturation, and value/hue, saturation, brightness, as well as HSL, which stands for hue, saturation, and lightness. As an example, four colors are listed with their Hex Color code. For each of the colors there is a list of the associated values in the RGB, the CMYK as well as HSB color spaces.

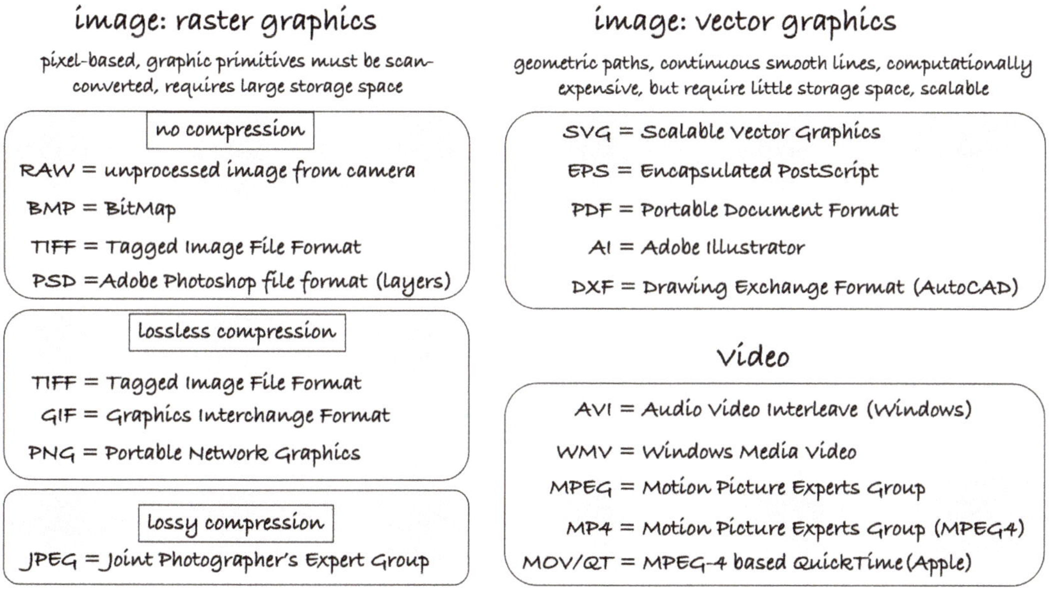

Figure 6.12 File formats: Raster graphics, vector graphics, video. The main two categories for image file formats are raster graphics and vector graphics. Raster graphics are pixel-based, thus graphic primitives (such as lines, circles, etc.) are represented as pixels (using anti-aliasing). Raster graphics (e.g., RAW, BMP, TIFF, PSD) typically have large storage space requirements. Therefore, compression schemes have been developed, some of which as lossless (TIFF, GIF, PNG) whereas others are lossy (e.g., JPEG). Vector graphics images on the other hand are based on geometrical paths, which ensure smooth lines (without the need for anti-aliasing as needed in raster graphics). Computational representation may be computationally expensive, but typically data storage is smaller than with raster graphics and it is easy to scale to larger size. Prominent examples are SVG, EPS, PDF, AI, and DXF. Video file formats, such as AVI, WMV, MPEG, MP4, and MOV or QT typically use a large amount of compression.

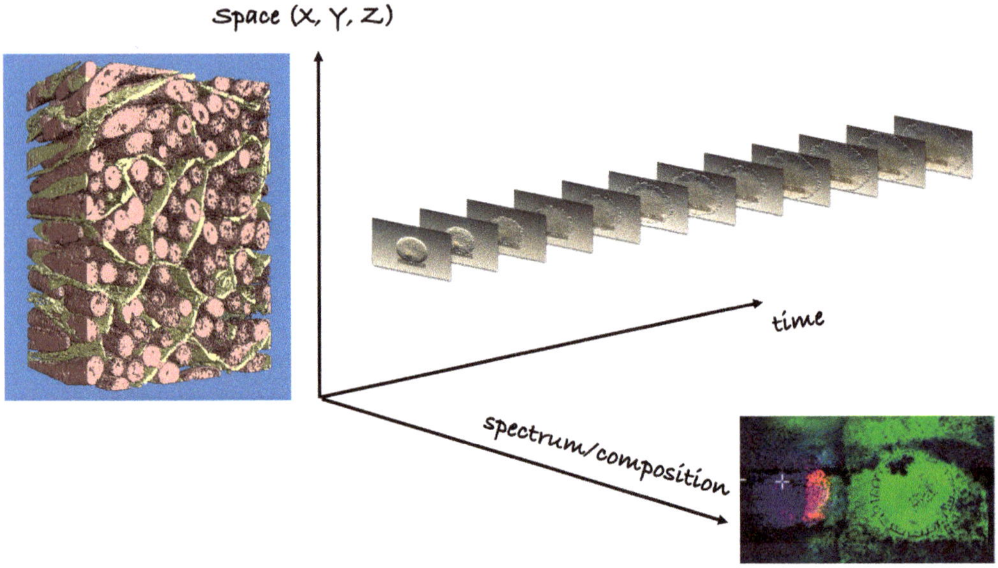

Figure 6.13 2D, 3D, 4D, and 5D images. A single image is two-dimensional, with X- and a Y-axis. For volumes we need add another (third) dimension (Z-axis). Alternatively, time or spectral information may be the third dimension if added to a two-dimensional image. If time or spectral information is added to a three-dimensional image (volume), we speak of a four-dimensional image, if volume, time and spectral information are combined, we have a five-dimensional data set.

is that to read these formats one needs to use their proprietary software; hence the format is often not easily portable. However, there exists some plugins that allow reading of such file formats by non-commercial, freely available image displaying and processing software packages such as FIJI and its predecessor program ImageJ.

3D Data and Higher-Dimensional Data

A picture traditionally has two dimensions. If one wants to store three-dimensional images, a third axis (the *Z*-axis) needs to be added. As we enter the 3D world, a pixel is referred to as a voxel (or volume element) instead of the pixel (picture element). 3D volume data is often stored as a stack of 2D-images. In principle, any series of 2D images (of the same type and dimensions) can be written into a 3D image stack, and vice versa, 3D image stacks can be written out as a series of 2D images. Often a 3D volume is at least initially inspected slice by slice, often in form of a video-loop.

Time may add another axis/dimension, and chemical signatures in terms of intensity values as a function of a spectrum (wavelength or frequency) adds yet another dimension for each single *X*,*Y*- or *X*,*Y*,*Z*-position (Figure 6.13). Chemical imaging is often also referred to as hyperspectral imaging.

6.3 Compression of Image Data

Depending on the amount of information that needs to be stored, file sizes can become quite large. With storage space always being at a premium, there are many approaches to compress image data, with some compression algorithms such as the popular JPEG (Joint Photographic Experts Group) format leading to loss of information, which is not problematic for consumer digital photography, but can be detrimental for scientific data imaging.

JPEG compression works by dividing the image into blocks of 8×8 pixels and calculating the discrete cosine transform (DCT), which then operates in the frequency space, followed by quantization of the DCT (Figure 6.14). Note the similarity of DCT to Fourier transforms, but in DCT only the real axis is considered. DCT is widely used in signal processing and is not restricted to image data.

Quantization is the process of taking a dataset, dividing its values by a matrix of numbers, rounding down to its nearest integer, and then multiplying the value again by the same certain number. Through quantization, regions with small variations in intensity values will have the same intensity value, and thus can be stored in a very efficient way, which in turn allows significant compression (Figure 6.15). The larger the numbers used in quantization, the coarser the intensity values in the histogram are being sampled, and the more compression is achieved, but also image artifacts will become more noticeable. Images compressed by lossy compression algorithms cannot be restored to their original state as some information is lost during compression.

Besides lossy compression algorithms there exist also loss-less compression algorithms (e.g., JPEG-LS), where compressed images can be restored to their original state. One way that lossless compression can be accomplished is by using previous pixels (and pixels in close proximity) to predict the value of the pixel of interest, then calculate

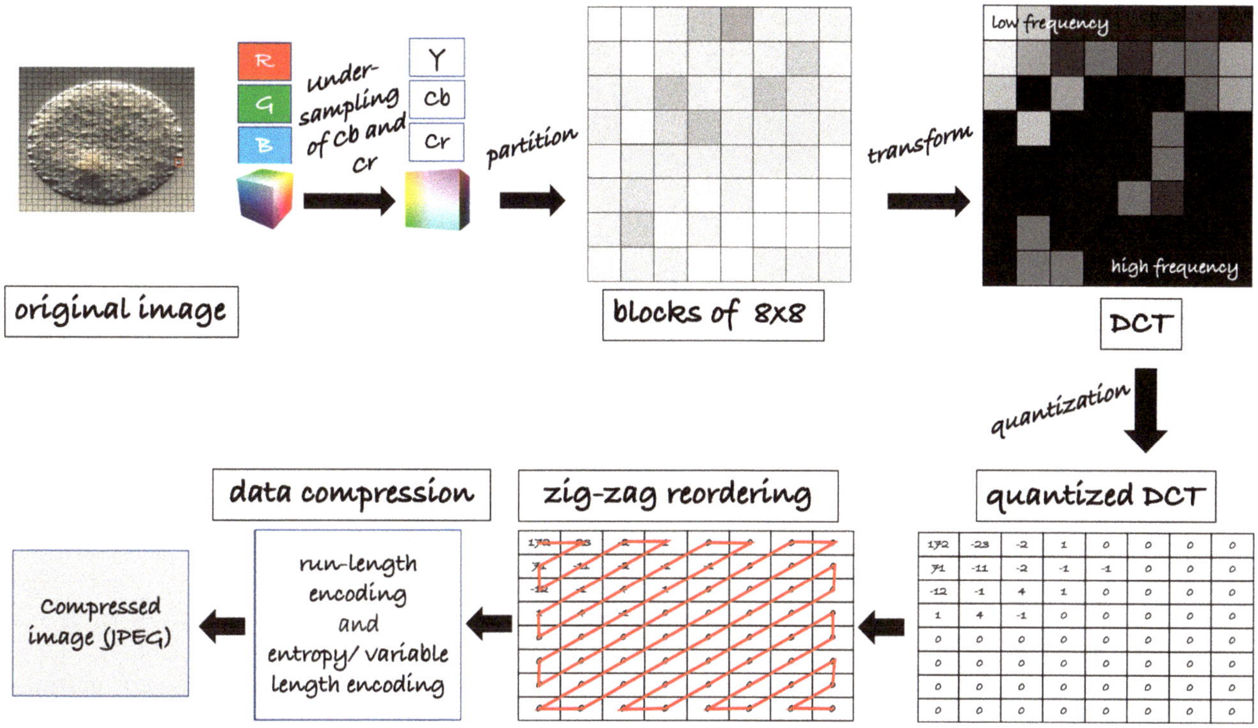

Figure 6.14 JPEG-compression of image data. The first step of JPEG compression of image data is to divide the image into blocks of 8 × 8 pixels, and to perform a discrete cosine transform (DCT) on the 8 × 8 pixel area. The resulting transform will have low- and high-frequency terms. Upon quantization of the DCT and subsequent zig-zag-reordering the data is being compressed using run-length encoding as well as entropy coding/variable length encoding, resulting in a compressed JPEG image.

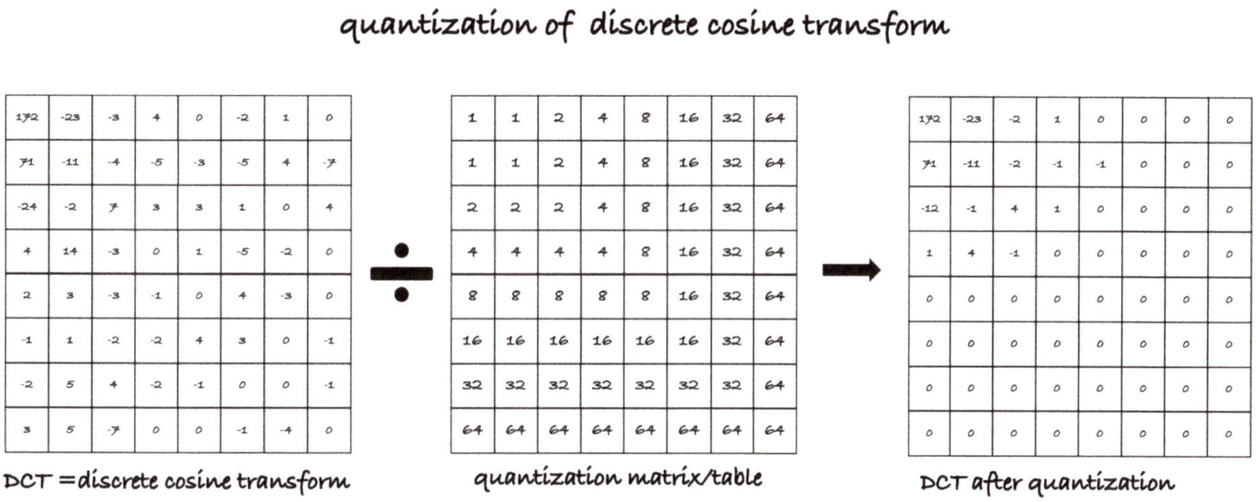

Figure 6.15 Quantization. Quantization starts with a discrete cosine transformed (DCT) 8 × 8 block of an image. The values in the DCT are divided by a quantization matrix (table), which after rounding down the nearest number leads to a quantized matrix and multiplication with the same values leads to a quantized DCT.

the error and encode the error. Assuming not much changes in an image region, one can get good prediction and thus small errors, which then through Huffman coding (one of several variable length coding strategies) can be efficiently stored, resulting in good compression without loss of information. In variable length coding, the code (how many combinations of 1 and 0 are needed for encoding a certain number) depends on the probability (fraction) of the value being found, with values at high probability needing a short code, and values at low-probability needing a longer code. Other variable length coding approaches, also known as entropy coding, are Lempel–Ziv (LZ) coding or arithmetic coding. Run length coding can be another way for compression, where one determines at which pixel a certain intensity value exists and for how many more pixels this value propagates.

Scientific images typically contain a much larger pixel-to-pixel variation of intensity than a typical landscape photograph does, thus it is advisable to stay away from lossy compression algorithm for as long as possible in scientific data processing. If there is a high level of noise, with data showing significant pixels to pixels variations (as is often the case for scientific data), there is little compression possible without compromising information. It is advisable, when planning the scientific imaging experiment, to be aware of the amount of imaging data that will be created to have sufficient space available for data storage.

Video data (images with an additional time component) poses a challenge, as storing video-rate imaging data (e.g., 30 frames per second) as a series of individual full-size images is storage-space prohibitive. Thus, video data typically requires some form of compression. Intra-frame coding exploits the spatial similarity of adjacent pixels as the basis for compression (as done in JPEG-format image compression), whereas inter-frame coding achieve compression by examining changes in the time domain. The program makes a prediction in time for each pixel and keeps track of the error (Figure 6.16).

Key frames are complete images in a video image sequence, whereas the frames in between key frames are defined by the frame-by-frame changes that occur. If there are few changes from frame to frame, one can greatly reduce the amount of information that needs to be stored, and hence the data can be significantly reduced without compromising information. A variety of video formats exist, such as MPEG (Motion Picture Experts Group), MP4, AVI, MOV, and others, all of which carry out some form of compression of the data.

6.4 Metadata

In addition to all the actual information that form the 2D (image), 3D (volume), 4D (volume and time), or even higher dimensional data sets, there is additional information that can and should be stored, such as experimental sample preparation and microscope imaging conditions, including laser settings, microscope focus settings, date- and time-stamps, to name a few. This kind of information is often referred to as metadata, and for many commercial microscopes this metadata is stored along with the actual image information, unfortunately often in file formats that are proprietary to each manufacturer (Figure 6.17).

This metadata is becoming increasingly important, particularly for data that is uploaded to imaging databases, and particularly when the goal is to allow the comparison of images that were taken at different time points, in different labs, under slightly different experimental conditions. There are a variety of solutions to the challenges of metadata capturing and data "warehousing," including the Open Microscopy Environment (OME) (www.openmicroscopy.org), to name just one.

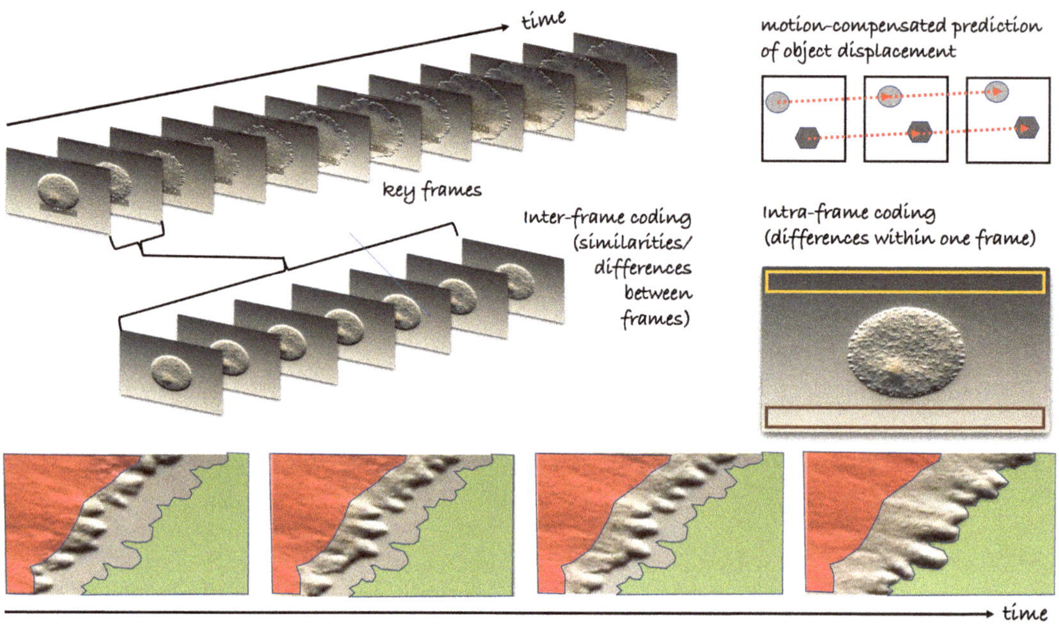

Figure 6.16 Video compression. For video compression there are different types of compression schemes, one is intra-frame coding where the content of each key frame is compressed not unlike JPEG compression for still images. If there are linear movement of objects from frame to frame, one can predict the position of the object (and thus pixel values) for future frames. One important form of video compression is the inter-frame coding, where there are key frames that act like anchoring frames, with frames in between key frames being encoded in terms of similarities and differences (changes) from frame to frame. If in a video sequence significant portions of the frame do not change, one can obtain significant size reduction. The algorithm predicts the value for each pixel and encodes the error from the prediction.

image metadata

sample:
- experimental system/setup
- details of sample preparation/processing

instrumentation and image acquisition:
- pixel image information: pixel size, channels, time points, focal planes, etc.
- microscope: modality, hardware, and configuration, including illumination and detector calibrations, mechanical stage calibrations, etc.
- data acquisition parameters

image data analysis:
- image restoration, image correction/enhancement, denoising
- segmentation/feature extraction
- quantitative analysis

Figure 6.17 Metadata. Metadata typically contain information about the sample and its preparation, about the data acquisition process, including the instrumentation and the settings used for data acquisition, and about any data processing that may have occurred such as image restoration, enhancement, etc.

6.5 Spatial, Temporal and Spectral Resolution

The maximally obtainable resolution is limited according to the Nyquist–Shannon sample theorem, with the Fourier transform of an image showing the highest resolution information near the edge of the Fourier transform. The resolution cannot be better than at least 2 times but typically more like 2.5 or 3 times the minimum sampling distance (the pixel size/dimension value). Hence, it is important to plan ahead what instrument settings are needed to obtain a desired resolution, and whether resolution should be traded for larger coverage. Higher resolution typically results in a smaller field of view and/or requires much longer data acquisition time, and thus more instrument time and larger data storage. Apart from spatial resolution, there is also temporal resolution, which defines the number of frames one can gather in a certain amount of time, as well as spectral resolution, which determines how finely the radiation spectrum (typically wavelength or frequency) can be sampled (Figure 6.18).

6.6 Image Intensity Values

6.6.1 Contrast

The contrast of an image is the difference in brightness of objects in the same image, with the maximum contrast reflecting the dynamic range of the image. The human eye

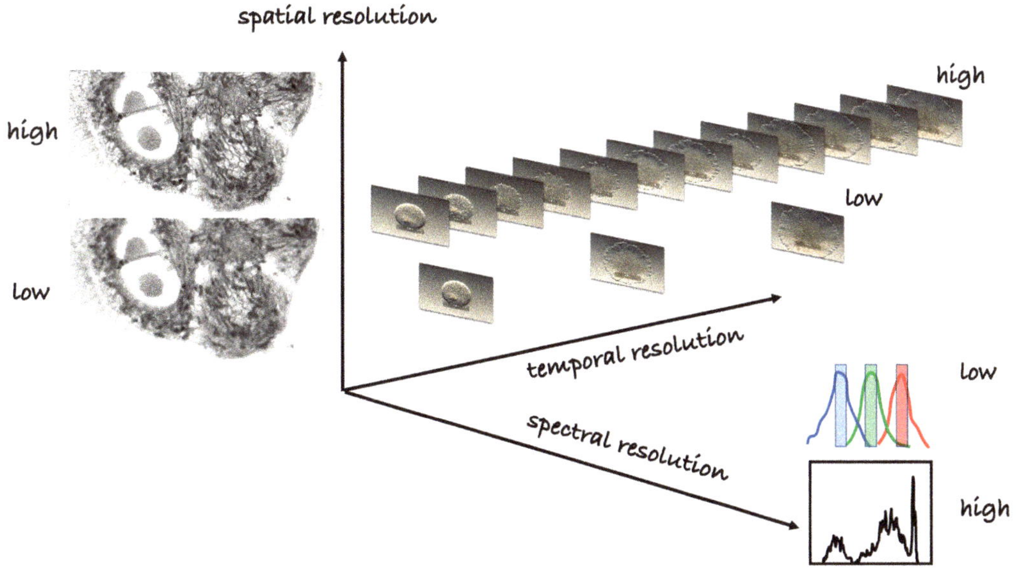

Figure 6.18 Spatial resolution, temporal resolution, spectral resolution. Spatial, temporal, and spectral resolution is the minimum increment that two objects/events can be distinguished as separate entities in space, time or in terms of their spectral characteristics, respectively.

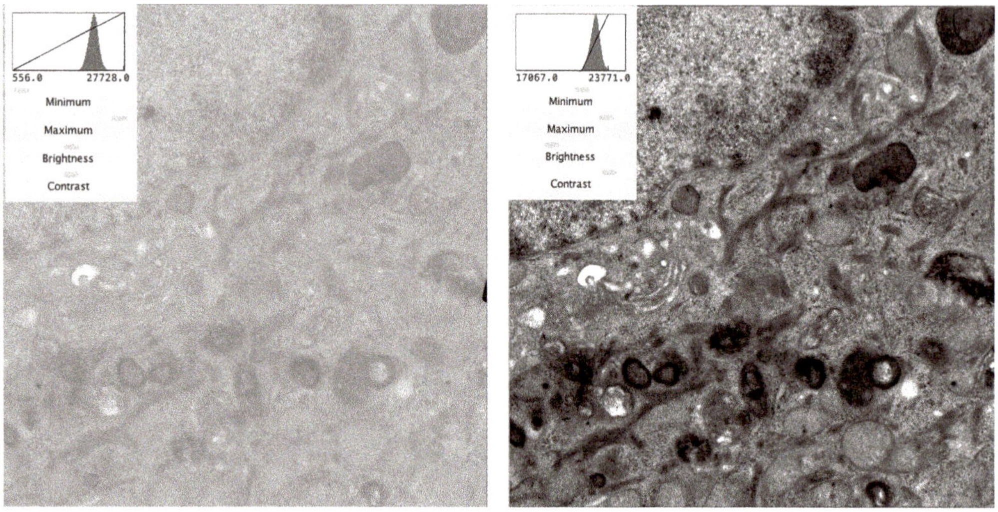

Figure 6.19 Contrast adjustment. Density values in images often do not cover the entire dynamic range but occupy only a small region of the histogram. As displays for gray values are often 8 bit, all the 27,172 values in this image (ranging from 556 to 27,728) are resorted into the 256 gray bins of the 8-bit display, which means that a little more than 100 gray values in the image are displayed as one gray value on screen. By adjusting the contrast from to 17,067 as the minimum value and 23,771 as the maximum value, the binning of image gray values to screen gray values goes from 100 to 26. As a result, more fine details can be appreciated in the contrast-adjusted image compared to image on the left.

(and brain) is much more sensitive to contrast than to the absolute brightness value. Hence, it is important to optimize contrast and use the whole dynamic range for displaying the features over the background levels (Figure 6.19). Adjustments of what should be considered the minimum and maximum value in the image are helped by histograms.

So far, we have just assumed a linear relationship in intensity scaling. However, there can be instances where one would like to emphasize certain parts of an intensity spectrum, like highlights or shadows. In such cases, one can scale data in a non-linear fashion. This is called gamma-correction, where a gamma value below one is good to brighten up dark regions of an image without losing the information in the bright regions, and a gamma value above 1 darkens the overall image without losing the information in the high intensity range.

6.6.2 Histogram

A histogram is diagram that lists the number of pixels (*Y*-axis) for each gray value (*X*-axis). Histograms can be useful to see in which intensity range the relevant image information lies. For example, there may be a large amount of bright or dark regions in a 16-bit image, which are irrelevant to our biological imaging goal, with the actual relevant information being a rather narrow peak of gray values. Since gray scale values in computer monitors typically come in 8 bit, therefore, it may be very useful to rescale the image by trimming intensity regions with no relevant information, and instead allocate the full 8 bit of the monitor to the actual gray scale value range of our features of interest. Setting the minimum and maximum to the lower end and higher end of the relevant data distribution results in higher image contrast.

This histogram-based minimum/maximum setting approach is most useful (and essential) when the original data being 16-bit is converted to 8-bit, as otherwise many different grayscale values in 16-bit would be placed the exact same bin of an 8-bit image. Most importantly, without setting the minimum and maximum correctly, upon conversion from a 16-bit to an 8-bit image, subtle intensity differences and thus information may be lost. Let us assume a 16-bit image, where the microscope camera captured image intensities for our features of interest ranging from ~8,000 to ~9,000, hence there are ~1,000 different intensity values captured. The histogram of such a 16-bit image would likely look like a Gaussian distribution of intensity values, centered around the gray value ~8,500, with a width on either side of ~500. There would likely be very few intensity values from 0 to ~8,000 or from ~9,000 to 65,535. If one now simply takes the entire dynamic range of the 16-bit data (65,536 bins) and converted that into an 8-bit data format, those 1,000 different gray values would now be put into 4 or 5 out of the 256 gray scale bins available in 8 bit. All the data would reside in bin number 31 through 35 or 36, with bin number 1–30 and 37–255 being empty. Setting the minimum and maximum to 8,000 and 9,000 would mean that 1,000 gray values are now stored as 256 gray scale values (Figure 6.20). Often, we may even find that the relevant information for the objects of interest may even lie in a narrower range, in which case there is even less or no loss.

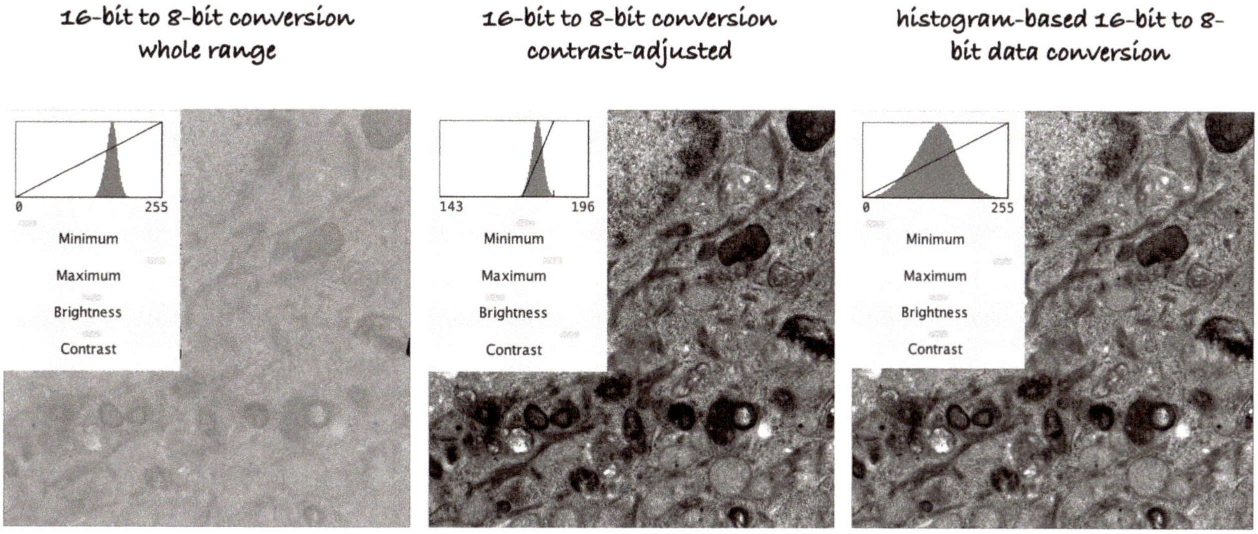

Figure 6.20 Histogram-based 16-bit to 8-bit conversion. The entire 16-bit imaging data shown on an 8-bit screen results in images with little contrast (left). Adjustment of contrast of the 16-bit image results in a much higher contrast with many features being now appreciated that were not visible before (middle). 16-bit to 8-bit file format conversion of the image leads to a high contrast image at 8-bit (right).

Histogram equalization and histogram matching are not just for display purposes but can also be used for intensity transformation with the goal of comparing images taken under different (lighting) conditions by making the images more similar to one another. It can also be used for non-uniform illumination correction. Histograms can also play a prominent role in image segmentation, with different regions of the histogram possibly depicting different features in an image. Histogram-based segmentation is often used in combination with other criteria for distinguishing features of interest.

6.6.3 False-Color Representation and Lookup Tables

Since the grayscale dynamic range of a computer screen is typically 8-bit, it can display 256 gray scale values, which is more than a regular human being can discriminate. To appreciate subtle intensity differences, it can be advantageous to display the grayscale data as colors, since the human eye can distinguish many more colors than grayscales. Hence, different gray values can be assigned different colors by lookup tables (LUT). LUT do not alter the data in any way, they simply can be helpful for display of subtle differences (Figure 6.21).

Such false-color representation of grayscale data can also be used to identify different objects in an image, but if it is not solely based on intensity differences, it may indicate that some manual or semiautomated segmentation (and thus interpretation/annotation) has been performed. In such cases colors do not represent intensity differences but simply allow one to allocate different colors to different objects.

6.7 Raster Graphics Versus Vector Graphics

It should be pointed out that an image does not necessarily be stored as an array of pixels, as a matter of fact, if image content is created based on geometrical objects (such as by various presentation software packages), an image may not be stored as a pixel-by-pixel X,Y representation but as geometric objects with an origin, type of object (e.g., circle, square, triangle), as well as the respective parameters such as radius, length dimensions, angles, etc. Of course, one may argue that such drawings do not constitute true images, however it seems prudent to be aware of vector-space representations, as they will become important when discussing geometric/volumetric model building. It might be worth mentioning that vector-based images often require substantially (several orders of magnitude) less storage space, as a simple instruction about the center, radius and line thickness, e.g., of a circle is all that is needed in vector-based imaging, whereas pixel-based imaging would require all pixels in an image with their appropriate grayscale or color values.

There are many software packages that will accept both data types (pixel-based and vector-based) side-by-side. Note that a circle in a vector-based program is described by its origin and its radius, whereas in a pixel-based data format, a circle is approximated as a pixelated object with lighter and darker values. This attempt to make the object

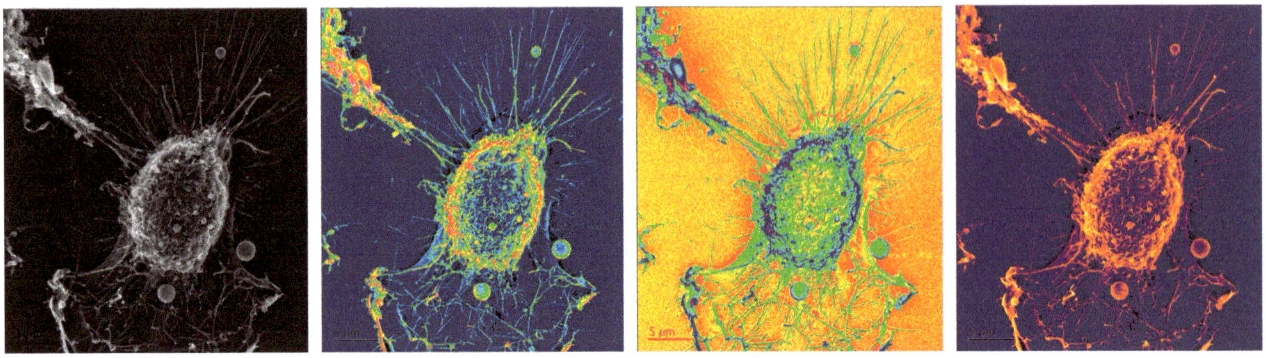

Figure 6.21 False color representation, look-up tables (LUT). 8-bit screens can display 256 different levels of gray. However, humans can discriminate far fewer shades of gray, whereas they can perceive and distinguish many more colors. Using various predefined lookup tables one can false-color-code gray-scale images and thus emphasize different parts of an image.

such as a circle appear round by different forms of shading is called anti-aliasing. Anti-aliasing is not easily recognized if the image (and the display) is at sufficiently high resolution, and hence one may not realize the difference between a pixel-based and vector-based images. But as one zooms in to the point where individual pixels in the image can be distinguished, the difference becomes obvious (Figure 6.22).

Note that pixel-based images rotations in X,Y require a resampling of the image data, which changes the grayscale values for each pixel, hence the details of our features of interest may be slightly altered due to resampling. Resampling of the image at a finer grain (hence larger image size) prior to rotation might help in retaining important spatial information, but one cannot completely avoid changing the features upon rotating the sample. Hence it may be advisable to analyze quantitatively the image in its unrotated state, and only rotate later for presentation purposes. Vector-based objects on the other hand can be rotated without any loss in resolution.

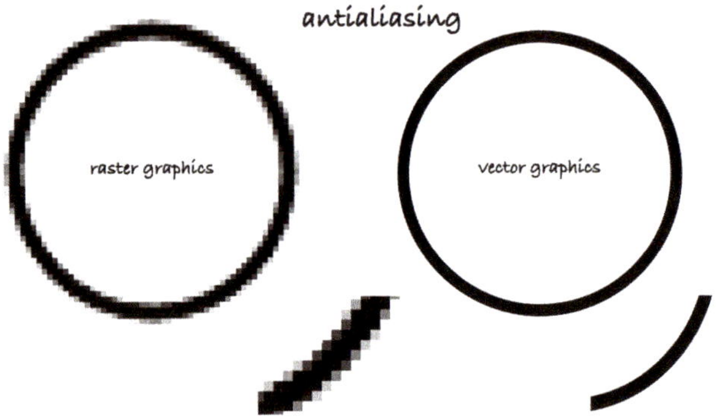

Figure 6.22 Pixel-based raster image versus vector-graphics and anti-aliasing. If a geometrical object such as a circle is drawn and displayed at high magnification (and insufficient resolution), the curvature of the circle is no longer visible as a smooth object with sharp boundaries (left) unlike it is the case in vector graphics (right). Anti-aliasing is used to smooth out the boundary between the object and its background. Note that computer screens are always raster images with individual pixels, even when they display vector graphics. Vector graphics is easy to scale, whereas scaling of raster graphics always requires interpolation.

6.8 Simple Image Processing Operations

Resizing Images and Binning

Resizing an image means either making the image smaller or bigger. In the former case adjacent pixels need to be averaged to create a new pixel, whereas making the image bigger just magnifies the area that one pixel occupied. It does not create more detail, which is why one often speaks of empty magnification in an enlarged image. Practically there is some interpolation going on, to ensure that the object does not appear obviously pixelated and clunky, yet the information content in the image is certainly not going up, which is why starting with a sufficiently large image size is important. Binning by a factor of 2 is frequently done in microscopy, in part to save space, but also to reduce noise, given that image features in adjacent pixels usually are not completely independent from one another, whereas noise may vary in individual pixels, and thus noise may average out upon binning (Figure 6.23).

Cropping

It is often useful to crop the image to an area or 3D image volume to a subvolume, which contains the features of interest but no unnecessary surrounding areas/volumes. Note that once the data is cropped it is not possible to go back, so always keep the original larger image stored. Cropping should always be carried out only after rotation of an image, as rotation of cropped images may result in blank corner areas of the rotated image.

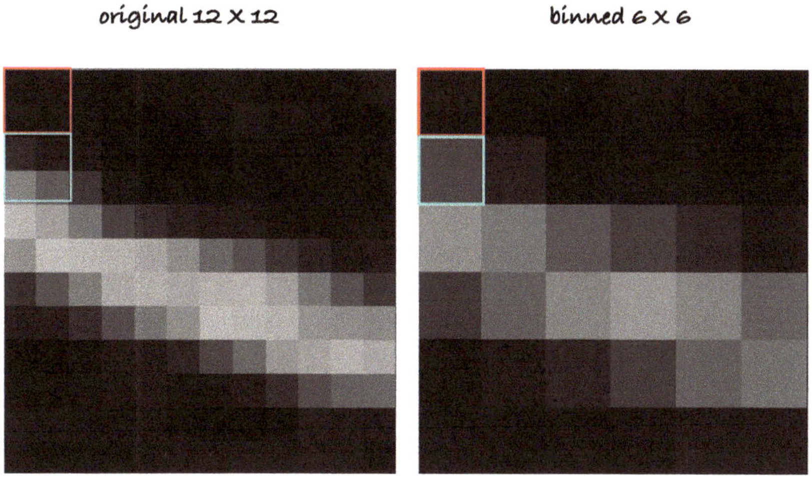

Figure 6.23 Resizing images and binning. When resizing images, one needs to calculate each pixel value. When binning, adjacent pixels are combined and the individual pixel value for each of the four smaller pixels is averaged into one number for a now larger pixel. Near boundaries where there are significant variations in value between these four pixels, the change in value for the new pixel can be quite significant (cyan box), whereas regions that were homogeneous show little change upon binning. For these reasons, binning can also be viewed as form of smoothing and noise reduction, but note that once the data is binned, one no longer can get back the original image at higher resolution.

Contrast Inversion

Inverting image contrast can be helpful, e.g., for visualization purposes. Our history with black-and-white photography has taught us that the exposure of the photographic emulsion by photons leads to silver grains, and thus a darkening of that image area in what we call a film negative. However, we associate the presence of photons with brightness, which is why in the photographic process, we create a positive print by exposing the negative again to light. In traditional transmission electron microscopy of heavy metal-stained samples, the stain (which represents a feature) prevents electrons to penetrate, which in a film negative would stay light, whereas regions where the electrons would penetrate without obstruction would appear dark on the negative. However, since we associate stain as being dark, we create a print with inverted contrast, with dark being a feature and light being background (Figure 6.24).

However, as cameras count electrons hitting the camera, a signal is usually bright over a dark (non-irradiated) background, which in our experience then looks more like a photographic negative. So, while processing and analysis should be carried out on the original contrast image, visual inspection may require contrast inversion to appear more familiar to us. Some visualization programs will allow (or by default will do) the contrast inversion, but one should

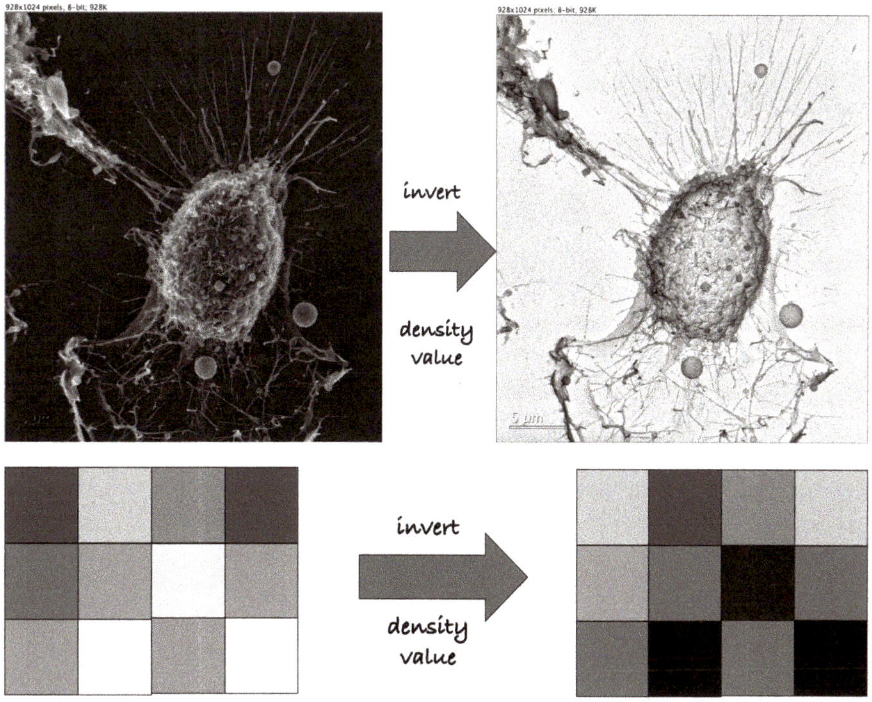

Figure 6.24 Contrast inversion. Contrast in a scanning electron micrograph of a cancer cell (left) is inverted by turning all dark density values into light values and vice versa. The contrast-inverted cell (right) looks more familiar to us.

always make sure to understand which portion of intensity distribution is signal and which one is background, which is not always so obvious. Paying attention to whether a biological membrane or a gold fiducial (in the case of electron tomography) appear dark or light in the image can help in interpreting the data. Note that different programs will display the data in a different way, so always make sure to understand whether the signal is bright on a dark background or vice versa.

Good Practices

It should be clear by now that the exact same data can be viewed and presented in different ways, and thus it is important to disclose any kind of changes being done to the original image, particularly non-linear (e.g., gamma) corrections. Brightness and contrast adjustments are usually acceptable, if they are applied to the whole image and do not suppress or eliminate any background signals. It would seem self-evident that cutting and pasting of regions within an image (such as eliminating or adding, e.g., individual cells) is never justified. One might argue that it is always good practice, when presenting data, to provide an overview image at low resolution to provide some sense of coverage as well as possible spatial relationships of regions (clustering of certain phenotypes or lack of phenotypes in certain parts of the image) along with selected examples at higher resolution, with these examples being representative and not simply a "best-of" selection that closest matches expectations or a desired outcome. Whatever adjustments are made to the images, make sure that the experiment and control data are treated the exact same way.

6.9 Image Restoration

A visual inspection of the image data is always a first step to evaluate the data and to detect possible artifacts or imperfections. While many arithmetic operations such as density inversion, resizing, and rotation of images are carried out on a pixel-by-pixel basis, many techniques described in this section take into consideration the immediate surrounding of individual pixels. Thus, each pixel is re-evaluated in the context of its surrounding environment.

The goal of image restoration is to correct for the degradation of the image due to instrumentation, detection- and sampling-imperfections. One example is the removal of vertical or horizontal stripes with a different contrast from its surroundings. Such de-striping may be necessary for Focused Ion Beam Scanning Electron Microscopy data sets. Histogram equalization may be used for contrast adjustments, e.g., in the case of non-uniform illumination correction.

Deblurring

A frequently found degradation function of images is the blurring of features in an image, where the image is convoluted with specimen movement during data collection This can be corrected for separating the motion component and multiplying the images and the motion correction in Fourier space. Wiener filtering is a frequently used approach, with the main idea being that Wiener filters minimize the mean square errors between the reconstructed and the original image.

Histogram-Based Data Scaling

With respect to image enhancement, histograms can be used for optimizing the relevant image information and ignore irrelevant information, e.g., by setting minimum and maximum values to fully utilize the entire 8 bit for image processing, or for emphasizing brighter or darker regions in the image, e.g., through gamma-correction. Furthermore, histogram normalization can be used for comparing images taken under different imaging conditions, which can be very useful for transmission electron microscopy serial sectioning imaging to name just one example.

Non-uniform Illumination Correction

The first step in image restoration may be to correct for imperfections in the data collection, e.g., due to illumination or detector imperfections. For example, if illumination was non-uniform, meaning that the image is overall brighter in center than at the periphery or there is a linear gradient in the image, one might want to apply shading correction (Figure 6.25), e.g., by recording a blank image under the exact same condition and then subtracting it from the current image. Variations in brightness may also occur when image montages are tiled together from smaller images. Also, cameras may have a non-zero offset or there may be a non-specific background signal, e.g., due to autofluorescence. Histogram equalization can be a powerful tool for such corrections.

6.10 Image Enhancement

Image enhancement prepares the image for analysis, e.g., by optimizing the relevant information content of the images. Image enhancement may include applying filters to the image for smoothing, denoising, sharpening, or to detect and preserve edges. Denoising can be carried out in the frequency domain (Fourier space), such as in a low-pass filter or in the spatial domain (real space), where a filter kernel with defined shape and size is swept pixel-by-pixel over the image in a process often referred to as convolution. It should be pointed out however that filters change

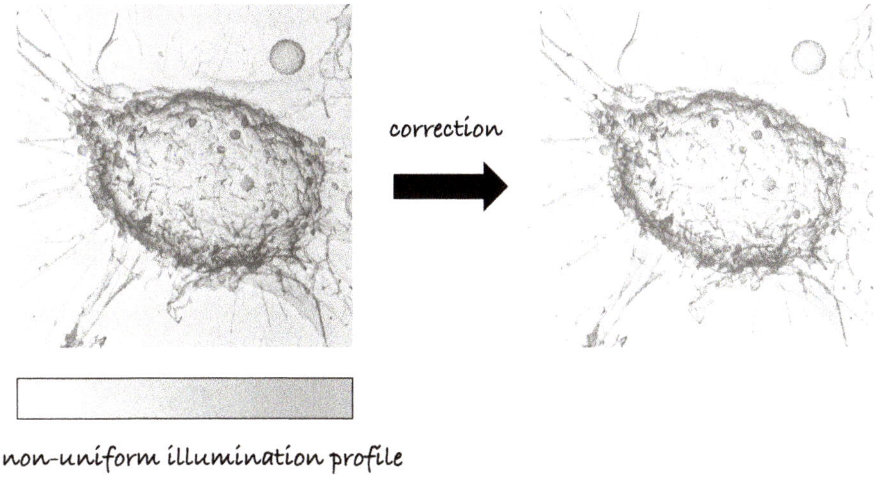

Figure 6.25 Non-uniform illumination correction. Non-uniform illumination correction is an image restoration technique that determines a non-uniform illumination profile and corrects the image accordingly.

the density map, and when applying multiple filters, it may be important to pay attention to the order in which the filters have been applied as applying the same filters in a reverse order may lead to a different result.

Smoothing Filters for Noise Reduction

Noise reduction is a common goal in image enhancement, as it improves the signal-to-noise ratio of the data, and often is essential for adequate visualization and subsequent segmentation results.

There are different types of noise, including Gaussian noise, Raleigh noise, gamma noise, exponential noise, uniform noise, and impulse noise. While Gaussian noise is rarely found in actual real images, the Gaussian noise model is widely used, in part because from a mathematic point it can be dealt with easily, and it often serves as a good model for other types of real noise.

Noise may not only arise from the instruments used for data acquisition, but also can be introduced during image processing steps, such as quantization and predictive coding noise, both of which may arise in data compression. So-called salt and pepper noise (referring to pixels that are either white or black, hence called salt and pepper, respectively) are classical examples of faulty pixel response in detectors. Histogram analysis may hint what kind of noise the image is suffering from, when focusing on small homogeneous image regions.

There are noise removal methods which rely on local neighborhood operations where a kernel (a 3×3 or 5×5 matrix with appropriate weights) is convoluted with each pixel in the data. There is also "non-local means" denoising, which averages pixel intensities from pixels that reside in different parts of the image but face a similar local neighborhood intensity distribution.

There are many noise reduction filters available, each with their own advantages and disadvantages, including lowpass filter, Gaussian filter, maximum, minimum or mean filters, median filter, non-local means filter, wavelet filter, non-linear anisotropic diffusion (NAD) filter, bilateral filter, and other filters. While all these filters will suppress noise, their performance for feature preservation can be very different, hence it may be valuable to explore multiple filters in parallel, and carefully evaluate the smoothing result (Figure 6.26).

Filtering in Fourier Space: Bandpass Filter

Lowpass filtering cuts off high resolution signal variation, as one assumes noise to affect individual pixels and thus high-resolution signals. Filtering in Fourier space allows to restrict the data to the lower-resolution shells, which means that high-resolution noise is filtered out, however, any high-resolution data will also be eliminated (Figure 6.27).

Filtering in Real Space: Gaussian Filter

In Gaussian noise removal, each pixel is changed from its original value by a small amount by using kernels that resemble a Gaussian distribution (Figure 6.28). Gaussian filtering will blur the information, and thus may not be the first choice, but Gaussian filtering is computationally much cheaper than more sophisticated approaches such as non-linear anisotropic diffusion (NAD). A Gaussian filter is similar to a mean filter but offers gentler smoothing while at the same time better preserving the edges of a feature. Gaussian smoothing is often used prior to edge detection, which is very sensitive to noise.

Filtering in Real Space: Maximum, Minimum, and Mean Filters

In the maximum, minimum, and mean filters, a pixel value is replaced by either the maximum, minimum, or mean value of its neighboring pixels, respectively (Figure 6.29). These approaches are designed to smooth

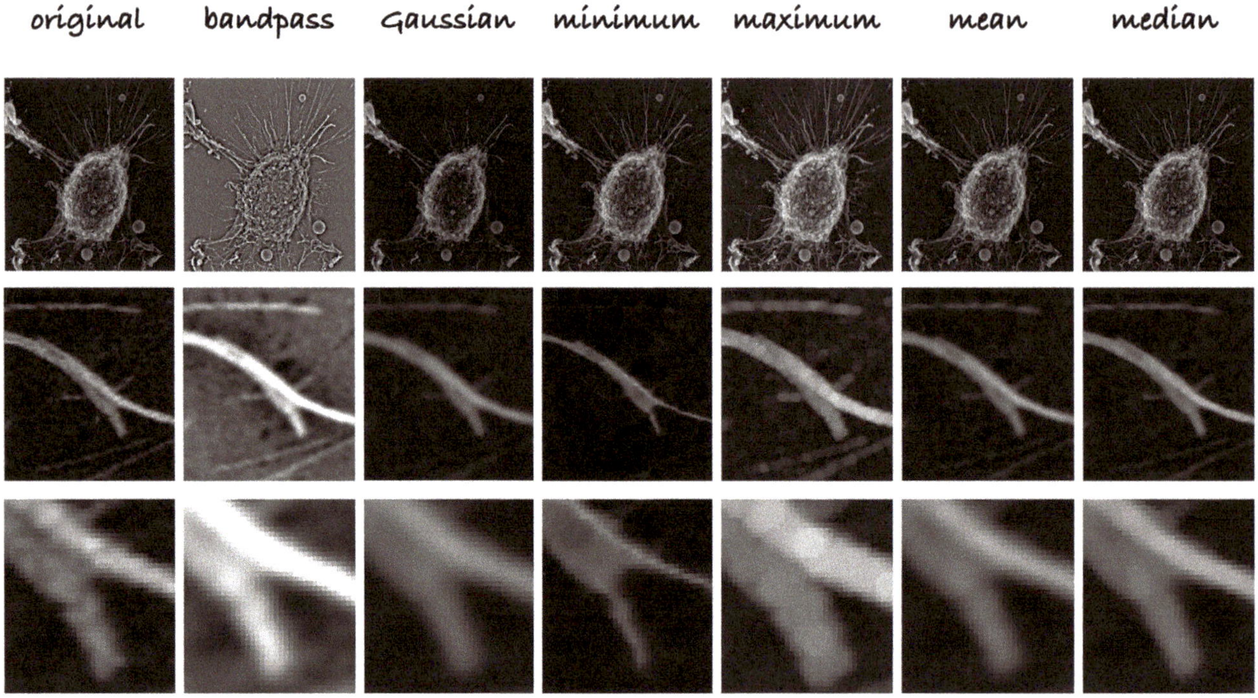

Figure 6.26 Noise reduction – Smoothing filters. Top row shows the entire image of a cancer cell as recorded by scanning electron microscopy. Middle row shows a protrusion from the cell at intermediate magnification where the overall organization of the feature can be appreciated. The bottom row further zooms into the feature and shows a small portion at the level of individual pixels. The effect of different filters for noise reduction can be seen, with the original image being shown as the first column, followed by bandpass-, Gaussian-, minimum-, maximum-, mean-, and median-filtered images. Note how much a simple feature such as these filamentous protrusions can be altered by application of these smoothing filters.

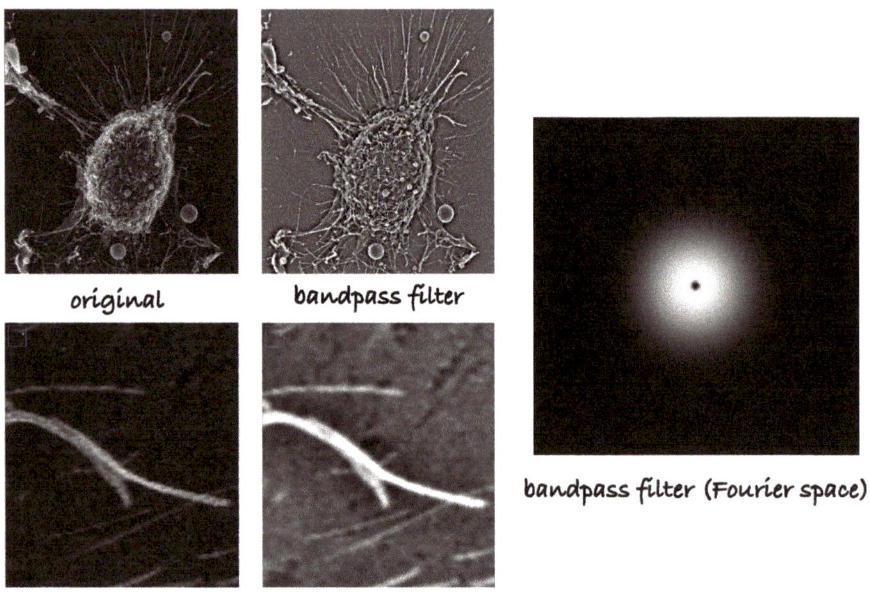

Figure 6.27 Noise reduction in Fourier space – Bandpass filter. Bandpass filtering occurs in Fourier space, where high frequencies are cut off, and lower frequencies are emphasized. The rationale behind this approach is that local pixel to pixel variations of density represents noise, whereas densities belonging to the same object will be more similar to one another and form an underlying (low frequency) structural feature.

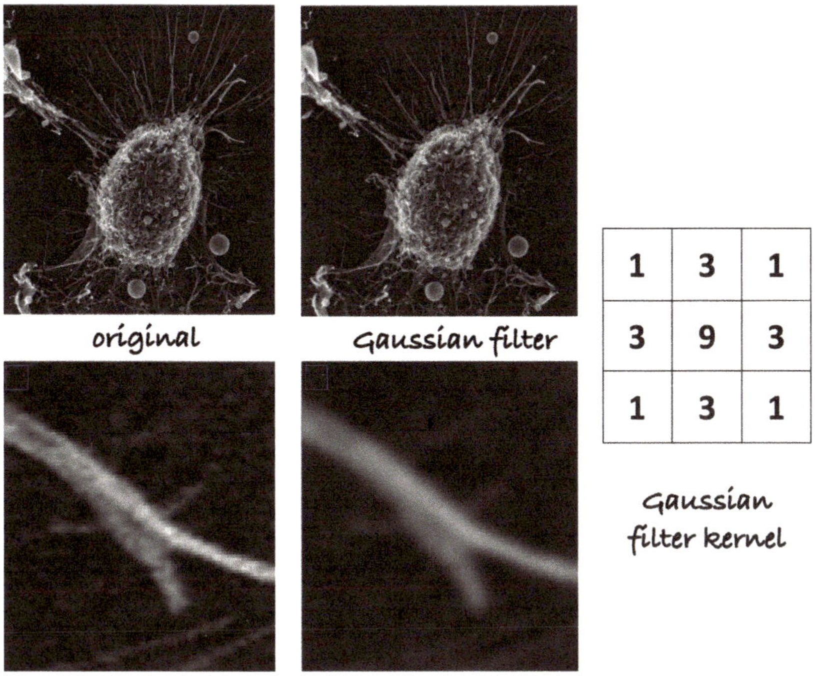

Figure 6.28 Noise reduction in real space – Gaussian filter. Applying a Gaussian filter kernel (the kernel resembles a Gaussian distribution) results in the local smoothing (blurring) of the image data. However, Gaussian filtering is computationally cheap and can be very useful to apply prior to edge detection which is very sensitive to noise.

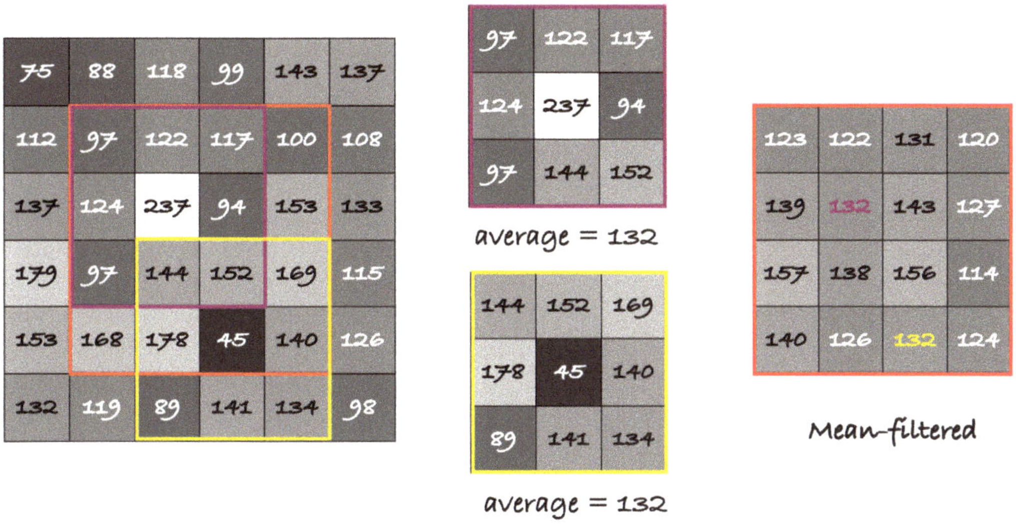

Figure 6.29 Noise reduction in real space – Mean filter. When applying the mean filter, the pixel of interest is replaced by the average of its immediate neighboring pixel environment, resulting in the elimination of salt and pepper noise (individual very bright and very dark pixel outliers).

out non-representative pixels, and thus reduce pepper noise (Maximum filter) or salt noise (Minimum filter). However, while the non-representative pixels will be smoothened out this way, the value if its neighboring pixels will be significantly affected, a problem also encountered near feature edges where there is a sudden jump in image pixel value.

Filtering in Real Space: Median Filter

Salt and pepper noise is effectively reduced by median filtering, which corrects individual pixels that are either way too bright (salt) or dark (pepper) compared to their surroundings. Median filtering rejects outliers and replaces with the expected values without blurring the image in a significant manner. The median filter is similar to the

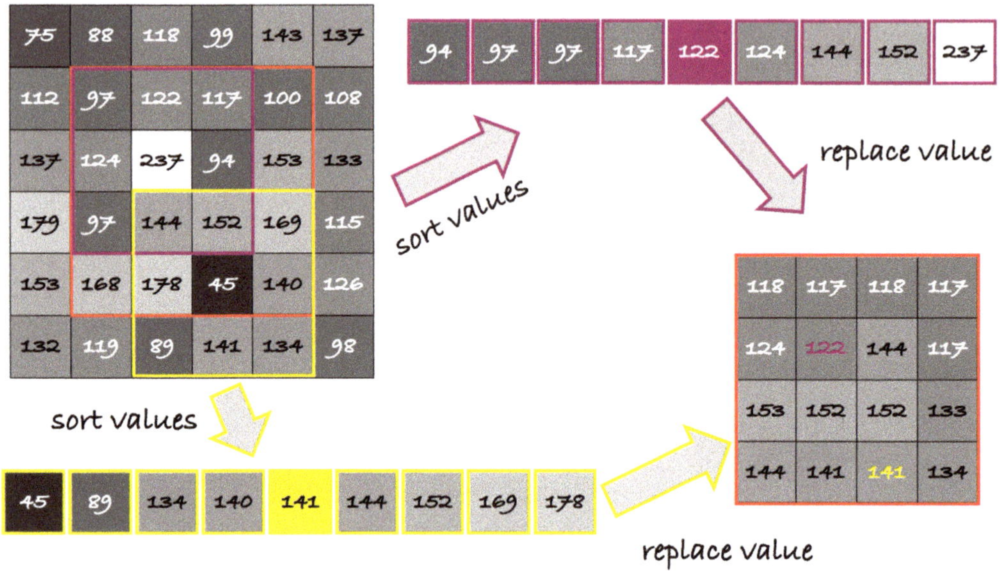

Figure 6.30 Noise reduction in real space – Median filter. The median filter is another effective filter to eliminate salt and pepper noise by replacing an outlier pixel value with the median value of its immediate surrounding pixel neighborhood. Median filtering does not lead to image blurring and is more robust toward single pixel outliers and performs better near edges.

mean filter in that it replaces the pixel value of interest with a value derived from its immediate neighboring pixels (Figure 6.30). However, instead of replacing it with the mean, it will replace it with the median of those values, which makes the filter more robust toward single pixel outliers (as is found in salt and pepper noise). It also performs better near feature edges.

Filtering in Real Space: Non-local Means Filter

The non-local means filter will determine the mean value of a group of pixels surrounding the target pixel, however, as the name implies, it does so over the entire image, by not only examining the target pixel and its neighbors but all pixels in the image, weighted by the degree of similarity they share with the target pixel. Non-local means filtering is often a good choice for smoothing noisy images.

Filtering in Real Space: Wavelet Filter

Wavelet filtering relies on the calculation of a wavelet transform, which in turn yields wavelets that correspond to features in the image. Wavelets are commonly used for filtering one-dimensional data, but the concept can be easily extended to 2D images, as edges (boundaries of an object) are simply places where the image brightness changes rapidly. Like it is the case in Fourier space, noise will be jitters on the wavelets, which can be effectively filtered out. However, edges will be preserved, unlike it is the case in low pass filtering where edges may be smoothed. Wavelet-based methods can be used both for noise reduction (by distinguishing signal from noise) as well as for feature extraction/image segmentation.

Filtering in Real Space: Non-linear Anisotropic Diffusion Filter

The non-linear anisotropic diffusion (NAD) filter is based on a generalization of a diffusion process. Local averaging mathematically is closely related to diffusion equations describing heat flow, and thus partial differential equations (PDE) form the basis of this iterative filtering technique. One key point however is that the diffusion process must be stopped at the appropriate point, otherwise the diffusion will even out all intensity differences eventually. One strategy is to systematically vary the number of iterations (and other parameters that can be controlled) and stop the diffusion process when the filtering process appears successful.

Isotropic diffusion (which resembles closely a heat-diffusion process) would smooth the image across a boundary and thus blur edges, whereas NAD (also known as Perona–Malik diffusion) recognizes the presence of a steep gradient and thus a boundary. As a result, NAD will only smooth parallel to the boundary but not across, and therefore is very effective in noise removal without blurring edges (Figure 6.31).

Filtering in Real Space: Bilateral Filter

Like the NAD algorithm, the bilateral filter is a non-linear, edge preserving noise-reducing algorithm, by replacing the

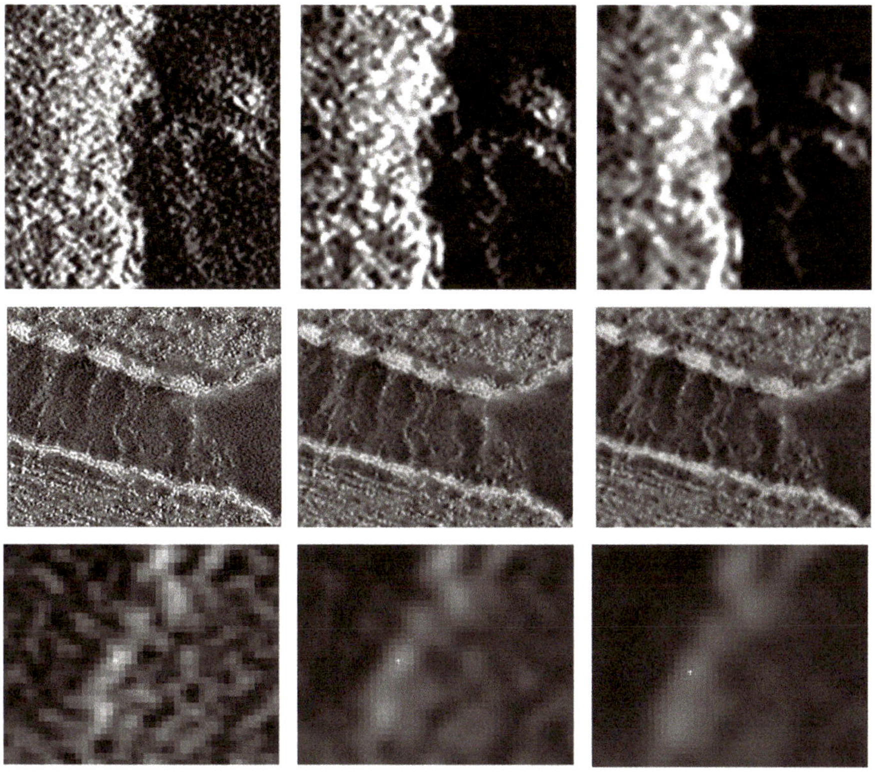

Figure 6.31 Noise reduction in real space – Non-linear anisotropic diffusion. Non-linear anisotropic diffusion is a noise reduction technique that is based on partial differential equations similar to calculating isotropic heat diffusion. One key difference is that it recognizes steep gradients as boundaries and thus the algorithm is anisotropic and will only smoothen parallel to such boundaries but not across feature boundaries. Thus, noise is efficiently reduced without edges being blurred. Note that what constitutes sufficient smoothing is somewhat in the eye of the beholder and depends both on the features of interest and its surrounding areas.

intensity of each pixel with a weighted average of intensity values of nearby pixels while preserving sharp edges. Together with the non-local means filter, the bilateral filter can be considered a good starting point for image smoothing/noise reduction.

6.11 Image Reconstruction

Image reconstruction describes the process to reconstruct a 3D volume. It includes image registration and alignment as well as reconstruction of 3D volumes from 2D images. There are fundamentally two different ways to reconstruct a 3D volume from 2D images. First, 2D images constitute adjacent frames that simply need to be registered (by translation in *X* and Y), as is the case for confocal fluorescence microscopy or 3D volume scanning electron microscopy. Second, 2D images are projection views of samples that have been rotated and thus imaged in different orientations, as is the case for electron or X-ray tomography as well as single-plane illumination microscopy.

Alignment is aided by fiducial markers or is carried out by simple cross-correlation. In some cases, such is the case for serial section transmission electron microscopy, even for 3D reconstruction from untilted adjacent sections it may be necessary to make rotational corrections and/or small magnification changes, due to physical changes upon sectioning (Figure 6.32). For electron tomography, projection images recorded at different tilt angles need to be aligned, which can be challenging and require sophisticated software. Once all images in a tilt series have been properly aligned, a 3D volume can be calculated (Figure 6.33), e.g., by weighted back-projection or by iterative reconstruction techniques.

6.12 Visualization

6.12.1 Introduction to Scientific Visualization

The goal of scientific visualization is to enable scientists to get a deeper insight from their data. Prominent examples are the dot map, used in 1855 to identify the source of the contaminated water in a cholera outbreak in London's Soho district, and the flow map of Napoleon's march on Moscow (Figure 6.34).

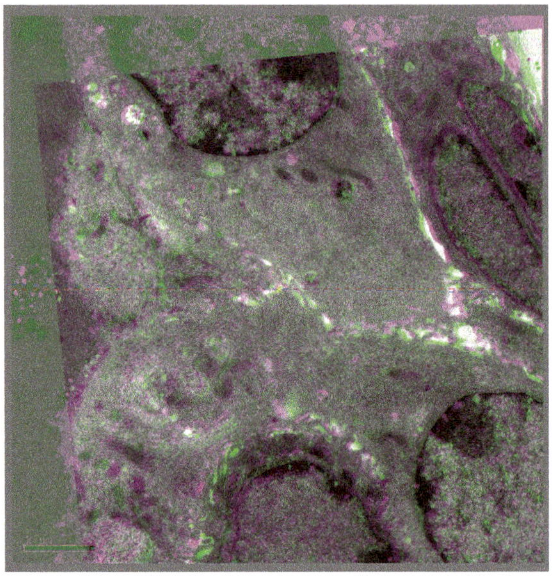

Figure 6.32 Image registration – Serial section transmission electron micrograph alignment. Image registration is usually straightforward if there are few changes between adjacent image frames that make up a 3D volume. This is usually the case in confocal fluorescence light microscopy or focused ion beam scanning electron microscopy, where the features are typically bigger than the *Z*-step size chosen. However, a more challenging examples is shown here where images (one shown in magenta, the other one shown in green) of serial resin sections of ~70 nm thickness are superimposed onto one another. Black are regions where the images superimpose well, whereas magenta and green mark regions where the fit is poor. Among the challenges are that the images can be rotated with respect to one another, and there may be slightly different compression artifacts at work that result in small changes in magnification, all of which makes it difficult to find the best fit.

Hence scientific visualization goes beyond simple displays of a grayscale or color image. It often includes computer graphics and visualization. Interestingly, one of the earliest visualization examples of 3D scientific data was a sculpture in clay prepared by James Clerk Maxwell in 1874 to provide a visual model of a thermodynamic surface.

The roots of computer visualization and computer graphics go back to the late 1950s and 1960s with the founding of the Hewlett-Packard company in the Greater San Francisco Bay Area, also known as Silicon Valley, and with the invention of a light pen that together with the Sketchpad software developed by Ivan Sutherland allowed interaction with images on a screen. Furthermore, it was the starting point of creating vector-based objects on a computer screen, and thus this time marks the beginning of early day modeling and the development of computer games, which became one of the big driving forces for computer graphics development going forward.

By the mid 1960s companies like Lockheed, General Electrics, and IBM invested in computer graphics, which led to the first graphic terminals. In 1968, David Evans and Ivan Sutherland (both Professors of Computer Science at the University of Utah) founded the first computer graphics company, called Evans & Sutherland, and their students later went on to found Pixar film studios with their 1995 landmark animated movie "Toy Story," Silicon Graphics computer company, which dominated the computer graphics industry until the mid 1990s, and Adobe Photosystems, which brought the world the first sophisticated 2D image processing/photo editing program Adobe Photoshop. Its PostScript format had a major impact on the publishing

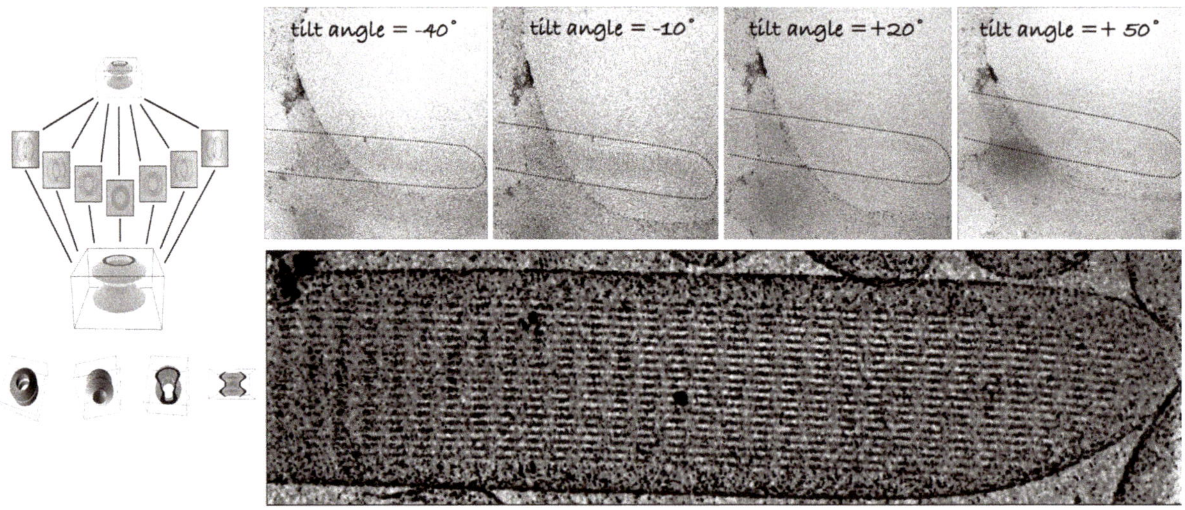

Figure 6.33 Alignment of tilt series image for 3D reconstruction. As shown on the left, a 3D object can be projected in different orientations to obtain 2D projection images. Upon alignment of such a tilt series and knowledge about the tilt angle, an 3D volume can be reconstructed. Top row: Four low-contrast cryo-electron tomography projection images of an unstained, vitrified mouse hair cell stereocilium at four different tilt angles. The dotted line indicates the outline of the stereocilium in each image. Bottom: Slice through 3D reconstruction of the hair cell stereocilium, showing a regular actin filament array.

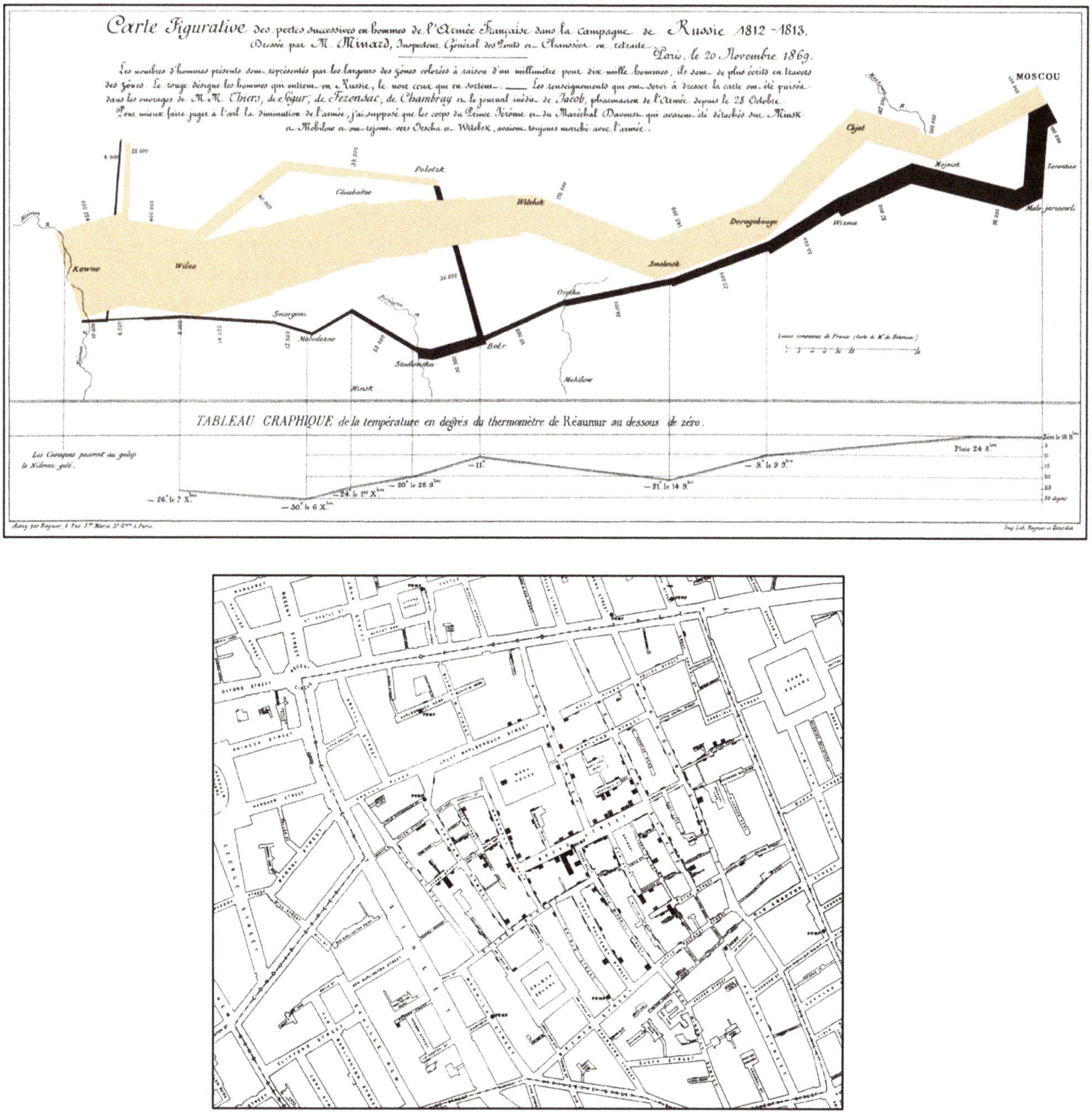

Figure 6.34 Famous examples of scientific visualization. Top: Flow map of Napoleon's march on Moscow showing among other things the weakening of his troop numbers; Bottom: Dot map of known cholera cases during the 1855 London Soho district cholera helped identify the source of the contaminated water.

and printing industry. In 1966, Ivan Sutherland had invented a head-mounted display system, the precursor of modern-day stereo-glasses, which allows depth perception in 3D rendering, essential for atomic model building in X-ray crystallography. Other milestones in computer graphics were ray casting (tracing of virtual light rays), texture mapping (wrapping of a patterned piece of paper around an object), hidden surface determination (coming up with what part of an object is behind other objects and thus needs to be hidden for rendering), shading (using darker colors as shadow for 3D perception), as well as bump mapping (the simulation of uneven surfaces).

With respect to visualization of an electron density map in two dimensions one can use contour maps to display different levels of density, non unlike a geographic topographic map shows terrain elevation as contour lines, with the spacing between contour lines signifying the gradient (the steepness) of contour map level changes.

This has been one of the earlier concepts in structural biology when computer graphics were at their infancy. Contour maps could be printed (or drawn) on paper or overhead transparency sheets. 3D electron maps could be modeled by using balsa wood, a soft yet strong material that could be easily cut as a thin slice according to the shape of the contour map. Different slices representing the contour maps at different *Z*-height can be glued together into a physical 3D model of the density map and thus the shape of the macromolecule for which the 3D contour maps were obtained. An alternative to balsa wood models are transparencies with the contour maps drawn or printed on overhead plastic film sheets that are spaced by plexiglass plates of an appropriate thickness. Once higher resolution structures became available, a physical model of the atomic structure could be built, with atoms being represented as balls and the bonds in between as sticks. With the help of a grid of thin rods, such ball-and-stick model could be supported in space.

As computer graphics matured, algorithms such as marching cube, marching tetrahedra, and surface nets algorithms became available for 3D rendering. Nowadays, there are many visualization packages available in combination with powerful computer workstations. Density maps can be viewed in volume rendering mode, in mesh mode or surface rendering mode (Figure 6.35). Volume rendering projects through all the layers of voxels of the respective (sub)volume of the density map, adding up the density along the viewing direction. High density features are depicted as light gray to white and low density are increasingly transparent, which on a black background appears as dark gray to black. This is the most direct form of visualization as it directly depicts the value in a density map. However, it appears somewhat pixelated and more importantly it is rather difficult to make out individual components of the scenery. In many ways it feels like standing in a heavy fog, where one can imagine the objects but cannot truly see them very well. Surface rendering on the other hand requires the choice of a defined map density threshold at which the map is rendered as solid objects, depicted in color with highlights and shadows further augmenting a "realistic" depiction of objects.

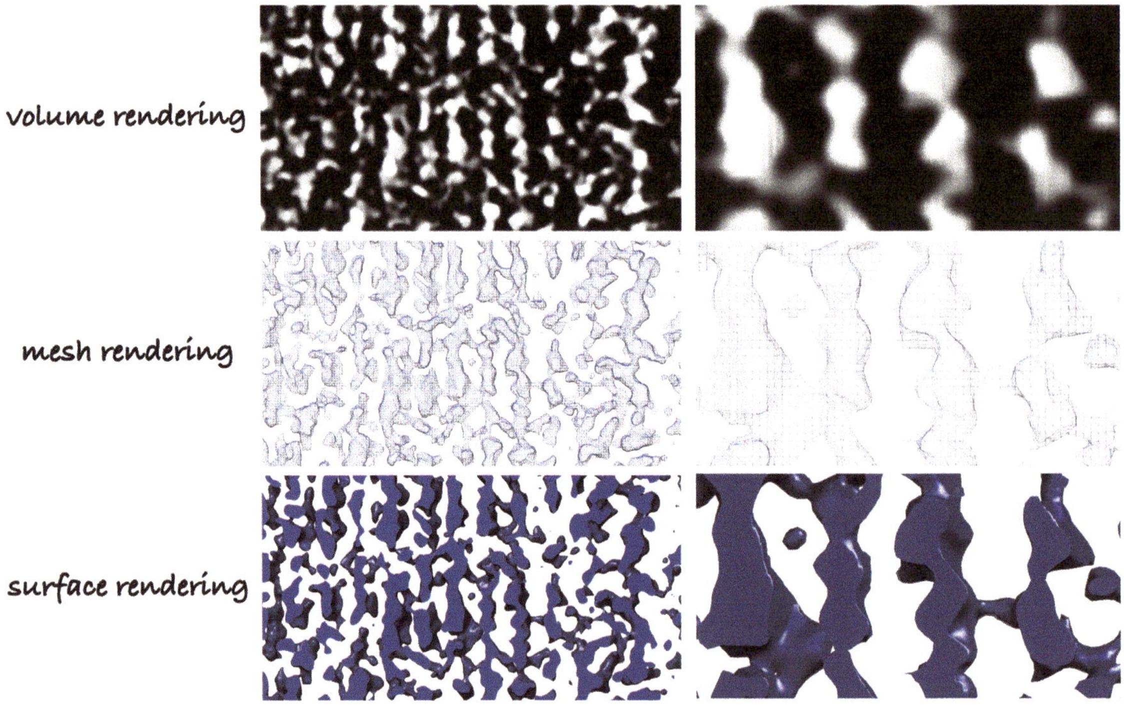

Figure 6.35 Macromolecular density maps are visualized by volume rendering, mesh rendering, or surface rendering. The density shown is a 10 nm-slab of a 3D volume of inner ear hair cell stereocilia, with a single layer of cross-connected actin filaments. Volume rendering adds up the density along the direction of view. High density appears as light gray to white, whereas low density along the viewing direction shows up as dark regions. While being the most direct form of visualization, volume rendering has a fog-like or ghost-like appearance and can be challenging to comprehend when thicker volumes are studied. Mesh rendering depicts density maps as meshes (often referred to chicken wire), with the meshes allowing ball and stick models to be placed into the meshes. Surface rendering depicts the density maps as solid objects (although transparency settings may allow to see through the solid object boundary). Note that both mesh rendering and surface rendering require a certain density threshold to be chosen for rendering. Surface rendering is effective once different features have been identified and can be color-coded according to the identity.

Noise is particularly detrimental in the surface rendering of objects, as objects seem to be immersed in an ocean of tiny rocks. Furthermore, objects in front of other objects will obscure them and without color-coding the various features it can be very difficult to comprehend the scenery one is visualizing. Mesh representations often present as compromise, they have the clarity of the solid surface rendering, while allowing objects obscured by another object to be somewhat visible. Mesh-rendering (also sometimes referred to as chicken wires) are widely used in high-resolution structure determination, in part also because they allow atomic models to be fitted to the density map.

Solid surface rendering with raytracing as well as mesh rendering can be quite effective for visualization of macromolecules and even supramolecular complexes such as a 10 nm thin slab of cross-connected parallel actin filaments residing in inner ear hair cell stereocilia (see Figure 6.35). Here the surface rendering and the mesh rendering provide a more three-dimensional depiction of this single layer of actin filament density compared to volume rendering.

However, the usefulness of mesh and surface rendering for raw cellular 3D volume, that had not undergone substantial denoising and/or segmentation, is questionable as it indicated by Figure 6.36. Not only is rendering at a single threshold very challenging, but also, different features such as mitochondria, the endoplasmic reticulum and the nucleus (depicted in the surface rendering of the segmented volume as yellow, salmon, and blue, respectively), cannot be easily discriminated in the unsegmented volume.

6.12.2 Visualization Software Examples

There are a variety of visualization software packages available, some of which are proprietary, such as Zen, Amira, Metamorph, or Imaris (and many more). They are often part of a larger software package, which also controls microscope operation and data acquisition as well as subsequent data analysis.

Below is a list of popular free open-source image analysis programs, some of which are for general image analysis use, or more specialized for certain purposes, e.g., optimized for handling of very large datasets, for comparison of many images, or for tracking a signal or cells through a video or time-lapse series, to name a few. Obviously, this

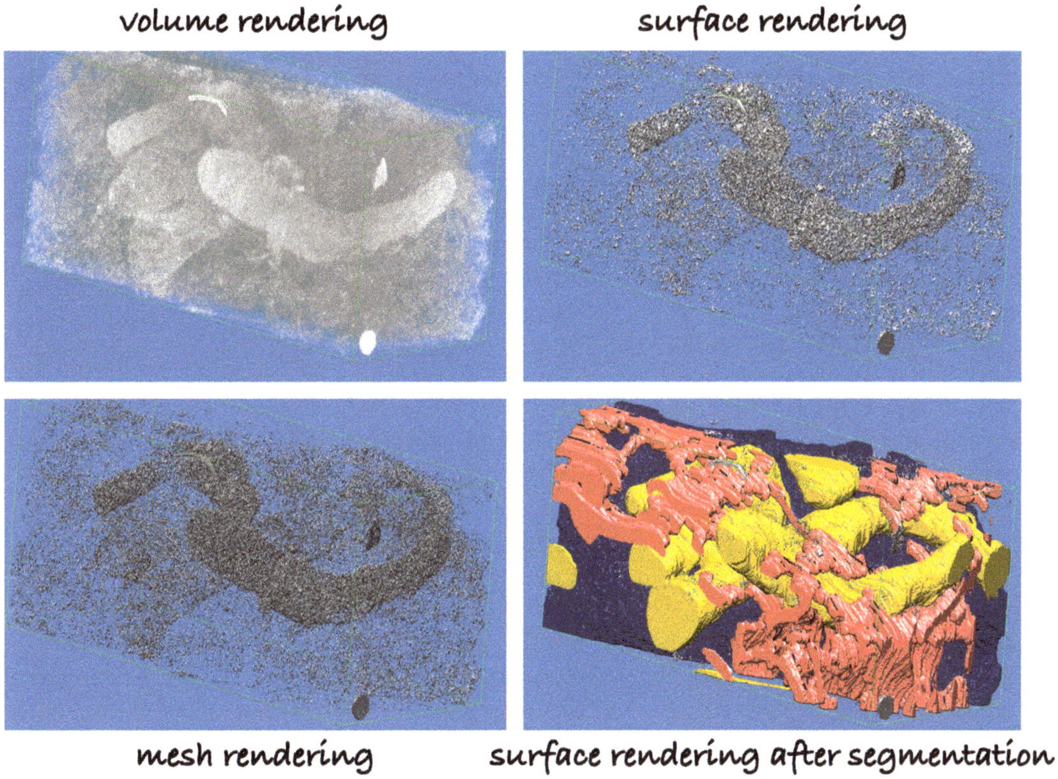

Figure 6.36 Subcellular region of a cell imaged as 3D volume by Focused Ion Beam Scanning Electron Microscopy (FIBSEM). Electron density as depicted by volume rendering, surface rendering, mesh rendering. Note that the features and their 3D organization is difficult to comprehend, particularly if a single threshold is chosen. Surface rendering after segmentation and annotation of densities being either nuclear envelope membrane (blue), endoplasmic reticulum (salmon) or mitochondria (yellow) renders this cellular scenery much more interpretable. Hence, segmentation and annotation of the different subcellular features is key to an understanding of cellular electron microscopy imaging data.

list is just an incomplete snapshot of current visualization software packages.

Some programs are best suited for fluorescence microscopy, digital pathology, chemical imaging data or electron microscopy. No program is ideal for all applications, but many programs can be adapted for all sorts of image data (e.g., by downloading specialized plugins modules), and thus can handle both a large number of fluorescent images and very large electron microscopy grayscale data. Most packages have noise reduction and segmentation capabilities, and many have recently been updated to capitalize on recent advances in machine learning/deep learning (ML/DL).

The Java-based ImageJ and more recently Fiji (which is also known as "FIJI Is Just ImageJ") is one of the best-known and longest-lived open-source program packages that was originally developed for image analysis of biological/biomedical images by a collaboration between the U.S. National Institute of Health and the Laboratory of Optical and Computational Instrumentation at the University of Wisconsin. Its original scope has been extended over the years with a variety of plugins that have been developed by individual researchers often for their own image analysis needs, and then subsequently made available to the wider scientific community. Given the nature of its history and its community structure, the GUI is simple, and using the program (while being relatively simple) does require some knowledge on when and how to use the different modules, and/or where to find appropriate plugins. However, a wide array of tutorial and help pages (including a user community forum) are available for any potential users to answer specific questions. Fiji is well-suited to handle large electron microscopy datasets, including segmentation and annotation tools, and due to its organization and sorting of capabilities into different categories, Fiji may be a little easier to use than ImageJ. Fiji and ImageJ are examples of software packages that allow non-expert users to simply use what presently exists but also allows experts with programming skills to create new plugins.

CellProfiler (http://CellProfiler.org) is another popular open-source program that allows quantitative measurement of cell phenotypes (size and shapes of objects) for thousands of images in an automated batch-process manner. It was developed at the Broad Institute of the Massachusetts Institute of Technology and Harvard University and has a MATLAB-based flexible modular design that allows a user to create a pipeline of image correction, noise filtering, segmentation, and quantitative analysis tools in combination with a user-friendly GUI. CellProfiler can also track cells through time-lapse images series. Parameters in the pipeline can be easily adjusted, new modules can be easily added or subtracted, allowing for high versatility und user-friendliness, particularly users without extensive prior knowledge in image analysis. CellProfiler analyst add-on software goes beyond image analysis and can provide deeper analysis of the data provided by CellProfiler.

Cytomine (http://cytomine.com) is an open-source web-based tool designed for or the collaborative management, segmentation, semantic annotation, and quantitative analysis of large image data by multidisciplinary teams. Image data is uploaded to and stored in the cloud.

Orbit (http://www.orbit.bio) is another free open-source software for quantifying large image data (such as whole slide images of tissues), that are either stored locally or on the OME image server (OMERO). Like other packages, Orbit offer tools for segmentation and classification based on supervised ML approaches. Regions of interest (tiled sub-regions) can then be processed via CellProfiler or ImageJ, and the results can be read back into Orbit for visualization.

Similarly, OMERO (http://www.openmicroscopy.org/omero), which is part of the OME image data management platform, enables access, processing, sharing and analysis of image data and metadata. OMERO can read over 140 file formats, and view both 2D image data (including high content screening image data) as well as volumetric (3D) image data, either locally on a desktop computer or via a web browser, with data being stored in the cloud. Analysis in OMERO relies on tools from other packages and libraries, such as ImageJ, MATLAB, and other tools.

In addition, there exists a fair number of other packages, which are used in various specialized fields of biological and medical imaging. Presented here is only a small set of programs, which may provide a starting point and serve as examples to illustrate the capabilities typically found in such programs.

6.12.3 3D Volume Image Data

It is remarkable how much of a challenge it can be to visualize a 3D volume data set. (Note that the term 3D volume is redundant as all volumes are three-dimensional. However, we use the term 3D volume to emphasize the 3D nature of the data and contrast with the 2D nature of the recorded images from which 3D volumes are reconstructed.)

We all are used in our daily life to the idea that we live in a 3D world, and thus visualization and comprehension of 3D data should come easy to us. But this turns out to be a misconception: in reality, we only experience 2D images of our surrounding world, our brain then synthesizes a 3D world out of these 2D images. This becomes clear if one takes a walk through a dense forest. Not only can one only see what is directly around us, our brain has difficulties to remember what the scene was like a minute ago, and we likely would not be able to draw a 3D map of a forest from

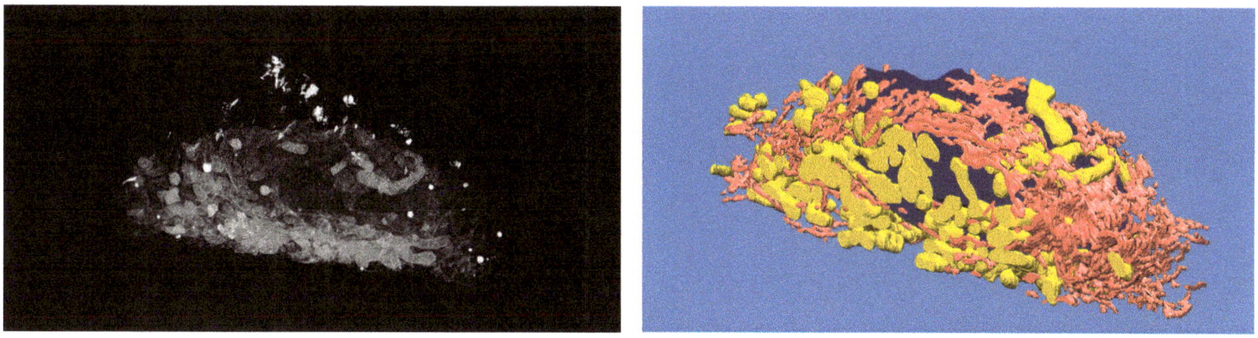

Figure 6.37 Visualizing 3D (sub)cellular data. Left: Mesh rendering of a cellular scenery. Note that the organelles can hardly be recognized, and details of their organization are almost completely lost, due to the high complexity of the cellular volume; Right: Surface rendering after segmentation. Mitochondria, endoplasmic reticulum (ER) and a nuclear envelope are depicted as yellow/golden, salmon, and blue, respectively. While the rendering on the right is a little easier to comprehend, the details of the organization of the ER and the mitochondrial network remain obscure unless one focuses on small regions.

memory. Navigating through a cellular volume is a bit like navigating through a dense forest. There are many objects in our path that may obscure our view, and thus simple volume rendering (adding up the grayscale values along the line of sight) can be very confusing. Surface rendering on the other hand, provides a view onto the surface of an object, but obscures everything that is hidden behind this surface. So-called chicken wire mesh allows to peak through this first layer, but also can get very confusing, even if one works with different colors for displaying different objects. Likewise, using different colors and rendering thresholds, in combination with surface transparencies for different objects can be helpful but for a complex system, none of such approaches is ideal (Figure 6.37).

6.12.4 Visualizing Macromolecular Imaging Data

The first representation of John Kendrew's myoglobin 3D structure in 1958 was a brass-model that was supported by 2,500 vertical rods. When the high-resolution 3D structure of myoglobin became available in 1960, a detailed physical ball and spoke (stick) model was built that detailed the position of most atoms in the polypeptide chain and the heme group. The position of each the atoms were recorded and stored in extensive lists, and the *X*,*Y*-position (as well as the position in *Z*) was reflected in the resulting 3D atomic model. While a picture of this model documented its existence, little detail could be derived from such pictures due to the complexity of its 3D structure. A white ribbon depicted the position of the polymeric backbone and thus revealed some overview of the macromolecular organization. Replica of the physical models were built and sold to interested labs around the world.

The next step for visualization of myoglobin was the creation of stereoscopic drawings in 1966, a strategy further refined and used for many decades for the publication of atomic 3D structures of macromolecules. Another approach was to create so-called Corey–Pauling–Koltun (CPK) space-filling models, but such space-filling models make it difficult to appreciate molecular interactions in the macromolecule's interior. Yet another approach to make physical rather than computational models of 3D structure was pursued in the early 1970s in the lab of Jane Richardson, where a machine was developed by Byron Rubin to bend wires to create a physical representation of protein backbone traces, which lead to the realization that proteins with little sequence identity can adopt similar protein folds. Other physical representations were tiny laser-induced fractures within glass blocks that provided 3D structures of macromolecules (e.g., proteins or DNA). 3D printing is the latest incarnation of creating physical models of computer graphics maps.

The first system for interactively displaying protein molecular structures on a screen was developed by Cyrus Levinthal in the mid 1960s at the Massachusetts Institute of Technology, where an oscilloscope showed a wireframe-like representation of the backbone of the protein. The 3D effect was accomplished by rotating the model, with the user being able to control rotation speed and direction. Upon reprogramming, molecular details of smaller regions could be displayed with this approach. Stereoscopic drawings with a pen-plotter became available in 1965.

In the late 1960s, the "Richards Box" (also referred to as Fred's Folly) created a physical model of electron densities by printing the values of the density map onto paper and connecting areas of similar density values to create contour levels (Figure 6.38). Such contour levels were then traced onto transparent plates, which were stacked accordingly to create a 3D density map. Such density map depictions could be superimposed onto atomic models using half-silvered mirrors.

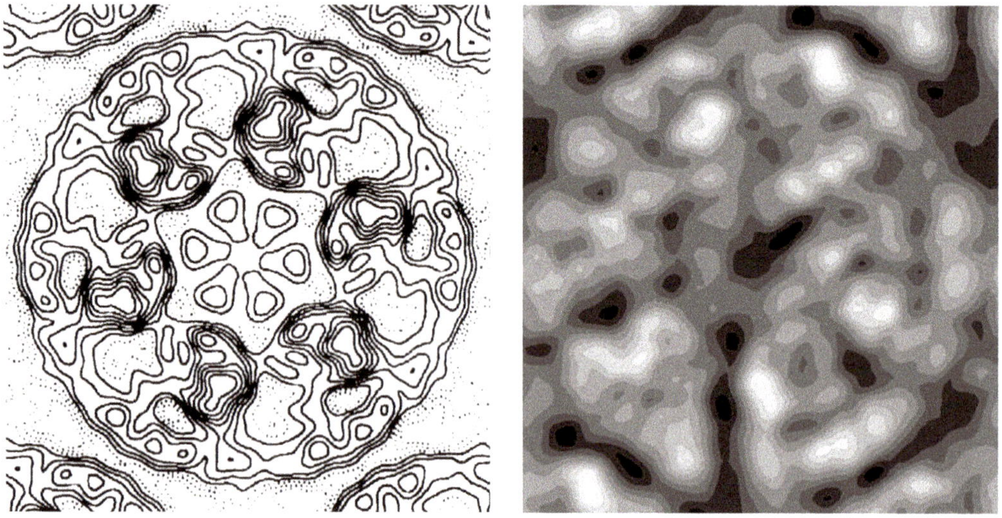

p6 p321

Figure 6.38 Contour levels for visualizing macromolecular structures. Projection density single-layer and double-layer maps of a P-type ATPase hexamer obtained by electron crystallography of 2D crystals. Left: Single layer 2D crystal with p6 symmetry depicted as contour lines connecting points of equal map density. The closer the lines the steeper the map gradient. Right: Double-layered 2D crystal with p321 symmetry shown as contour levels, areas of different gray shading, with dark color showing regions of low density and light areas regions of high density.

The rendering of contour levels in computer graphics was an electronic equivalent of Richard boxes. Also, the list of atomic coordinates were kept as an electronic record, making distance measurements much more straightforward.

X-ray crystallography early adopted computer graphics, capitalizing on the computer raster graphics revolution of the 1980s by Evans & Sutherland and SGI (Silicon Graphics) computer companies, which included the development of 16-bit central processing units (CPU) as well as the first graphics processing units (GPU), allowing parallel processing that dramatically sped up rendering of 3D objects. Such graphics computers were extremely expensive, costing a quarter of a million dollars in 1985.

The earliest 3D visualization tool in macromolecular structural biology was FRODO. Both FRODO and its successor O ("O is the end of FRODO") were developed by the group of T. Alwyn Jones at Uppsala University in the late 1970s. FRODO capitalized on these high-end graphics computers using scalable vector graphics to display electron density maps into which atomic 3D models based on the amino acid sequence could be built (Figure 6.39). Note that map density voxels were not displayed in volume rendering mode (which amounts to a fog-like depiction of density) but displayed as (chicken wire) meshes. Such meshes were interpolations of the voxel density and often appear as higher resolution as the voxel representation. Such meshes have become a prominent form of representing macromolecular density maps.

KINEMAGES, developed by David and Jane Richardson in 1992 at the Massachusetts Institute of Technology, allowed lower-end computer to display selected views of protein structures, but it did not allow an independent interactive exploration of protein structures. RasMol, developed by Roger A. Sayle in 1993, filled this void, and allowed lower-end computer users to visualize 3D structures in a more abstracted alpha-helices/beta-sheets/turns format, rather than as an exact 3D structure, which is very confusing to look at and computationally very demanding.

More recent packages have been the Python-based program PyMol and the UCSF Chimera software package. Chimera is still frequently used in X-ray crystallography, single particle cryo-EM as well as in electron tomography and has extensive model building capabilities. Also, UCSF Chimera has been very valuable for cellular data visualization, including the generation of ball-and-stick models and volumetric quantitative analysis of lower resolution (e.g., electron tomography) data.

6.12.5 Visualizing Cellular Imaging Data

Commercial packages are often more user-friendly and very powerful, but require a substantial financial investment, which is beyond reach for many labs around the world. Such commercial packages often offer sophisticated tools for segmentation of complex cellular sceneries, including interactive tools for (semi-automated) manual

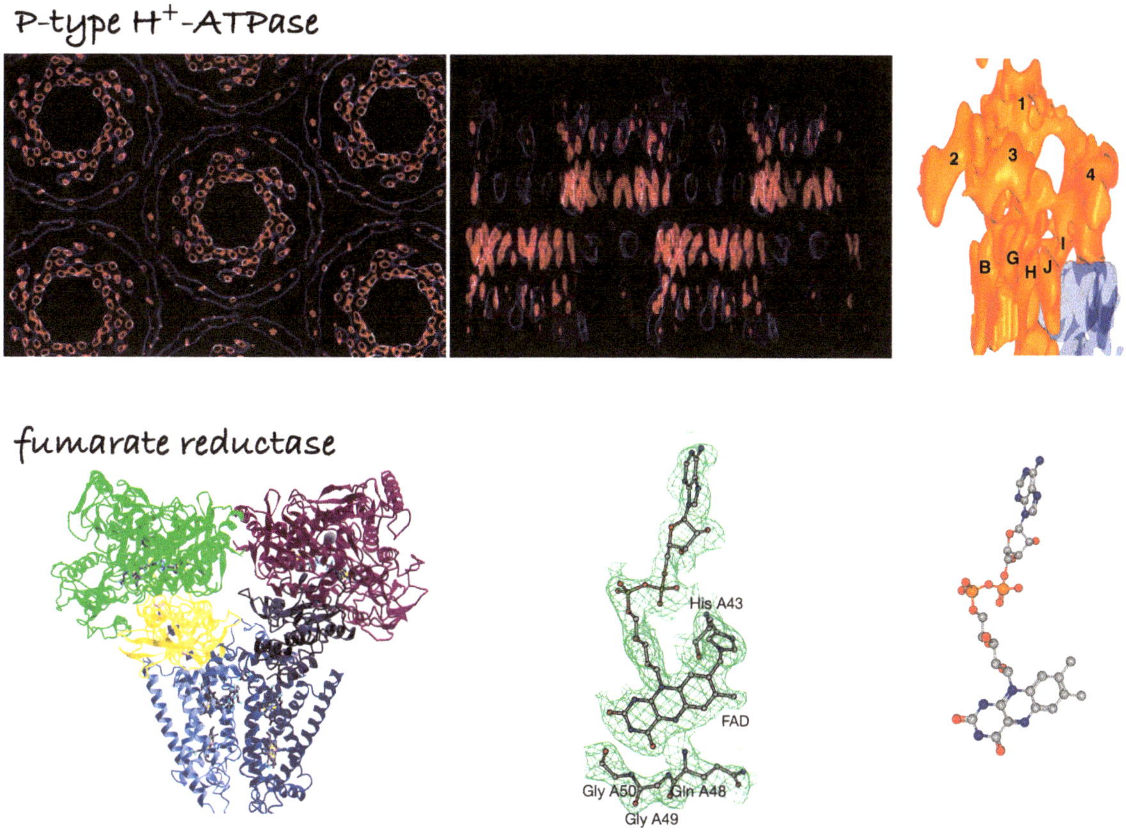

Figure 6.39 Visualizing macromolecular structures. Examples of different representations of macromolecular structures of P-type proton-ATPase (top row) and fumarate reductase (bottom row), obtained by electron crystallography of 2D crystals and X-ray crystallography of 3D crystals, respectively. Top left: Thin slice through the 3D mesh rendering of the ATPase hexamer membrane region, revealing the cross-sectional organization of the transmembrane alpha-helices; Top middle: View perpendicular to the plane of the membrane revealing the longitudinal organization of the transmembrane helices as well as the p321 symmetry of the two-layered 2D crystal. The density map was shown at high threshold which emphasizes the transmembrane alpha helices. Top right: Surface rendering of an ATPase monomer with its transmembrane helices (labeled as B, G, H, J, and I), a detergent ring (blue) and its cytoplasmic regions (labeled as 1, 2, 3, and 4). Bottom left: Ribbon diagram of the 3D structure of fumarate reductase, depicting the overall fold of the protein sequence backbone. Transmembrane alpha helices are shown in blue; Bottom middle: Electron density map, rendered as mesh, of a small portion of the 3D structure with a flavin adenine dinucleotide (FAD) prosthetic group being fitted to the density. Bottom right: Ball-and-stick model of FAD. Note that the 3D structure of the ATPase was determined only at intermediate resolution of 8 Å in *X*,*Y* direction, whereas the structure of fumarate reductase was at near-atomic (2.2 Å) resolution.

feature selection and extraction, as well as support for Deep Learning-based feature classification and segmentation. Note that cellular sceneries can be highly complex and in terms of scale are much larger than macromolecular volumes (see Figure 6.40).

Advanced Visual Systems (AVS) was one of the earliest commercial visualization packages in the 1990s for macromolecular 3D structures and allowed high-quality surface rendering of any kind of density maps.

Amira, developed by the company FEI (now part of Thermo Fisher Scientific corporation) is a stand-alone visualization package, ideally suited for electron microscopy data such as electron tomography, but it is very expensive, and one often needs to pay for extra modules, such as handling of large data sets or ML/DL. Likewise, the microscope company Zeiss promotes its own software (Arivis Vision 4D). There is much ongoing development, as microscope manufacturers recognize the need to offer integrated software solutions from data collection over cross-modality workflows to visualization, segmentation and quantitative analysis.

ORS Dragonfly is a particularly powerful package with similar capabilities as Amira. Upon registration ORS Dragonfly is cost-free for academic users and allows visualization of cellular 3D datasets, segmentation, quantitative analysis as well as ML/DL. Unlike many academic packages, Dragonfly is developed by a professional company, hence does not rely on the uncertainties of

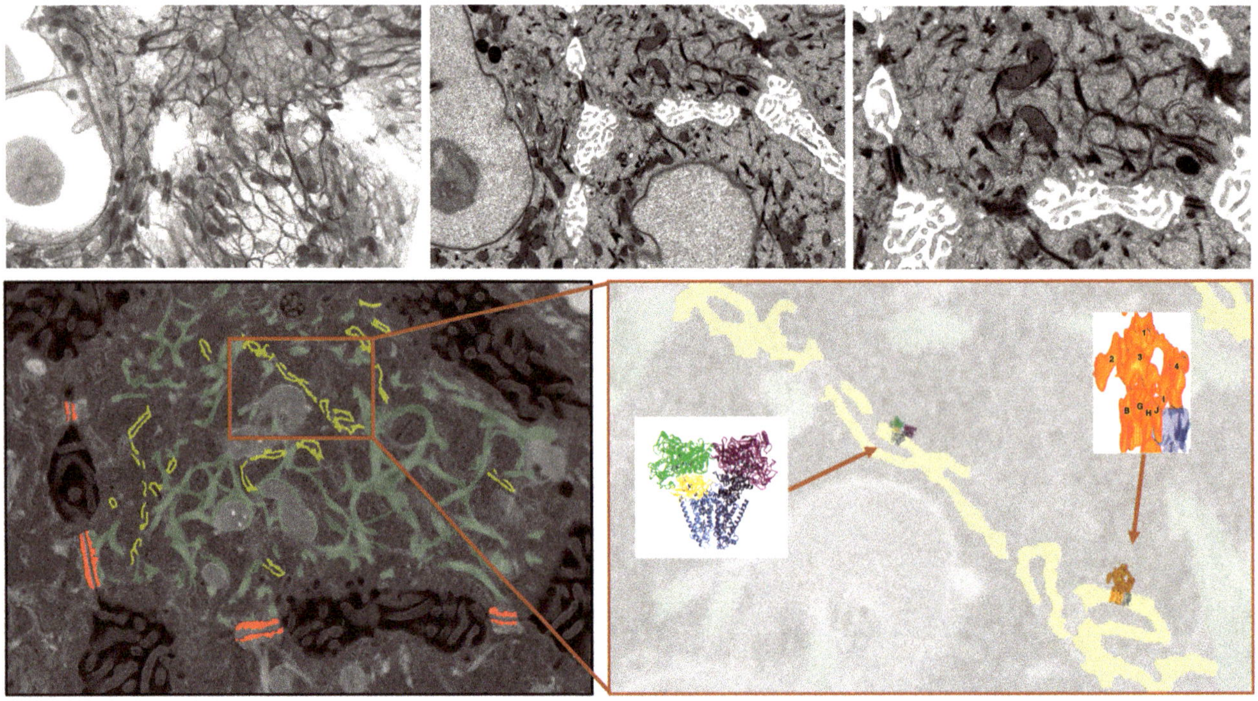

Figure 6.40 Visualizing cellular imaging data – Scale and complexity. Cellular imaging data can be rather large in dimensions (microns in *X*, *Y*, and *Z*) and highly complex. This volume represents a ~1 μm thick portion of a human mammary gland acinus, cultured in a collagen-rich 3D matrix, fixed, heavy-metal stained and resin-embedded before being imaged by dual beam/focused ion beam scanning electron microscopy. Such acini range in size from ~20 to ~40 μm in diameter and contain a few dozen cells. In this volume there are portions of 4 different cells, connected to one another by cell–cell adhesion complexes. Note the plasma membrane protrusions into the space in between the cells. Top left: Projection view through a ~1 μm thick 3D volume; Top middle: Single 5 nm thick slice through the 3D volume. Top right: Zoomed-in view of single 5 nm slice. The complex organization of the cytoskeleton, mitochondria, as well as cell–cell adhesion complexes is clearly visible. Bottom left: Single slice segmented into cytoskeleton (green), cell–cell adhesion complexes, and internal membrane systems (possibly the endoplasmic reticulum) shown in yellow. Bottom right: Close up view with the yellow-colored membrane system. For reference, the structures of the ATPase and fumarate reductase are superimposed onto the membrane to give an idea about the difference in scale between individual proteins and subcellular volumes.

funding cycles, and thus can react more quickly to community user needs.

More generalized and free 3D visualization packages have emerged since the 1990s, with the Visualization Tool Kit (VTK), created and supported by the Kitware team, being one of the first open-source software systems for cross-platform 3D computer graphics, consisting of a variety of graphic libraries for scientific visualization. VTK uses scalar, vector, tensor, texture and volumetric methods for visualization and a variety of approaches for advanced modeling. Being rooted in a companion software to a book called "The Visualization Toolkit: An Object-Oriented Approach to 3D Graphics," VTK was further developed by researchers around the world. VTK forms the core of such successful biomedical computing applications as 3DSlicer.

3DSlicer is a very powerful free open-source software for 3D visualization, segmentation, and analysis of volumetric image data, as well as of diffusion tensor imaging data as is found in Magnetic Resonance Imaging (MRI). It also allows tracking of devices in image-guided surgery and is widely used in clinical settings. It is built on the VTK graphical library pipeline and the ITK framework of image registration and image segmentation.

Another popular free open-source 3D image visualization and analysis software is VAA3D (3D Visualization-Assisted Analysis), which can handle 3D, 4D, and 5D data, that is further enhanced by plugins for data acquisition, data management and statistical data analysis. VAA3D excels in the analysis of data at very large (massive) scale (up to Tera voxels) 3D image stacks (as well as surface data) and allows cell segmentation, neuron tracing, brain registration, annotation, and quantitative statistical analysis. It is widely used in brain connectome mapping and provides interactive local and global 3D views at different scales.

NeuronStudio is another interesting tool, developed for the tracing the 3D structure of neurons and neural connections from confocal fluorescence microscopy image stacks, and allows deconvolution of the image data, skeletonization as well as quantitative morphological measurements (including diameter estimation) of Dendritic spines. The software is no longer supported but the Windows source code and documentation can be still found via the Internet Archive. This example illustrates an important point, namely that software packages often come and go, and that they often are particularly well-suited for very specific problems. Since they are developed by academic labs, they are vulnerable to changes of the academic environment and/or funding pressure, which results in platforms that contain a wealth of highly powerful and highly useful routines but may not be user-friendly and/or require a significant amount of expert knowledge to reap the maximal benefit of such program.

There are also packages that are more specific to certain communities such as the example of 3Dmod by the University of Colorado, which is well-known and widely used in the field of electron tomography. 3Dmod (formerly known as Imod) is highly sophisticated when it comes to the generation of 3D electron tomographic volumes from 2D projection images tilt series, but has only modest 3D visualization, 3D rendering, image segmentation and model building capabilities.

6.12.6 A Few More Points Worth Noting

It is still common for many researchers to visualize their 3D image stack as looped movies of consecutive Z-sections before attempting 3D visualization. They hope (and to some degree correctly) that by scrolling through the 3D volume slice-by-slice, their brains create a 3D volume and thus an expectation for subsequent analysis.

Raw data in its pixel of voxel format looks very rough and clumsy. Most 3D visualization programs will use interpolation algorithms to smooth out the density map, with the result that the maps look better and appear more detailed than is apparent in the original data.

It should be kept in mind that the goal of rendering is to generate a 2D image of an 3D object by means of a computer program, so it can be displayed on the 2D surface of a monitor. Hence the result is not always intuitive. One typically chooses between volume rendering or surface rendering, whereas in volume rendering the gray values of voxels projected on the 2D screen of the monitor are added up, so the projected path of dense regions appears white, empty regions appear darker. However, while volume rendering gives an accurate impression how much density there is in a certain direction (for a row of pixels along the line of sight), it is very difficult to make out any details of the object.

For surface rendering, pixels are turned into vertices that represent the shape of on object at a particular density value. Determining the correct density value can be tricky, and often there is a pragmatic approach, namely that the map density threshold used for rendering is at a value that gives the best visual result. Choosing too low of a value may connect densities that should appear as separate entities, choosing too high of a threshold may lead to a loss of features altogether. Just like it is the case for 2D contour maps (topographic maps), higher threshold maps will appear thinner and more closely to the object's center, whereas lower density threshold maps appear thicker and thus the feature of interest appears wider. It can thus be valuable to simultaneously display different maps in different colors at different density thresholds/cut-offs, with the higher density value map typically residing inside the envelope of a lower density value map. Both, chicken wire/mesh rendering or a surface rendering with sufficient transparency allow the different maps to be seen simultaneously.

6.13 Image Segmentation

The goal of image segmentation is the partition of an image into multiple segments, also referred to as image regions or objects, and to extract certain features of interest in an 2D image/3D volume for better visualization or further analysis. As a result of image segmentation, the data will be much easier to deal with and to analyze, as regions of interest and/or boundaries (such as lines and curves) are detected and thus localized. In essence, image segmentation leads to an assignment of labels to pixels, with the idea that pixels of the same label have some characteristics in common.

The features that will be extracted can be simple, such as individual cells like bacteria against a homogenous background, or they can be highly complex with respect to shape, signal strength/density and contrast with respect to its immediate environment. An example of the latter would be supramolecular complexes residing in a crowded cell environment.

There are different ways how computer programs deal with an extracted feature. For example, one may simply set the background to 0 and the map density/grayscale value in the extracted feature to 1 (or to 255 to create a black and white image). This clearly serves the purpose of distinguishing the feature from the background, but one loses all internal details such as map density/grayscale pixel or voxel variations within the segmented feature. Alternatively, one can opt to keep the value as it was for each pixel/voxel for the segmented object (e.g., by creating a mask for the segmented feature with the value 1 and multiplying the mask with the original image), while setting the region immediately outside of the feature to 0. Furthermore, once segmented features of interest have been identified, one can manipulate the features through a process of dilation or erosion, where the boundary of the object is either increased or decreased by a pixel, respectively. Also, holes inside the feature can be filled.

6.13.1 Map Density Value-Based Segmentation

Thesholding

Thresholding is the simplest form of segmentation, as its only criterium for feature selection is a threshold intensity value above which the pixel/voxel is considered feature (of foreground) and below which the pixel/voxel is considered background (Figure 6.41).

For thresholding to work, the intensity value of the feature should be well above background and ideally features should be surrounded by background. This is often the case for fluorescence microscopy images. In any case, as noise smears out the grayscale value distribution, noise reduction is recommended prior to thresholding. But all too often, simple thresholding is not sufficient for adequate segmentation particularly in high noise environments and/or when the image is very complex, as is often the case for electron microscopy data. Also, thresholding eliminates all pixel density information as it categorizes the pixels either as having a value of 0 or of 1 (or 255) to create a black and white image. Thresholded images can be used as a mask for multiplication with the original data, and thus the density values for the non-zero pixels can be restored.

Histogram Region Selection

Histograms are an excellent source of information about the image. One can define only certain intensity regions of the histogram to be considered as a feature whereas areas above and below the minimum and maximum settings will be treated as background or to be precise as intensity regions that are not of interest (Figure 6.42). This is particularly interesting if the histogram shows a distinct bimodal distribution, with no overlap between the distribution of foreground (feature) and background pixel values. Based

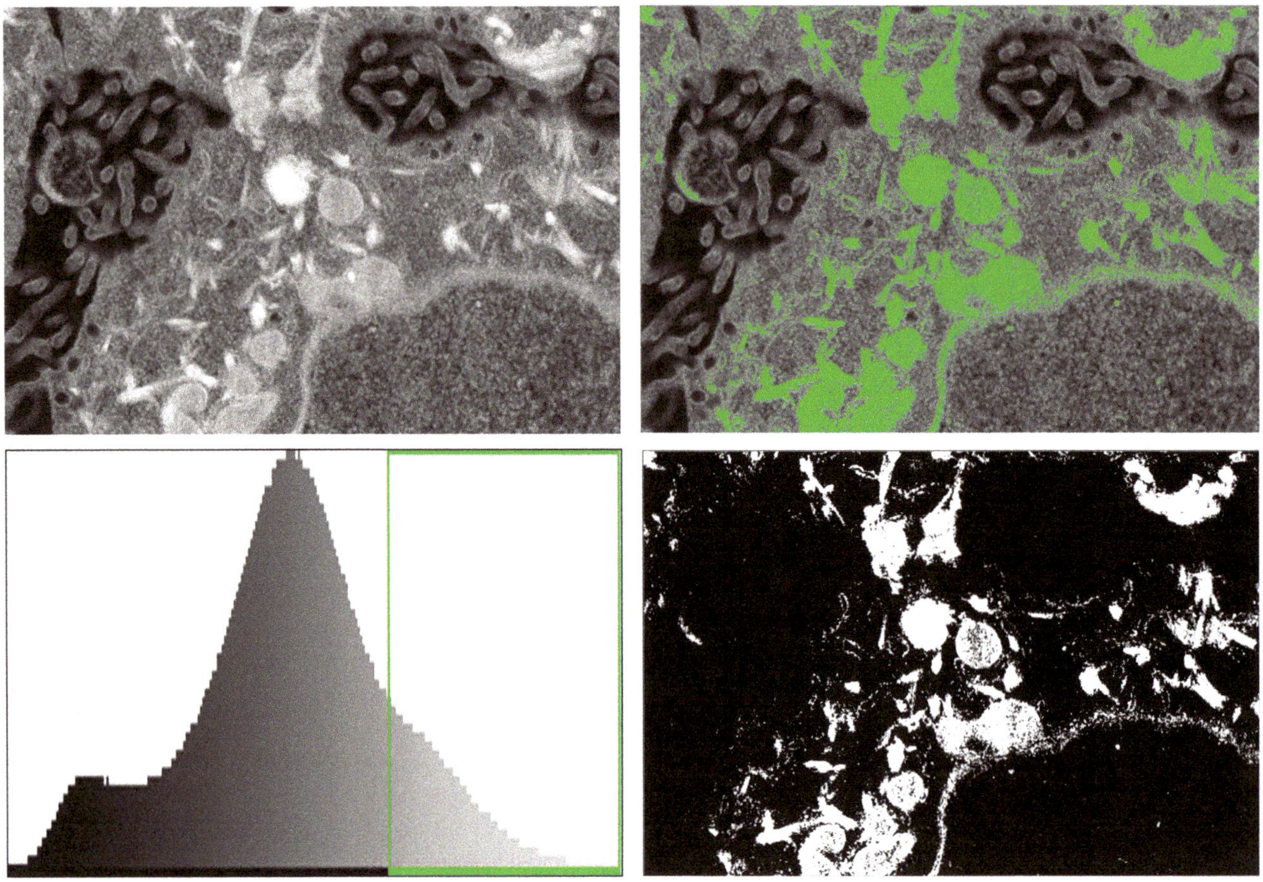

Figure 6.41 Thresholding. In this case, a cellular volume was recorded by dual beam/focused ion beam scanning electron microscopy. Bright features (pixels with a value higher than the threshold, as indicated by the green box in the histogram) are selected (green labels in top right panel). Thresholding leads to black and white images (bottom right) with white being pixels above the threshold and black being the background. Note that thresholding is particularly vulnerable to noise in the data.

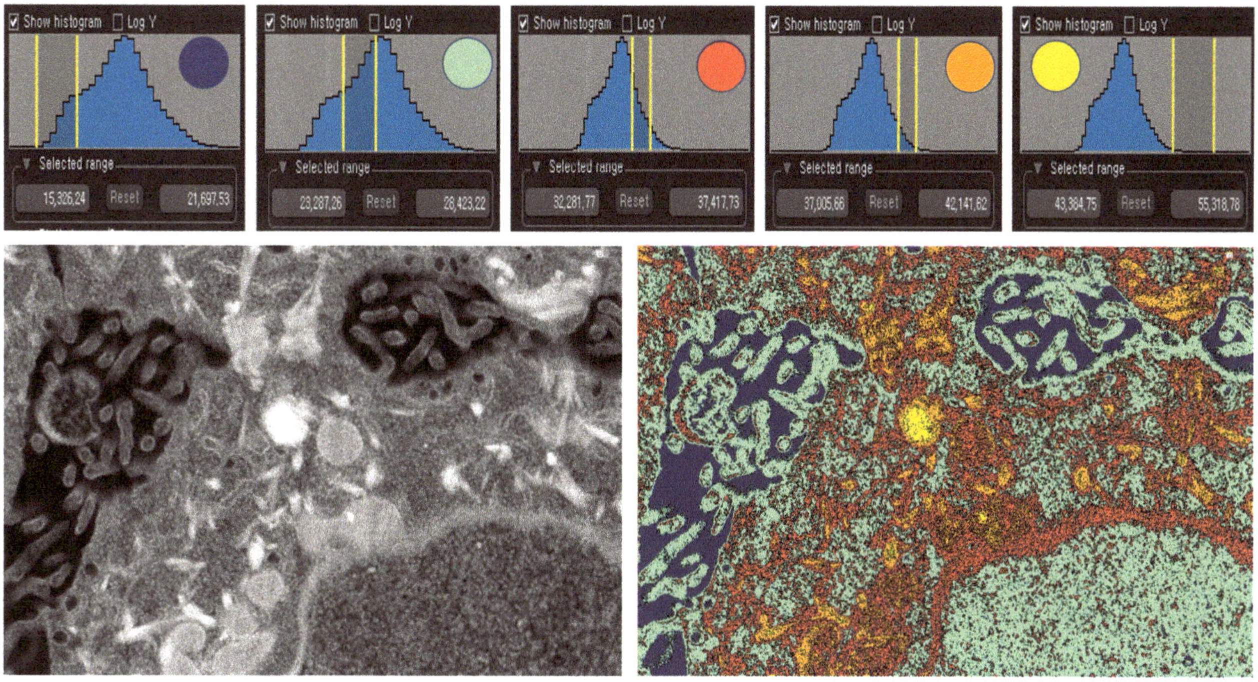

Figure 6.42 Histogram region selection and thresholding. Top row: Different intensity regions in the histogram are selected and color-coded; Bottom left: Original image; Bottom right: Thresholding of the image at different histogram values. Note that noise in the image data compromises the success of histogram-region-based selection and thresholding.

on this principle is the so-called Otsus segmentation, which essentially is a thresholding algorithm. For a successful histogram-based segmentation it may be useful to apply smoothing filters prior to segmentation.

6.13.2 Manual Segmentation – Creating Regions of Interest

The decision which pixels belong to the features of interest (objects) or reside outside the boundary of the objects can be taken interactively by an expert user, who has extensive knowledge about the features. The user interactively decides what is of interest and applies judgment of what features should be included in the selection, which can be based on regions of similarity, boundaries, and texture. Many visualization and segmentation packages offer brush tools with different diameters and either circular or square shape that a user can use for pixel selection.

Regions can be identified that belong to the same biological category, whether that category being a cell, an organelle, or a supramolecular complex in their respective image environment. Manual segmentation is a very labor-intensive endeavor and thus is only feasible for small datasets/regions. Furthermore, it is always vulnerable to the criticism of being subjective, meaning that the user may only select what conveniently fits with prior expectations, however, the brain is unsurpassed in detecting patterns and in considering larger region trends, which has proven helpful for filament selection in a high-noise environment.

Hybrid approaches exist that combine manual painting with computer-assisted detection of regions of feature similarity and edges, and thus highly sophisticated programs allow a combination of multiple segmentation approaches to be used simultaneously or sequentially to extract the features of interest and to curate the pixel selection until the best segmentation result has been accomplished (Figure 6.43). Brush tools can be of great help for including active contours, graph cuts, or region-growing approaches (including level sets), as the brush provides seed points, which can serve as starting points for the automated algorithms.

Also, a brush can be used to select regions that have been determined by the computer software package as similar to one another (by watershed segmentation and/or by edge detection). Brushes can also be used to correct local mislabeling by the automated approaches. The higher the magnification, the smaller the regions, and hence regions are broken up into several smaller regions, which then can be selected. The curated selection can then be considered the ground truth for ML approaches or are the benchmark against which all other automated forms of pixel selection must be compared.

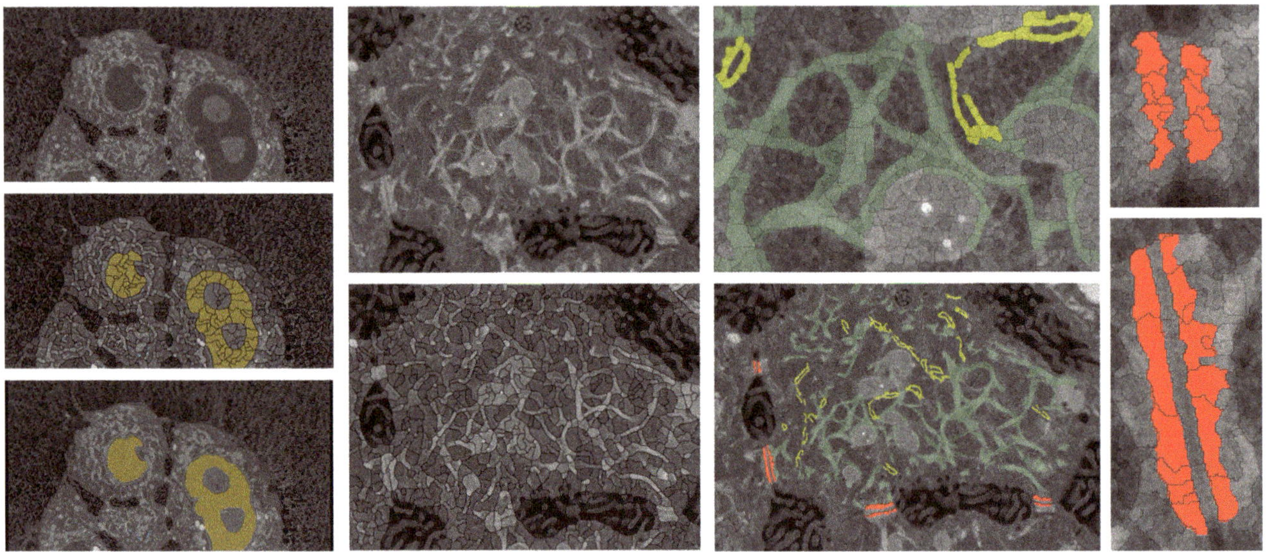

Figure 6.43 Image segmentation – Manual painting combined with watershed segmentation. Effective segmentation of a 3D volume of a human mammary gland acinus by a combination of manual painting and watershedding. Left column: Segmentation of the nucleus (golden), Middle panels: Original image, watershed segmentation of different regions. Manual segmentation of such regions of the cytoskeleton (green), internal membrane system (yellow) and cell–cell adhesion complexes (red). Right column: Close-up view of cell–cell adhesion complexes. Note the object boundaries are identified automatically by the ORS Dragonfly visualization package based on water shedding, whereas the the decision, which regions to be chosen for segmentation is taken interactively by an expert user.

6.13.3 Automated Segmentation

Automated segmentation is still one of the hardest tasks in the field of image processing/analysis. Most classical approaches are procedural in nature, meaning that algorithms with specific instruction for the detection of region, edges, and texture have been developed.

Most segmentation approaches are based on either similarity of pixels inside a region or discontinuities between different regions, which would correspond to region-based or edge-based segmentation approaches, respectively. Many of these approaches compare pixels only locally, and once a similarity criterion is satisfied, the pixels are grouped together. Texture-based approaches take larger regions and their higher-level occurring patterns into consideration. Some region-growing segmentation approaches require seeds from which the region can grow. Regions are iteratively grown by comparing pixels to the mean of their neighborhood's pixels, so they can be assigned to a region. This process is repeated until all pixels are allocated. It should be noted that noise is the enemy of such clustering and region-growing algorithms, as it may be hard to establish an appropriate similarity criterion. Commonly used methods are based on a combination of region growing and region merging, including clustering, as well as of edge detection and active curve/surface motion (active contours) (Figure 6.44).

Region-Growing: *k*-Means Clustering

The process of grouping data points that fulfill certain characteristic similarity criteria (such as a combination of pixel intensity value, color, texture, location) is called clustering, and can be used for segmentation. Clustering approaches do not require seeds to be provided, but clusters organize themselves according to criteria of similarity.

k-means clustering assumes random cluster centers in a feature space, and then goes through an iterative process separating samples into groups of equal variances, minimizing a criterion known as the inertia or within cluster sum of squares. After conversion of the algorithm *k*-means can be used to divide an image into a defined number of meaningful regions (Figure 6.45). Success depends on the correct choice of the initial set of clusters. Note that the number of clusters has to be specified a priori. Mean shift clustering does not require such specification and can provide clusters with irregular shape.

Region-Growing: Graph Cut

Graph cut/partition methods borrow tools from graph theory. Graph partitioning approaches allow the identification of regions in an image, which are homogeneous with respect to texture and contrast. Images are represented by graphs with nodes and edges, and pixels are then associated with such nodes and edges (Figure 6.46).

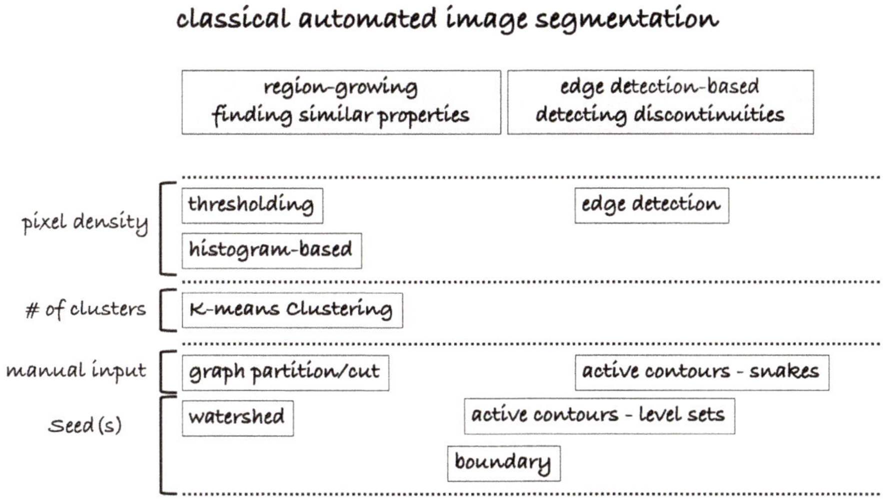

Figure 6.44 Classical automated image segmentation. There are a variety of classical approaches for automated segmentation that are either based on region growing for pixels with similar properties or on edges/boundaries, where discontinuities are being detected. Simple thresholding or histogram-based approaches, as well as K-means clustering, or graph partition/cuts fall in the first category as does watershed segmentation. Examples for the detection of discontinuities are edge detection, active contour snakes. Active contour level sets and boundary segmentation use elements of both strategies.

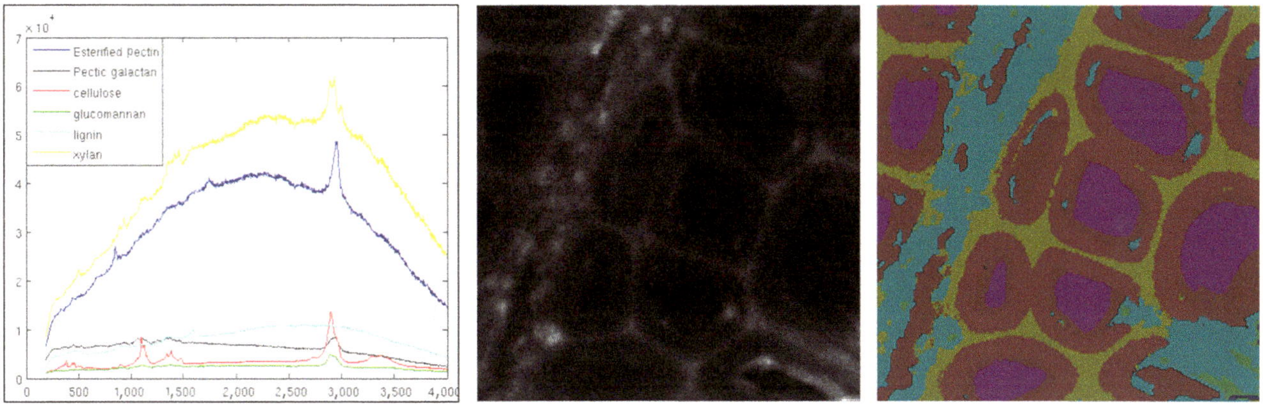

Figure 6.45 Clustering methods. Left: Raman spectrum of pure compounds known to reside in plant cell wall; Middle: Raman image of thin sections of plant tissue; Right: Regions of self-similarities in the Raman spectrum of the Raman image using k-means clustering and graph cut.

Spatial features of interest are usually marked up by a user, who will mark up certain image regions with a simple stroke. The computer then uses the information of the pixels that were selected by these simple strokes to assign a probability for all other pixels to belong to the selected category (which is then called foreground) or to be part of the background. Those pixels that fall into the category foreground are then grouped together, and the background pixels are cut away, which then also defines the boundary of the segmented object. There can be several categories defined by the user for which the user provides simple stroke examples. Texture features can also be extracted by a bank of Gabor filters, which are linear filters for texture analysis. Regions of self-similarities are detected in this approach and used for segmentation.

Edge-Based Segmentation

As an alternative to region-based approaches one can also utilize the fact that the different regions are separated from one another by some sort of boundary, a discontinuity in whatever was used as a similarity criterion in the region-based approach. Two different regions corresponding to two different objects may have distinct intensity values, color, or texture. Hence rather than focusing on what pixels in a region have in common, edge-based approaches focuses on describing the boundary between two different regions.

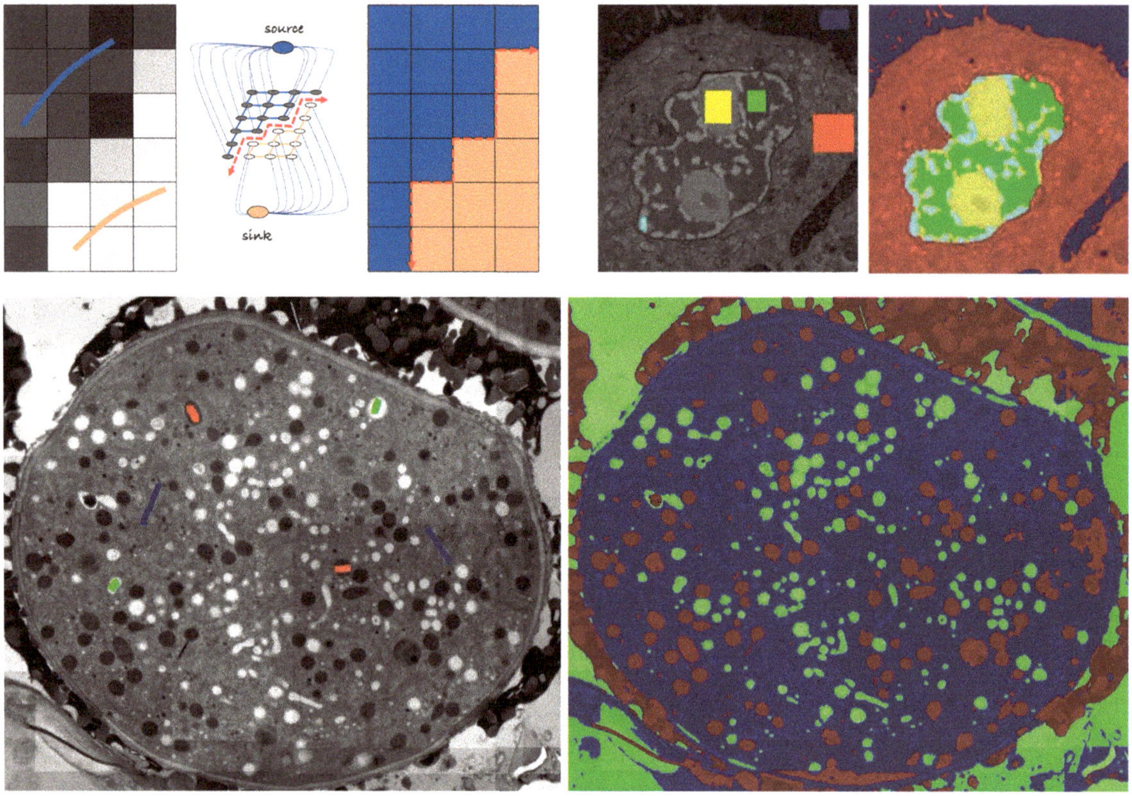

Figure 6.46 Region growing: Graph cut. Top row, left panels: Schematic depiction of graph cut. After manual assignment of different regions, other pixels are predicted to either belong in the same category (foreground) or they are considered background; Top row, right panels: Graph cut segmentation of a eukaryotic cell: yellow, green, and cyan annotations of different regions of the nucleus, annotation of a large portion of the cytoplasm (red) leads to a categorization of three regions of the nucleus as well as the cytoplasm: Bottom row: application of graph cut to a yeast cell, with the cytoplasm being depicted in blue, dark features as red and light features as green.

Edge-detection filters have been a classical way to detect boundaries. Due to the nature of the edge detection algorithm, edges that are detected are local (neighboring pixels), and they may also be disconnected. In other words, they do not fully enclose a region, which may render the delineation of a region solely based on the detection of its edges somewhat difficult.

The Hough transform is an efficient way to detect straight lines, circles and other simple shapes that can be easily parameterized. Line segment detection then leads to coherent curves. Edge integration is the process of combining local edges with long edge curves for segmentation, whose length is then minimized.

Algorithms that can detect gradients can also discriminate propagation across a gradient from propagation along a gradient. They lay at the heart of active contours (curve/surface motion) with snakes and level sets as their mathematical implementations.

Edge-Based Segmentation: Edge Detection

Regions are characterized by boundaries, where intensity sharply changes. The detection of such edges with a steep gradient of intensity value changes can be used for segmentation, as edge detection provides location, direction, and strength of such local steep-gradient positions (Figure 6.47). Sobel edge detection is a widely used algorithm. Two other prominent edge detection algorithms have been proposed by Canny and Prewitt.

Active Contours: Snakes

Active contours are widely utilized image segmentation approaches that produce regions with continuous boundaries, whereas for example Sobel edge detectors often produce disconnected boundaries. Active contours use numerical algorithms for solving PDE, which are used for the evolution of curves/surfaces. Typically, a cost function is optimized, i.e., by using an energy minimization scheme, to determine curve evolution.

Snakes are predefined parametrized curves/surfaces which are pulled toward boundaries such as lines and edges by image forces, while simultaneously resisting deformation by internal forces. As a result, active contours attach themselves to the objects' boundaries. This works best when the contours are already placed near such

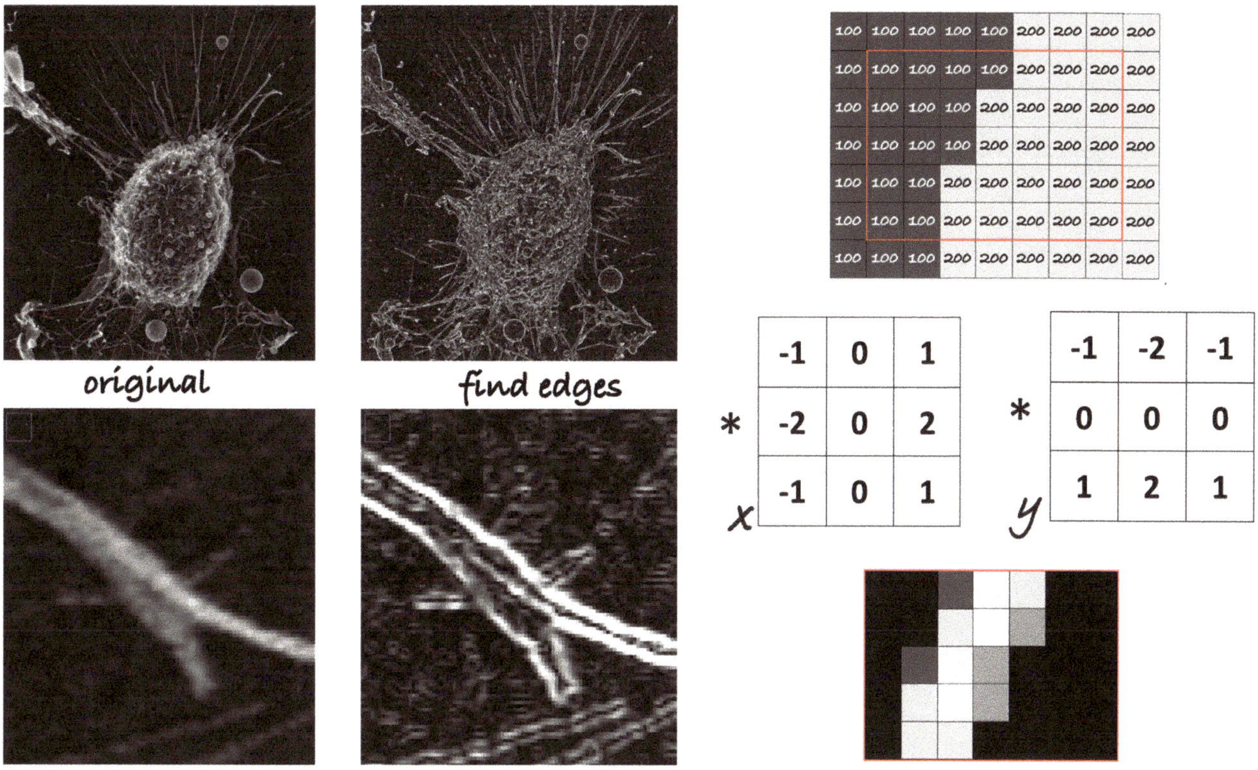

Figure 6.47 Edge detection. Edges are regions in an image where there is a steep gradient of the pixel intensity value. By applying suitable kernels in *X* and in *Y*, one can emphasize such boundary regions. Note that edge detection significantly alters the image, and thus should only be used as a diagnostic tool to find edges and not part of an image processing pipeline.

boundaries (Figure 6.48). The algorithm may start with a very coarse outline of the object, which then moves toward the object of interest in the form of active contours (contour evolution). Such contours are iteratively modified by shrinkage or expansion using traditional region-based approaches, or they are based on PDE energy cost function optimization.

Looking for big intensity jumps (steep gradients) in an image can be an effective way to find the boundary of an object. However, defining what constitutes a big jump is more difficult, as too small of a value will find too many boundaries, whereas too large of a jump will not detect any boundary. This is even more complicated if there are large noise spikes. In the Mumford–Shah segmentation approach

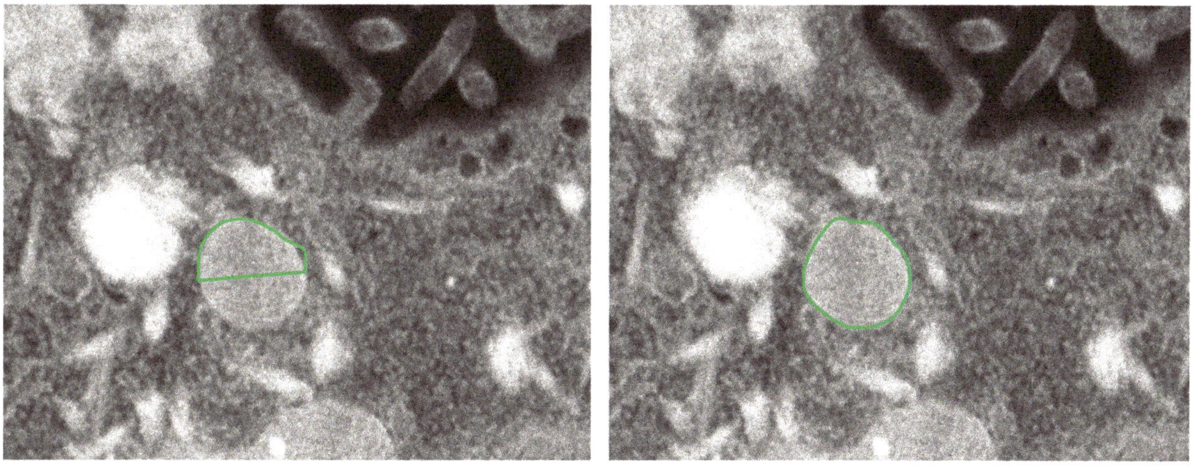

Figure 6.48 Active contours. Active contours are curves being placed somewhat near the edge of an object. By contour evolution they attach themselves to the boundary and allow the object to be selected for segmentation.

a compromise is reached by penalizing many errors as well as penalizing too many edges, hence obtaining a reasonably accurate depiction of the object of interest without many tiny details.

Snakes move open or closed 2D curves/surfaces explicitly, whereas level sets are implicit 3D surfaces and move contours implicitly as a particular level (zero-level). Snakes can segment one component, whereas level sets can segment multiple components and allow more flexibility and convenience in the implementation of active contours. Compared to classical feature extraction, snakes have the advantages that they search for a minimum state, however, among the shortcomings of snakes are that they are sensitive to local minima, and that they tend to ignore small features since the energy minimization occurs over the entire contour. Also, snakes do not react well to sudden changes in curve changes.

Active Contours: Level Sets

The level set approach, first proposed in 1988 by Osher and Sethian is one of the more frequently used approaches for image segmentation. From a small area (seed) inside the region of an object, e.g., a circle (a balloon) is allowed to grow outwards until it reaches a boundary, between the inside and the outside of an object. So, while it has some elements of region-growing, the main aspect is the detection of a boundary that slows and possibly even stops the expansion. The basic idea is that level sets are curves or surfaces as the zero-level set of a higher dimensional hypersurface. There is no change along the level set and maximal change perpendicular to the level set, which allows the filling of a curve as an envelope of the object of interest (Figure 6.49). Level set approaches have numerous advantages over other approaches, e.g., it is parameter-free, implicit and provides a direct way to determine the geometric properties of an evolving structure.

The "Fast Marching" method is a simplified and faster variant of the traditional level set method. Once a seed has been chosen, a contour is allowed to grow until a certain stopping condition is reached. However, the algorithm does not have an explicit stopping criterion, which is why the computationally more expensive level set method is used for finalizing the segmentation.

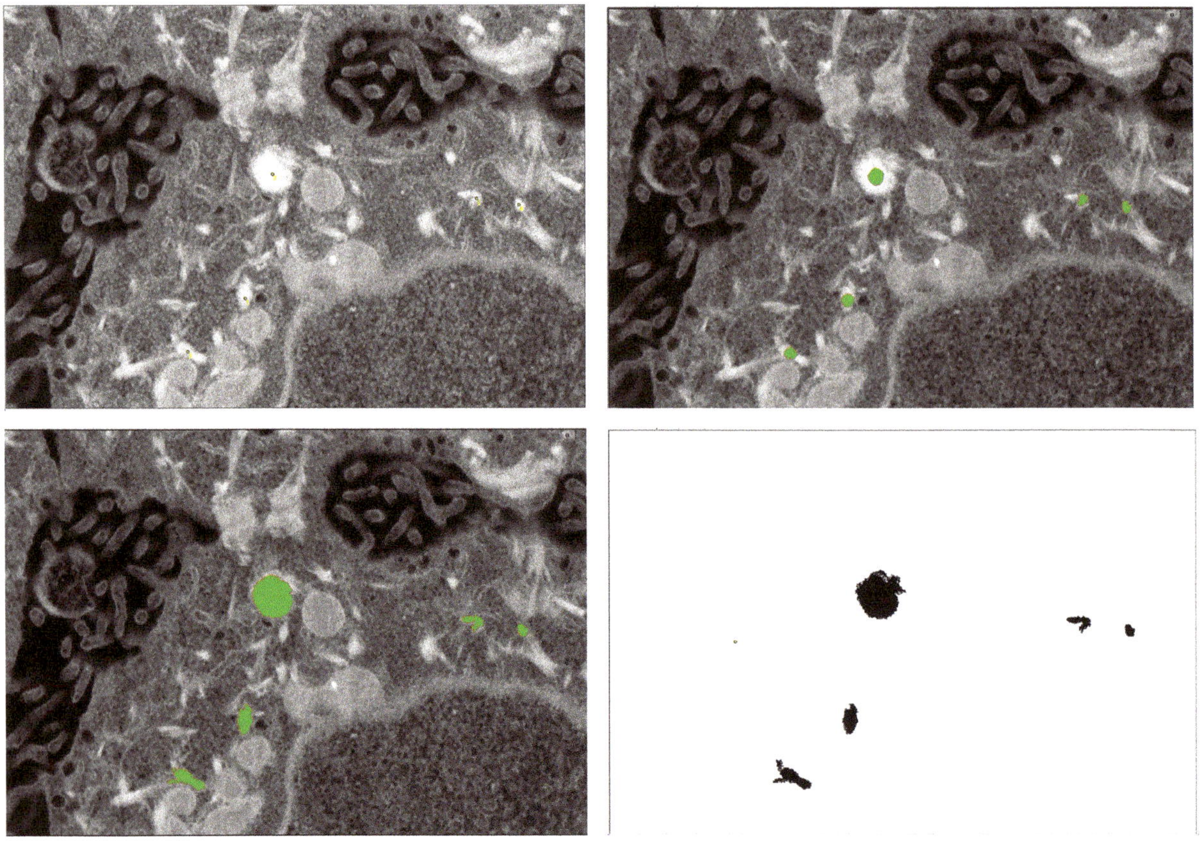

Figure 6.49 Level set method. In the level set method, a user identifies seeds within regions (objects) for segmentation. In the popular Fast Marching method, these seeds will expand with the expansion slowing down near the object's boundary. Once the boundary has been reached a level set is established as the curve where one crosses from the inside of an object to the outside, which stops the expansion process and leads to the segmentation of the object. Note that in this example, dark color in the bottom right panel refers to the segmented volume, whereas white refers to the background of the segmentation.

The speed function of the "Fast Marching" method depends on the image gradient, where initially contours expand fast in places where the image gradient is small and slows down its expansion where the image gradient becomes large (near the boundary). At the boundary one establishes a level set that defines the curve where one crosses from the inside of the object to the outside of the object. While the concept was initially invented for 2D images, it has been easily extended to 3D, as one simply replaces curves by surfaces that are then evolved (propagated) in 3D instead of 2D.

Watershed-Based Segmentation

A watershed refers to a drainage divide, which separates adjacent drainage basins. Watershed segmentation can be understood in terms of a topographic terrain map (profile), with the intensity/density map's high and low values representing peaks and valleys. If one now assumes that the topographic profile is put upside down, then the peaks become the depressions in the terrain (Figure 6.50).

Let us now assume that it rains, and the holes are filling up with water, there will be a point where the water from two neighboring holes would merge, at which point a wall (watershed) is erected that will prevent the waters to mix. Instead, the two regions will retain their separate identities, which forms the basis of segmentation. Where such watersheds are erected depends not only on the profile but also on how much water is allowed to fill the hole before one decides to erect a watershed. Too little rain will result in too many different segments, and thus to over-segmentation, whereas choosing too coarse of a step size will produce only a few regions of flooding, with many peaks being combined into one region.

Boundary Segmentation

Boundary segmentation works with gradient vector fields rather than actual grayscale intensities. Boundary segmentation is based on the fast-marching method for curve/surface propagation. Seed points (so-called critical points) are chosen by finding maxima and minima of the gradient vector field, where surrounding vector points point toward or away from these critical points. Also saddle points are determined where surrounding vectors from both sides point toward these points along one direction, whereas in other direction they point away from these points. This results in three classes of critical points, namely feature seed points (high intensity), background seed points (low intensity), and saddle points. In comparison, watershed segmentation only uses one type of seed points (maxima), from where contours propagate. In boundary segmentation, we start with dual contours, one starting from feature seeds and one starting from background seeds. Both contours propagate until they encounter one another at a boundary, an idea that is similar to the multi-label fast marching method for motion analysis in video image processing. Meeting of the dual contours provides a convenient

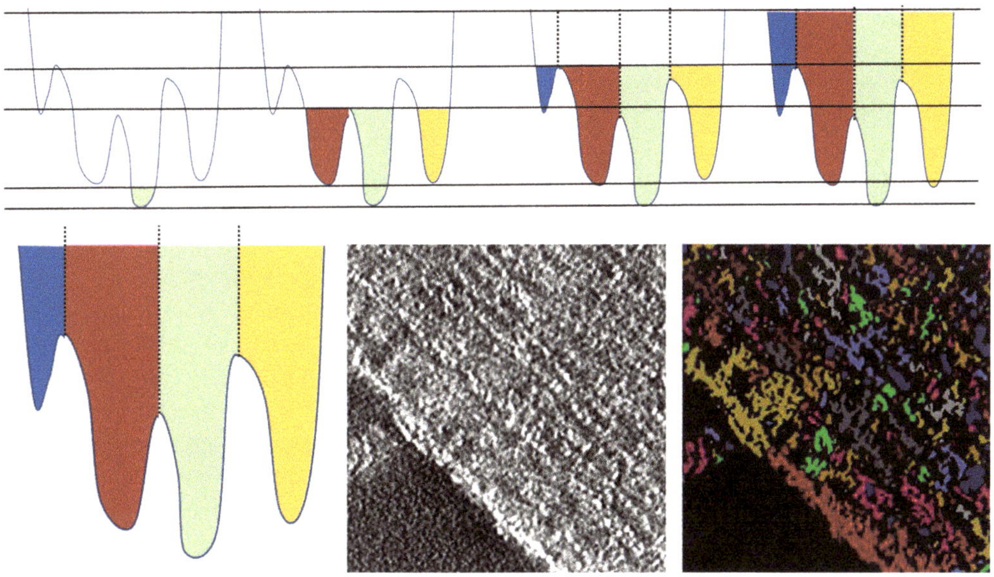

Figure 6.50 Watershed segmentation. Watershed segmentation starts with the highest peaks of grayscale intensity (displayed upside down) and assigns each of them an identity (color). As the intensity threshold is lowered additional peaks emerge, which will also be assigned a unique identity. Further lowering of the intensity threshold will result in two regions with different identity to meet, at which point a watershed is erected that will keep the two neighboring regions as regions with different identity (color). As a result, the volume is segmented. Note that choosing the correct step size for lowering of the intensity threshold is important as too small of a step size results in over-segmentation (too many regions), whereas too big of a step size results in few segmented volumes of large size.

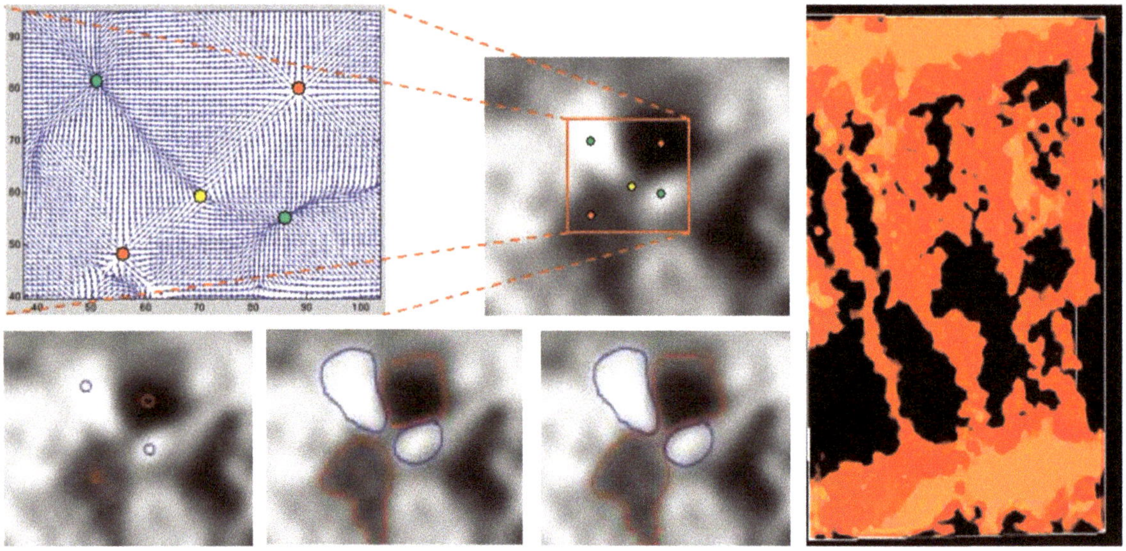

Figure 6.51 Boundary segmentation. Prior to boundary segmentation on needs to determine the intensity gradients in the image, which leads to seed points (high intensity points, shown in green/blue), background seed points (low intensity points, shown in red) as well as saddle points (shown in yellow). From these seed points, regions are allowed to grow until they meet another region. When regions grown from seeds points meet one another they are allowed to merge, whereas a boundary is erected where regions grown from feature seed points meet with regions grown from background seed points. An example of boundary segmentation is shown on the right depicting kinociliary links in sacculus frog inner ear hair bundles.

stopping criterion, namely at a boundary with maximal image gradient (Figure 6.51). The marching process used in boundary segmentation is analogous to the immersion process in watershedding, but the additional feature of the image gradient is taken into account. In addition, boundary segmentation allows merging of similar contours that started from different seeds at the saddle points, which helps to reduce the issue of oversegmentation, which is often found in the watershed immersion method.

Machine Learning- and Deep Learning-Based Segmentation

A whole different category for segmentation is ML which is part of the more general term artificial intelligence (AI). AI goes back to the late 1950s and the 1960s, with ML starting to flourish by the 1990s.

ML programs can perform tasks such as image segmentation, without being given explicit programming instructions (also referred to as feature engineering). Instead, ML algorithms build data models and learn the rules needed for the task by being given many annotated images, known as ground truth. Based on those learned rules, it can classify data based on these data models created and make predictions for data that were not part of the training set.

ML approaches are divided into supervised learning, where a user provides inputs and desired outputs, and unsupervised learning, where the learning algorithm perform cluster analysis in the images without prior training input by a user, based on the similarities of regions detected in the image. Care must be taken to provide sufficient variation of the feature to obtain a robust classification tool.

Supervised ML approaches learn what works best for segmentation by iteratively comparing their segmentation results with user-provided examples of desired segmentation outcome (ground truth), which trains the neural networks. The more examples can be provided, the more sophisticated the learning result and thus the more accurate the predictions will be.

Classical Neural Networks (including Random Forest models) with their feedforward neural network architecture have no understanding of the relationships of pixels in their vicinity. One popular free software package for ML is "Weka" (Waikato Environment for Knowledge Analysis) that was developed at the University of Waikato in New Zealand. Weka was the companion software to the book "Data Mining: Practical Machine Learning Tools and Techniques." The Weka software features a variety of algorithms for data analysis and predictive modeling as well as some visualization tools. Figure 6.52 shows the Weka software applied to a large volume electron microscopy data of a bacterial biofilms, which contains bacteria and extracellular metal deposits of various shapes. The Weka was able to classify these features and discriminate them from the background.

As an example of how classification can work for determining orientation of a feature, one can devise

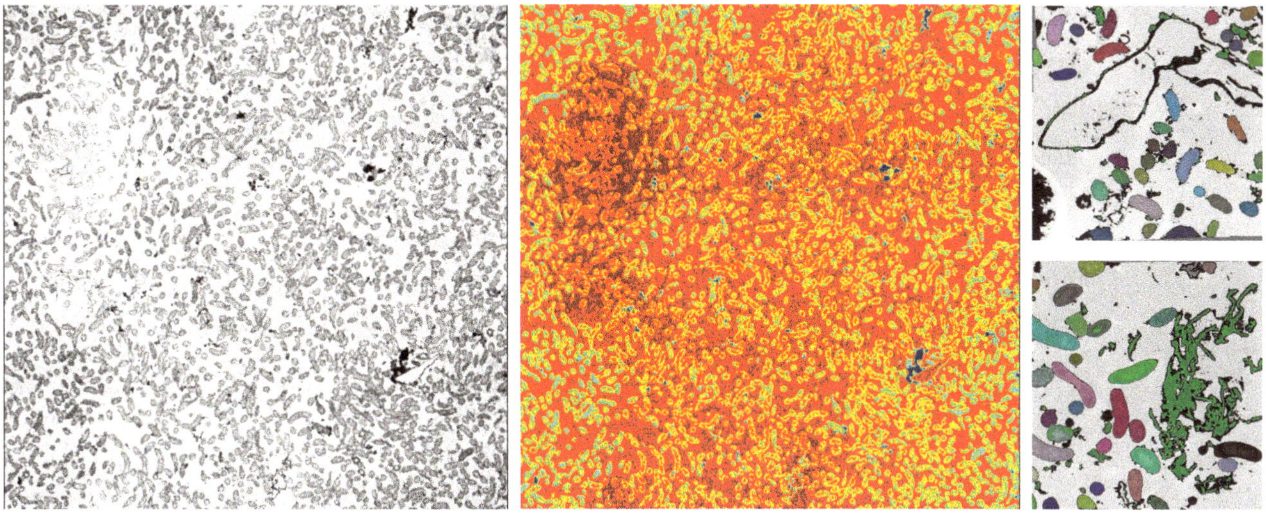

Figure 6.52 Machine learning – Large volume of a *Desulfovibrio vulgaris* (bacterial) biofilm analyzed by Weka. A large volume of ~5,000 × 5,000 × 10,000 voxel volume depicting a bacterial biofilm with extracellular metal deposits was analyzed the Waikato Environment for Knowledge Analysis (Weka) software package. Weka learns from the examples given and develops a probabilistic model for all other features, and thus predicts to which category (bacteria, background or metal deposits) they belong. This allows an automatic segmentation of the large volume. It uses several linear filters and shape parameters such as area, *k*-means and distances.

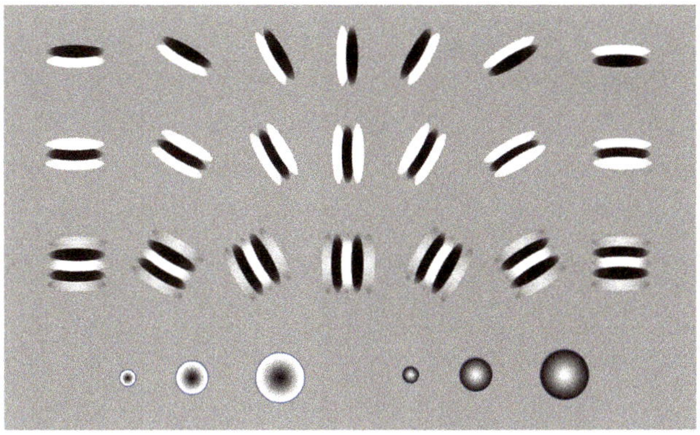

Figure 6.53 Machine learning – Orientation classification model. By providing different kernels (with the algorithms being presented here graphically), one can create an orientation classification model that allows detection of orientation for different features in an image.

algorithms that lead to an orientation classification model (Figure 6.53). Application of the orientation classification model to features of an image allows features with different orientation to be detected and classified.

Deep Learning (DL) refers to ML techniques with a deep, multi-layered architecture of neural networks that learn effective representation of data at multiple levels of abstraction. In contrast to ML, where representations are manually designed (feature engineering), DL chooses its own set of functions that best allow the differentiation of the objects of interest from its surroundings. Many computer architectures for CNN have a large variety of presets of functions for pixel-based and region-based training, which allows the CNN to learn what constitutes the best segmentation result.

Neural networks lie at the heart of DL, and they were introduced to mimic the way a human brain would process information, with neurons being organized into a variety of layers, with each layer performing a different kind of transformation of its input. Such neural networks are often referred to as artificial neural networks (ANN), and specifically convolutional neural networks (CNN) or deep neural networks (DNN), consisting of multiple layers of inter-connected nodes that are parameterized by weights between 0 and 1. In CNN, each layer of processing uses the data representation created by the previous layer and affect subsequent layers (Figure 6.54). Typically, the first set of layers in the CNN identifies lower-level features whereas the last set of layers can lead to a higher-level understanding of image features and texture. As a result, DL can find non-linear, complex correlations between pixels, which is needed for object detection. Therefore, DL is in many ways superior to classical ML, leading to a higher accuracy for segmentation.

U-net was the first and remains one of the better-known CNN used for image segmentation of biological imaging data. Originally developed to detect cell borders in biological imaging, U-net and DeepCell (another DL package) classify objects in an image at the pixel-level and assigning a probability prediction for each pixel of the input image (e.g., by labeling a pixel as belonging to the cytoplasm, cell membrane, mitochondria, or nucleus). Figure 6.55 shows the result of a U-net-based deep learning segmentation of a

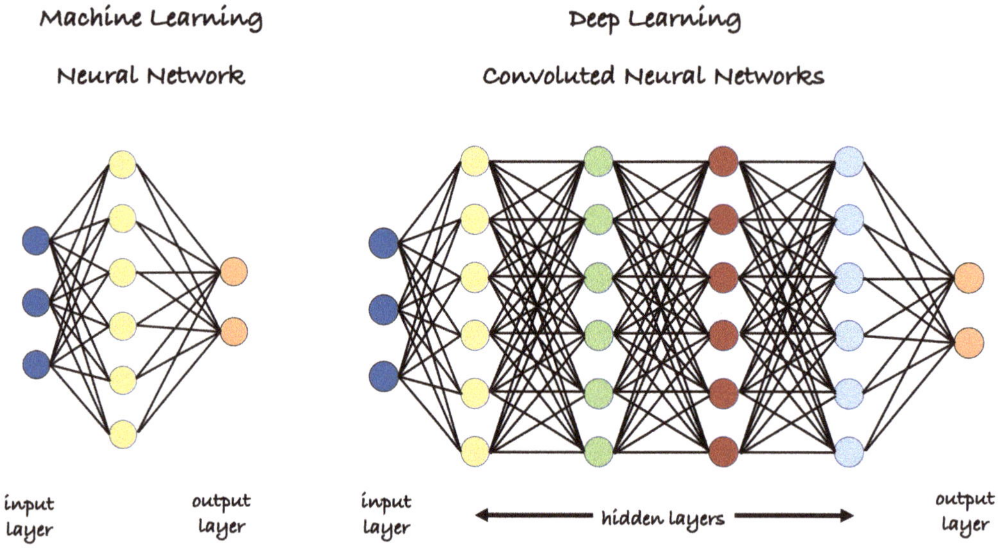

Figure 6.54 Machine learning and deep learning. Machine learning refers to the ability of computer programs to learn from experience without being explicitly programmed. DL, which is one form of machine learning, has many hidden layers of algorithms in convolutional neural networks (CNN). CNN, which are inspired by signal processing in the human brain, are much more complex than conventional neural networks used in classical machine learning approaches. Due to their complexity, CNN allow a higher-level understanding of image features, and thus often show better performance.

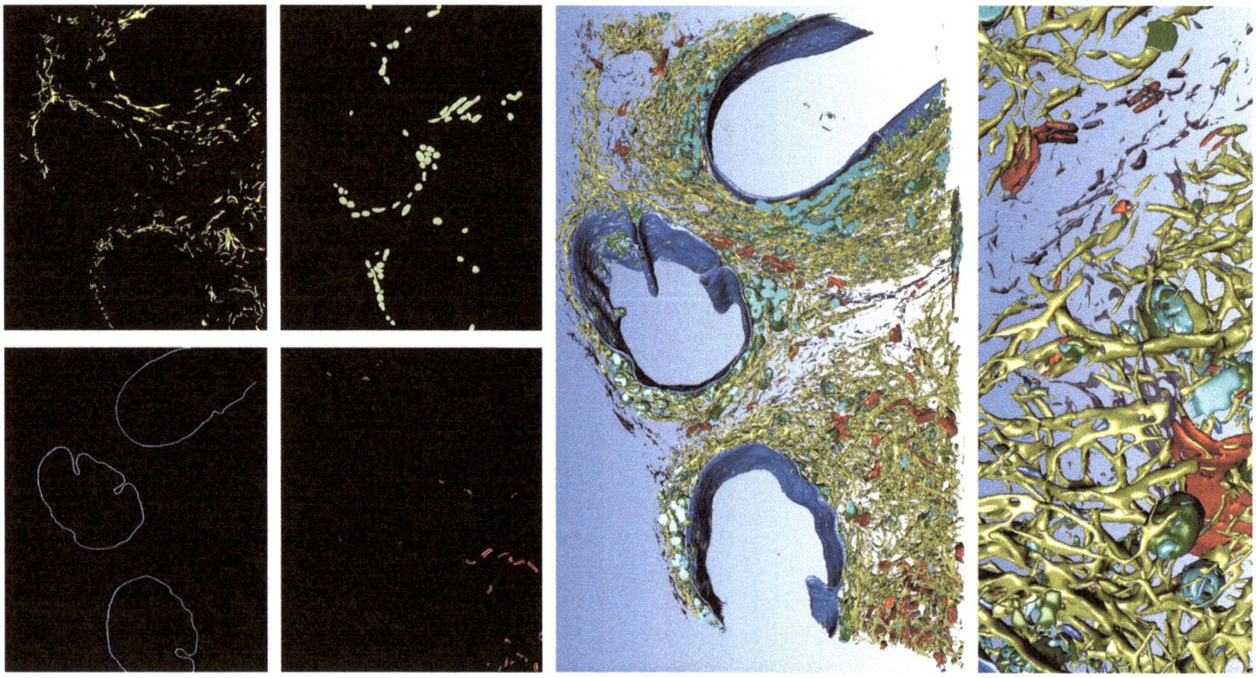

Figure 6.55 Deep learning – U-net based segmentation of large cellular 3D volumes. Based on a relatively small training dataset of manually segmented individual slices, a U-net based segmentation algorithm as part of the ORS Dragonfly deep learning module was able to automatically segment a 3D volume of the human breast cancer progression model system S1-acini.

cellular large volume dataset, recorded by focused ion beam scanning electron microscopy of premalignant human breast cell acini.

DL requires less human intervention to learn as it can learn from its own mistakes. However, DL requires a large training datasets, whereas classical ML can train on smaller datasets. Furthermore, DL is computationally more demanding as it trains on GPU, where ML usually can train in a CPU.

Results from classical automated image segmentation approaches as well as ML need to be compared to the so-called ground truth (typically obtained by an expert's manual segmentation). Criteria for comparison are accuracy (the fraction of pixels that were classified correctly), false/true positive (incorrectly/correctly predicted positive class) as well false/true negative rates (incorrectly/correctly predicted the negative class). Model accuracy is calculated from precision (true positive divided by the number of all positive) versus recall (true positive divided by the number of all that should have been positive). Precision is also referred to as positive predicted value, whereas recall is referred to as sensitivity.

Like it is the case for any other approach in computer science, attention must be paid to the generalization (the ability of an algorithm to perform well on data that has not been part of the training data set), the problem of overfitting and underfitting of parameters, as well as its performance, typically referred to precision versus recall.

The following list serves as a starting point for researching and choosing the appropriate DL packages, such as U-Net, CellProfiler, Cell Cognition Explorer, DeepCell, CDeep3M, Mask R-CNN, DeepLabCut, uTrack, TrackMate, but undoubtedly many more packages are available and/or will become in the future.

Another application of DL, besides image classification and image segmentation, is object tracking, which is the task of following objects through a series of time-lapse images. This requires object detection and object linkage.

Motion-Based Segmentation

Segmentation is an ill-posed problem in computer science, and besides the approaches discussed above, there are additional ways an object can be distinguished from its surrounding, including motion of an object versus a static (or slower moving) background, in which case compression-based approaches can be used for segmentation. In this approach, a comparison of adjacent frames of time-dependent image series and thus the difference between image pairs will discriminate objects that are moving with respect to their surroundings.

6.14 Making Changes to Object Selection: Dilation, Erosion, Closing, Filling Holes

Once a region of interest has been selected, and the outline for a feature of interest has been determined by any of the methods described above, there are additional tools that allow a user to further make changes to the suggestions made by the various algorithms. A user may decide to further expand (using dilation) or shrink (using erosion) the envelope of the object to better fit the envelope to the densities (Figure 6.56). Also, a combination of dilation and subsequent erosion can be used to fill small internal holes in an object, that the user knows not to be an actual significant feature of the object but instead an artifact. Furthermore, an expert on the biological topic may recognize that certain features that have been identified as separate objects are part of the same object and thus the segmented densities should be merged.

6.15 Measurements/Quantitative Analysis

Frequently, visualization of a segmented volume is the last step in a long pipeline of image processing. Much care is spent on using photorealistic rendering and ray-tracing tools of high-end visualization packages to create figures for publication and movies as supplemental material, often with the object being shown from multiple orientations, and/or spinning around one or several axes. The idea seems to be that the nicer the rendering and the more sophisticated the movie, the higher the chance to be chosen as the journal cover art, and the more impressive seem the results for other researchers and the lay public.

However, over the last decade efforts have increased to go beyond the pretty pictures (and movies), and to use images not just as eye candy to support a foregone conclusion, but to take images as the source for measurements and for phenotype classification. Certain properties of segmented 2D and 3D images (volumes) are straightforward to quantify, such as number of bacterial colonies on a culture plate, the number of cells in solution or on a surface, or the number of speckles in an image, as one simply need to count the segmented objects. Likewise, intensity minimum, maximum and mean, as well as area, volume, or center of mass for the segmented objects can literally be counted and analyzed measured pixel by pixel.

Other measurements require the fitting of a geometric (2D) or volumetric (3D) model to the segmented object (Figure 6.57), which then can yield perimeter length, diameter length, major and minor axes ratios, surface area, and thus some information about shape. However, shape information can be more complicated to assess quantitatively and may require additional tools used in statistical shape analysis.

Often, the segmented pixel/voxel data alone is insufficient to get to the higher-level analysis. There are other types of phenotype classification, including the study of intensity patterns, of branching behavior, of spatial relationships, including object distribution, co-localization, as well as the study of texture is needed.

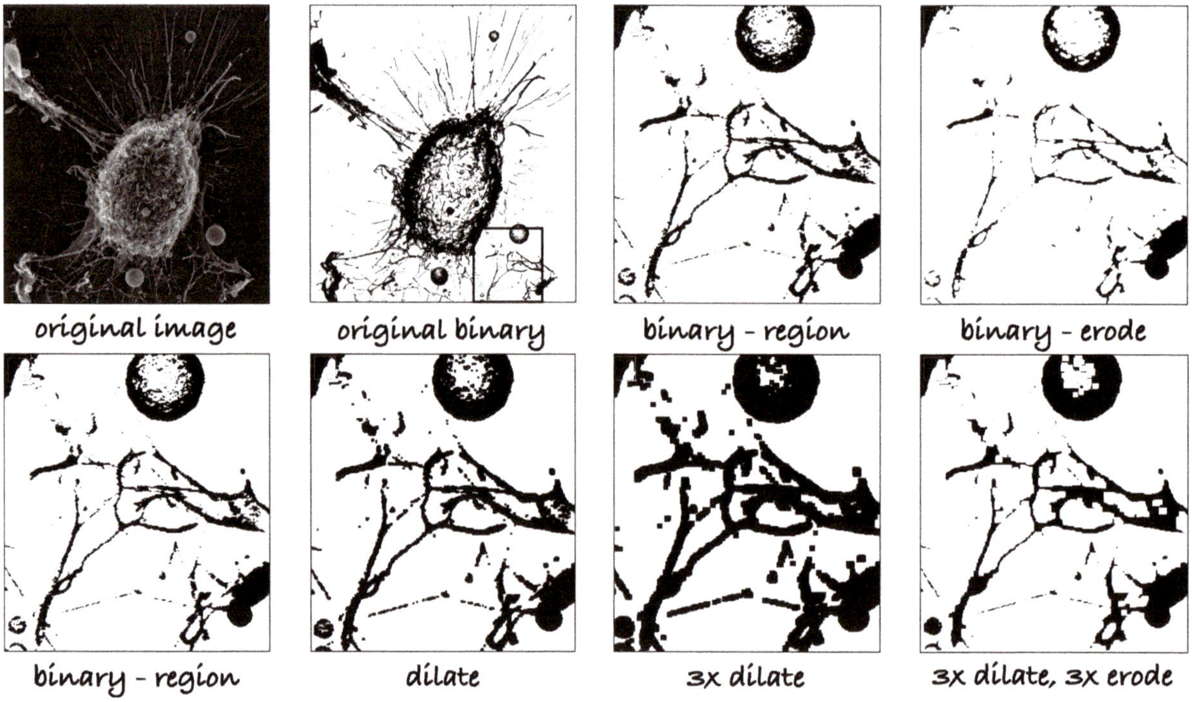

Figure 6.56 Making changes to the object selection. Top: Thresholding an image leads to a binary representation of features of interest (above a certain density threshold value). Zooming in on a smaller region, reveals continuous feature strands. On the right, the binary image was eroded, which leads to the loss of connections between certain regions that were formerly connected; Bottom: Dilation of the binary region, results in thick connections, repeated dilation even in thicker connections. A combination of three times dilation followed by three-times erosion is shown, which seems like a fair (but not identical) representation of the original binary region. Note that the order in which dilation and erosion are carried out matters, as three times erosion followed by three times dilation would have resulted in the near complete loss of features (not shown).

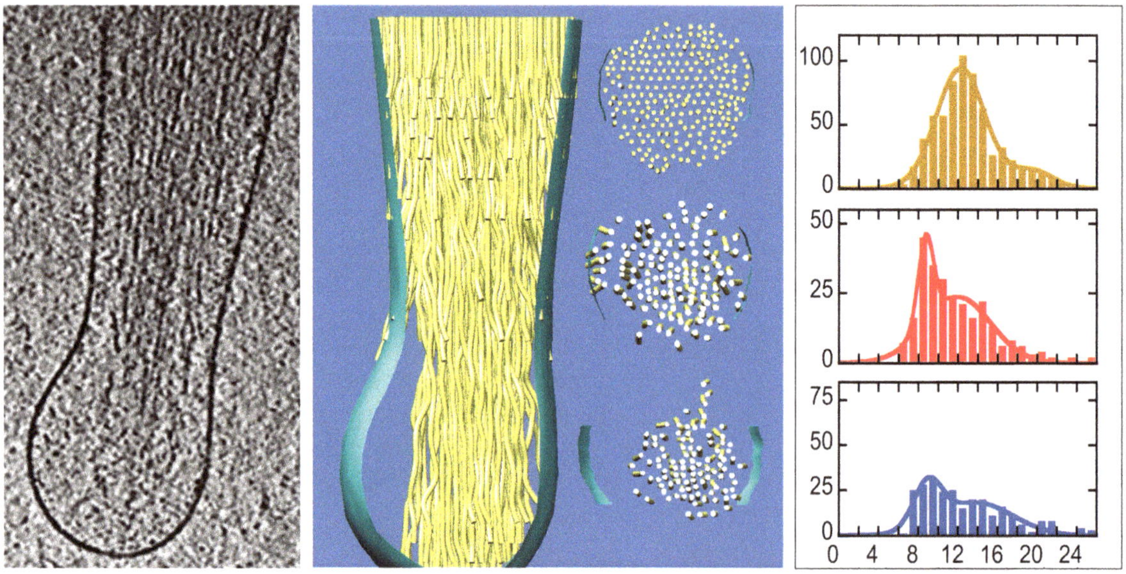

Figure 6.57 Model building and quantitative analysis. Quantification of some data sets require the building of a volumetric model that recapitulate certain features of the data. Shown here is a ball-and-stick model (yellow) that have been built into the actin-filament density map of a cryo-electron tomogram of the taper and rootlet region of mouse inner ear hair cell stereocilia. Once a volumetric model has been obtained, inter-filament distances (right) can be easily calculated, and their distribution can be statistically analyzed. Furthermore, the orientation and potential curved path of such filaments can be much better appreciated.

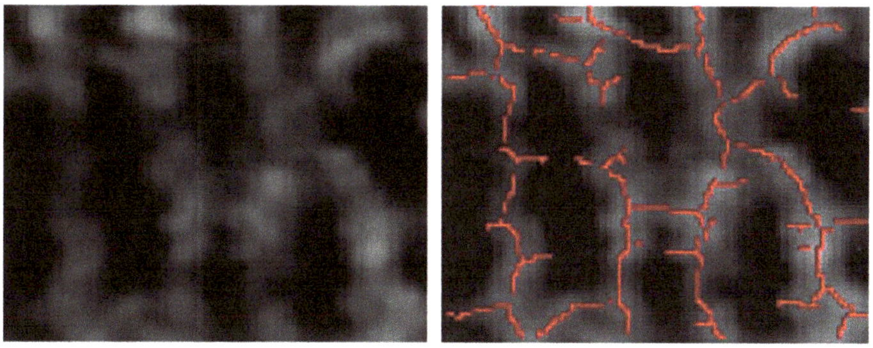

Figure 6.58 Skeletonization. After segmentation, skeletons of filamentous features can be automatically determined. Such skeletons are a highly simplified representation of the feature density and can help for quantification and further mathematical analysis.

Skeletonization of segmented objects provides a highly simplified representation of the feature density (Figure 6.58), which can also help in quantitative analysis, and may be accessible to further analysis such as graph theory.

Furthermore, semantic description, possibly via use of a controlled vocabulary may be necessary to describe tissue, cellular and subcellular organization. Additional analysis may include tracking (the following of moving objects over time), which relies on the identification of the objects of interest via segmentation and the connection of objects from frame to frame (linking). During this process it may be necessary to extract cluttered objects (untangling), based on their morphological properties and model their path during the time lapse series.

We are just at the beginning with respect to quantification of cellular volumes, with respect to shapes, interaction patterns and dynamics, and it seems safe to predict that this area will see enormous growth in the coming years and possibly decades.

7

Techniques – Macromolecular Structure Determination

Techniques discussed:

- X-ray crystallography
- Cryo-EM
- NMR spectroscopy
- SAX
- SANS
- AFM

We start in our discussion on specific techniques employed in bioimaging with methods used for macromolecular structure determination. Strictly speaking, only cryo-electron microscopy (cryo-EM) and atomic force microscopy (AFM) in this chapter use images to derive information about a biological system. X-ray crystallography relies on diffraction patterns, which technically may also be considered images (a distribution of intensities in a periodic pattern), although strictly speaking they are just intensity measurements at certain predicted locations and not continuous images.

The goal of macromolecular structure determination is also slightly different, as it is really about the building of an atomic model, with the exact knowledge of the position for every single atom, which then helps to understand an enzymatic activity or molecular interactions with another molecule in atomic detail. Figure 7.1 shows a comparison of the three predominant methods for macromolecular structure determination: X-ray crystallography, single-particle cryo-electron microscopy and nuclear magnetic resonance spectroscopy.

7.1 X-Ray Crystallography

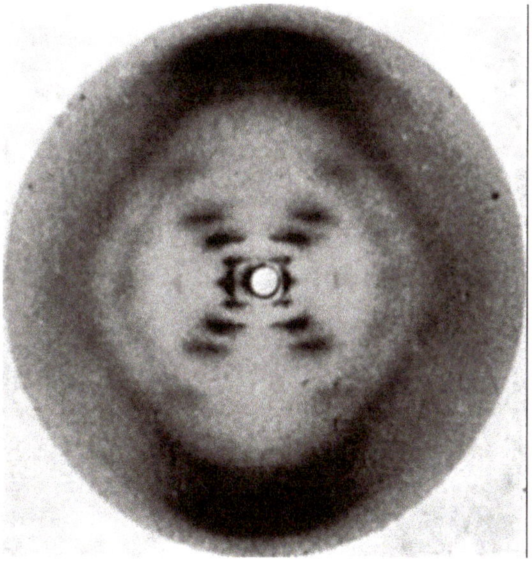

X-ray diffraction pattern of DNA, taken by Rosalind Franklin and Ray Gosling in 1952. *Source:* Raymond Gosling / King's College London.

7.1.1 Overview

The history of structural biology began in 1926 in Cambridge, UK, when William Thomas Astbury and John Desmond Bernal examined fibers (such as wool) and crystals by irradiating them with X-rays.

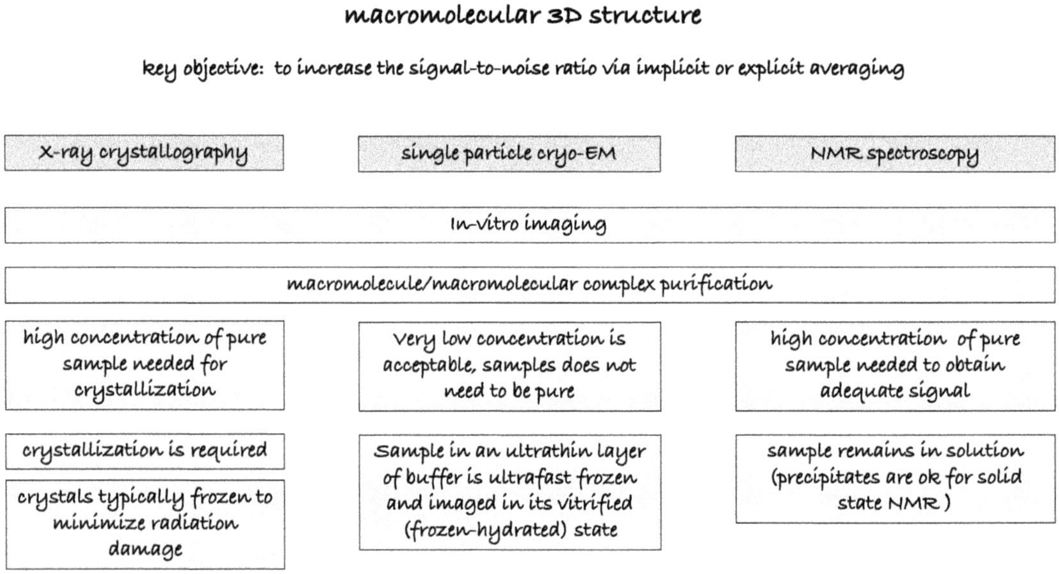

Figure 7.1 Macromolecular 3D structure. X-ray crystallography, single particle cryo-EM, and NMR spectroscopy are all in-vitro imaging approaches that rely on the purification of macromolecules/macromolecular complexes. X-ray crystallography typically relies on high concentrations of highly pure and crystallized samples, whereas single particle cryo-EM can be carried out with samples at a much lower concentration and purity (although compositional and conformational homogeneity certainly helps a lot). NMR spectroscopy requires high concentration of pure samples but allows imaging of macromolecules in solution.

X-ray diffraction is the oldest technique for structural determination, and X-ray crystallography for the longest time was considered the "gold standard" for structure determination of biological macromolecules, including nucleic acids, peptides, individual proteins and macromolecular machines. Given the scale of distances between neighboring atoms of ~5–10 Å (0.5–1 nm), X-ray radiation is the part of the electromagnetic spectrum that is needed to resolve neighboring atoms. X-ray crystallography relies on the periodic arrangement of macromolecules in form of a three-dimensional crystal, which then diffracts X-rays, resulting in discrete reflections (diffraction spots) at a high signal-to-noise ratio. The position of the spots in the diffraction pattern depends on the crystal geometry and internal symmetry as well as the rotation angle of the sample. It can be predicted with high precision. While the intensity for each reflection (and thus its amplitude) can be determined with high accuracy, the phase information, which is critical to determine the structure factor for each reflection, is lost upon detection of the diffraction spots. This is commonly known as the "phase problem" in X-ray crystallography. For structure determination to be successful, one needs good phase estimates, as they are more important than good amplitude measurements.

The use of heavy atom derivatives for multiple isomorphous replacement (MIR), multi-wavelength anomalous diffraction (MAD) phasing or molecular replacement (MR) methods have largely solved the phase problem. MAD phasing has become the dominant approach to obtain an initial phase estimate for each reflection, due to the ease of genetic engineering of protein sequencies and the tuneability of synchrotron radiation. The combination of an initial phase estimate and a high accuracy intensity (and thus amplitude) measurement leads to structure factors for each reflection with their respective h, k, and l indices, which upon Fourier transformation results in an electron density distribution as a function of the fractional XYZ coordinates of the unit cell. This electron density map is then interpreted by building an atomic-level model into the density map. It is important to opt for an incomplete model over an incorrect model, as model bias is difficult to overcome in the refinement process. From the atomic model being created one can calculate a diffraction pattern, which is then compared to the observed diffraction pattern. In this iterative process the phase estimates are being refined, resulting in improved density maps to which a better atomic model can be fitted.

Among the challenges in X-ray crystallography is the fact that the macromolecule of interest must be crystallized and that such crystals must be ordered to a high degree. Crystallization often requires the availability of tens of milligrams of highly purified and conformationally homogeneous proteins, concentrated to 1–10 mg/ml, which can constitute another difficulty for proteins that cannot be expressed at high levels or are notoriously challenging in terms of biochemical handling, such as, e.g., membrane proteins. However, as smaller crystals can be nowadays used for diffraction, sample amounts can be reduced.

Also, posttranslational modifications may be important for protein function but can also increase heterogeneity and interfere with the formation of highly ordered crystals. While the crystal structure of a protein is an exquisite starting point for determining its mechanism of function, the protein is locked into a particular conformation, and the packing into the crystal lattice can lead to conformations that are rarely adopted in solution. Hence, it is always a good idea to examine different crystal forms and ideally trap the protein into different conformations (e.g., by co-crystallization with substrate, activators, inhibitors, or macromolecule interaction partners).

Sensitivity to radiation damage upon X-ray irradiation has been largely overcome by freezing 3D crystals, allowing multiple datasets being collected from single crystals. Furthermore, the brightness of synchrotron X-ray radiation typically ensures high-quality diffraction patterns even for rather small crystals. Finally, the process of structure determination has been largely automated, which allows rapid interpretation and model building for most proteins (Figure 7.2).

7.1.2 Historical Perspective/Milestones

Discovery of X-Rays

In 1895, while experimenting with electrical discharge in partially evacuated glass tubes (also known as Crookes tubes), Wilhelm Conrad Röntgen found a new form of radiation. This radiation was able to pass through black cardboard that surrounded his Crookes tube and produced a faint green glow on a barium platinocyanide-painted screen located 1 m away. He began systematically studying this new type of radiation, which he termed X-rays. To this day, X-ray are referred to as Röntgen rays in many countries. He found that X-rays were able to penetrate a variety of materials that light could not penetrate. Most notably he created an image of his wife's hand, showing her wrist and finger bones, as well as a ring on her ring finger.

As it turns out, X-rays had been unwittingly observed for many years by several scientists that used Crookes tubes to carry out cathode ray experiments. Even images have been created as early as in 1893 by a process referred to as "electrical photography." However, the discovery of X-rays is attributed to Röntgen, which earned him the 1901 Nobel Prize in Physics "in recognition of the extraordinary services he has rendered by the discovery of the remarkable rays subsequently named after him."

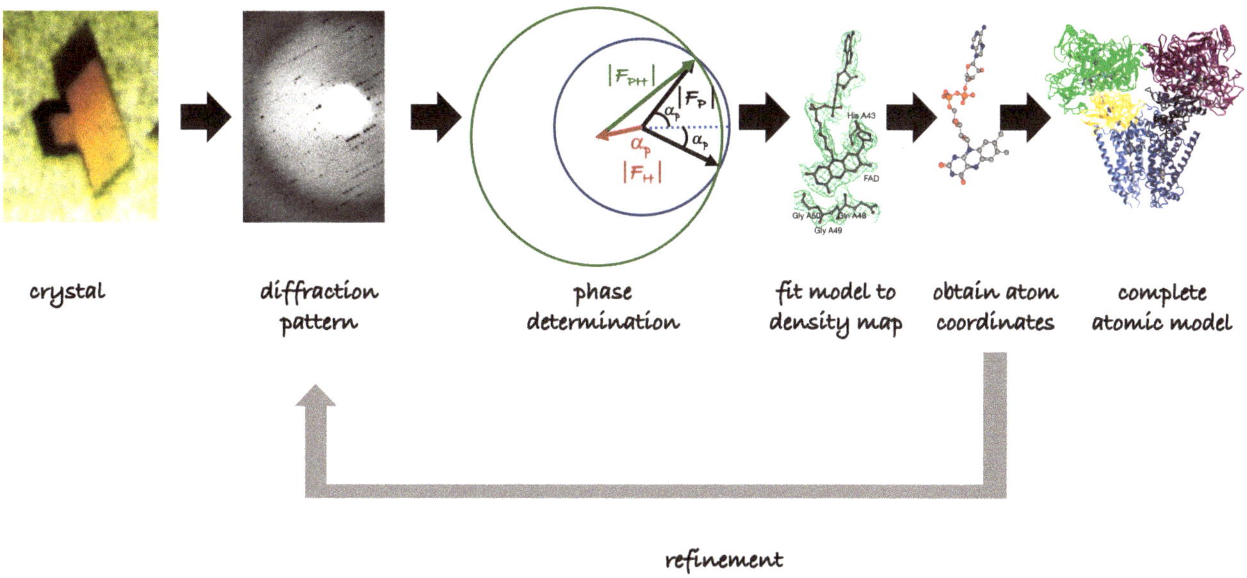

Figure 7.2 X-ray – Overview. X-ray crystallography relies on the formation of 3D crystals from high concentrations of purified macromolecules. Upon X-ray irradiation, diffraction patterns provide accurate amplitude information for a Fourier transform calculation. By overcoming the phase problem either by multiple isomorphous replacement, multiple anomalous diffraction or molecular replacement, initial phase estimates can be obtained, leading to the calculation of initial electron density maps into which atomic models can be built. A comparison between a calculated diffraction pattern based on the atomic model with the actual diffraction data leads to a refinement of the density map and thus an improved atomic model. The final result is then an atomic level detail model of the protein structure, which can subsequently be abstracted as ribbon diagrams, from which an overall fold can be determined.

First X-Ray Diffraction Experiments

Initially, it was controversial whether X-rays should be considered as electromagnetic radiation, given their particle-like property to ionize gases. However, in 1912 Max von Laue used crystals to perform X-ray diffraction experiments, which confirmed that X-rays were indeed electromagnetic radiation, a finding that earned him the 1914 Nobel Prize in Physics in recognition of "his discovery of the diffraction of X-rays by crystals."

William Lawrence Bragg in 1912–1913 developed what is now knowns as Bragg's law that relates the discrete reflections in a diffraction pattern to the spacing of planes within a crystal. Together with his father William Henry Lawrence he went on to solve the structure of inorganic compounds, such as diamond, table salt, and copper. In 1915, both father and son, shared the Nobel Prize in Physics "for their services in the analysis of crystal structure by means of X-rays."

X-Ray Crystallography for Structure Determination

X-ray crystallography became the method of choice for structure determination of minerals, metals, and organic molecules, including hexamethylenetetramine (in 1923), long-chain fatty acids as well as close relatives of porphyrins. Among the important biochemical structures that were solved by Dorothy Crowfoot Hodgkin was cholesterol (1937), penicillin (1946) as well as vitamin B12 (1957), which earned her the 1964 Nobel Prize in Chemistry "for her determinations by X-ray techniques of the 3D structure of important biochemical substances." In 1969, Dorothy Crowfoot Hodgkin was also able to solve the structure of insulin, crowning her 35-year efforts on the structure determination of this peptide. The first crystal structures of proteins, namely myoglobin and hemoglobin, emerged in the late 1950 by John Kendrew and Max Perutz, respectively. Myoglobin was smaller than hemoglobin and was solved to 6 Å resolution in 1957, whereas a 5.5 Å resolution map of hemoglobin was only published in 1959 by Max Perutz, along a 2.8 Å resolution map of myoglobin by John Kendrew (who was Max Perutz's student). They both shared the 1962 Nobel Prize in Chemistry "for their studies on the structures of globular proteins." It was the same year that the Nobel Prize in Physiology or Medicine was awarded to Francis H.C. Crick, James D. Watson, and Maurice H.F. Wilkins "for their discoveries concerning the molecular structure of nucleic acids and its significance for information transfer in living material." Watson and Crick had built a model of DNA that was consistent with the high-quality X-ray images that Rosalind Franklin had recorded in the laboratory of Maurice Wilkins, to which Watson and Crick had gained access to without her permission.

X-ray crystallography has arguably had the biggest impact as a technique when it comes to understand biochemical processes. For a large number of Nobel Prizes, the atomic 3D structure provided a framework to fully understand the (bio-)chemical mechanisms that underly protein function. For a more complete list see Table 7.1.

7.1.3 Theoretical Background

Concept of Studying Crystals

X-ray crystallography is based on the diffraction of X-ray electromagnetic radiation by atoms, ions or (macro-) molecules that are arranged in a highly ordered, crystalline manner. Such 3D crystals are defined by the arrangement of the atoms within a repeating unit cell, and by the translation vectors, also called lattice constants or lattice parameters.

The symmetry aspect of crystals had been known and appreciated for centuries, and the theoretical foundations of crystal symmetry has been worked out in the late 19th century. A crystal is the periodic repetition in 3D of a group of atoms/macromolecules. The smallest repeating unit is called the unit cell, with its three axes defined by the vectors a, b, and c and the corresponding angles alpha, beta, and gamma (with alpha being the angle between vectors b and c, beta being the angle between vectors a and c, and gamma being the angle between vectors a and b). Depending on whether axis parameters are different or the same, and whether the angles are 90° or different, crystals can be grouped into the seven crystal systems (Figure 7.3). In addition, crystals can have internal symmetry, with symmetry operators relating the (macro)molecules to each other by a combination of rotation, translation or mirror symmetries.

For some of the seven crystal systems, there can be primitive (P), base-centered (C), body centered (I), or face-centered (F) organization, which brings the number of possible unique crystal lattices to 14, the so-called Bravais lattices.

The Bravais lattices describe the translational aspect of crystal symmetry, whereas rotation, mirror (reflection) and inversion symmetries are described by the crystallographic point groups, of which there are 32. The total number of space groups is 230, which includes screw axes and glide

Table 7.1 Nobel Prizes involving X-rays and crystallography.

Year	Laureate	Prize category	
1901	Wilhelm Conrad Röntgen	Physics	In recognition of the extraordinary services he has rendered by the discovery of the remarkable rays subsequently named after him
1914	Max von Laue	Physics	For his discovery of the diffraction of X-rays by crystals an important step in the development of X-ray spectroscopy
1915	William Henry Bragg William Lawrence Bragg	Physics	For their services in the analysis of crystal structure by means of X-rays
1946	James Batcheller Sumner	Chemistry	For his discovery that enzymes can be crystallized
1962	Max F. Perutz John C. Kendrew	Chemistry	For their studies of the structures of globular proteins
1962	James D. Watson Francis H.C. Crick Maurice H.F. Wilkins	Medicine	For their discoveries concerning the molecular structure of nucleic acids and its significance for information transfer in living material
1964	Dorothy Hodgkin	Chemistry	For her determinations by X-ray techniques of the structures of important biochemical substances
1972	Stanford Moore William H. Stein	Chemistry	For their contribution to the understanding of the connection between chemical structure and catalytic activity of the active center of the ribonuclease molecule
1976	William N. Lipscomb	Chemistry	For his studies on the structure of boranes illuminating problems of chemical bonding
1985	Jerome Karle Herbert A. Hauptman	Chemistry	For their outstanding achievements in developing direct methods for the determination of crystal structures
1988	Johann Deisenhofer Hartmut Michel Robert Huber	Chemistry	For the determination of the three-dimensional structure of a photosynthetic reaction center
1997	John E. Walker	Chemistry	For the elucidation of the enzymatic mechanism underlying the synthesis of adenosine triphosphate (ATP)
2003	Roderick MacKinnon Peter Agre	Chemistry	For discoveries concerning channels in cell membranes [. . .] for the discovery of water channels
2006	Roger D. Kornberg	Chemistry	For his studies of the molecular basis of eukaryotic transcription
2009	Ada E. Yonath Thomas A. Steitz Venkatraman Ramakrishnan	Chemistry	For studies of the structure and function of the ribosome
2012	Brian Kobilka	Chemistry	For studies of G-protein-coupled receptors

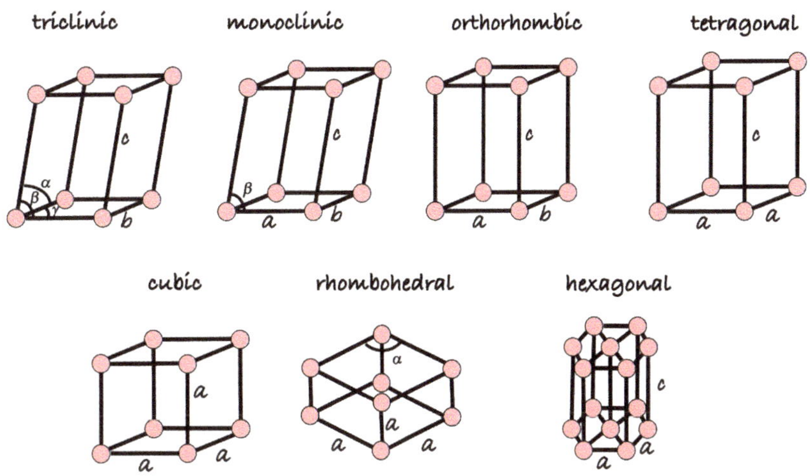

Figure 7.3 Crystal lattices. There are seven crystal systems that differ in whether the unit cell parameters are different from one another or whether two or all three are identical, as well as in whether the angles between the axes in the unit cell are 90° or not. In addition, systems can be primitive (P), base-centered (C), body-centered (I), or face-centered (F), which brings the total number of unique crystal lattice arrangements to 14 lattices, also known as the Bravais-lattices.

planes. However, in biological samples atoms are chiral and usually only one enantiomer of a chemical group is found (L-amino acids, D-saccharides), and thus inversion is not allowed as a symmetry operator. Thus, only 65 space groups need to be considered for X-ray crystallography of biochemical (macro)molecules.

It should be noted that the symmetry considerations discussed here only serve a practical purpose in data collection and analysis, e.g., reducing the angle of coverage and thus the amount of data that need to be collected. They are not needed to comprehend the theoretical concept of structure determination from diffraction patterns.

Physical Principles

Now let us consider a coherent X-ray beam with all X-ray photons originating in phase from the same point source with the same wavelength/energy, reaching the atoms in the crystal. Upon interaction with the electron cloud surrounding each atom's nucleus, the X-ray photons are scattered elastically (meaning without loss of energy) in form of a spherical wave. These regular arrays of spherical waves will cancel each other out in most directions through destructive interference, however for each crystal with its unique unit cell dimensions and geometry, there are certain angular directions, where these spherical waves will interfere constructively. Hence, only in these directions the detector will register a signal as diffraction spots.

Another (perhaps more intuitive) way to think about X-ray diffraction is described by Bragg's law. In this model one can think of a regularly spaced 3D array of particles (a crystal of macromolecules) that form sets of evenly spaced planes running through the center of each particle. Each plane is defined by a coordinate system, which is defined by the three so-called Miller indices (h,k,l) and has a plane-to-plane distance spacing d. One can imagine the X-rays as bouncing off such planes as if they were bouncing off a mirror. In such an experiment there will be angles θ where $2d \sin\theta$ equals an integer multiple of the wavelength λ (i.e., $2d \sin\theta = n\lambda$). In other words, beams bouncing off from neighboring parallel planes will be in phase ($2d \sin\theta = n\lambda$) and thus will constructively interfere at certain angles (Figure 7.4).

Given that the lattice parameters of biologically relevant (macromolecules) are in the tens to hundreds of Ångstroms length range, X-rays with wavelengths of ~1 Å are well-suited for such diffraction experiments. X-rays are primarily scattered by the electron density in an atom, with the contribution of the nuclei being negligible. The interaction of X-rays with the electron cloud can be modeled as an interaction of an electromagnetic ray with a free electron (Thompson scattering), which also describes the polarization of the scattered radiation.

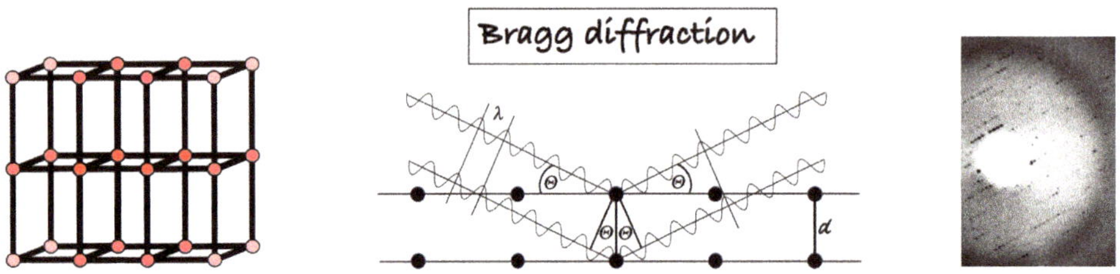

Fourier methods

$$\rho(xyz) = \frac{1}{V}\sum_{hkl\;-\infty}^{+\infty} |F(hkl)| \cdot e^{-2\pi i[hx+ky+lz-\phi(hkl)]}$$

$$F(hkl) = \sum_{j=1}^{n} f_j \; e^{2\pi i[hx+ky+lz]}$$

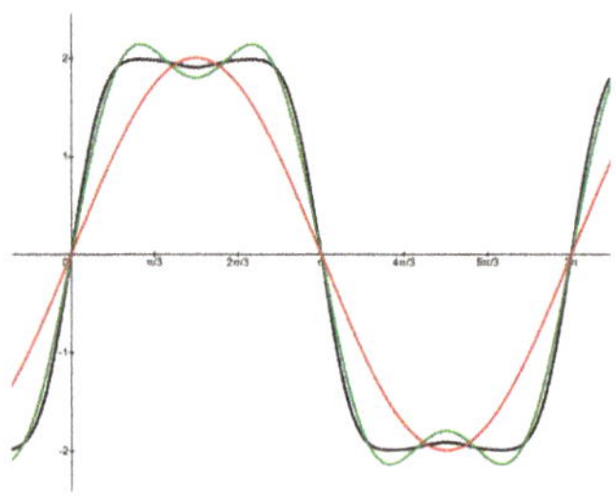

Figure 7.4 X-ray – Bragg diffraction and Fourier methods. A crystal is a regular array of a unit cell (of a macromolecule). Bragg diffraction be thought of as X-rays bouncing off a crystal lattice planes, interfering constructively, leading to a discrete diffraction pattern. Fourier methods are very useful to transform between the real space with *XYZ* coordinates and an electron density and the reciprocal space of a diffraction pattern with its Miller indices *hkl* (frequency space). Corresponding structure factors $\vec{F}$ as a function of *hkl* (as a vector) consists of an amplitude at *hkl* that can measured and a phase at *hkl* that needs to be experimentally determined.

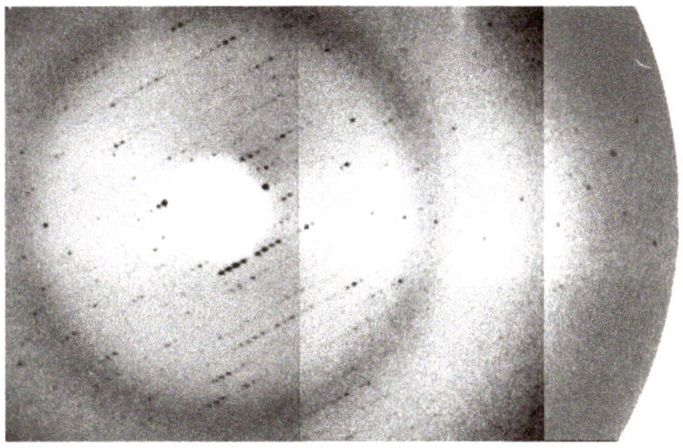

Figure 7.5 X-ray diffraction pattern. The diffraction pattern of fumarate reductase shows discrete spots (reflections). Note the difference in spacing of reflections in orthogonal direction, reflecting differences in the axis dimension of the unit cell. Three regions of the diffraction pattern have been contrast adjusted to show all the spots.

Diffraction patterns consist of discrete diffraction spots, also known as reflections. As one slowly rotates the crystal, many of such diffraction patterns can be recorded as a function of the rotation angle (Figure 7.5). As there are many atoms in the unit cell, the information from all atoms in the unit cell contributes to each of these discrete spots. This means in turn that all the data from all these spots needs to be collected and analyzed to reconstruct the electron density distribution in a single unit cell.

Deviations from perfect crystal morphology, such as small amounts of local disorder or other crystal imperfections, as well imperfections in the X-ray irradiation lead to the widening of the diffraction spots. The intensity of the spot can be obtained by integrating the signal for each pixel of the diffraction spot, which should be above the surrounding noise level. Each reflection of a diffraction pattern is indexed, which means that each reflection is categorized according to its Miller indices. Also, the space group of the crystal and the unit cell parameters (unit cell lengths and the lattice angles) need to be determined. Note that depending to which space group the crystal belongs, a unit cell does not need to be based on an orthogonal coordinate system. From the intensity of the spot with the indices h, k, and l the amplitude $|F|$ of the structure factor $\vec{F}$ (h,k,l) at the position h,k,l can be obtained as the square roots of the spot intensity. The structure factor $\vec{F}$ (hkl) is the essential component in the Fourier analysis to determine the electron density distribution (the arrangement of atoms) within the unit cell. Note that the structure factor $\vec{F}$ is a vector and thus can be written as complex number, and thus as an amplitude $|\vec{F}(hkl)|$ and a phase φ (hkl).

The relationship between the electron density within the unit cell (with its coordinates x,y,z) and the structure factor $\vec{F}$ of the reciprocal lattice (with its coordinates h,k,l) is described by a Fourier transform (FT). In the Fourier analysis one determines the electron density (ρ) for each point in real space (x,y,z) by integrating over all structure factors $\vec{F}$ (h,k,l), meaning the sum of all structure factors at each combination of h, k, and l. The phases φ (h,k,l) cannot directly be determined from the diffraction patterns, due to the fact that the phase information is lost when X-rays hit the detector. This is also known as the phase problem and constitutes the major hurdle in the process of molecular structure determination by diffraction. Different approaches have been developed over the decades to overcome this problem, the most prominent are isomorphous replacement, anomalous dispersion, and molecular replacement.

Until the early 1990s MIR was the method of choice for solving the phase problem, until MAD phasing became widely available. In MIR a heavy metal atom (typically in form of a heavy metal salt) was introduced into the crystal lattice, either by co-crystallization or by soaking an existing crystal in a heavy metal compound solution. A key requirement for this approach to work is that the crystal lattice parameters aren't affected by the introduction of the heavy metal atom, hence the word isomorphous. MIR requires data collection from a crystal without heavy atom, as well as datasets of at least two different heavy atom derivatives.

The heavy atom derivative structure factors are the vector sum of the native protein structure factors and the structure factor of the heavy atom; hence the three structure factors form a triangle. If one of the structure factors can be determined, the other two structure factors can be determined, with a phase ambiguity remaining.

Single isomorphous replacement (with only one heavy atom) produces two phase values for each reflection, only one of which can be correct. This ambiguity is resolved by adding data from a second heavy atom derivative. A so-called Harker diagram illustrates this phase-relationships and offers a visual explanation how the phase ambiguity can be resolved with the second derivative dataset (Figure 7.6).

In a heavy atom derivative, the large number of electrons of the heavy atom will produce disproportionally large scattering amplitudes, which in turn then dominate the diffraction pattern of the heavy atom derivative crystal. The first step in structure determination is then to find the position of the heavy atom within the unit cell, by calculating a Patterson function, which is essentially an autocorrelation function. The Patterson function is equivalent to the FT of the intensities rather than the structure factors, with a setting of all phase values to zero. The resulting contour map will show heavy atom vector distances as peaks, thus providing a starting point for phase determination.

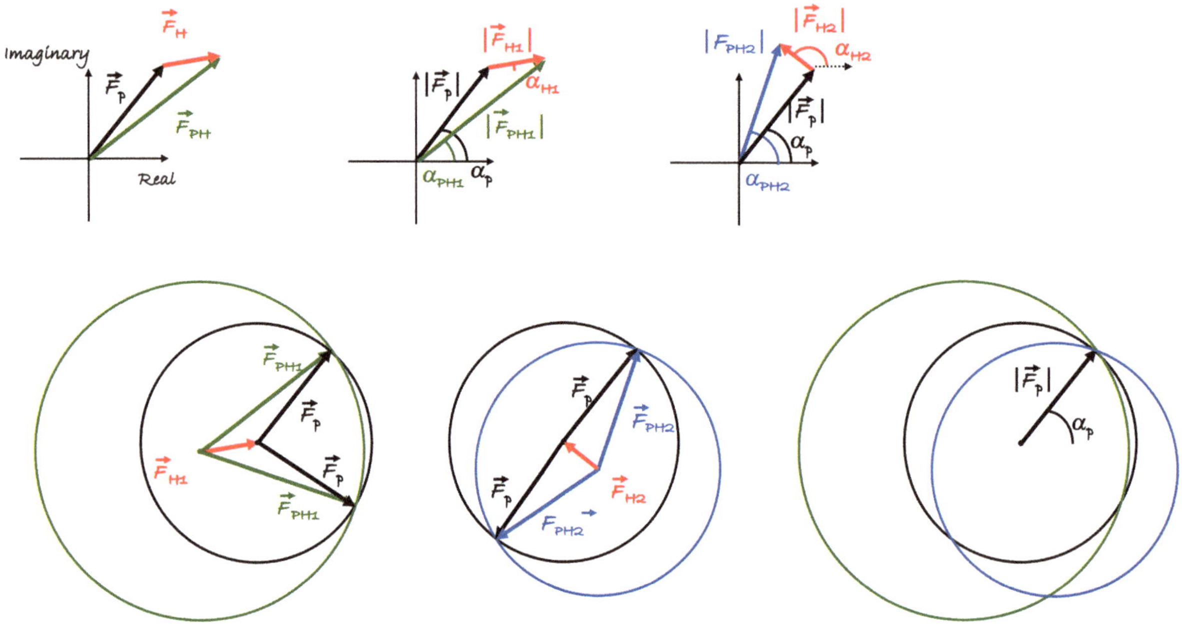

Figure 7.6 Isomorphous replacement – Harker diagram. For each *hkl*-index there is a structure factor with an amplitude $|\vec{F}\ (hkl)|$ and a phase α (which is the same as φ). The amplitude is the length of the vector, and the phase is the angle with the *x*-axis. For a dataset of the protein only crystal, the structure vector is $\vec{F}_P$, whereas for the heavy atom derivative, it the structure factor is $\vec{F}_{PH}$. Since these are vectors, one can use the vector sum to determine the structure factor of the heavy atom alone is $\vec{F}_H$. In a Harker diagram, a circle with the amplitudes can be drawn around the origin of the structure factor. For each heavy atom derivative there will be two locations where these circles will intersect. If one uses two derivatives the circle of the protein structure factor and the two derivatives structure factors will meet in a single point, thus the solution is unambiguous.

The Practical Side of Studying Crystals: Sample Preparation and the Growing of Diffraction-Quality Crystals

One of the major hurdles in X-ray crystallography is to obtain a high-quality crystal that diffracts X-rays to high resolution. Since a crystal consists of periodically arranged (macro-)molecules, the diffraction signal is much stronger the larger the size of the crystal is. However, larger crystals are more likely to show defects such as twinning, which may complicate structure determination. With synchrotron radiation the need to grow large crystal is lower as the X-ray beam is much more intense, compared to laboratory X-ray sources.

To grow 3D crystals, one first needs to obtain significant amounts of protein at high concentration (typically several milligrams of protein per milliliter) in a highly purified state. The higher the amount of contamination, the less likely is it that the protein of interest will crystallize (adopt a periodic arrangement). Crystallization in organic chemistry has been used as a way of achieving and demonstrating compound purity. However, proteins even at high concentration rarely just crystallize spontaneously, instead if the point of protein insolubility in solution is surpassed, the protein may precipitate instead of forming a crystal, and in the process the protein is denatured, often irreversible.

Hence, care must be taken to keep the protein in solution at high concentration in its native conformation by adjusting for example the pH and the ionic strength of the solution. From such highly concentrated protein solutions, one can obtain crystals (Figure 7.7) by very slowly reaching a supersaturated state, e.g., by controlled evaporation (e.g., in form of a hanging drop or sitting drop equilibrating against a higher-concentration reservoir) or controlled concentration (e.g., in form of a microdialysis experiment).

Successful crystallization is a two-step process where first crystal nuclei are formed (typically dozens to hundreds of molecules adopting a periodic arrangement), which then need to slowly grow into a crystal of macroscopic size (~50 to ~500 μm). Conditions must be chosen that favor formation of only a few crystal nuclei and promote slow crystal growth.

While there are some general conditions that can serve as a starting point (there are commercially available screens), each protein tends to crystallize optimally at one or several of its own certain fine-tuned conditions, and thus typically a fair amount of time and precious protein is spent in this process prior to X-ray diffraction data collection and structural analysis.

Once crystals are obtained, they need to be mounted for irradiation by X-rays. Traditionally, glass capillaries have

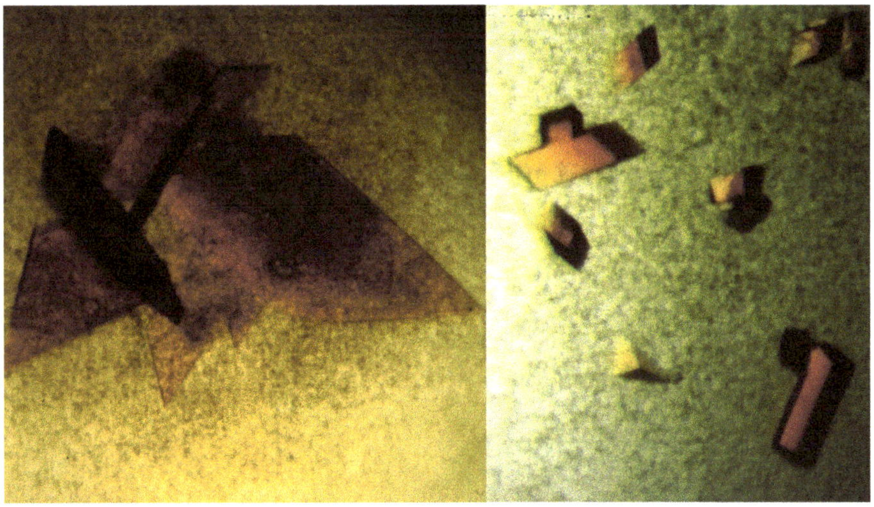

Figure 7.7 3D crystals. Fumarate reductase grows as 3D crystals under slightly different conditions into two different crystal forms with different crystal morphology thin sheets and thicker cuboids. The red color of the crystal is due to the prosthetic groups essential for electron transfer.

been used to mount crystals. In this approach, crystals are aspired into the capillary tubes with a small amount of the crystallization buffer (the mother liquor), then immobilized against the capillary glass wall by minimizing the liquid around the crystal. To maintain a humid atmosphere in the capillary, often some more mother liquor was placed on either side of the crystal, and the capillary was sealed to avoid drying out of the crystal, prior to mounting the crystal inside the capillary on a goniometer that will allow X-ray data collection. Alternatively, crystals have been soaked in a cryo-protectant, picked up by a nylon-loop and subjected to fast freezing (e.g., in a cold nitrogen stream, near liquid nitrogen temperature). Frozen crystals are more resistant to X-ray irradiation, as radicals that are created during bombardment of atomic bonds by X-rays are immobilized and thus cannot cause further damage to other macromolecules in the crystal. This allows crystals to withstand a higher dose of X-ray irradiation, and thus reduces the number of crystals needed for data collection. Soaking in a cryo-protectant prior to freezing is usually needed as un-soaked crystals may crack in the freezing process due to formation of water–ice–crystals. However, sometimes the process of soaking the crystal in a cryo-protectant can itself lead to the break-up of the crystal, and thus freezing of crystals may require yet another optimization process.

7.1.4 Instrumentation/Experimental Setup

Radiation Source: X-Ray Generation by Rotating Anode

X-rays are generated when electrons that were emitted from a heated cathode and accelerated by strong electrical field (e.g., 50 kV) collide with a metal anode material (often copper), thus the German word Bremsstrahlung (deceleration radiation) as X-rays are also often referred to. If the anode is stationary, the setup is known as a Crookes tube (the type of X-ray generators Wilhelm Röntgen experimented with). More commonly are water-cooled rotating anodes, which have been widely used as laboratory X-ray sources before synchrotrons became widely available. Copper-based rotating anodes produce two strong peaks at ~1.54 Å and ~1.39 Å, corresponding to Kα and Kβ lines, a result of copper inner-shell electron excitation (Figure 7.8). If one uses Molybdenum instead of copper as the rotating anode material, X-rays of ~0.71 Å and ~0.63 Å can be obtained.

The emitted X-ray spectrum is then typically filtered to one wavelength to obtain monochromatic X-ray radiation, and using a long collimator tube or a system made of mirrors the rays are collimated into a beam with a small cross-section, which then irradiates the crystal.

Radiation Source: X-Ray Generation by Synchrotron Radiation

X-rays are a by-product in synchrotrons, which are particle accelerators that accelerate electrons to nearly the speed of light, while forcing them by magnetic fields on a roughly circular loop. This causes the electrons to give off broadband radiation, including X-rays, which then can be used for irradiation of protein crystals. Synchrotrons are gigantic storage rings with several dozen user stations (Figure 7.9). Such synchrotrons can be the size of a football field or even bigger.

A large portion of the electromagnetic spectrum can be produced by synchrotrons. Synchrotrons were developed for high energy physics applications, but many such national facilities worldwide are now dedicated to biological imaging, and within that discipline to a large extent to

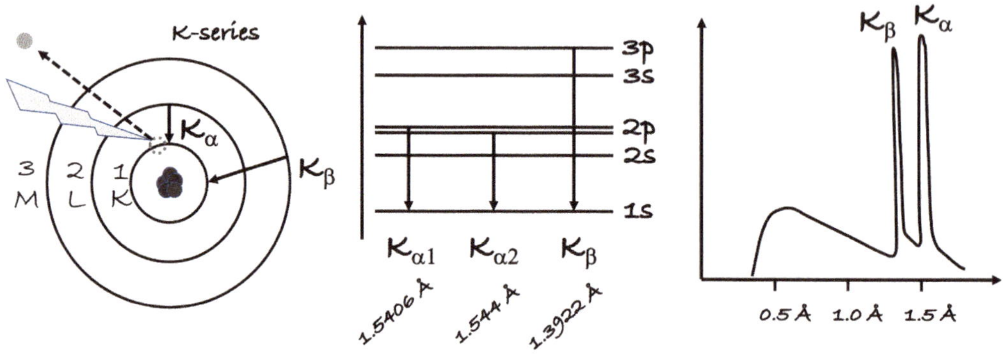

Figure 7.8 X-ray generation. Accelerated electrons hit a rotating copper anode, resulting in the ejection of a 1s inner shell electron. Electron transitioning from a 2p or 3p orbital to the 1s orbital leads to the emission of Kα and Kβ X-ray photons at 1.54 Å and 1.39 Å, respectively. Note the two spikes of intensity at 1.39 Å and 1.54 Å.

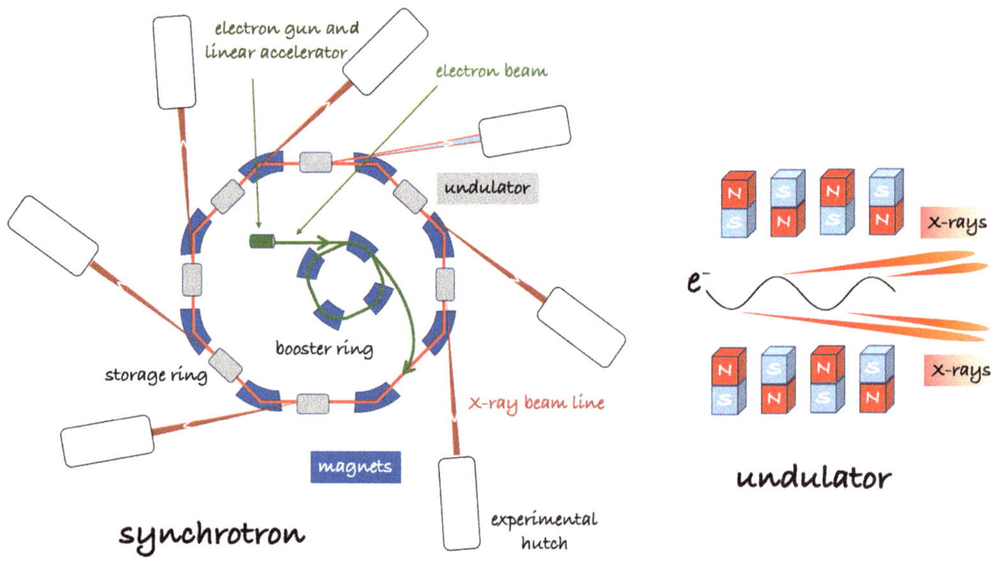

Figure 7.9 Synchrotron radiation. Synchrotron radiation is given off by high-velocity electrons in a particle accelerator storage ring, where electrons are forced on circular orbits by electromagnetic fields. The journey for the electrons starts in an electron gun with a linear accelerator before they enter the booster ring. The booster ring then feeds the storage ring, typically twice a day. With the help of undulators, electrons give off X-rays that are then channeled into an X-ray beamline. These X-rays are used in the experimental hutches for a variety of scientific experiments, among which X-ray diffraction features prominently. Apart from X-rays other parts of the electromagnetic spectrum is also utilized, such as the strong infrared radiation used for FTIR imaging.

X-ray crystallography. There are two main advantages of synchrotron radiation for structural biology: one is the high intensity of the X-ray beam, allowing the imaging of rather small crystals in a short period of time. The second advantage is that synchrotron radiation is tunable, meaning that different wavelengths can be selected, which is very convenient for multiwavelength anomalous diffraction (MAD), which allows to obtain phase information without the need for a heavy atom derivative.

Radiation Source: X-Ray Generation by Free-Electron Laser

Free-electron lasers emit extremely bright X-ray sources as femtosecond bursts. With such short intense burst, individual tiny (sub-micron) crystals in random orientation can be irradiated, yielding a diffraction pattern, while being destroyed in the process. Combining the data of hundreds of thousand such diffraction patterns, on can obtain high-resolution structures.

Detector Types

For decades X-ray films were used for the detection of X-rays. However, the process of film development is slow and tedious, and the X-ray dose could not be adjusted in real time. Furthermore, the films needed to be digitized for computational analysis, a process that again was slow and tedious.

Sensitivity was increased and thus the necessary dose for data collection could be lowered by using photographic film in combination with a scintillator material. The scintillator absorbs the energy of incoming X-ray photons and re-emits it in form of fluorescence or phosphorescence in the visible light part of the electromagnetic spectrum.

Multi-wire area detectors became available in the mid-1980s and were based on gas ionization: incoming X-ray photons ionizes gas molecules, which are then detected by their neighboring wires. Ultimately, area detectors were limited by the area they could cover and their dynamic range.

The process of photostimulated luminescence allowed the replacement of film and/or multi-wire area detectors by a photostimulable phosphor plate (PSP), also known as image plates (IP), where irradiation by X-rays leads to the excitement of electrons in the phosphor material that remain trapped in this state until subsequent stimulation by a laser beam. The emitted phosphorescence light at that point is detected by a photomultiplier tube and digitized. After read-out by the laser beam the PSP can be reused, making it an ideal detector for automated data collection, however the readout is slow (minutes) compared to X-ray radiation exposure (seconds). Compared to area detector IP covered a much larger area and had a higher dynamic range, thus they could not be as easily saturated compared to area detectors.

Charge-coupled device (CCD) detectors are based on semiconductor technology, where X-rays directly or indirectly (via a scintillator) lead to charge accumulation in the CCD array, before they can be read out subsequently through a shift register mechanism. CCD detectors are based on metal-oxide-semiconductor (MOS) thin film transistor technology, which either directly or indirectly (through the mediation of a scintillator) detects X-rays in a photosensitive layer, converting them to electrons via the inner photoelectric effect. Electrons are then stored in "wells" (capacitors) before the accumulative charge is then subsequently read out for each well like a bucket brigade (Figure 7.10).

CMOS (complementary metal-oxide semiconductor) is another variant of the thick film layer MOS technology, widely used in computer design and operation, (e.g., as a

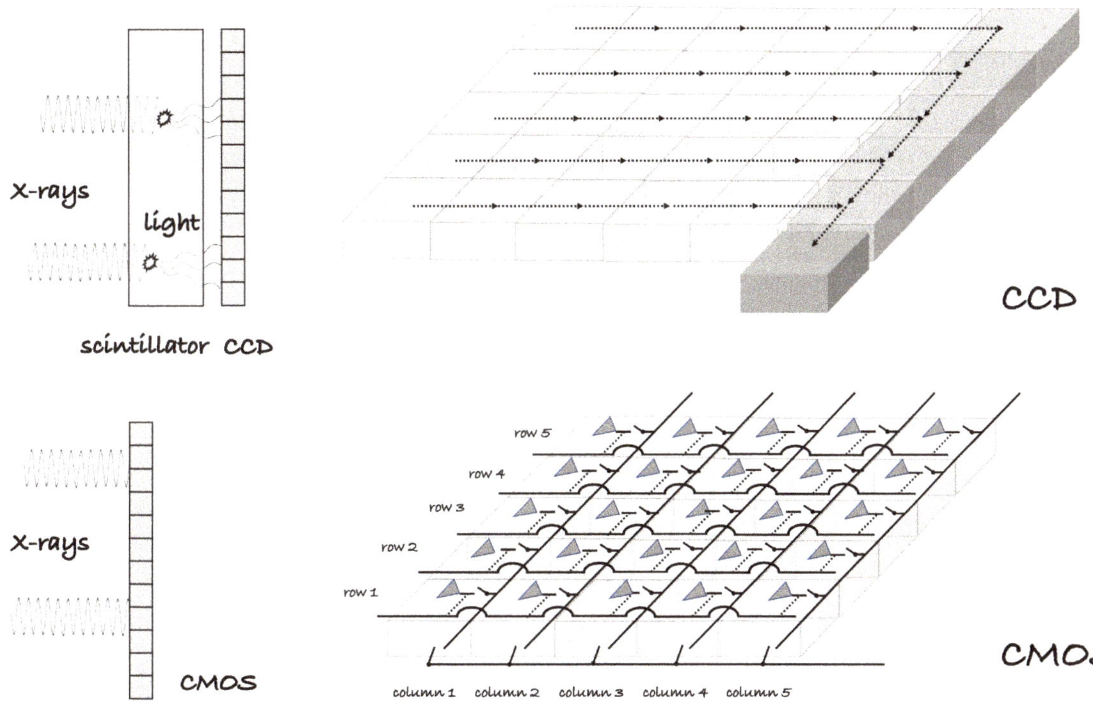

Figure 7.10 Detectors for X-ray crystallography – CCD and CMOS. CCD detectors for X-ray crystallography utilize a scintillator layer to capture X-ray photons and to emit light, which is then detected by the CCD camera. However, the read-out of CCDs is notoriously slow. Therefore, the current generation of detectors is the CMOS detector that does not require a scintillator layer and excels by low noise and fast read-out.

local small amount of memory on the motherboard) and can be run in a charge integrating or charge counting mode, as readout is much faster than with CCDs as it does not require a shift register read out mechanism. CMOS detectors have in the last decade replaced the older CCD technology and they are now characterized by very low noise, allowing individual photons to be counted.

7.1.5 Data Collection

Crystals need to be carefully chosen, as ideally they will be free from any obvious signs of imperfections, such as twinning or cracks. Since macromolecular crystals contain a significant amount of solvent, they must be prevented from drying out, either by sealing the crystal in a glass capillary with a small amount of mother liquor next to the crystal to keep the interior of the glass capillary moist, or by flash-freezing the crystal, followed by data collection at cryogenic temperature. Flash-freezing (e.g., by using a nylon loop) bears the risk of destruction of the crystal particularly in the absence of cryo-protectants. Flash-frozen crystals (kept frozen) have the advantage that they are more robust during data collection, as the consequences of radiation damage are minimized at ~100K, extending the amount of time that high resolution data can be collected from the same crystal. Also, it is much easier to store crystals at liquid nitrogen temperature for future data collection.

Once the crystal is mounted on the goniometer, care must be taken to ensure that the crystal stays centered when rotated during data collection. Once the crystal is mounted onto a goniometer head, it can be rotated at the center of an X-ray beam, typically at 0.2°–1° increments, resulting in diffraction patterns (Figure 7.11). From such images, the upper limit of resolution of the data can be estimated at which the 3D structure can be determined, with spots at a far distance from the detector center indicating high resolution. Spots only presenting themselves close to the detector indicate low-resolution data, most likely due to internal disorder in the crystal. Also, other crystal pathologies that would make it difficult or impossible to solve the structures can be assessed from the first few images.

Also, from the first few images, unit cell parameters and the likely space group can be determined, which helps to determine how many degrees the crystals need to be rotated before a complete data set can be collected. Crystals displaying higher symmetries require less data collection, which can be important if the overall dose of X-ray irradiation must be limited due to radiation sensitivity of the crystal.

Traditionally, multiple data sets were recorded from the same or different crystals, also depending on the method chosen of phasing. MIR require multiple crystals obtained under slightly different conditions, e.g., by soaking a heavy metal salt into the crystal or by growing the crystal in the presence of a heavy salt solution. MAD data can be collected from the same crystal, if the crystal is radiation-tolerant, by collecting data at least three different wavelengths. MAD phasing typically requires the introduction of selenium methionine, typically by using methionine-auxotrophic expression systems with selenomethionine being present in the growth medium.

The diffraction images recorded at each rotational increment (reflecting a particular crystal orientation) are merged/combined after scaling into a three-dimensional data set, with each of the diffraction spots being indexed, and its intensity peak profile being measured. This serves as input for the inverse FT, which serves as the mathematical link between the diffraction spots and the corresponding electron density.

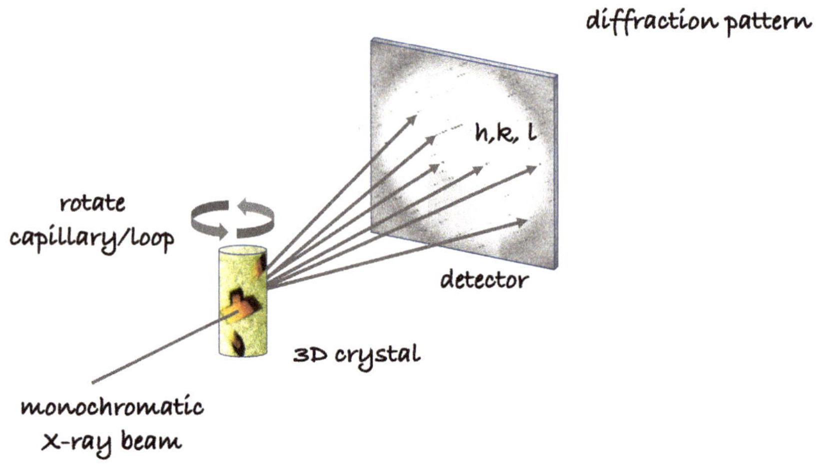

Figure 7.11 Data collection. For data collection in X-ray crystallography, the monochromatic X-ray beam hits a 3D crystal of suitable size mounted in either a capillary or in a loop. Small increments of rotation of the capillary or loop results in diffraction patterns that can be indexed and analyzed.

Indexing of the diffraction spots, determination of lattice parameters, intensity measurements and peak profiling are all done automatically these days, with the experimenter just briefly checking the statistics to ensure that data collection was completed successfully. However, it is not sufficient to only determine the amplitudes (as the square root of the measured reflection intensities) but one also needs to get a starting estimate for the phase information at each Miller-indexed spot of the 3D diffraction pattern. Often symmetry-equivalent spots are recorded multiple times which allows to judge the quality of the data.

7.1.6 Data Analysis and Phasing

The three-dimensional diffraction pattern is in essence a reciprocal space (Fourier space) representation of the crystal lattice, and each of the reflection contains information about the electron density distribution within each unit cell. Once the intensities for each of the reflections with their Miller indices has been measured, the amplitudes (as being proportional to the square root of the intensities) for each spot can be entered into the inverse FT for each of the Miller indices h,k,l. However, since the structure factor F for each reflection h,k,l is a complex number (and thus a vector), both the amplitude of the vector (i.e., the length of the vector), as well as the phase (direction of the vector) must be known. While the amplitude can be determined for each spot, the phase information is lost in a diffraction experiment, and hence the phase for each spot is unknown: it can assume any value between 0 and 2π (or in terms of an angle between 0° and 360°).

This is known as the phase problem in X-ray crystallography. As discussed earlier, there are different approaches that lead to a starting estimate of phases for each reflection, including single or multiple isomorphous replacement (SIR/MIR), anomalous dispersion (single-wavelength anomalous diffraction; SAD/multi-wavelength anomalous diffraction; MAD) or molecular replacement (MR).

For (single/multiple) isomorphous replacement methods (SIR/MIR), data sets of the protein without (native) and with (derivative) heavy atom bound to the protein are collected. The heavy atom derivatives must be isomorphous, which means that neither packing within the unit cell nor any unit cell parameters can change. For such heavy atom derivatives, the X-ray scattering of the heavy atom dominates. Using Patterson function approaches (autocorrelation), one can determine the position of the heavy atom in the unit cell and thus a structure factor for the heavy atom alone. By comparing reflections in the native and derivative datasets, one can get an initial phase estimate, which then subsequently gets further refined, i.e., by model building.

Ab initio phasing (direct methods), which exploits known phase relationships between certain groups of reflections, usually only works for relatively small molecules. While SIR/MIR phasing has been the traditional approach to solve protein structures, SAD/MAD phasing, which is based in anomalous scattering, has become the predominant method for phasing.

Anomalous scattering is a violation of Friedel's Law, which states that the reflections (h,k,l) and $(-h,-k,-l)$ have the same intensities. It is this very difference between the Friedel pair reflections that is the so-called anomalous difference (also known as the Bijvoet difference). The anomalous signal yields the positions of the anomalously diffracting atoms (similar in concept to isomorphous replacement), as it provides the starting phase estimates for the entire macromolecule. By collecting data at tunable X-ray sources (at synchrotrons), the anomalous signal of the selenium K-edge can be used for phasing. Similar to MIR phasing, collecting multiple datasets eliminates phase ambiguities (Figure 7.12).

However, MAD phasing can be challenging for larger proteins as there could be too many selenium atoms per protein structure to interpret the anomalous difference. Also, since MAD data collection occurs at the absorption edge, energy is absorbed (taken up) by the macromolecule, which in turn can lead to radiation damage.

Overall, it should be said that in the case of MAD phasing one must deal with a substantially smaller signal difference compared to MIR phasing. Improvements in the signal-to-noise ratio in X-ray diffraction experiments have made it possible to use sulfur instead of selenium, which can be important for proteins that cannot easily be expressed in methione-deficient bacterial expression systems. Furthermore, proteins containing metal ions or metal clusters are ideal for MAD phasing and do not need the introduction of selenium.

Besides SIR/MIR and SAD/MAD, molecular replacement (MR) is a powerful tool for initial phasing, if a closely related structure or a substantial part of the structure is known. Homology modeling based on primary sequence similarity can be a starting point for obtaining a search model. Starting with an appropriate model cuts short the process of obtaining initial phases, but as discussed earlier, it is important to be careful what model is used in this process, as model bias is hard to overcome in the phase refinement process.

Nowadays, statistical concepts such as maximum likelihood methods integrate over probability distributions rather assuming one single optimal value for the phase of each reflection, as was done in conventional least-squares approaches.

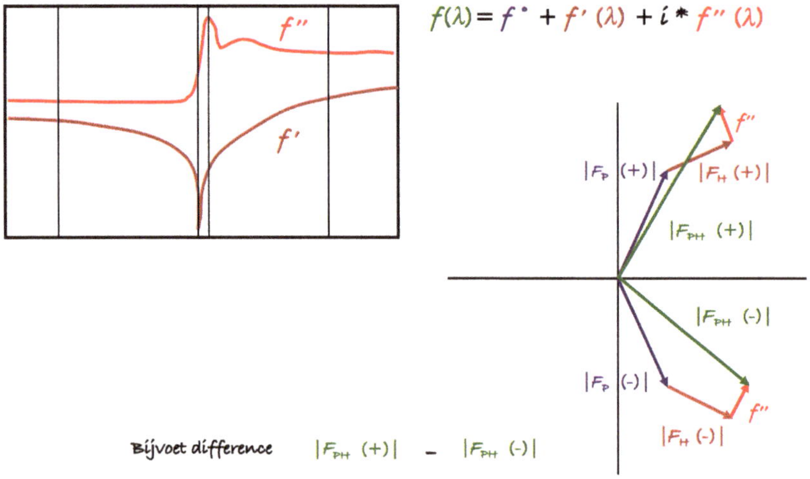

Figure 7.12 Multi-wavelength anomalous diffraction (MAD) phasing. For MAD phasing diffraction data is recorded by tunable synchrotron radiation at different wavelengths near the absorption edge of selenium (or other suitable atoms), where the atomic scattering factor are significantly different from one another as there are additional phase shifts due to anomalous scattering. This results in differences of the structure factors due to the violation of Friedel's law. The difference is known as the Bijvoet difference.

7.1.7 Map Calculation and Model Building

Only when amplitudes and phases are known, can a final electron density distribution of a unit cell be calculated via a mathematical operation known as the inverse FT.

In turn, with a known density distribution, meaning a density value at any position x,y,z of the unit cell in real space one can obtain via FT the structure factor $F(h,k,l)$ in reciprocal space of the diffraction pattern, with $\vec{F}$ being a vector with an amplitude and phase. As $\vec{F}$ is a complex number, it can be written using an exponential or a sine/cosine expression. For the electron density at each position x,y,z, the FT can be thought of a gigantic summation of all the information that resides in each of the reflection (amplitude and phase) over all combinations of h,k,l. Likewise, a structure factor, and thus amplitude and phase, can be calculated for each reflection, by summing for each h,k,l the electron densities over all x,y,z positions.

Once initial phase estimates for each structure factor $\vec{F}$ at each h,k,l position has been obtained, one typically starts the process of model building, where an atomic model is fitted to the emerging density map (Figure 7.13). Dependent on the quality of the first phase estimates, model building can either be a straightforward process, and these days it can be done automatically by sophisticated computer programs, or it may require substantial human intervention, e.g., the manual tracing of the polypeptide backbone into the somewhat diffuse density map.

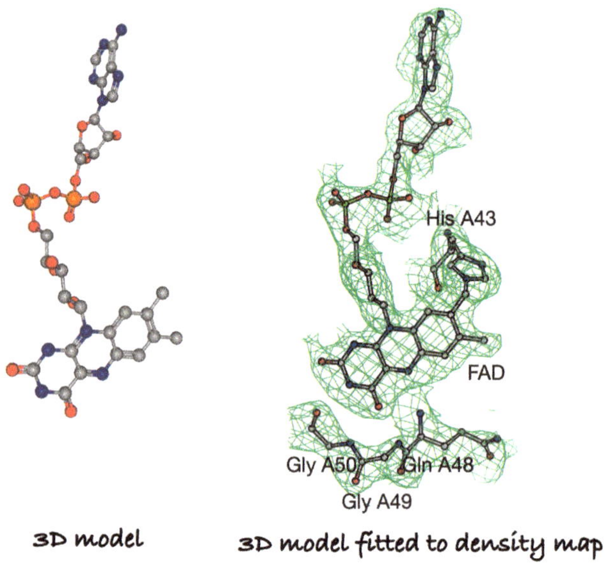

Figure 7.13 Atomic model building. Atomic models can be placed into the experimental density map. Once the fit seems appropriate, the atom positions of the model are used to iteratively calculate an electron density map.

Several steps help in this process, namely the definition of the molecular boundary by-so-called solvent flattening, the identification of the asymmetric unit, and exploitation of non-crystallographic symmetry to improve map quality. This typically allows an initial placement of C-alpha positions of the polypeptide backbone into the density map. Bulky amino acid side chains of the primary amino acid sequence can serve as guides for accurate tracing. However it must be emphasized that errors in tracing should be avoided, and when in doubt those parts of the density map should not be fitted in this round and left to a later stage when the density maps becomes clearer.

7.1.8 Refinement and Validation

With an initial model, one can calculate a new version of all structure factors for each reflection, and the newly calculated structure factors can be compared with the experimentally determined values. Iteratively new maps of increasing quality can be calculated, to which atomic models can be fitted. Maps are typically calculated at different thresholds (as multiples of the standard deviation), with higher thresholds reflecting stronger portions of the map, but also showing less connectivity, whereas lower threshold maps may not allow accurate tracing. Multiple maps at multiple thresholds can be displayed simultaneously (e.g. as different colors), which can help with model building.

Through this process of model building (fitting of atoms into the density map) and by comparison of the structure factors obtained from the model with the experimentally observed data, the reciprocal space phases (and thus structure factors) for each reflection are refined, which results in an improvement of the real space electron density map. As an accurate knowledge of phases is much more important than an accurate description of the amplitudes, early errors in the tracing of the density map (model building) will lead to wrong phase estimates that will propagate through the refinement process and are hard to get rid of. For each of atom a so-called B-factor or temperature factor (also known as Debye–Waller factor) is assigned, which indicates an uncertainty for the atom in that position, often interpreted as a flexibility of the atom or vibrational motion.

There are objective criteria for the quality of the model/data, such as the R-factor or the R-free (referred to as residual factor or reliability factor), which measure the agreement of the model with the experimental data. The R-factor is calculated from a subset of the reflections, which were not included in the structure refinement and monitor the quality improvement of the density map during the process of refinement.

Once a model has been found that agrees well with the experimentally observed data, molecular dynamics calculation, often referred to as simulated annealing, are carried out. In simulated annealing, atoms in the structure are computationally heated up, meaning atoms are allowed to move locally from their original position, and then computationally cooled down to allow for local force fields to guide the atoms to a low-energy state position. The final atomic model also needs to satisfy molecular chemical bond length and angle geometries restrictions (stereochemistry), to be free of clashes atoms, and be within typical value region in a Ramachandran plot (polypeptide backbone angles). One also assesses the presence of hydrogen bonding, which in enzymes often are critical for the catalytic mechanism. Note that in some cases, an atomic model cannot be built for certain parts of the density map, as local disorder of the molecule in the crystal may smear the electron density in that region. Furthermore, sometimes there is more than one way how an amino acid side can be fitted to the density map, for example if there is more than one defined conformation that the side chain can adopt.

7.1.9 Visualization

The end result of a structure determination is an atomic model, which is a file – also referred to as a PDB (protein data bank) file – where each atom is listed with its identity, *x,y,z* coordinates, as well as other information, such as temperature factor. Visualization of these atoms can be challenging, as detailed atomic models are often very complex, and very confusing to look at. For this reason, 3D structures are often shown in a cartoon-like depiction by so-called ribbon diagrams, also known as Richardson diagrams (as they were first introduced in the 1980s by Jane S. Richardson). The ribbon diagrams depict alpha helices as thick rods or coiled ribbons and beta-strands as arrows. Ribbon diagrams are also very useful to detect so-called protein folds and thus allows 3D structures to be compared by their overall organization and thus classified using their 3D fold organization.

7.1.10 Outlook

The enthusiasm for X-ray crystallography has veined a little in recent years, as the "resolution revolution" in single particle cryo-EM has taken place, courtesy of advanced detector technology that over the last decade has allowed correction for beam-induced specimen movement. Many X-ray crystallography labs have converted to single particle cryo-EM or at least have extended their structure determination portfolio to include cryo-EM.

Furthermore, electron diffraction of tiny (submicron) 3D crystals, a technique also known as cryo-EM microcrystal electron diffraction (MicroED), has now become a routine method to determine the high-resolution 3D structure of (macro-)molecules.

High hopes have been placed on free-electron lasers, which uses high-dose X-ray pulses of femto-second duration to study small 3D crystals without the need for cooling, as irradiated samples are quickly destroyed but yielded sufficient information. Millions of extremely weak patterns can be collected and combined in this way, requiring automated approaches to rapidly replenish the sample into the beam while generating the lowest possible background. Therefore, the method is well suited to conduct time-resolved measurements from below picoseconds to several seconds, however it is unclear whether the ab initio structure determination of individual macromolecules in their soluble state is a realistic goal. Time-resolved studies of changes of structurally known macromolecules using the free-electron laser have already been successful.

7.2 Macromolecular Cryo-Electron Microscopy

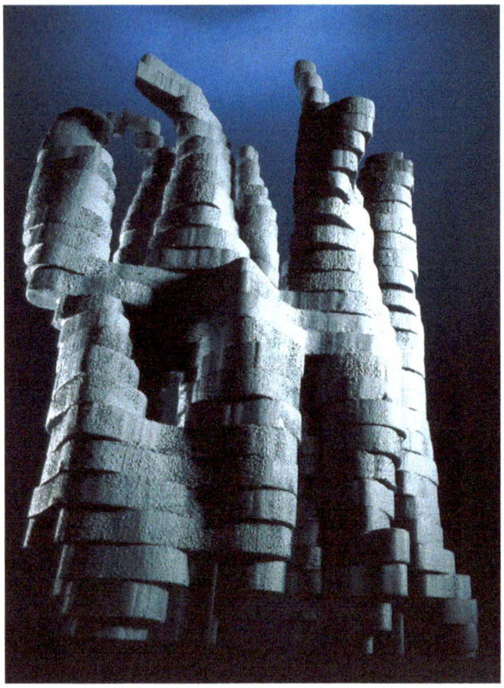

A 7 Å model of very first membrane protein – bacteriorhodopsin – solved in 1975 by Richard Henderson and Nigel Unwin using electron crystallography of purple membrane 2D crystals. *Source:* With permission from MRC Laboratory of Molecular Biology.

7.2.1 Overview

Cryo-EM has recently overtaken X-ray crystallography as the method of choice for structure determination of individual proteins and macromolecular complexes. Improvements in CMOS detector technology have allowed researchers to overcome beam-induced specimen movement, a fundamental barrier to high-resolution data collection that has plagued transmission electron microscopy (TEM) for decades. With the "resolution revolution" (as it was dubbed) that has taken place over the last 10 years, it is now possible to solve the structures of individual proteins and macromolecular complexes at high resolution in a matter of days (sometimes even hours). This can be accomplished with small amounts of purified protein without the need for crystallization. Furthermore, since cryo-EM provides images (instead of diffraction pattern as is the case for X-ray crystallography), there is no phase-problem that needs to be overcome, and thus high-quality density maps are now attainable from 2D projection images of particles in random orientation. Boxed images of individual macromolecules/macromolecular complexes are sorted into 2D class-averages, with different classes representing different viewing directions of the macromolecules. The combination of such class averages allows the reconstruction of a 3D volume density distribution, into which an atomic model can be built.

TEM has had a long tradition as a method to determine high- and intermediate-resolution structures of individual macromolecules, macromolecular complexes (also known as macromolecular machines) and supramolecular assemblies. Some macromolecules arrange in a planar 2D crystalline manner, in a tubular and filamentous assembly with helical symmetry, or into a complex with icosahedral symmetry (as is typical for viruses). In such cases, the internal symmetry relationship of the macromolecules can be exploited to increase the signal-to-noise ratio and thus to determine the macromolecular 3D structure. Other macromolecules may still assemble into larger complexes (such as the ribosome contains a number of RNA and protein subunits), that do not form regular arrays and thus must be averaged explicitly as single particles. In electron tomography, the exact same sample is imaged multiple times under different tilt angles before being reconstructed into a 3D volume (Figure 7.14). Unlike X-rays, electrons can be focused to high resolution, resulting in images of an object instead of diffraction patterns.

Since its inception, macromolecular electron microscopy faced a number of challenges arising from the strong interaction of electrons with matter and the fact that transmission electron microscopy can only yield 2D projection view from which 3D structures need to be calculated (Figure 7.15). However, since electrons interact strongly with matter (i.e., with the nuclear field of the atoms), a few millimeters of air would stop the electron beam completely. Therefore (biological) samples need to be studied in the high vacuum of an electron microscope. Samples that can be studied in an electron microscope must be rather thin (typically less than 1 μm for an intermediate voltage electron microscope). Furthermore, radiation damage encountered by the light element biological specimen cannot be fully avoided, but they can be minimized by lowering the dose for imaging, which in turn results in poor signal-to-noise images. Close-to-native preservation of the sample in amorphous ice at very low temperature, combined with low-dose imaging at low temperatures, has led to the success of cryo-EM.

Ultra-rapid freezing of the specimen is achieved by plunging the sample as a thin film on an electron microscope grid surface into liquid ethane, which is kept at liquid nitrogen temperature. This results in a non-crystalline, glass-like state of frozen water, also known as vitreous ice. During the transfer of the grid with the specimen into the

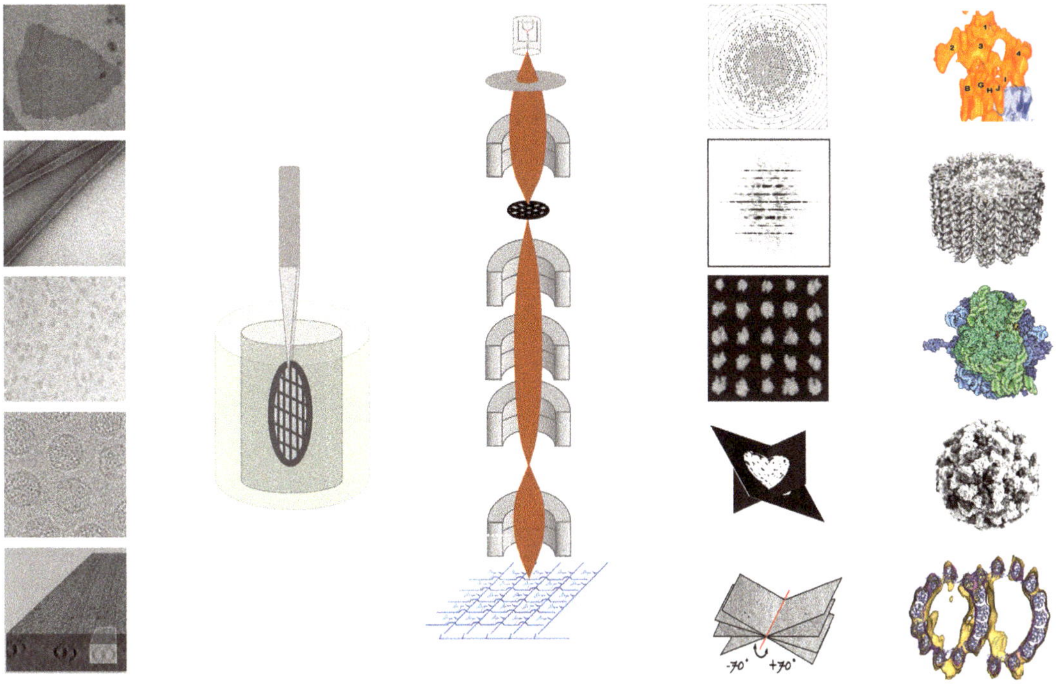

Figure 7.14 Overview – Cryo-EM. Thin films of different kind of samples such as 2D crystals, filaments and tubes with helical symmetry, virus particles with icosahedral symmetry or supramolecular complexes/single particles with no symmetry, are plunge-frozen and subjected to transmission electron microscopy imaging, The images are analyzed, and 3D structures are obtained using implicit or explicit averaging.

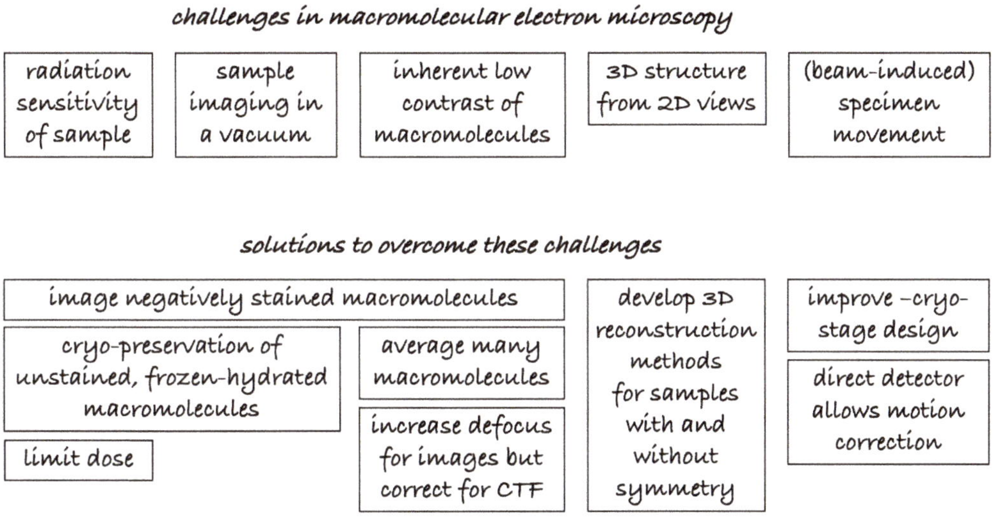

Figure 7.15 Cryo-EM: Challenges and solutions. A variety of challenges need to be overcome ranging from radiation sensitivity of biological samples in the electron microscope and sample hydration stability in the vacuum of the electron microscope to low inherent contrast of unstained biological samples. They can be overcome in different ways ranging from sample staining to freezing and limiting radiation dose. Low inherent contrast and obtaining 3D structure from 2D view can be overcome by implicit or explicit averaging and 3D reconstruction of particles. Last but not the least important, (beam-induced) specimen movement could be overcome by improved stage design and direct detector motion correction.

grid holder and the transfer of the holder into the electron microscope, the temperature of the samples needs to be kept below −140 °C, otherwise vitreous ice will phase-transition into crystalline (cubic and then hexagonal) ice, which could destroy the samples and lead to unwanted background signal of the ice.

Cryogenically preserved samples can only be subjected to a minimal dose to limit radiation damage, which can lead to free radicals, cause further damage in the macromolecule's vicinity, and alter the 3D macromolecular structure. Imaging at low temperature at minimal dose prevents free radicals from diffusing from their place of generation and keeps broken pieces of the macromolecules in place. However, low-dose/minimal dose imaging also leads to images that are characterized by low contrast and thus low signal-to-noise.

The information in such low-dose images can be significantly improved by implicit or explicit averaging techniques, in some cases taking advantage of sample symmetries. Implicit averaging is possible for images of macromolecules that form planar or helical 2D crystals (tubules), helical filaments, or particles with icosahedral symmetry, such as many viruses. For specimen with helical or icosahedral symmetry, each image contains multiple views of each macromolecule, and for this reason 3D reconstructions from 2D images can be obtained from untilted specimen, as each image provides views of the macromolecules in different orientations. Planar 2D-crystalline specimen on the other hand need to be tilted in the electron microscope. However, tilt angles for electron microscopy (EM) support grids are limited to about ±70°, and beam-induced specimen movement is typically more detrimental to image quality at high tilt angles. As a result, density maps from planar 2D crystal are usually anisotropic, with a far better *X*,*Y*-direction compared to the *Z*-direction. A similar situation arises in tomographic imaging, which also requires the collection of a tilt series, which also results in a much better *XY* versus *X* resolution.

Until about 10 years ago, cryo-EM was the domain of intermediate resolution structures. Hence the art and science of cryo-EM also earned the nickname "blobology." Yet, while resolution was limited, cryo-EM often was able to provide a density envelope, into which higher resolution structure could be fitted, which is known as the hybrid approach for 3D structure determination.

Currently the most widely used approach of cryo-EM imaging of individual macromolecules and macromolecular machines is single particle cryo-EM, which is based on explicit averaging of individual particles with no assumption of symmetry in the reconstruction process. Difficulties can arise in this approach if the particles show preferential orientation (e.g., top view versus side view), in which case tilting may be necessary, or if the particles are highly inhomogeneous in terms of conformation, shape or size.

However, single particle cryo-EM has become the dominant form of macromolecular EM and has rendered most other disciplines in macromolecules TEM such as 2D crystallography, helical reconstruction, and icosahedral 3D reconstruction more or less obsolete. A recent application of cryo-EM is the electron diffraction of tiny 3D crystals, where the TEM (being operated in diffraction mode) replaces X-ray generators as the radiation source.

7.2.2 Historical Perspective/Milestones

The TEM is the successor of cathode ray oscilloscope measuring devices and was invented by Ernst Ruska in the early 1930s. A variant of this approach, using electron imaging in a reflected mode, was invented by Manfred von Ardenne in 1939. The TEM initially had a resolution of 10 nm, which by the mid 1940s was improved to a theoretical resolution value of 2 nm, and thus 100 times higher resolution than diffraction-limited optical microscopy. Ernst Ruska was honored in 1986 with a share of Nobel Prize in Physics for his fundamental work in electron optics, and for the design of the first electron microscope (Table 7.2). The other half of the award went to Gerd Binnig and Heinrich Rohrer for their design of the scanning tunneling microscope, a scanning probe microscope, whose successful performance was demonstrated in 1981, while building on earlier work of the 1960s. The 2017 Nobel Prize in Chemistry was awarded to Joachim Frank, Richard Henderson and Jacques Dubochet for developing cryo-electron microscopy for the high-resolution structure determination of biomolecules in solution.

Advances in Instrumentation

Improvement in resolution, which was the main objective in the early years of TEM, was the result of better and brighter electron guns, increased acceleration voltage, improved electron lens performance (minimization of aberrations) and better vacuum technology. In terms of brighter and more coherent electron sources, microscope manufacturers switched from heated tungsten filaments to heated lanthanum hexaboride (LaB_6) crystals as the electron source, and in the early 1990s field emission guns (FEG) became the new state-of-the-art, with filaments no longer needed to be heated. Thermionic electron guns have an electron beam with a much broader spectrum of kinetic energy. With cold emitter FEG technology, electrons are extracted from a sharply pointed tip with a high field strength, before they get accelerated by a large voltage gradient of typically 160–300 kV. This results in an electron beam that is not only up to 1,000-fold brighter compared to

Table 7.2 Nobel Prizes involving macromolecular electron microscopy.

Year	Laureate	Prize category	Reason for award
1917	Prince Louis-Victor Pierre Raymond de Broglie	Physics	For his discovery of the wave nature of electrons
1982	Aaron Klug	Chemistry	For his development of crystallographic electron microscopy and his structural elucidation of biologically important nucleic acid–protein complexes
1986	Ernst Ruska	Physics	For his fundamental work in electron optics and for the design of the first electron microscope
2017	Joachim Frank Richard Henderson Jacques Dubochet	Chemistry	For developing cryo-electron microscopy for the high-resolution structure determination of biomolecules in solution

thermionic electron sources, but also shows higher spatial and temporal coherence (hence, smaller relative energy spread).

Along with the development in electron source performance, there were other technological improvements over the years to improve electron microscope performance, including building better and more stable electron lenses with less hysteresis, advances in vacuum technology, which not only enabled the introduction of FEG electron sources, but substantially reduced contamination of the microscope column and specimen. Reduction in specimen contamination was crucial for the latest development of cryo-electron microscopy (cryogenic-EM) (or as it correctly should be called electron cryo-microscopy). What was required was the development of temperature-stable cryo-stages and surrounding cryo-shielding (including cold-forks and other shielding) in order to keep the specimen at nearly liquid nitrogen-temperature during specimen loading of the sample stage, during transfer of the stage into the vacuum of the electron microscope, and also to keep the specimen temperature the same in the microscope, all while minimizing drift and vibration during data collection.

Biological samples imaged by macromolecular EM typically fall into one of four categories: Either they show icosahedral symmetry, as many viruses do, helical symmetry as many filaments or tubular structures do, planar symmetry as 2D crystals do or they have no symmetry at all that can be exploited. The latter category is also known as single particles. Samples with icosahedral or helical symmetry inherently display multiple views of the macromolecule, hence a somewhat coarse 3D reconstruction can be obtained from a single image (Figure 7.16).

For samples with planar symmetry or no symmetry, one typically needs to tilt the specimen in the EM to get additional views. The requirement for images of tilted samples of single particles has loosened as 3D reconstruction algorithms have become more sophisticated.

The posterchildren for these categories are (1) tobacco mosaic virus (TMV), the first biological sample with helical symmetry to be studied by EM; (2) a variety of icosahedral viruses including the tomato bushy stunt virus (TBSV) and the human papilloma virus, but also Semliki Forest virus, rotavirus, herpes viruses and others; (3) 2D crystals such as bacteriorhodopsin; and (4) single particles such as the ribosome (Figure 7.17).

As protocols for imaging 2D crystals or single particles/cellular sceneries required tilting of the specimen in the microscope for 3D data collection, tilting stages and motorized goniometers, built for (semi-)automated data collection at minimal vibrations, became available.

Apart from improvements in instrument specifications, major objectives for microscope manufacturers became user friendliness of the TEM and robustness, as after all the microscopes were used by scientists in the biological, biomedical, and material science fields. Recovery from one's own or previous users' microscope operation mistakes could mean hours of painful lengthy realignment of the electron optical path. Low-dose imaging, with its cycling through a variety of very different microscope settings (such as search for suitable grids areas at low magnification or in defocused diffraction mode, high magnification focusing mode and intermediate magnification data collection mode) often resulted in lens hysteresis. Nowadays, lens settings can be restored digitally, simply by pressing a button on a computer instead of manual setting of lens currents.

Perhaps the most impact had the development of detector technology. Originally, film was the medium of choice for data collection, but data collection on film meant that only 50–100 images could be taken in a working day, as only a

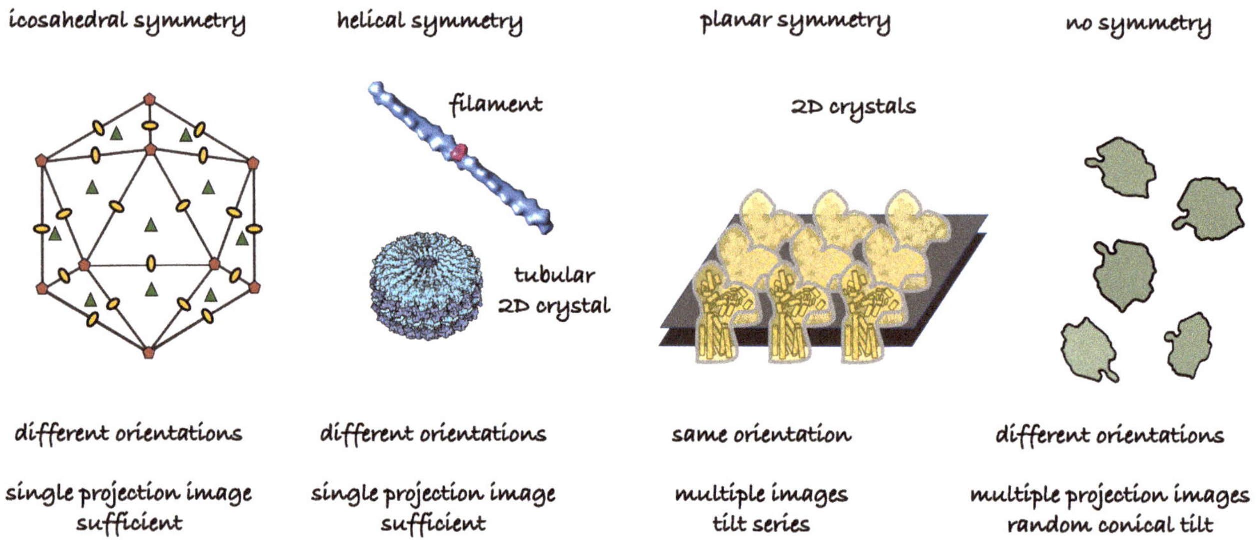

Figure 7.16 Macromolecular EM: Biological samples with icosahedral, helical, planar, or no symmetry. Biological samples that displayed either icosahedral, helical, or planar symmetry played an important role in the history of macromolecular electron microscopy, as such symmetry could be exploited to either obtain multiple views from single images and to obtain a much stronger signal due to implicit averaging. 2D crystals with planar symmetry needed tilting to obtain different views that could be combined for 3D reconstruction. Single particle averaging has been the latest and currently is the most impactful method for structure determination by cryo-electron microscopy. Single particles without internal symmetry need to be recorded in different orientation, which at least initially required tilting of electron microscope grids (e.g., in the context of random conical tilt reconstruction).

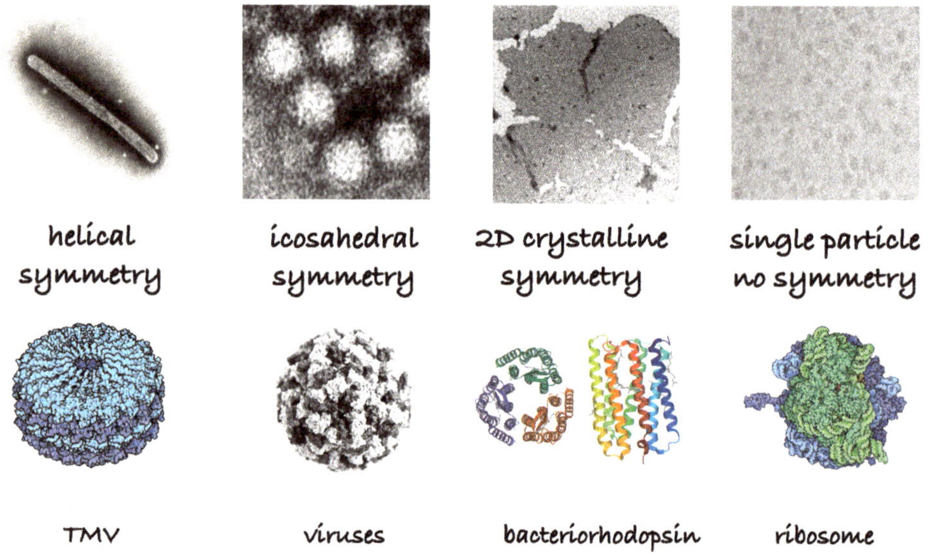

Figure 7.17 Prominent examples of specimen types for 3D-EM. There are several prominent examples for samples used for 3D electron microscopy: (1) tobacco mosaic virus (TMV) with its helical symmetry; (2) several icosahedral viruses, including tomato bushy stunt (TBSV), papilloma, herpes, and rotaviruses; (3) purple membrane bacteriorhodopsin, the first membrane protein to be studied to intermediate resolution; and (4) the ribosome, a well-defined multiprotein/RNA single particle with no internal symmetry.

few magazines of photographic plates could be loaded into the microscope. After each change of film plates the microscope vacuum needed to recover, which could take an hour or longer, even though the film plate magazines had been stored overnight under vacuum in a heated desiccator and thus contained only minimal moisture.

Furthermore, film plates needed to be chemically developed and dried, visually inspected for quality and then digitally scanned. Hence the time from the moment of data collection to having an adequate image for computational processing could be several days of work, which severely limited throughput.

CCD cameras, introduced in the late 1990s and becoming popular in the early 2000s, had a lower performance with respect to resolution and dynamic range, but allowed the acquisition of large amounts of data, and allowed fast feedback on the adjustments of experimental variable. Hence, while initially not being sufficient for high-resolution data collection, CCD cameras played an important role, as they led to the development of automated data acquisition.

Among the challenges of CCD cameras was the presence of a scintillator between the arrival of electrons and the detection of photons, which blurred the signal due to multiple scattering of the electron in the scintillator layer, resulting in limited sensitivity and resolution. Also, the long signal integration time of the CCD camera meant that stage position drift and beam-induced specimen movement blurs the image, resulting in the loss of high-resolution information.

The introduction of the CMOS direct detectors in the early 2010s has revolutionized macromolecular imaging. These direct electron detection devices (DDD) were developed by several different labs, including Henderson and Faruqui at the Medical Research Council – Laboratory of Molecular Biology at Cambridge, Denes and Agard at the Lawrence Berkeley National Laboratory and at the University of California at San Francisco, respectively, as well as Xuong and Kleinfelder at the University of California at Irvine. These DDD no longer needed an intermediary scintillator layer. DDD clearly outperformed CCD cameras (and even film) with respect to detective quantum efficiency (DQE), and thus showed high sensitivity. High sensitivity and high speed of data collection (frame rate) allows DDD to detect single electrons. Hence, unlike it is the case for CCD, where large number of electrons needed to be integrated for one final picture to emerge, dozens of frames with a low electron count can be collected. Thus, instead of one final image, one can obtain many frames, not unlike a movie. Particles in such frames can be aligned to high precision, which allows for correction for beam-induced specimen movement, and thus significantly sharper images. This in turn further improves particle alignment, and together with better image processing algorithms, leads to higher resolution structures.

More recently, development of phase plate technology has led to significant improvements in image contrast in focus, whereas before contrast was generated by collecting images at a certain amount of defocus (underfocus). A small amount of defocus preserves higher resolution but provides little contrast for alignment of particles, whereas larger defocus allows a stronger signal contrast and thus good alignment but at the cost of losing the fine details in the data. The shape of the contrast transfer function (CTF) depends on the defocus value chosen, and the defocus value must be determined with high accuracy to allow for CTF corrections and thus avoidance of using incorrect phase values in map calculation.

Electron phase plates promise to overcome the issue of CTF correction as with an ideal phase plate, contrast can reach 100% throughout the entire resolution range. A variety of designs have been proposed, but commercially successful so far has been the so-called "Volta phase plate" design, featuring a thin carbon-film placed in the back focal plane of the microscope's objective lens, which adds a phase shift to the CTF and thus allows imaging samples (particularly small proteins) with good contrast at near focus settings.

Sample Preparation

The use of an electron beam requires the sample to reside in a vacuum while being irradiated, which for water-based biological samples constitutes a problem: the water will evaporate in the microscope's vacuum, and thus the biological sample can only be examined in its dehydrated state. While environmental electron microscopes, which allow retention of some residual water in the sample chamber, became available in the 1980s, the technology never caught on.

Furthermore, given the strong interaction of the electron beam with matter, radiation damage quickly leads to the disintegration of the sample, unless the sample is imaged at very low temperature.

Last, but not least, given that biological samples are predominantly hydrogen-, carbon-, oxygen-, and nitrogen-based, there is little specimen contrast variations to be expected throughout the sample. Despite these limitations, the first electron micrographs of unstained biological samples were published in 1938 by Bodo von Borries, Ernst Ruska, and Helmut Ruska, and revealed an overall shape of a variety of bacteria and viruses without much detail but at unprecedented magnification.

The initial solution to all the aforementioned problems of imaging biological samples in an electron microscope (dehydration, radiation sensitivity, lack of inherent contrast) was the use of heavy metals to cast a shadow (shadowing) using evaporation of a metal (e.g., platinum) at an angle onto a sample before examination in an electron microscope (Figure 7.18). Shadowing was first applied in 1945 to the study of the TMV protein. While the sample underwent radiation damage and was destroyed upon imaging, the heavy metal cast remained stable and was readily observable. This allowed the exact dimensions and shape of a macromolecule (macromolecular complex) to be determined. This concept was further refined in the late 1950s with the carbon replica technique, where after metal shadowing and subsequently

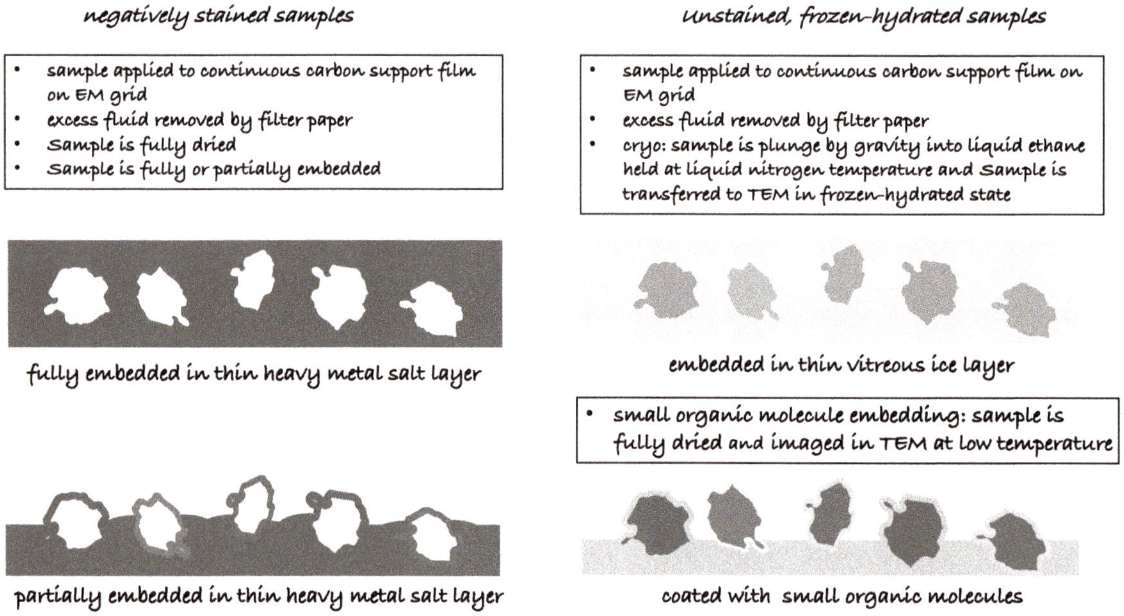

Figure 7.18 Sample preparation for macromolecular electron microscopy. Macromolecular structure determination by electron microscopy either relies on contrasting agents such as negative stain or uses the macromolecule's own inherent contrast with no stain altogether. For negatively stained approaches, samples are either fully or partially embedded depending on how much of the heavy metal salt solution is being left. Frozen-hydrated samples are usually fully embedded in a thin vitreous ice layer, but at least initially high-profile samples were merely coated with a small layer of organic molecules such as sucrose, trehalose or tannic acid. Those samples can be considered as dried down but with a thin layer providing a hydration shell to the macromolecule of interest.

carbon layering, the biological sample was digested away or otherwise dissolved. This resulted in a replica of the sample that could be studied in the electron microscope. However, replica creation was a lengthy process and did not provide instant feedback on the sample.

Positive staining and negative staining techniques became popular in the 1950s and 1960s, where the biological macromolecular samples were exposed to diluted (1–2%) heavy metal salt (uranyl acetate or phosphotungstic acid) solutions, before they were either washed in distilled water (or not), before being applied to an EM grid support film. The excess liquid was typically removed by the capillary forces exerted to the sample by filter paper. While in positive staining, contrasting metal was applied to the sample itself, in negative staining the contrasting metal was applied to its immediate surrounding resulting in a negative imprint of the macromolecule. In reality however (particularly if not done correctly), negative staining can be a mixture of positive and negative contrast, and thus one needs to be careful with interpretation of the resulting images. Compared to shadowing and replica formation, negative staining was very fast, and provided more details about the internal structures of macromolecules, and thus it has been used for several decades as the method of choice, even though the resolution has been limited to ~15 Å (~1.5 nm) resolution due to stain granularity. Furthermore, samples may be flattened due to the strong capillary forces during blotting of the grid.

In 1975 Henderson and Unwin imaged purple membranes, which naturally occurs as a 2D crystal of the light-driven proton pump bacteriorhodopsin, in its unstained state. Embedding the sample in a thin layer of sucrose, which presumably takes the place of water molecules, they prevented the dehydration of the specimen in the electron microscope's vacuum. Using low-dose imaging, they were able to obtain the first 3D structure of a membrane protein at 7 Å resolution.

In 1971 Glaeser demonstrated that radiation damage limited resolution for biological samples, and in 1974 Taylor and Glaeser showed that freezing of crystals of the protein catalase preserves the structural integrity to better than 3 Å and thus at atomic level. In 1976, using electron diffraction, Taylor and Glaeser showed that cryo-protection was able to overcome the effects of radiation damage.

The notion that cooling biological samples to liquid nitrogen (or possibly liquid helium temperature) could overcome radiation damage led to efforts by Dubochet and his team to search for methods that would preserve biological samples in their native, unstained frozen-hydrated state for EM imaging at low temperature.

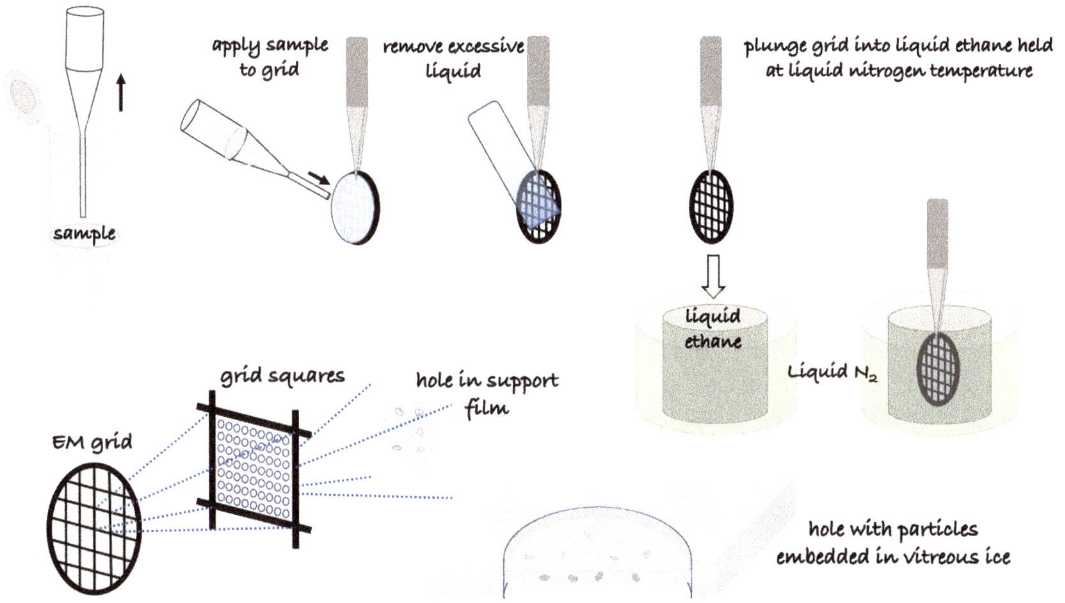

Figure 7.19 Sample preparation for cryo-EM. Plunge-freezing of a thin biological sample on an electron microscopy grid in liquid ethane, held at liquid nitrogen temperature had become the leading method for cryo-EM sample preparation. The electron microscope grid with its many grid layers featured a holey carbon film, with holes containing particles in various orientations embedded/ suspended in vitreous ice.

Adrian, McDowall, and Dubochet in the early 1980s developed a simple technique for obtaining vitreous ice-embedded sample by plunging a grid into liquid ethane, held at liquid nitrogen temperature (Figure 7.19). In 1984, they presented images of unfixed and unstained adenovirus suspensions obtained by cryo-EM in a frozen-hydrated (vitrified) state.

In the early 1990s, using electron micrographs and electron diffraction patterns of 2D crystals of purple membrane, Henderson, Downing and colleagues were able to obtain a near-atomic 3.5 Å map of bacteriorhodopsin. The power of cryo-EM for high resolution structure determination was further confirmed in 1994, when the near-atomic 3.4 Å map of the first eukaryotic membrane protein (Light Harvesting Complex-II) was published by Kühlbrandt, Wang, and Fujiyoshi.

The advantages of cryo-EM imaging of unstained, frozen-hydrated samples were not only obvious for the imaging of flat 2D crystals but also yielded important biological insight into the structure of other samples with either helical symmetry, icosahedral symmetry or without any symmetry. For example, in 1993 the group of Ron Milligan solved the structure of a rigor state actin filament-myosin head complex using a hybrid approach, by fitting higher resolution X-ray structures into lower resolution EM density maps. Also, in 1993 Steve Fuller and his group determined the structure of the adenovirus at 25 Å. In 1995 Nigel Unwin determined the 9 Å structure of the acetylcholine receptor in the open state using time-resolved cryo-EM of acetylcholine-stimulated helical 2D crystals. In 1997 the icosahedral Hepatitis B virus core was solved for the first time at sub-nanometer resolution independently by the groups of Anthony Crowther and Alasdair Stevens, showing for the first-time alpha helices. In 2008 Hong Zhou and his group, studying the Cytoplasmic Polyhedrosis Virus (CPV), for the first time reached a near-atomic (~4 Å) resolution structure of the icosahedral virus capsid, allowing backbone model tracing into the cryo-EM map.

Since the 1980s the groups of Joachim Frank and Marin van Heel studied the structure of ribosomes, a particle with no apparent symmetry that could be exploited for structural analysis. At first, samples studied were negatively stained, but in the 1990s cryo-EM of unstained, frozen-hydrated ribosome samples resulted in 3D reconstructions of *Escherichia coli* 50S ribosomal large subunit at 25 Å and the *E. coli* 70S ribosome at 23 Å resolution, respectively. Further advances in CTF correction led to a report in 1999 by the van Heel's group of the *E. coli* 50S ribosomal large subunit at 7.5 Å resolution, followed in 2000 by a 11.5 Å map of the *E. coli* 70S ribosome published by Frank's group. Atomic models of the ribosome at ~2 Å resolution were finally published in 2019 and 2020, but the dream of obtaining atomic structures from single particles in solution by cryo-EM came true as early as 2013, when Cheng published the high-resolution structures of the TRP channel in three different functional states.

Computation

Apart from progress in instrumentation and sample preparation, advances in computational approaches and algorithms were critical for the success of cryo-EM in the structure determination of macromolecules and macromolecular complexes.

Thin unstained biological samples behave in the electron microscope as weak phase objects, which means that scattered electrons will experience a 90° phase shift, whereas the transmitted (non-scattered) electrons experience a negligible phase shift when traveling through the 2D Coulomb potential of the specimen atoms. For structure determination, only phase contrast needs to be considered, as for thin unstained samples amplitude contrast can be neglected. In other words, the electrons are scattered elastically. However, biological samples are radiation-sensitive and will only tolerate a minimal dose before being damaged beyond recognition. As a result, images recorded in low-dose imaging mode will be characterized by a low signal-to-noise ratio. Even when imaged at a low dose the sample experiences some radiation damage, which may alter the structure of individual particles slightly. This in turn implies that averaging over a larger number of particles can overcome both problems. Another problem that needs to be dealt with is the large focal depth of the electron microscope: a 3D sample will be recorded as a projection image with the information of all the atoms in the *Z*-direction being overlaid on top of one another at the level of the detector. Hence, to reveal the 3D nature of an object, one needs to combine projection views of the object recorded at different angles.

Aaron Klug was a key figure in the early days of image processing of electron micrographs, working with Donald Caspar and Anthony Crowther on negatively stained spherical viruses with icosahedral symmetry such as TBSV, and with David DeRosier on negatively stained viruses with helical symmetry such as TMV and the tail of bacteriophage T4.

DeRosier and Klug demonstrated in 1968 the projection theorem for helical assemblies, that showed that a 3D image can be calculated from 2D image projections using FTs as the central mathematical approach for 3D reconstruction. The projection theorem states that the 2D FT of a plane projection of a 3D density distribution is the same as the corresponding central section or slice of the 3D transform normal to the viewing direction (Figure 7.20).

Thus, a 3D FT can be built up by Fourier space information (the different central sections) calculated from the different views of the object. Once the Fourier space is populated with information calculated from the real space images, a 3D density map in real space can be calculated by Fourier inversion (synthesis). An important feature of this approach is that one can predict how many different views need to be collected for a given resolution target, with any internal symmetry of the particle reducing the number of different views that must be collected. For icosahedral symmetry in viruses this means that 60-fold averaging can be applied.

The approach taken by Klug and colleagues is similar to the approach taken in 3D map calculation in X-ray crystallography, which starts with diffraction patterns, which are essentially providing directly the 3D information in the

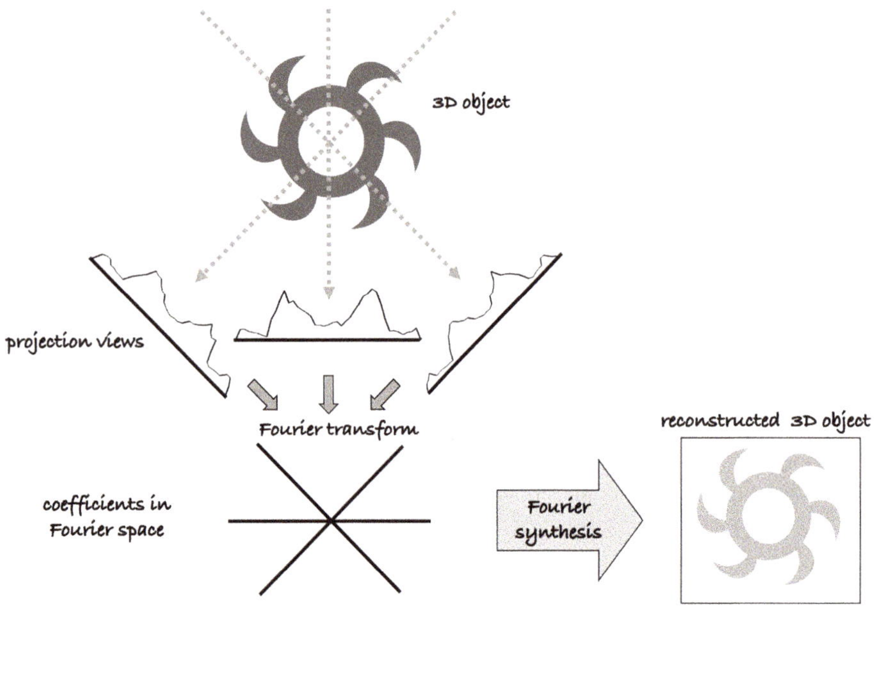

Figure 7.20 The projection theorem. The projection theorem states that a 3D image can be calculated from 2D projection images of an object, which can be thought of sections through the center of the 3D Fourier space. Thus, to calculate a 3D volume, one records projection views at different angles (viewing directions), calculates their Fourier transform and determine the orientation of these different transform to build up/fill the Fourier space with data. Another Fourier transform will then yield the 3D volume density of the object.

Fourier space. The advantage of EM data over X-ray data is that the phases in the Fourier synthesis are readily available from digitized electron micrograph images. The Fourier method is just one way to solve the problem of 3D reconstruction, but it has the distinguished advantage that working with periodically arranged molecules in Fourier space renders noise filtering straight forward.

Since helical symmetry offers views of the different subunits in many different orientations, samples with helical symmetry do not need to be tilted. Therefore, reconstructions can in principle be obtained from a single specimen.

This concept was adapted to particles with icosahedral symmetry by Anthony Crowther, Linda Amos, John Finch, David DeRosier, and Aaron Klug. The method by Crowther is known as the common-line approach for determination of orientation and center parameters, which then in 1970 led to the 3D reconstruction of the icosahedral TBSV via Fourier–Bessel series synthesis.

Aaron Klug received the 1982 Nobel Prize in Chemistry "for his development of crystallographic electron microscopy and his structural elucidation of biologically important nucleic acid-protein complexes."

Many structures have been solved by helical reconstruction, with microtubules being a prominent example. After the high-resolution structure of the tubulin dimer was solved by Eva Nogales, Sharon Wolf, and Ken Downing from zinc-induced sheets, an 8 Å resolution envelope of microtubules, determined by helical reconstruction could be fitted with the atomic model of the tubulin dimer (Figure 7.21).

The projection theorem also holds for flat 2D crystals, where different views of the samples need to be obtained by tilting the sample in the electron microscope. This was demonstrated in 1975 by Richard Henderson and Nigel Unwin, who determined the 3D structure of bacteriorhodopsin (bR) to 7 Å resolution from unstained purple membranes membrane with its naturally occurring bacteriorhodopsin 2D crystals. Embedding the sample in sucrose avoided dehydration in the electron microscope vacuum. They took images at minimal dose as well as diffraction patterns from samples that were tilted up to 60°. This 3D structure was also the first structure of a membrane protein and revealed the packing of the seven transmembrane helices.

Advances in sample preparation such as freezing of 2D crystals in liquid ethane, combined with data collection at low temperature and improved computational analysis, including crystal lattice unbending and CTF correction, allowed in 1990 the publication of a 3.5 Å resolution 3D map of bR and thus the first 3D map of a biological sample obtained by EM at atomic resolution. Several other membrane protein structures at atomic resolution were published in the 1990s. While at a lower resolution (8 Å) the *Neurospora crassa* proton ATPase may serves an example for 2D crystalline data processing (Figure 7.22).

It was grown directly on a continuous carbon-support film forming a two-layered 2D crystal. After Fourier filtering a 2D projection map could be obtained from untilted and tilted samples, which after CTF correction was the merged into a 3D data set. Determination of lattice lines allowed an interpolation of phase values, resulting in the calculation of a map density. From the hexamer a monomer was extracted, and models of alpha helices were placed into the density map.

By the early 2000s, it became clear that X-ray crystallography got the upper hand when it came to structure determination of membrane proteins. Also, it turned out to be very difficult to obtain 2D crystals diffracting to high-resolution, and to obtain adequate image data sets for samples at high tilt angles due to beam-induced specimen

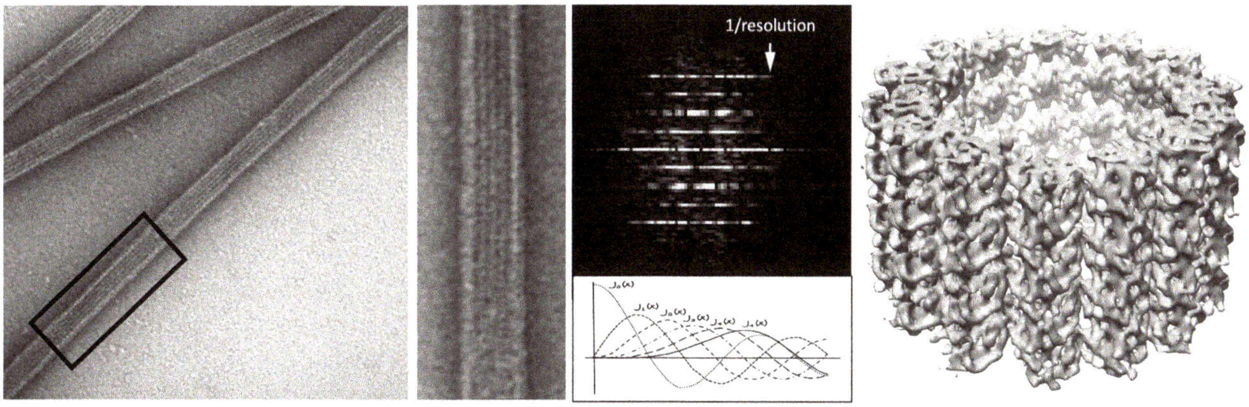

Figure 7.21 Helical reconstruction – Microtubule. After straight portions of microtubule helical filaments are Fourier transformed, and the helical lattice has been indexed, Bessel functions are being assigned to these spots. This resulted in a real space density map of microtubules, to which the structure of tubulin could be fitted.

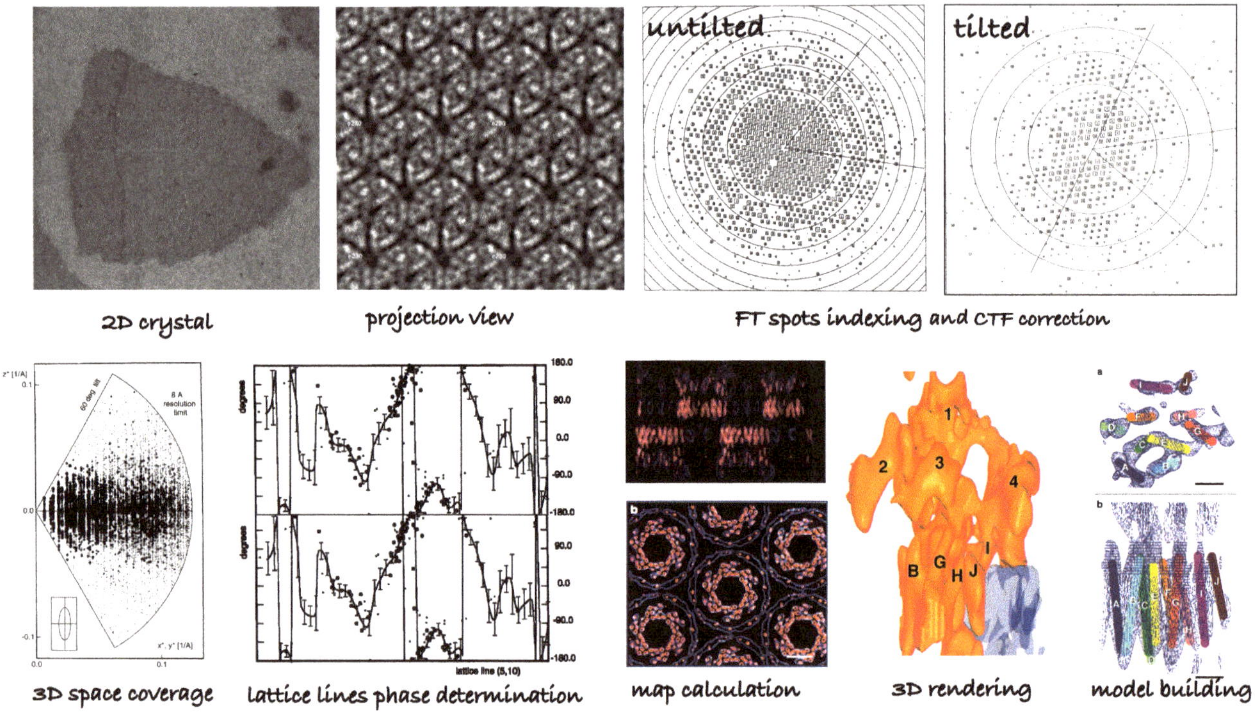

Figure 7.22 2D crystalline symmetry – P-type H^+ – ATPase. 2D crystals of the *Neurospora crassa* P-type ATPase were grown directly on a continuous carbon-support film, resulting in a two-layered crystal with p321 symmetry. Projection views from untilted and tilted specimen were recorded, Fourier filtered and subjected to unbending (which accounts for crystal imperfections and thus results in stronger diffraction spots), before amplitudes and phases were extracted to fill the 3D Fourier space. For individual lattice lines (the third dimension for each 2D diffraction spot), experimentally determined phases lead to continuous function which allows interpolation of phases. After calculating the Fourier transform one obtains a map density (shown here in longitudinal and cross-sectional orientation). From the hexamer a monomer was extracted, and models of alpha helices were placed into the density map.

movement, which is even more severe for tilted than for untilted samples. These challenges led to the demise of 2D crystallography, which was once a highly promising field in cryo-EM.

While helical, icosahedral and 2D crystallographic Fourier-based approaches pioneered the field of EM-based structure determination, it is the field of single particle analysis where cryo-EM has had its biggest impact.

As the projection theorem also holds for projection views of single particles without internal symmetry, it should in principle be possible to obtain 3D reconstruction from a single particle. However, radiation sensitivity of biological samples does not allow multiple images to be taken from a single object.

Low-dose imaging results in high noise levels, and thus a large number of images of individual particles must be recorded to improve the signal-to-noise ratio, and also to average over a large number of molecules with some of them possibly being damaged by the electron dose encountered.

Furthermore, particles ideally are in random orientation, and when recording tens to hundreds of thousands or millions of particles, each projection must be categorized and sorted into class averages. Finally, such class averages need to be combined into a 3D reconstruction, by finding the relative angular relationships between these class averages. The map is iteratively refined with respect to individual particle orientation and CTF correction (Figure 7.23).

For single particle reconstruction to have the success it currently enjoys, many computational advances were needed, and thus many people/groups contributed to the success of single particle cryo-EM, which culminated in the 2017 Nobel Prize in Chemistry. The single particle analysis effort was initially spearheaded by the group of Joachim Frank and later also by Marin van Heel and colleagues. Joachim Frank was a student of Walter Hoppe, who is seen by many as the founding father of electron tomography. In 1975 Frank proposed that averaging multiple different projection views could lead to 3D reconstructions of individual particles without internal symmetry, and in 1978 he published with Timothy Baker a projection map of glutamine synthetase using computer averaging from 50 particles embedded in negative stain. In 1981, Marin van Heel and Joachim Frank used multivariate

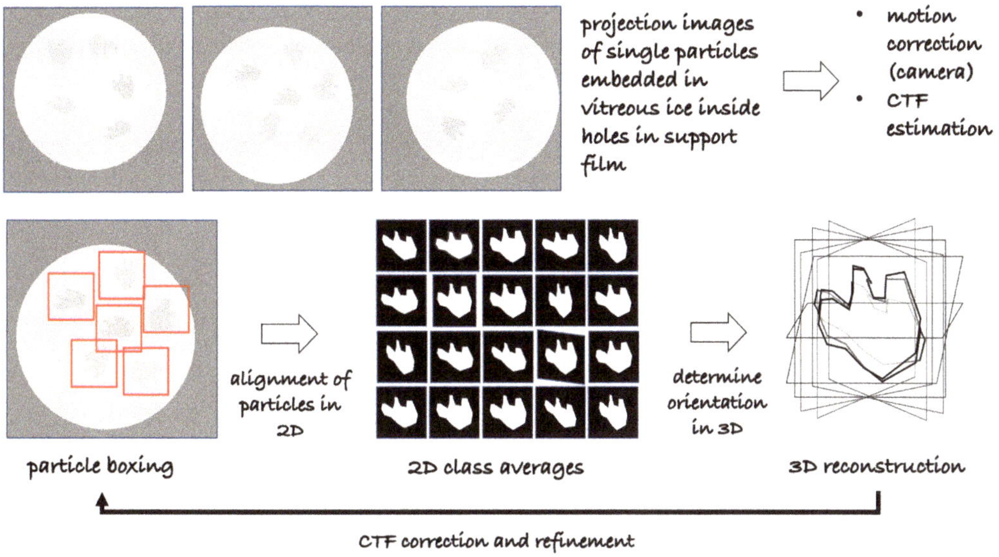

Figure 7.23 3D structure of particles with no internal symmetry. For single particle analysis each cryo-EM image contains multiple single particles embedded in vitreous ice, which after motion-correction at the CMOS camera level and an initial CTF estimation need to be individually selected, aligned and classified into 2D class averages. After determination of their orientation, a 3D reconstruction can be calculated, and a final map can be obtained after iterative CTF correction and refinement.

statistical analysis (i.e., correspondence analysis) for 2D classification of images of negatively stained images, to address heterogeneity in the data sets, and to obtain class averages, which significantly improved the signal-to-noise ratio of the image data.

However, determining a resolution for class averages was not straight forward. One solution was to split the data set in half and measure the reproducibility for different resolution ranges. The Fourier Shell Correlation (FSC), which is directly related to the alignment error, is commonly used as a measure of resolution of single particle analysis. Strictly speaking, the FSC is a measure of self-consistency of the data.

In the early 1980s Michael Radermacher joined Frank's lab and developed the random conical tilt reconstruction method, which in 1987 led to the 3D structure of the large ribosomal subunit from *E. coli*, which was the first particle without symmetry that had been reconstructed in 3D by EM. Jose Maria Carazo and Pawel Penczek in Frank's lab were instrumental in 3D projection alignment and angular refinement, as well as use of Wiener filtering for merging data with different CTF profiles. 3D refinement was carried out either in real space or in Fourier space.

A maximum likelihood approach was introduced in 1998 by Fred Sigworth, which takes into consideration the uncertainty of the particle orientation and instead of assigning a single best orientation, the maximum likelihood approach integrated over the probability distribution of all possible orientations. This approach has also proven powerful with respect to distinguishing subpopulations of particles in different conformational structural states. There are several image processing packages that were developed over the years by the different groups active in the field of single particle analysis, such as SPIDER, IMAGIC, EMAN, and more recently RELION (as well as other software packages).

In 1995, Richard Henderson, examined how many views were needed to obtain high-resolution structural information, assuming a perfect imaging situation, while considering radiation damage. He predicted that averaging 10,000 (asymmetric) particles should be sufficient to obtain a 3 Å (and thus atomic) resolution map, 5,000 particles particle should reach 4 Å resolution, 1,500 particles to reach 6 Å and 800 particles to 10 Å resolution. However, the 25 Å cryo-EM map of ribosomes, published in 1995 was based on ~3,600 particles, and the 11.5 Å cryo-EM map, published in 2000 was based on ~73,000 particles. In retrospect, the discrepancy was resolved when CMOS direct detectors replaced CCD detectors, which addressed some of the non-ideal imaging conditions. In the light of recent developments, Henderson's prediction may even be considered conservative. The history of cryo-EM may also serve as an excellent example of how a large variety of advances in different fields, such as instrumentation, sample preparation and image processing were needed to come together at the right time to accomplish an ambitious goal in science.

The 2017 Nobel Prize in Chemistry was awarded to Jacques Dubochet, Joachim Frank, and Richard Henderson "for developing cryo-electron microscopy for the high-resolution structure determination of biomolecules in solution."

7.2.3 Theoretical Background

Contrast Formation in the Electron Microscope

The de Broglie hypothesis states that accelerated electrons – just like photons – have wave-particle duality and therefore are characterized by a wavelength (and energy) that depends on the voltage by which the electrons have been accelerated. For an acceleration voltage of 120 kV, 200 kV, and 300 kV the corresponding wavelengths are 0.033 Å, 0.025 Å, and 0.020 Å and thus well below the scale of inter-atomic bonds. Even taking into considerations that electronic lenses, needed to focus the electron beam, are not nearly as good as optical lenses, an electron microscope should allow the structure determination of macromolecules at atomic resolution (~2 Å).

The weak phase object approximation states that nearly all electrons travel through the Coulomb field of the atomic nuclei and hence will emerge with no appreciable energy loss, in other words: most electrons that are scattered are scattered elastically. Elastic scattering is the source for the signal in cryo-EM image formation (Figure 7.24).

However, a small but non-negligeable portion of the electrons will be scattered inelastically, which means that they transfer part of their energy to the molecules, leading to bond breakage, free radical formation, and ionization. Free radical formation can start a chain reaction of radiation damage, which means that their effect needs to be curtailed, e.g., by keeping them frozen in place through cryogenic sample immobilization and by imaging at liquid nitrogen temperature. Unscattered electrons will show no change in phase, whereas scattered electrons will experience a phase shift of 90° (a quarter of the wavelength). When scattered and unscattered electrons are combined to form an image, this 90° phase shift will be of significance.

When electrons are scattered, they can be either scattered at a small angle (as is expected for lighter elements in unstained biological samples) or at a large angle (e.g., when entering a heavy/high molecular weight atom). So, if one blocks the electrons scattered at a large angle – e.g., by putting an aperture in the back focal plane – such large angle-scattered electrons can be filtered out, which can be a way of contrast generation, e.g., for heavy-atom-stained biological samples. For unstained samples – if imaged near focus – there is little contrast as the phase shift of the unscattered and the scattered electron wave only differ by 90°, hence there is little constructive or destructive interference, and thus little contrast. However, there are two ways contrast

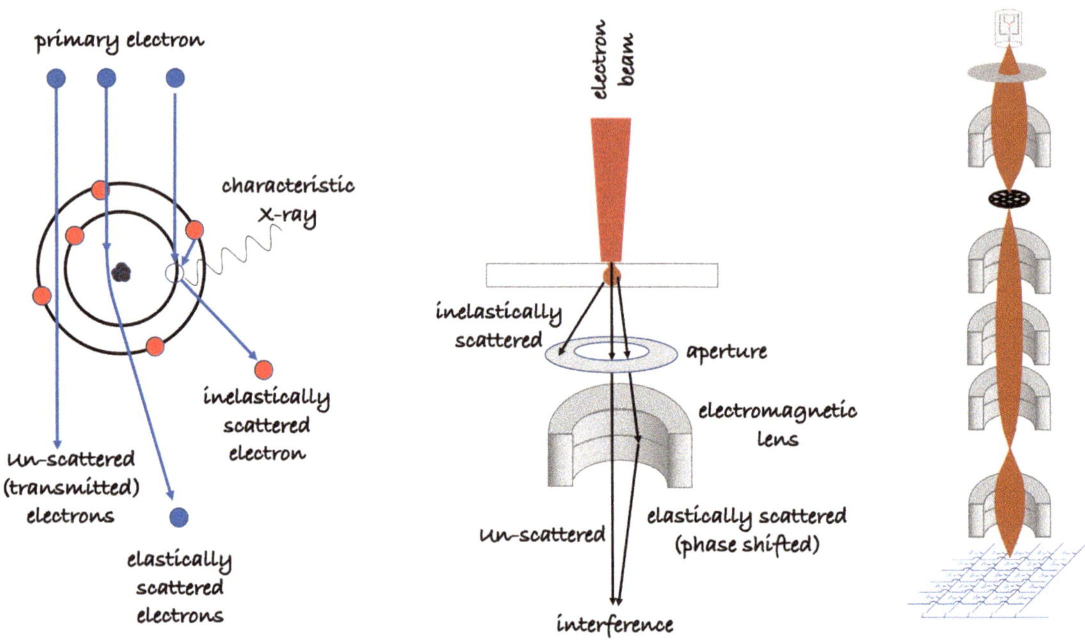

Figure 7.24 Contrast formation in cryo-EM (TEM). Electrons traveling through the Coulomb field of the atom nucleus either experience elastic or inelastic scattering, or simply pass through without any scattering. The unscattered electrons experience a negligible (close to zero) change in phase of the electron particle wave, whereas elastically scattered electrons undergo a 90° phase shift without loss of energy. Inelastically scattered electrons knock out electrons from the atom, and the resulting electron loses energy in the process. Since inelastically scattered electrons typically emerge at a larger angle, they can be filtered out using an aperture, which is how amplitude contrast is being generated. Elastically scattered electrons (that have undergone a 90° phase shift) typically emerge at smaller angles and are refocused by the electromagnetic lenses to combine with the unscattered electrons to create phase contrast. Phase contrast can be enhanced by either using a phase plate or by imaging the sample at small underfocus, both of which will introduce an additional phase shift for the scattered electron.

could be increased, one is using phase plate technology (which has recently become commercially available) or to record images out of focus, which has been the predominant way of contrast generation for over five decades.

Phase plates can be in design as simple as a thin amorphous carbon film with a hole in the center (Zernike phase plate) or hole-free carbon film that is slowly charged by the beam (Volta phase plate), but much more complicated designs have been proposed and prototyped. In a Zernike phase plate, the scattered beam that travels through the carbon film experiences an additional 90° phase shift, whereas the unscattered beam, which passes through the hole at the center, will not experience a phase shift. Hence, the scattered beam will have a total phase shift of 180° and thus destructively interfere with the unscattered beam, which in turn generates contrast.

The other approach has been to take images at underfocus (instead of imaging at focus), which apart from slightly blurring the image creates a phase shift of the scattered electrons that varies in a predictable manner for different frequency ranges according to the CTF. The CTF can be thought of as the microscope's power spectrum and is a periodic function, whose exact shape depends on the spherical aberration (C_s) of the microscope's objective lens (thus is a constant for each microscope) and the amount of defocus chosen. The images are best taken at underfocus (not overfocus), since the sample as a phase object already possesses some scattering contrast. Underfocus simply enlarges this contrast, whereas overfocus would counter it and thus complicate interpretation of the image. The pattern of the CTF can be seen if one takes a FT of the image and for pure carbon it will be characterized by concentric bright/gray rings that are separated by dark rings. This pattern is also known as Thon rings. The bright areas show frequency ranges where the contrast is well transferred by the microscope, whereas dark regions indicate frequency bands where the CTF is near zero, and thus little to no contrast is being transferred by the microscope. Hence in such frequency ranges (for a particular defocus setting) the microscope can be thought of as having a blind spot. These regions are equivalent to the minima in the point spread function in optical microscopes. It is important to note that in adjacent bright regions the contrast is inverted, hence restoration of the true image must take this fact into consideration, a process known as CTF correction. Also, since the frequency position of these blind spot regions depends on the amount of defocus chosen while recording the image, these blind spots can be filled by recording additional data at different defocus settings. There two additional characteristics of the CTF that one should be aware of, namely that the function oscillates faster and faster as a function of frequency, hence it is important to determine the exact amount of defocus, as a small mistake in defocus determination can lead to the assumption of the wrong sign of the contrast. This determination is complicated by the second additional characteristic of the CTF, which is that the oscillating signal gets weaker the higher the frequency/resolution, or in other words there is an envelope function that dampens the signal toward higher resolution. Also, noteworthy is that tilted samples show a different defocus in different regions of the image.

Phase plate technology can be combined with small amounts of defocus to obtain optimal contrast, which is particularly powerful for imaging small proteins and for tomography applications.

3D Reconstructions from 2D Projection Images

The TEM projects a 3D object onto the 2D surface of the detector, in part due to the large focal depth of the microscope. In other words, this mean that all atoms along the path of the electron beam are projected onto the same spot on the detector, and thus information about the third dimension (along the Z-direction) is lost in this projection process. However, according to the projection theorem, a 3D object can be calculated from a series of projection images, by treating every 2D projection in Fourier space as a central slice through the 3D FT, with that respective slice being normal (orthogonal) to the viewing direction of the object. In other words, each of the FTs of each of the different projection views of an object, recorded for different orientations of the object, constitutes a central slice of the 3D Fourier of an intact 3D object, with each central slice being in a different orientation with respect to the 3D FT.

So, if one knows how the different orientations of the object relate to one another, one also knows how the Fourier space central slices, relate to one another, and one can fill in the Fourier 3D space by adding more and more central slices, each obtained from a 2D projection view of the object in a particular orientation. Once the Fourier space is filled in, a simple inverse FT will yield the 3D structure of the object in real space (Figure 7.25).

Radiation damage, due to inelastic scattering of electrons and thus bond-breakage, ionization and/or free radical-formation, limits the dose that can be tolerated by light element-based biological structures. The inherently weak scattering properties of unstained biological macromolecules combined with low-dose imaging results in a poor signal-to-noise ratio of the images, which further complicates the analysis. Furthermore, each image will contain particles that upon radiation have suffered some damage and thus their 3D structure could be slightly altered. For all these reasons it is not practicable to obtain an entire dataset from a single particle, even if it could be

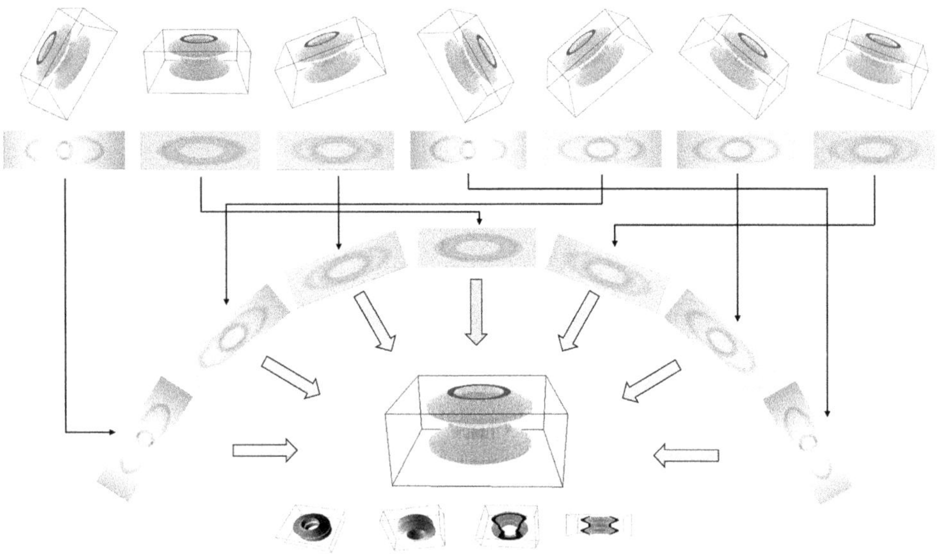

Figure 7.25 3D volumes from 2D images – Particles in random orientation. Zero-degree tilt projection views of particles can be sorted into their respective orientations. Once the respective angles of orientation of the particles are known one can calculate a 3D reconstruction.

imaged in all different orientation. Instead, it is much more advisable to average over a large number of particles, which not only will strengthen the signal but also average out alterations of the 3D structure due to radiation damage.

Macromolecules that arrange into an assembly with helical symmetry such as for filaments or tubular 2D crystals have the advantage that the sample does not need to be tilted in the electron microscope, as a single image of such helical structure offers a variety of different views of the macromolecules, where each subunit is in a defined orientation given by the helical lattice parameters.

Likewise, particle with icosahedral symmetry such as many viruses, offer views of the subunits in multiple orientation without the need of tilting the sample, and given the repeating nature of subunit arrangement, icosahedral symmetry allows 60-fold averaging.

Planar 2D crystals offer the advantage that a large number of molecules are arranged periodically and reside in the exact same orientation, which allows discrete diffraction patterns being calculated from the 2D images. This makes noise-filtering in Fourier space particularly straight forward. One disadvantage however is that for 3D structure determination the sample needs to be tilted in the electron microscope. High angle tilting can be detrimental due to beam-induced specimen movement, particularly for image data while the collection of diffraction patterns is not affected by beam-induced specimen movement. Given that samples in the electron microscope cannot be tilted more than 60–70° (due to EM grid holder and EM grid geometries and thickness), the attainable resolution will be anisotropic. This means that the density map will appear "smeared" out in the *Z*-direction (the direction normal to the 2D crystal plane).

In the case of single particle analysis, one cannot exploit symmetry relationships between macromolecules within an assembly (implicit averaging), but instead needs to explicitly average over many particles. In absence of a good 3D model, the challenge also lies in determining in how a particle projection view is orientated with respect to other particle projection views.

There are two approaches to obtain an initial 3D model that differ in the way the data is being collected: either all data is recorded in at 0° tilt and particle orientation is determined by the common line approach, or pairs of images are collected with a known geometrical relationship of particle orientation.

In the first approach, all particles are in random orientation. With a sufficient number of views that one can bootstrap the orientations of the particles and create an initial 3D model via angular reconstruction. While this approach is elegant, it can be difficult to implement in practice, as angular reconstruction assumes the correct classification of all particles. This can be particularly challenging if the particles display some preferential orientation or some degree of conformational variability.

The second approach to obtain an initial model is based on collecting a pair of images, either at 0° and at 60° (or any high tilt angle), which is known as the random conical tilt reconstruction approach, or more recently at +45° and −45° tilt angle, which has been dubbed as orthogonal tilt reconstruction. This second approach is well suited for samples that show preferential orientation, and it also has

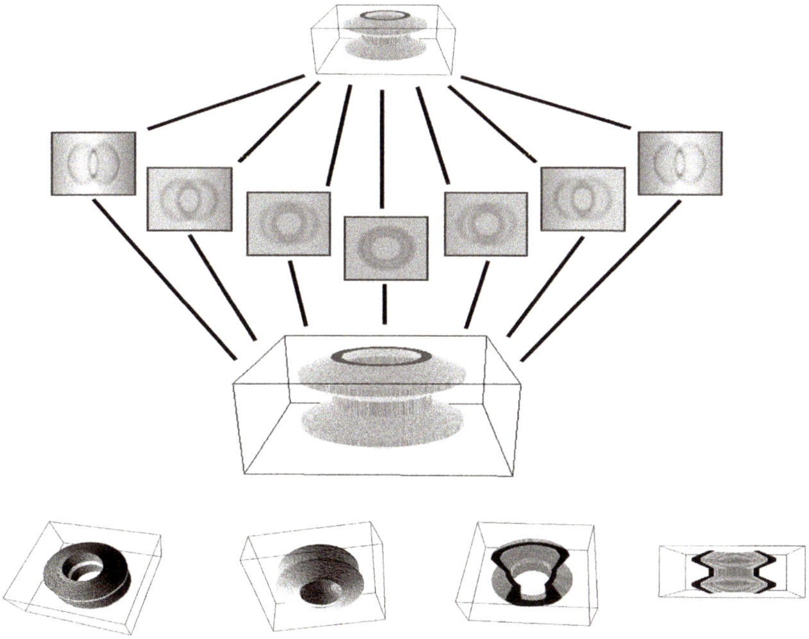

Figure 7.26 3D volumes from 2D images – Tilt series data collection and back-projection reconstruction. The approach of tilt series data collection (controlled rotation of an object around an axis) is particularly well suited for electron tomographic imaging. If the resulting tomogram contains many equivalent particles, they can be extracted and subjected to subvolume averaging in 3D.

the advantage that it allows for multiple starting models to be created, which is particularly useful for samples where conformational variability is encountered.

While electron tomography (cryo-ET) is more typically used for structure determination of subcellular volumes (and will be discussed in more detail in Chapter 8), it can also be used for structure determination of macromolecular complexes. Briefly, instead of taking single or pairs of images of particles, one can collect an entire tilt series of the sample (typically from +70° to −70° tilt angle) either in one direction or two perpendicular directions. Given the limited tilt angle range, this results in a missing wedge or missing pyramid of data, and thus to resolution anisotropy in the *X*,*Y*- versus the *Z*-direction. Through this approach one can obtain a 3D reconstruction of each macromolecule in the reconstructed tomographic volume (Figure 7.26). These structures can be averaged directly in 3D (also known as subvolume averaging). However, one should keep in mind that the electron dose allowable is spent over all the images of the tilt series, hence each individual projection image shows a poor signal in a high noise environment. Also, the recording of tomographic tilt series is time consuming, hence regular single particle data acquisition from projection images is the preferred approach for structure determination of macromolecular complexes.

7.2.4 Instrumentation/Experimental Setup

An electron microscope consists of an electron gun (source and accelerator), a condenser lens (with aperture), a (cryo-) sample stage (that can be tilted), an objective lens (with aperture), as well as an image recording system, all of which is maintained under a high vacuum.

Electron Gun

In the most basic setup for a TEM, one may encounter a tungsten filament that is heated to produce free electrons, not unlike a light bulb. Most such thermionic tungsten filaments TEM sources have been replaced with either a single crystal source of lanthanum hexaboride (LaB_6) or by cold field-emission technology that avoids heating of the filament and instead extracts electrons by applying a strong field near the sharp filament tip. The freed electrons are focused into a beam (e.g., by a Wehnelt cylinder) and accelerated by a voltage gradient of between 80 kV and 300 kV (Figure 7.27).

Electron Optics – Condenser Lens, Objective Lens, and Projector Lens

After the electron beam leaves the electron gun, it reaches the (electromagnetic) condenser lens system which allows focusing of the beam to a desired size. Upon encountering the specimen, scattered electrons are collected by the objective lens the beam is refocused onto the back-focal plane before a projector lens expands the beam to form an image at the level of the detector (Figure 7.28).

Electrostatic fields can be used to deflect the beam path off the center, a feature which is used in low dose imaging, where the focus is found at high magnification in a location near but outside the area from which image data will be recorded. Also, deflection of the beam is used in spot-scan imaging.

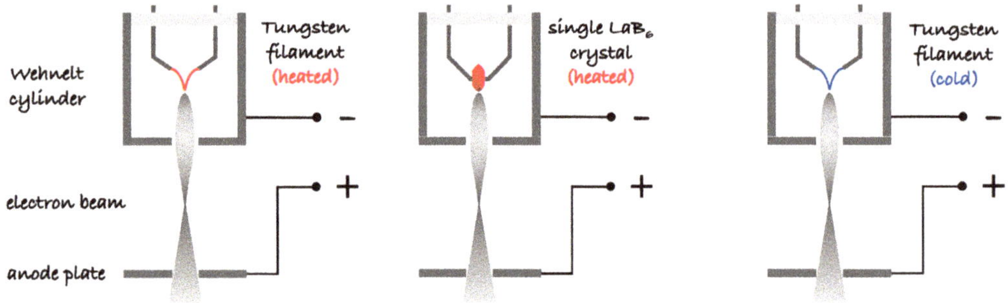

Figure 7.27 Electron guns. Electron guns consist of an electron source residing in a high vacuum. The source is either a thermionic (heated) tungsten filament, a thermionic lanthanum hexaboride crystal, or a cold field emitter. Once free electrons are obtained, they will be accelerated and focused into an electron beam by a Wehnelt cylinder.

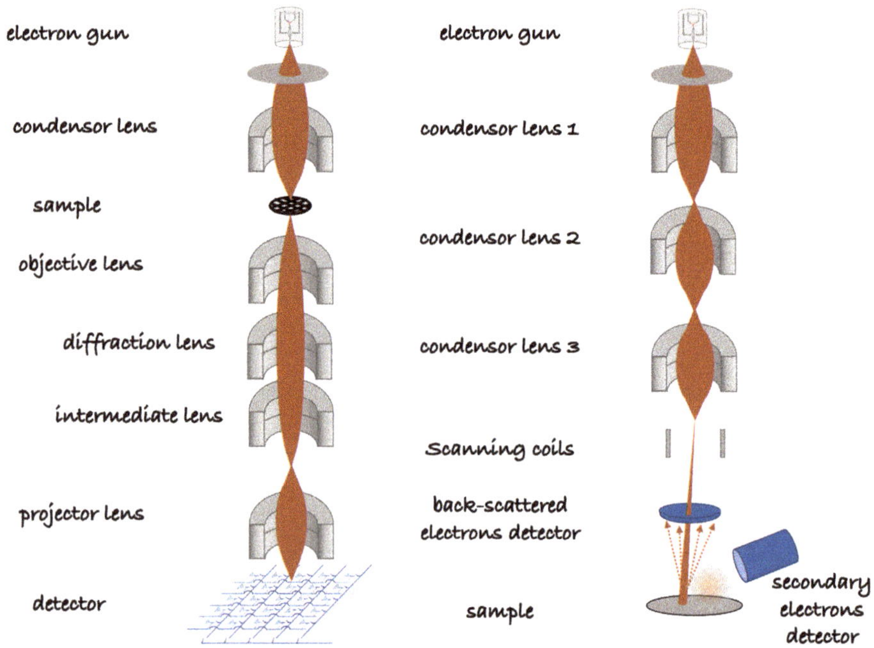

Figure 7.28 Electron optics – System of lenses for transmission (TEM) and scanning electron microscopy (SEM). The electron optics of TEM consists of several electromagnetic lenses, such as condenser lens, objective lens, and projector lens. For SEM neither objective lens nor projector lens are needed, but typically the condenser lens system consists of several electromagnetic lenses. Apertures, while being important components in the electron optics of an electron microscope, are not shown here. Their role is to keep unwanted electrons (e.g., at large scattering angle) from reaching the detector. The mode of detection of electrons varies significantly, with TEM typically have an area-detector, whereas in SEM, point detectors measure the response of the sample, when illuminated by a spot-sized beam.

Electromagnetic lenses are typically solenoid coils surrounded by ferromagnetic materials, whose fields can be changed quickly depending on the lens current settings, hence, one can go quickly between high and low magnification, only limited by lens hysteresis, which is typically avoided in low-dose imaging by going through a defined cycle of lens settings for finding an area of interest at low magnification, then finding focus at high magnification nearby the area of interest and then recording an image at intermediate magnification. Electromagnetic lenses require cooling, most frequently by water, which in turn then requires a water chiller, typically located along with the pumps of the vacuum system in a room adjacent to the microscope (to minimize noise and vibration that could compromise microscope performance).

Apertures are another important part of the lens systems as they can enhance contrast by blocking electrons that have been scattered at a wide angle. However, if one chooses a too small aperture, one runs the risk for not including high resolution image data. Stigmators are correction coils that can compensate for lens imperfections and aberrations, which are causing astigmatism (i.e., directionally uneven lens focal strength). There are commercially available microscopes with spherical aberration correction as well as energy filters that allow chromatic aberration correction.

Electron Detector

A TEM image of the sample is being formed on a detector device, which in current days is either a CCD camera or a CMOS camera, while photographic film is no longer used (Figure 7.29).

Vacuum System

As electrons interact strongly with molecules, the mean free path of the electrons is vastly extended by operating the inner working of the microscope under high vacuum. FEG technology requires a particularly high vacuum, whereas thermionic electron guns can tolerate a lower vacuum. Since photographic film is no longer used in TEMs, it has become much easier to maintain a high vacuum, as the exchange of film cartridges often resulted in hours of microscope downtime for the vacuum to recover to acceptable level, even when the film cartridges themselves had been placed in a heated desiccator for days prior to insertion into the microscope. The vacuum in a TEM is maintained by a series of vacuum pumping systems (including a combination of rotary vane pumps, diaphragm pumps, turbomolecular pumps and/or diffusion pumps) and airlocks that seal off different microscope compartments. High-voltage electron guns need additional vacuum pumping systems such as ion getter pumps, that already require a high vacuum to accomplish vacuums up to 10^{-9} Pa.

Specimen Stage and Holder

Biological samples for macromolecular structure determination by cryo-EM are typically a suspension of macromolecules frozen in vitreous ice in the holes of a thin film. The support film adheres to a metal (copper, molybdenum, gold, or platinum) grid, typically 3.05 mm in diameter with a mesh size of ~50–100 µm. The grid is mounted in its frozen-hydrated state in a specimen holder that is kept at liquid nitrogen temperature, and the holder needs to be transferred to the airlock system of the specimen stage, where the holder is pumped down before it is fully inserted into the microscope vacuum. The specimen stage where the specimen holder is loaded is usually also cooled to liquid nitrogen temperature. Some cryo-holders, known as side-entry holders, have an outside Dewar that is filled with liquid nitrogen. However, the Dewar of the holder is rather bulky, and the liquid nitrogen boils off slowly. Stages with a side entry holder inserted are vulnerable to vibrations and thermal drift, which in turn degrades image quality in the TEM. The situation becomes even worse when the stage with the attached liquid nitrogen-filled Dewar needs to be tilted, e.g., during tilt series data collection for tomography. This somewhat older design is inferior to other designs (such as top entry holder or computerized detached tip

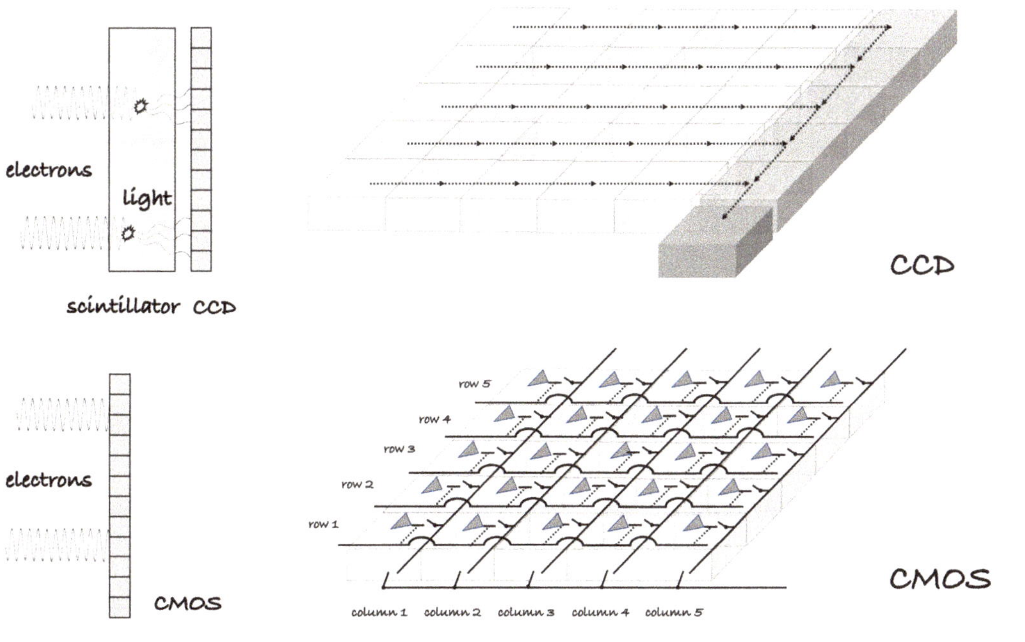

Figure 7.29 Transmission electron microscopy (TEM) detectors. Typical area detectors used for TEM imaging are the CCD camera as well as CMOS detector, which is also referred to as a direct detector. CCDs require a scintillator layer to convert incoming high energy electrons into visible light that is then detected by the camera.

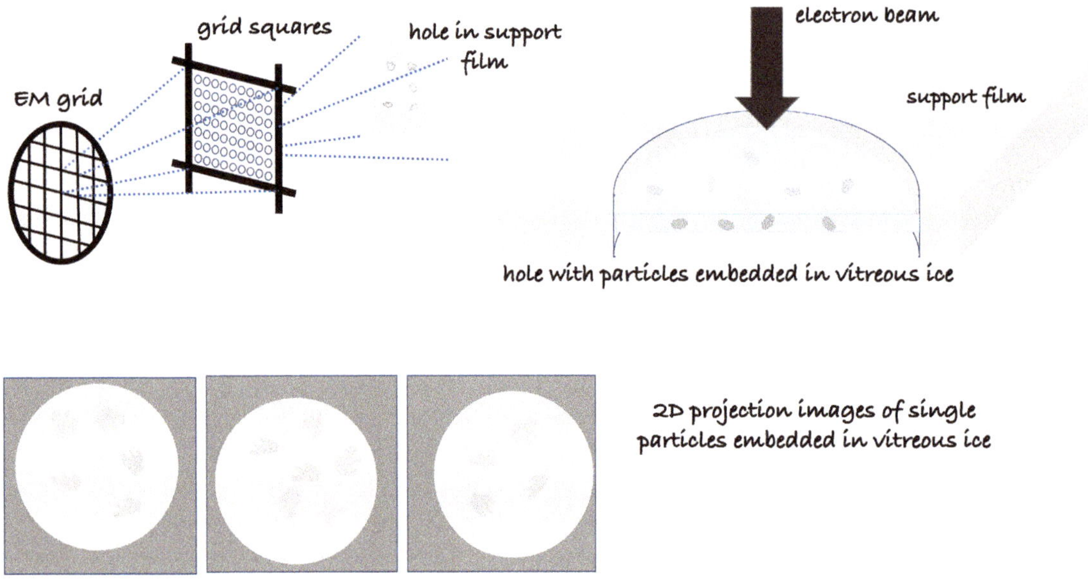

Figure 7.30 Cryo-EM – Sample preparation. EM grids with their metal bars support a thin film, with each grid square containing holes. Small droplets containing the samples are applied to the grid, with excess of liquids being removed by filter paper before the grid is being plunged into liquid ethane, held at liquid nitrogen temperature.

holder stages), where the sample holder or the grid is detached from the transfer device, which results in much better controlled thermal and vibrational stability of the sample holder. Needless to say that having the latest technology at one's disposal can make a huge difference in success or failure of good data collection, which of course is often costly and can only be afforded by a rather small number of well-equipped labs. However, many funding agencies have moved to a model that supports large EM centers that provide data collection as a service to the larger scientific community, an approach that is modeled after the success of synchrotron sources for X-ray crystallography.

7.2.5 Sample Preparation and Data Collection

Sample preparation and subsequent data collection in cryo-EM depends somewhat on what type of specimen is being imaged, but for most macromolecular suspensions there are number of similarities that are part of all sample preparation and data acquisition schemes.

First a droplet (a few microliters) of the sample is applied to the support film of an electron microscope grid, which has a pattern of holes varying in diameter between about one to several micrometers. Excessive liquid is blotted away with filter paper from the grid, which is held by a pair of forceps in a humidity-controlled chamber before being plunged into a liquid ethane-filled contained kept at liquid nitrogen temperature. This leaves a very thin film of frozen-hydrated single macromolecular or virus particles, 2D crystals, tubes, or filaments in a (frozen) suspension. The holes in the support film contain particles, ideally in random orientation, which are embedded in thin layer of vitreous ice, which then can be imaged to obtain 2D projection images (Figure 7.30).

Imaging the samples in the holes ensures minimal background and discourages preferential orientation (by adhering to a support film) or contact-induced alterations of the 3D structure. However, macromolecules also have been shown to reside near the air–buffer interface and hence partial particle denaturation/alterations cannot be fully ruled out even in suspension. Electron microscope grids containing vitrified samples are mounted in an EM sample holder submerged in liquid nitrogen with an overlaying cold nitrogen gas atmosphere. After mounting of the grid in the holder, the grid is protected by liquid nitrogen-temperature cold blades and the holder is transferred quickly to the sample holder stage of the microscope. The holder with the grid is inserted into an airlock and pumped down to an acceptable vacuum level before being fully inserted into the vacuum of the electron microscope. During the whole time of grid mounting and holder transfer the EM grid will be protected from building up ice contamination or warming up to temperature above minus 140 °C. This is the temperature at which point vitreous ice recrystallizes into either cubic or hexagonal ice, which would damage the sample.

Once the sample has thermally equilibrated in the microscope, areas of interest are identified, followed by

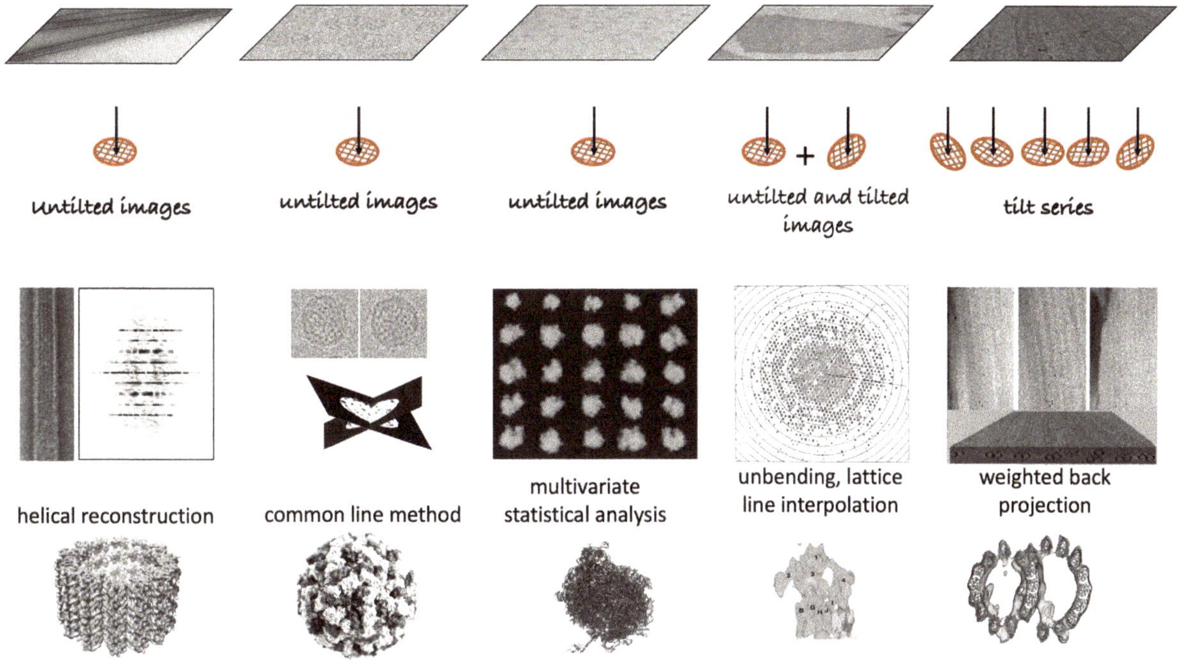

Figure 7.31 Cryo-EM – Data collection. Objects with helical symmetry or icosahedral symmetry do not require tilting. Depending on the approach taken, single particle may need some tilt images at least for initial 3D model generation. Planar 2D crystals will need the acquisition of both tilted and untilted samples, with data being merged in Fourier space before calculation of a 3D density map. Tomographic data collection of macromolecules or cellular sceneries requires the collection of a tilt series around one or two axes to create a 3D volume via weighted back projection.

low-dose data collection, where one finds a region of interest, finds focus at high magnification in an area close to the region of interest, and then records images. For 2D crystals, tomography data or orthogonal/random conical tilt reconstruction of single particles the sample holder may need to be tilted, whereas for other samples projection images at 0° tilt are sufficient (Figure 7.31). Images are taken as dozens of frames at a low electron count, and beam-induced specimen movement is diagnosed and corrected for before the frames are aligned and averaged to produce an image (or an image tilt series) for further analysis.

7.2.6 Data Analysis

The type of data analysis depends on the type of sample that has been imaged, and whether any internal symmetry can be exploited for implicit averaging.

Planar 2D Crystals

Planar 2D crystals are the two-dimensional equivalent of 3D crystals, which have been extensively discussed in Section 7.1. 2D crystals typically consist of either one or sometimes two crystalline layers of protein. Low-dose images, typically taken at low defocus, have a poor signal-to-noise ratio. The FT, which contains both amplitudes and phases, reveals discrete diffraction spots that form a lattice, which at lower resolution is readily detectable above the noise level. Fourier filtering of these diffraction spots eliminates noise, resulting in a Fourier-filtered real space image with vastly improved contrast.

The next step in image processing is the detection and correction of crystal lattice defects, which is done in real space by the so-called unbending routine through cross-correlation of a reference structure (typically a small portion of the image) with all image regions. The resulting scoring function and distortion map then allows the correction of such defects, which in turn strengthens the signal of higher resolution spots (Figure 7.32).

CTF correction allows correction of the phase value for each of the lattice indices, followed by the merging in Fourier space of the indices' amplitudes and phases from different data sets. It should be noted that typically image data at higher tilt angle is significantly worse than image data at low tilt angle, due to the challenges posed by beam-induced specimen movement at high tilt angles. Due to the limited tilt angle attainable in TEM, there is a missing cone of information, that along with the lower success rate at higher tilt angles, leads to a sparse population of certain regions of the 3D Fourier space. This in turn results in a resolution anisotropy in the direction perpendicular to the crystal lattice plane.

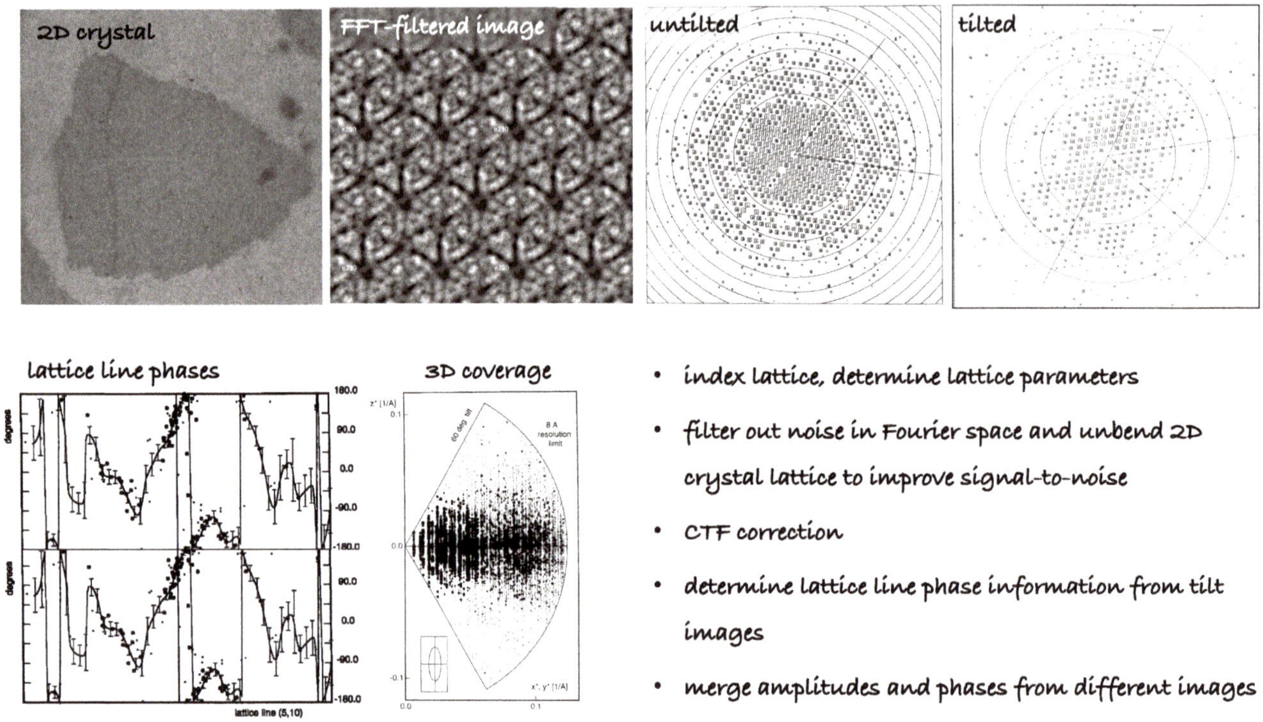

Figure 7.32 Data analysis – 2D crystals. Images of planar 2D crystals result in discrete diffraction patterns which can be Fourier filtered (by keeping the value at predicted spot positions while masking the space in between). Fourier-filtered images are then subjected to unbending which compensates for 2D crystal lattice distortions, which further improves the diffraction pattern for images of both untilted and tilted samples. After CTF correction and data merging from different images, data at known tilt angles is used to interpolate the lattice line phases and determine *hkl*-values for density map calculation. Note that data at high tilt is somewhat sparsely populated, which results in significant resolution anisotropy of the resulting density map.

Assemblies with Helical Symmetry: Filaments and Tubular 2D Crystals

Helical symmetry allows data collection without tilting of the sample in the microscope, as in a helical array all views of the subunits are present. Samples with helical symmetry can be thought of as 2D crystals wound around a cylindrical axis on a helical path. Such a helix can be described by the number of subunits for each helix turn (the number does not need to be an integral number but can be a fractional number) or by the angular and axial interval between the subunits. A helix can be also described by the radius of the helix and the repeat distance along the cylindrical axis (the helix pitch).

The FT of an assembly with helical symmetry is characterized by a series of horizontal layer lines. Such layer lines are analogous to diffraction spots in a 2D crystal lattice. However, each layer line represents a convolution of a reflection with a Bessel function (which is a direct consequence of the cylindrical nature of the helix). First, each layer line needs to be indexed correctly before inverse Fourier–Bessel transform can be applied to the layer line data to produce a real space density distribution (Figure 7.33). Among the challenges is the correct determination the handedness of the helix as there exist various ways for indexing the helical lattice. Correct indexing of the helical symmetry is crucial, as phase relationships in Bessel functions depend critically on it, but there is no objective way to verify that the assignment of Miller indices is correct. After recording of the image, the helix is reoriented, centered, and masked. After indexing, the Bessel order for each of the layer lines needs to be determined. In-plane rotation and out-of-plane tilt need to be corrected for before the amplitude and phase data along each of the layer lines can be extracted. This process produces two redundant data sets, often referred to as the near and the far side of the helical assembly, which reflects the two alternative 2D lattices used for indexing.

After CTF correction (which requires determining the value of defocus and astigmatism) these two data sets can be used as a resolution-dependent phase residual, i.e., a quality measure for phase statistics. If there is internal two-fold symmetry the near and far side data can be merged (and a phase residual is calculated by randomly splitting up data points into two different data sets). Data from multiple images can be averaged in Fourier space, assuming they all show the same symmetry. A final 3D structure can be

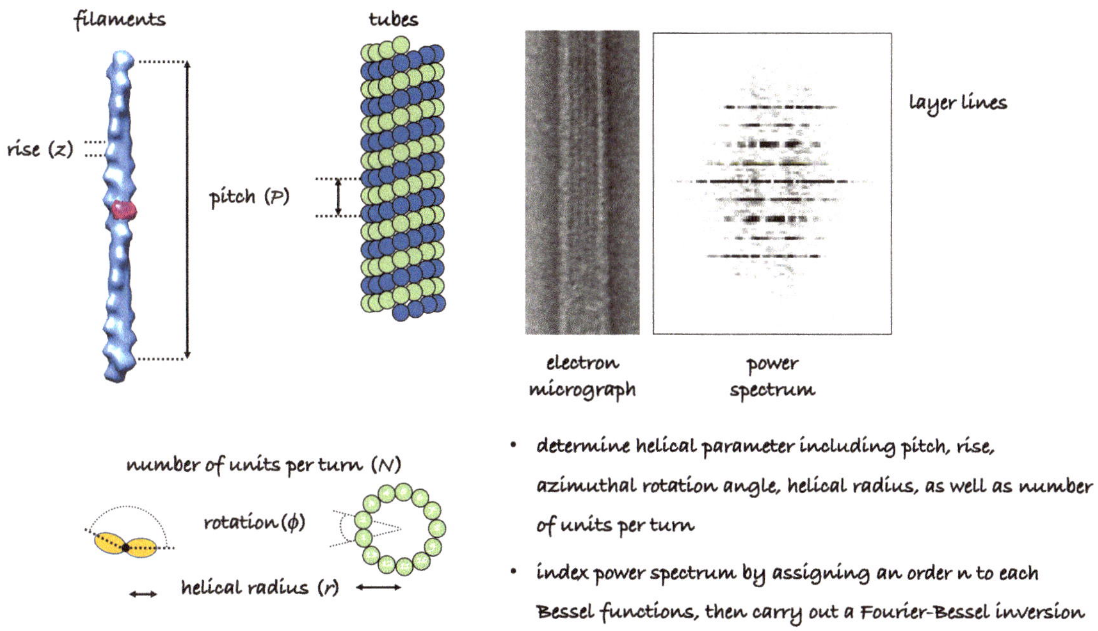

Figure 7.33 Data analysis – Tubular crystals and filaments with helical symmetry. The Fourier transform of electron micrographs of 2D crystals or filament samples with helical symmetry results in a diffraction pattern (power spectrum) with layer lines. After indexing of the helical lattice and determination of the helical parameters (including pitch, rise, azimuthal rotation angle, helical radius, und number of units per turn), Fourier–Bessel functions are assigned to each layer lines resulting in a 3D reconstruction (courtesy of Dr. Haixin Sui).

calculated from the information contained in the Fourier space layer lines via a Fourier–Bessel transform.

Specimen with helical symmetry (tubes or filaments) are rarely perfectly straight, but show some amount of bending, and require some unbending (straightening) for helical reconstruction methods to provide the highest resolution possible. There are two types of distortions that need to be considered, namely in-plane distortion and out-of-plane distortion. For in plane distortion one can reinterpolate in real space the image by finding the center position of the helix and thus determining the amount of distortion from a perfectly straight helix. This real space distortion correction approach is similar to the unbending procedure developed for planar 2D crystals. Out-of-plane distortions can be dealt with by dividing up the helix into shorter segments (with sufficient signal-to-noise ratio to allow reliable alignment) that can be processed separately and allow out-of-plane distortion correction.

An alternative to the above-described Fourier–Bessel reconstruction method is the so-called Iterative Helical Real-Space Construction (IHRSC) approach. One can think of this approach as a variation of the single particle analysis approach, where very short segments (typically much smaller than what is used for the out-of-plane distortion correction discussed above) are matched and averaged. This approach overcomes some of the challenges encountered in Fourier–Bessel approaches such as the correct layer line indexing and instead relies on projection matching to determine the relative orientations of individual segments of the helix. After alignment, a 3D structure is obtained by back projection, and helical symmetry can be determined through autocorrelation, and subsequently imposed, as a template for the next round of alignment and projection matching. This IHRSC approach has many advantages over traditional Fourier–Bessel methods and has led to a variety of high-resolution structures. Since it is an iterative refinement process, the choice of an initial model may seem important, but it turns out that starting with a solid cylinder is sufficient for an initial model (and can even be eliminated if one randomly assigns azimuthal angles to generate a starting volume). However, some estimates of helical symmetry (and knowledge of helical symmetry in general) are still required to succeed with this approach.

Assemblies with Icosahedral Symmetry Including Many Viruses

Particles such as viruses that display icosahedral (532) symmetry (which means 5-fold, 3-fold, and 2-fold symmetry) consists of 30 edges with 2-fold symmetry, 20 triangular faces with 3-fold symmetry, and 12 vertices with 5-fold rotational symmetry. In other words, the individual asymmetric unit is only 1/60th of the whole object or an icosahedral particle consists of at least 60 identical subunits that are related by icosahedral symmetry.

Viruses are often described by triangulation (T) symmetry, which is a pure mathematic concept concerning lattices. T-symmetry emerges from the 3D reconstruction, instead of being imposed during 3D reconstruction. The 3D reconstruction process presumes that in an icosahedral virus all subunits are identical and thus can averaged. After particles have undergone an initial CTF estimate (e.g., obtained from the Thon rings of the FFT), initial particle orientation and particle center are determined, resulting in an initial model.

The original way to build a model is based on the common lines approach, sometimes also referred to as the self-common lines, which derives from the projection theorem and states that two FTs of different views of the same particle imaged in projection will intersect in Fourier space and share a line where the two transforms intersect (Figure 7.34). For particles with internal symmetry there will be symmetry related views, and thus intersecting central sections, where the transform must have the same value in both sections. For each of the internal symmetry operators, such common lines exist, in the case of icosahedral symmetry there can be up to 37 pairs of such common lines. The angular positions of these lines are dependent on the orientation of the particle, hence by finding these common lines through comparison of the FT values along lines in different angular orientation through the center in the 2D FT of each particle, one can determine the orientation of the particle from a single particle without the need for a reference image. However, there are some shortcomings of the common line approach, such as clustering of views near symmetry axes, and the need to collect focal pairs to have high defocus images with sufficient contrast for the common line determination and low defocus image for higher resolution structure determination. Therefore, other approaches are nowadays preferred to build an initial model that that can be iteratively refined by adding more and more projection views at low defocus. One approach is to create a starting model by choosing particles that display twofold, three-foils, and fivefold symmetry, respectively, and then use those views for a crude 3D model for further refinement. Another starting point can be to build a synthetic model with an input of geometric information such as approximate size, angularity and shell thickness parameters or to use real particle images but to set the Euler angles (orientation parameters) to random values, which also results in an initial spherical average without any surface details. Such starting models are typically sufficient for iterative refinement and final convergence to a correct 3D structure.

Template matching works particularly well, if the general features of the structure are known or crude model can be generated, as discussed above. Particles that do not provide a good match should be excluded from further refinement, a process that can also be helped by visual inspection of the Thon rings of the FT, which can help to diagnose obvious problems such as beam-induced specimen movement or ice crystal contamination. The refinement of the 3D structure is an iterative process, not unlike the one used

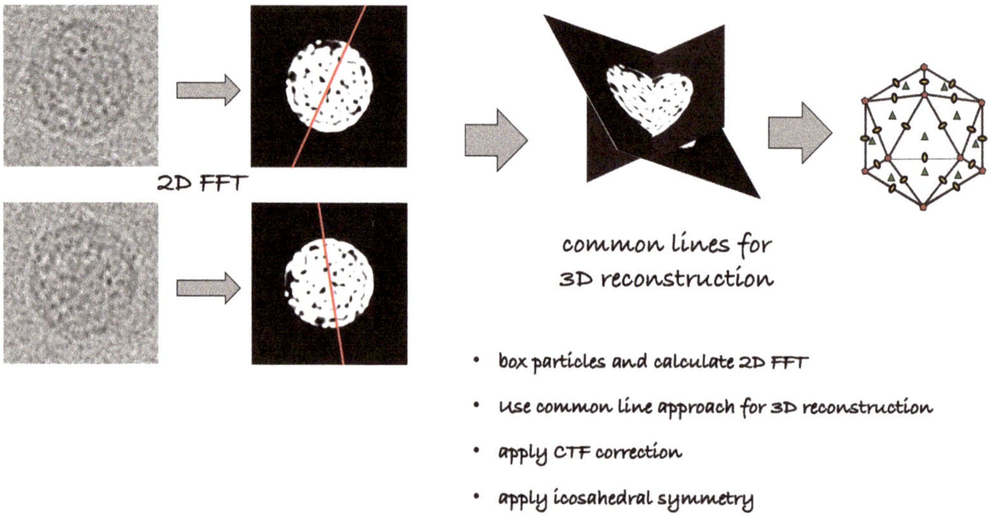

Figure 7.34 Data analysis – Viruses with icosahedral symmetry. Images of viruses in their frozen-hydrated state are boxed and a 2D Fourier transform is calculated. Lines of the Fourier transform through the center are then compared to such lines in other images until common lines can be found. This serves as an initial estimate of orientation of these two particles with respect to one another. By filling up the 3D Fourier space through the common line approach, and Fourier transform a real space initial model can be obtained. Further refinement is then carried out by adding more images and CTF correction. Furthermore, icosahedral symmetry can be explicitly imposed.

in single particle analysis. Here 2D projections of a 3D structure serve as a template to compare to and match with boxed projection images to refine the particle's orientation and center parameters.

The final map is calculated from CTF-corrected projection views of boxed particles, whose orientation and center has been iteratively refined. An estimation of resolution can be obtained by splitting the data set in half and carrying out the refinement independently for each of the two data sets, which leads to two independent 3D reconstructions, whose FSC can be calculated (often masking the non-icosahedral central portion of the particle which typically contains the nucleic acid).

It should be noted however, that in the process of icosahedral 3D reconstruction with its 60-fold averaging one averages out deviations from icosahedral symmetry. To study such symmetry-mismatches, one can relax the icosahedral symmetry to C1 symmetry for determination of particle orientation and carry out the 3D reconstruction without imposing icosahedral symmetry.

Single Particle Analysis

Single particle analysis has many similarities to the structure determination of particles with icosahedral symmetry as discussed above. However, determining a starting model is not as straightforward in the case of single particles due to the lack of self-common lines in the FT of individual particles. Initial 3D models can be generated from lower-resolution negative stain, a low-resolution-filtered X-ray model, an EM map of a homolog structure or even a random sphere. In an iterative process, for each particle its center and orientation are being determined, e.g., by projection matching, where a cross-correlation coefficient is calculated between the boxed particle image and a set of projections of the initial 3D model (Figure 7.35).

A coarser search saves computational time but results in less precision, hence an acceptable trade-off must be found. This task of a five-dimensional search can be divided into two tasks: First, to determine the x, y coordinates and a rotational in-plane angle, which leads to 2D class-averages of particle with similar orientation with a much-improved signal-to-noise ratio; Second, to determine two out-of-plane parameters (while simultaneously refining the three in-plane parameters). Another parameter to be considered is the amount of defocus used for data acquisition. Statistical clustering and maximum likelihood approaches are used for classification and parameter refinement.

Several user-friendly software packages exist to carry out all steps of the 2D classification and 3D alignments, some of the more popular packages are EMAN, RELION, and FREALIGN, to name a few. Like it is the case for icosahedral reconstruction, particles that do not show good correlation should be rejected, as they may hurt the 3D reconstruction more than they help.

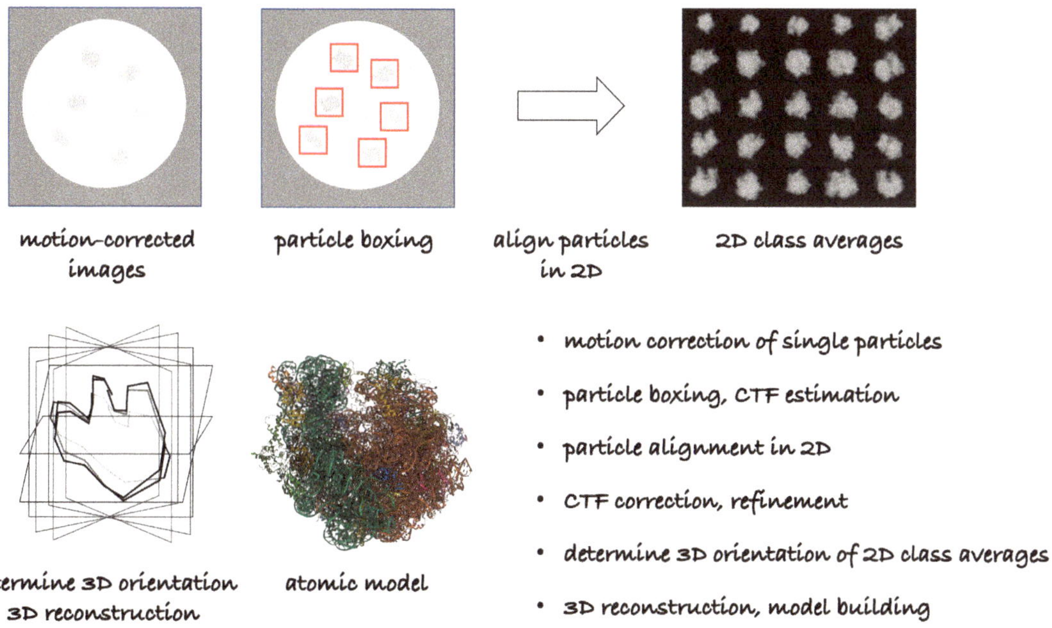

Figure 7.35 Data analysis – Single particles without internal symmetry. Single particle analysis starts with boxing of individual particles in electron micrographs (which ideally have been motion-corrected). Particles are aligned into 2D class averages, which will significantly improve their signal-to-noise ratio. The two out-of-plane orientation parameters and the amount of defocus need to be determined for each particle, using statistical clustering and maximum likelihood approaches. After refinement of the model, a high-resolution density map is obtained that allow the building of an atomic model.

Cryo-Single Particle Tomography – Subvolume Averaging

The strength of cryo-electron tomography (cryo-ET) lies in the visualization of cellular sceneries, and thus macromolecules in their native cellular context. This aspect of cryo-tomography will be discussed in more detail in Chapter 8.

Cryo-ET in combination with subvolume (subtomogram) averaging can be used to determine the structure of macromolecules as single particles, a somewhat recent approach known as cryo-single particle tomography (cryo-SPT). It differs from cryo-single particle analysis (cryo-SPA) since 3D volumes are created first by tomographic imaging followed by single-particle averaging of selected tomogram subvolumes, whereas cryo-SPA records 2D projection images that are then submitted to 2D class-averaging before reconstructing a 3D volume. Cryo-SPT overcomes a problem often encountered in cryo-SPA, namely the discrimination between changes in particle orientation versus changes in particle conformation in 2D images.

Subvolume averaging dates back to the early days of cryo-ET when Hanspeter Winkler and Ken Taylor in 1999 used multivariate statistical analysis to identify and average subvolumes of heavy-metal stained and resin-embedded insect flight muscle tomograms. In 2006, Haixin Sui and Ken Downing used cryo-tomography followed by subvolume averaging to study frozen-hydrated isolated microtubule doublets at a resolution of 29 Å (2.9 nm), which was sufficient to clearly resolve the protofilaments of tubulin monomers and other proteins and allowed the fitting of tubulin atomic models to the cryo-tomogram (Figure 7.36). In the last 10 years, several structures, such as the proteasome and the nuclear pore complex, have been determined at 20–30 Å resolution, and several others at subnanometer resolution. Florian Schur in the lab of John Briggs was able to obtain a 3.9 Å and thus atomic resolution 3D structure of a HIV-capsid protein from cryo-tomograms of immature HIV assemblies.

Since the total electron dose that can be used in cryo-ET is limited, the dose needs to be distributed over all images of the tilt series, which is known as dose fractionation. However, if well over 100 images are recorded per tilt series (e.g., at 1° tilt angle increments from +60° to −60°), each 2D projection image receives as miniscule electron dose, which makes alignment more difficult and thus 3D cellular volume rather noisy. As for cryo-SPT the goal is to average many subvolumes in random orientation, larger tilt angle steps can be tolerated and might even be preferable, as this speeds up data collection and results in higher-dose (and thus higher-contrast) images, with no negative impact on final averages, as long as enough subvolumes/subtomograms are averaged.

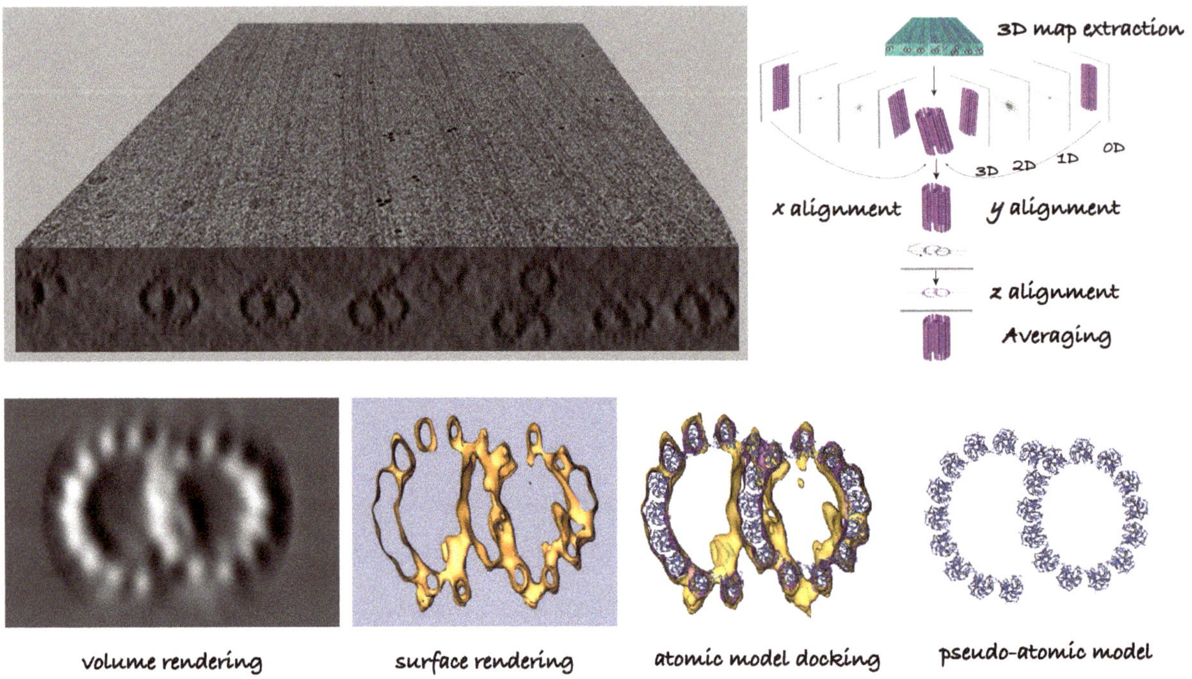

Figure 7.36 Data analysis – Electron tomography with subvolume/subtomogram averaging. In the case of the microtubule doublet structure, subvolumes were extracted, aligned, and averaged, which resulted in a density map to which an atomic model of tubulin could be fitted (courtesy of Dr. Haixin Sui).

One of the key challenges for subvolume averaging is the missing wedge, which is a region in the Fourier space devoid of data due to limitations of the tilt angles during data collection, and which leads to anisotropic resolution in tomograms. The missing wedge poses one of the most critical problems for alignment and classification of subvolumes/subtomograms, as care must be taken to prevent missing wedge bias that would lead to alignment of subvolumes according to their missing wedge (the strongest feature in a subvolumes) and not their underlying common features.

Another key challenge is CTF correction, as without CTF correction the resolution of subtomogram averages will be stuck at 20–100 Å (2–10 nm). If one wants to go beyond 20 Å (2 nm) one requires an accurate estimation of the CTF, and needs to correct for the CTF for each tomographic subvolume (particle), which is far from trivial and further complicated by defocus gradients in tilted views of the sample.

Electron Diffraction of Thin 3D Crystals – Micro-ED

While electron diffraction of one- or two-layered 2D crystals no longer has many followers, electron diffraction of thin but multilayered 3D crystals has recently become very popular for structure determination of small organic molecules and proteins. Electron diffraction features a parallel beam about 100-fold smaller in size than the X-ray beams at synchrotron microfocus beam lines and allows structure determination of crystals in the micrometer range. Strong interactions of the electrons with the atomic Coulomb field ensure strong diffraction signals even from rather thin samples and from lighter atoms (compared to X-rays). However, the strong scattering also can cause problems, as multiple scattering can occur.

Recent changes in the data collection strategy (including precession-assisted electron diffraction tomography, rotation electron diffraction and continuous rotation electron diffraction) together with improvements in the processing of the recorded diffraction patterns make this approach a very promising technique for high-resolution macromolecular structure determination. The approach for analysis is very similar to X-ray diffraction, with MR being a popular method used for phasing (Figure 7.37).

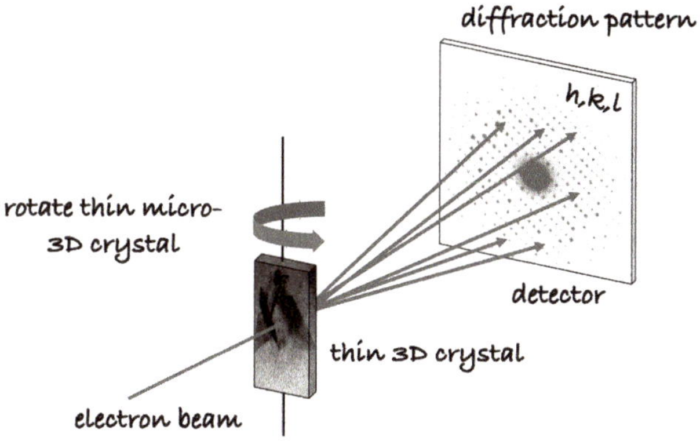

Figure 7.37 Electron diffraction – Thin 3D crystals. An electron beam irradiating micron-sized 3D crystals yields diffraction patterns due to the strong interaction of electrons with matter. A popular method for phasing used is Molecular Replacement.

7.2.7 Map Calculation and Resolution Estimates

Given the damping of the CTF at higher resolution, one needs to restore an appropriate balance of the signal at high resolution versus the signal at low resolution, i.e., by applying a so-called B-factor to the resolution shells to compensate for the amplitude decay. This process is called sharpening. Care must be taken not to simply amplify noise at high resolution. Hence, it is important to determine to which resolution the density map quality extends. In X-ray crystallography one determines the resolution as the highest spatial frequency range (i.e., in Fourier space) with an adequate coverage of diffraction spots that still contains interpretable information about the structure of interest.

In cryo-EM, the FSC has become the standard as a resolution criterium. The FSC curve is computed as the correlation coefficient between two independent 3D reconstructions and plotted as a function of resolution (spatial frequency). Typically, correlation is high at low resolution and drops close to zero at higher resolution when noise overtakes meaningful information. Several thresholds have been proposed, with the 0.143 FSC value threshold having become the standard for determining the resolution. Other values have been proposed in the past including the three-sigma significance criterion or the more conservative 0.5 FSC threshold that dominated the field for quite some time (Figure 7.38).

To make things even more complicated, different parts of a density map may be better defined as others (e.g., due to flexibility of certain residues or local particle heterogeneity), and the views may not be totally randomly distributed (i.e., preferential orientation) which could lead to a resolution anisotropy. This supports the notion that using a single number as a criterion for map quality may be somewhat limited anyway. It appears that the quality of density maps is better described by local resolution estimates than a single resolution value for the entire structure.

Ultimately, it is less important what exact number is given, but whether the final map can be interpreted in

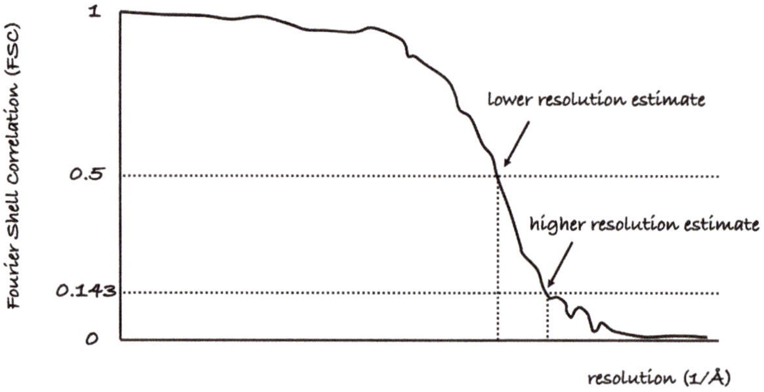

Figure 7.38 Resolution estimates – Fourier shell correlation. The Fourier shell correlation (FSC) is calculated as the correlation coefficient between two independent 3D reconstructions as a function of resolution. Typically, correlation is high at low resolution and low at high resolution. FSC values of 0.5 or 0.143 have been proposed as the cut-off values for determining the resolution.

Factors limiting resolution in the electron microscope

Instrumentation - Microscope:
- stability of sample stage (thermal drift, vibration)
- quality of electron optics (astigmatism, shape of CTF envelope function)
- imaging in underfocus (defocus) setting to generate sufficient phase contrast

Instrumentation - Detector:
- quality of detector (detective quantum efficiency DQE, modulation transfer function MTF)
- mode of detection (integration of signal versus direct detection)
- beam induced specimen movement requires motion correction which is feasible in direct detectors

Sample:
- unavoidable radiation damage even at low electron dose
- heterogeneity (conformational, damage)

Computation:
- very low signal to noise ratio (SNR) of data due to minimal dose imaging
- accuracy of alignment (due to low SNR) and image artifacts
- particle blurring due to beam-induced specimen movement (without motion correction)
- number of particles used for generation of class averages and 3D reconstruction
- averaging of particles with conformational heterogeneity
- accuracy of parameters used for the modeling of image formation (defocus, amplitude contrast, magnification)

Figure 7.39 Factors limiting resolution in the electron microscope. There are typically four factors that limit the resolution in cryo-EM. First, data may be limited by microscope performance, including vibration, thermal drift, quality, or settings of the electron optics. Second, detector type and performance may be limiting, particularly if motion correction (due to beam-induced specimen movement) cannot be compensated for. Third, the sample itself may be conformationally heterogeneous and/or be easily damaged by electron beam irradiation. Fourth, there may be a variety of challenges that prevent the computational signal-to-noise improvement and/or 3D reconstruction.

biological terms. These factors can limit the resolution in cryo-EM: First, microscope performance, including vibration, thermal drift, quality, or settings of the electron optics. Second, detector type performance (motion-correction). Third, the sample itself may be conformationally heterogeneous and/or be easily damaged by electron beam irradiation. Fourth, there may be a variety of challenges that prevent the computational signal-to-noise improvement and/or 3D reconstruction (Figure 7.39).

7.2.8 Visualization and Model Building

Density maps obtained by any of the 3D reconstruction techniques discussed above, must be inspected, and interpreted with an appropriate 3D visualization software package. Strictly speaking, the result of a cryo-EM 3D reconstruction is the Coulomb potential, not an actual electron density map like it is the case in X-ray crystallography. However, in first approximation they both describe the position of the atoms in a macromolecule, however negatively charged carboxy-groups of amino acid side chains tend to be weak in cryo-EM maps.

The density map is typically rendered as an isosurface (a surface representing a certain density threshold/cutoff that can be chosen by the user). Lowering the density threshold will result in bulkier features with less detail, whereas higher density thresholds will result in features being disconnected.

Depending on the resolution of the density map, one can see the structural shape of the macromolecule at ~15 Å, one starts to distinguish secondary structure elements such as alpha-helices and beta-sheets at 10 Å, which become increasingly more detailed as the resolution increases (e.g., at ~5 Å the beta-strands in the beta-sheets become resolved). At resolution of better than 5 Å one can see the polypeptide chain and trace the C-alpha backbone. As one nears 3 Å, one reaches (near-)atomic resolution, where (bulky) side chains become visible, and an atomic model can be built, by fitting the amino acid side chains into the observed density map. Water molecules can be seen at 2.5 Å and carbonyl groups on amino-acid side chains become visible at 2 Å resolution. Obtaining an atomic model is the ultimate goal for all methods in macromolecular structure determination.

7.3 NMR Spectroscopy

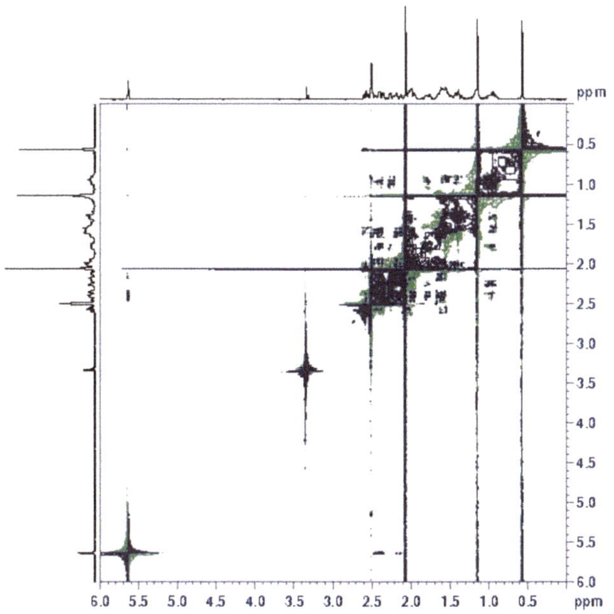

^{1}H–^{1}H NOESY NMR-spectrum of a protein.

7.3.1 Overview

Nuclear Magnetic Resonance (NMR) spectroscopy allows the study of proteins in solution, yet due to the relative low sensitivity of this technique, it requires comparably large amounts of proteins soluble at high concentration. Furthermore, the structure determination of large protein may require extensive isotope labeling, the biochemistry of which can be costly and time consuming.

NMR is different from the previously discussed methods for macromolecular structure determination, as it is not based on the scattering of photons or accelerated electrons, but on an entirely different principle, namely the resonance behavior of atomic nuclei with a half-integer spin (e.g., ^{1}H, ^{13}C, ^{15}N), when they encounter a strong magnetic field. The nuclei either can adopt a lower energy if they align with the magnetic field or adopt a slightly higher energy state when adopting a state where they are aligned in the exact opposite direction. The difference in energy between these two states will depend on the atoms under investigation and the external magnetic field, with a stronger field increasing the energy gap between both states. A radio pulse at the right resonance frequency will push more nuclei from the lower state to the higher state, from which the nuclei will eventually relax to adopt the energetically favorable lower state. Upon relaxation they will emit a radio pulse of the same frequency that can be detected with a suitable coil probe. The nuclei can be thought of as small magnets that can be manipulated by applying external magnetic field pulse sequences (Figure 7.40).

However, the exact energy gap between the low- and the high-energy state for each atomic nucleus varies slightly, depending on the local electron cloud environment that each atom experiences, such as the proximity through space of other atoms or the specific types and geometries of covalent bonds with neighboring atoms.

As a result, the resonance frequencies of the nuclei will experience a so-called chemical shift of a small fraction (typically 10–100 ppm), which lays the foundation for structure determination by this technique. These characteristic shifts depend on the precise chemical environment, and thus provide information about the nearest interaction partners.

One-dimensional- (1D-) NMR examines the exact frequencies of individual hydrogen atoms and their chemical shifts, two-dimensional (2D-) NMR probes for the transfer of magnetization of one type of nuclei to another type of nuclei, e.g., H–C or H–N, and three-dimensional- (3D-) NMR examines the transfer of magnetization between three different types of nuclei, e.g., H, C, and N. In 2D- and 3D-NMR transfer of magnetization (and thus the strength

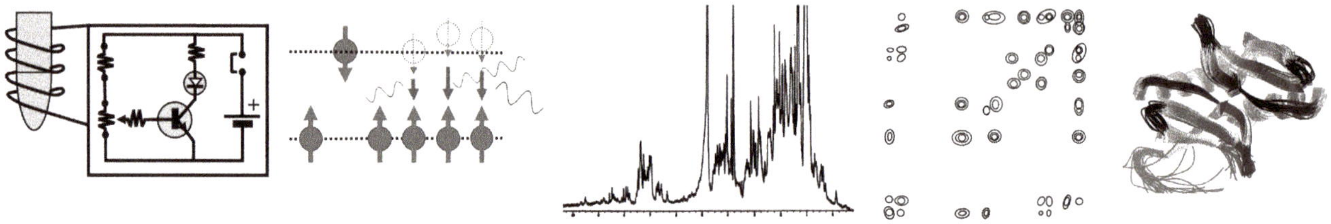

Figure 7.40 NMR overview. In ^{1}H-NMR spectroscopy, a macromolecular sample at high concentration is subjected to a high external static magnetic field, which leads to an alignment of the nuclei with the field either in a parallel (lower energy state) or antiparallel (high energy state) manner. The system is excited with a radio pulse sequence and allowed to relax. Upon relaxation radio signals are emitted, typically with small chemical shifts that depend on the precise chemical immediate environment. Resonance peaks are assigned to functional groups, and spin–spin interactions between pairs of nuclei are determined. Transfer of magnetization through covalent bonds (J-coupling) or through space (NOE) provides information about interacting atom partners and their distances. Such established distance constraints form the basis for structure determination. Atomic model building is based on the constraints provided, supported by molecular dynamics simulations, which then results in an ensemble of structure that is consistent with the experimentally determined constraints.

of interaction) between two or three nuclei either occurs through covalent bonds, also known as J-coupling, or through space, also known as the Nuclear Overhauser Effect (NOE).

J-coupling reveals angular information of bonded atoms, whereas NOE reveals proximity of two or three atoms through space up to a distance of 5 Å.

After assignment of the resonance peeks to atoms within the respective functional groups, determination of spin–spin interactions between pairs of nuclei, and assessment of chemical shift information indicating protein secondary structure elements, one obtains sufficient constraints for molecular dynamics calculations. Unlike X-ray crystallography or cryo-EM, NMR does not yield a density map into which an atomic model can be built but provides constraints for 3D structure model building.

Using molecular dynamics approaches, such as simulated annealing, and applying the constraints observed by NMR, a set of 10–20 structures can be found that are compatible with the experimental data. Often the spatial coordinates of some parts of macromolecules are in good agreement, whereas others differ widely, which is interpreted as conformationally stable or flexible protein domains, respectively. Determination of the structure of large proteins requires a very high magnetic field. For the longest time, proteins of molecular mass larger than 20–35 kDa were not accessible to solution NMR. However, developments in sample preparation, such as perdeuteration of proteins, along with new data collection schemes, such as transverse relaxation optimized spectroscopy (TROSY), have overcome this size limitation barrier. In addition, solid-state NMR also does not have a molecular mass limitation, but it suffers from a variety of other challenges so that it is not a routine technique for large protein structure determination and cannot be considered a high-throughput technique for atomic structure determination.

7.3.2 Historical Perspective/Milestones

The discovery of NMR goes back to the 1930s, when Isidor Isaac Rabi and his team at Columbia University developed an approach similar to the Stern–Gerlach experiment to confirm the existence of nuclear spin. With a much weaker magnetic strength than was necessary for the Stern–Gerlach experiment, and using an oscillating field, they accomplished nuclear resonance, and thus were able to determine the nuclear spin of sodium, lithium, deuteron (one proton, one neutron) and hydrogen, and by subtraction of the magnetic moment of hydrogen from deuteron the spin of a neutron. For his discovery of the principle of NMR, Rabi received the Nobel Prize in Physics in 1944 "for his resonance method for recording the magnetic properties of atomic nuclei."

NMR spectroscopy was independently developed by Felix Bloch and his team at Stanford University and Edwards Mills Purcell and his team at Harvard University in the late 1940s and early 1950s. They discovered that the exact resonance frequencies of nuclei depended on their chemical environment, which turned NMR spectroscopy into an analytical tool for the identification of the chemical structure of molecules. However, one big challenge was the relative low sensitivity of NMR spectroscopy. Bloch and Purcell shared the 1952 Nobel Prize in Physics "for their development of new methods for nuclear magnetic precision measurements and discoveries in connection therewith."

Until the mid 1960s NMR spectra were recorded by sweeping continuously across all frequencies, when Richard R. Ernst, then working at Varian in Palo Alto, California, the leading manufacturer of NMR instrumentation at the time, introduced FT NMR. Instead of a slow sweep, an intense short radio frequency (RF) pulse was applied that excites the entire spectrum. The resulting

Table 7.3 Nobel Prizes involving nuclear magnetic resonance spectroscopy.

Year	Laureate	Prize category	
1944	Isidor Isaac Rabi	Physics	For his resonance method for recording the magnetic properties of atomic nuclei
1952	Felix Bloch Edwards Mills Purcell	Physics	For their development of new methods for nuclear magnetic precision measurements and discoveries in connection therewith
1991	Richard E. Ernst	Chemistry	For his contributions to the development of the methodology of high resolution nuclear magnetic resonance (NMR) spectroscopy
2002	Kurt Wüthrich	Chemistry	For his development of nuclear magnetic resonance spectroscopy for determining the three-dimensional structure of biological macromolecules in solution

complex resonance pattern was then subjected to Fourier Transformation and led to higher sensitivity and higher resolution spectra.

He continued his work at the Swiss Federal Institute of Technology (Eidgenössiche Technische Hochschule, ETH) in Zürich, Switzerland, and collaborated there with Kurt Wütrich, resulting in the development of multi-dimensional NMR, which allowed distance measurements of certain atoms in a protein primary sequence and thus provided constraints for model building.

Ernst's work on FT-NMR was recognized with the 1991 Nobel Prize in Chemistry "for his contributions to the development of the methodology of high resolution NMR spectroscopy." Wütrich received a share of the 2002 Nobel Prize in Chemistry "for his development of NMR spectroscopy for determining the three-dimensional structure determination of biological macromolecules in solution" (Table 7.3). The ability to study proteins in solution rather than being bound in a crystal lattice is a major advantage of NMR-spectroscopy over X-ray crystallography.

7.3.3 Theoretical Background

Protons and neutrons possess a spin angular momentum, also referred to as spin, which is not the angular momentum of a spinning sphere from Newtonian physics but a quantum mechanics analogy. Protons and neutrons have a spin of ½, whereas nuclei made of an even number of protons and an even number of neutrons have a spin of zero. Typical spin numbers for elements relevant for biological imaging are ½ for ^{1}H and ^{13}C, 1 for ^{2}H and ^{14}N as well as 5/2 for ^{17}O.

As such spins create a magnetic moment, the presence of an external magnetic field will lead a spin ½ nucleus to adopt one of two spin states, either spin up or spin down. In the absence of an external magnetic field both spin states have the same energy and will be occupied equally. However, in the presence of an external magnetic field, these two states are no longer equivalent in terms of energy, as one spin state aligns with the external magnetic field, whereas the other one is antiparallel to the external magnetic field, resulting in a distribution that favors the lower energy state (Figure 7.41).

Radio wave irradiation of the sample will bias that equilibrium and excite lower energy state nuclei to the higher energy state. This is also known as the polarization of the magnetic nuclear spins by the constant (external) magnetic field B_0, the first of three steps in any NMR experiment.

The spin magnetization of the nucleus undergoes a precession movement (also known as Larmor precession) around the external magnetic field (not unlike the precession movement of a tilted spinning top in a gravitational field), resulting in a cone-shaped movement of the spin magnetization (Figure 7.42).

If an appropriate oscillating magnetic field pulse (or train of pulses) near the Larmor precession frequency is applied, spin magnetization flips from the longitudinal axis to a transverse plane at a 90° angle to the external constant magnetic field or to put it in different terms, the spin magnetization cone tilts sideways. This second of three steps in an NMR experiment is the perturbation of nuclear spin alignment by a short radio-frequency pulse (often referred to as a RF pulse), which consists of a range of frequencies in the neighborhood centered about the principal carrier frequency at the middle of the NMR spectrum, and which excites all nuclei (Figure 7.43).

The third and final step is the detection by a sensitive radio receiver of the electromagnetic wave that is emitted by the nuclei because of the perturbation. The signal, containing the sum of the NMR responses for all excited spins, is analyzed via a FT, resulting in a so-called 1D NMR spectrum. The transverse radio signal typically decays within seconds, also known as free induction decay (FID), with its relaxation time constant T2, due to nuclei falling out of alignment of their transverse orientation after the short RF pulse.

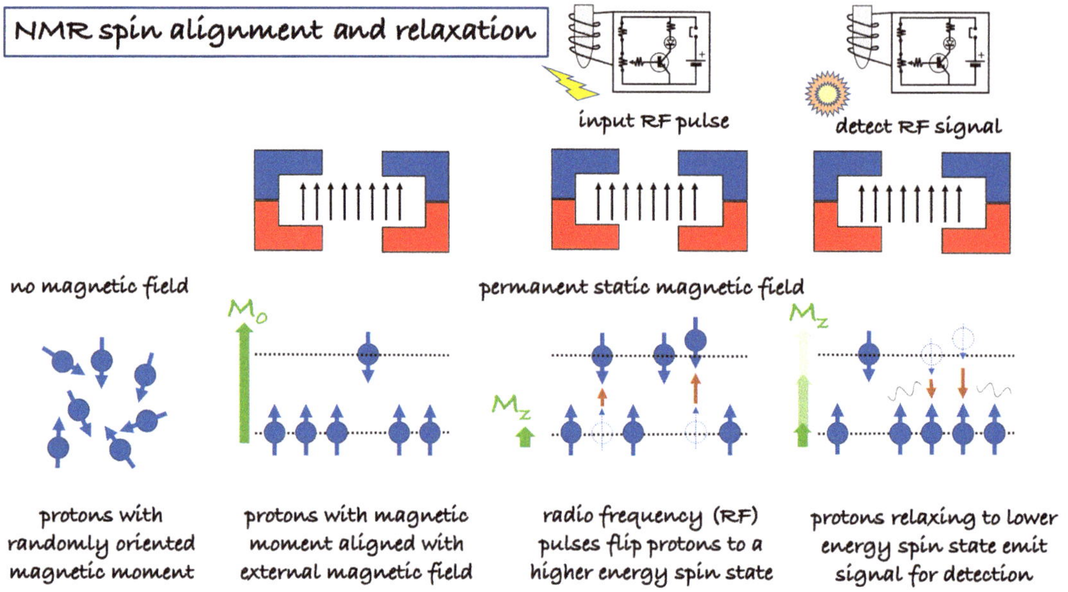

Figure 7.41 NMR – Spin alignment and relaxation. In the absence of a strong magnetic field, protons have a randomly oriented magnetic moment. In a strong magnetic field protons' nuclear spins align with the external magnetic field, with many nuclei adopting a parallel (lower energy level) and few adopting an antiparallel (higher energy level) orientation. A radio frequency pulse flips many of the spins to a higher energy level, from which they relax back to a lower state, emitting a detectable radio signal in the process.

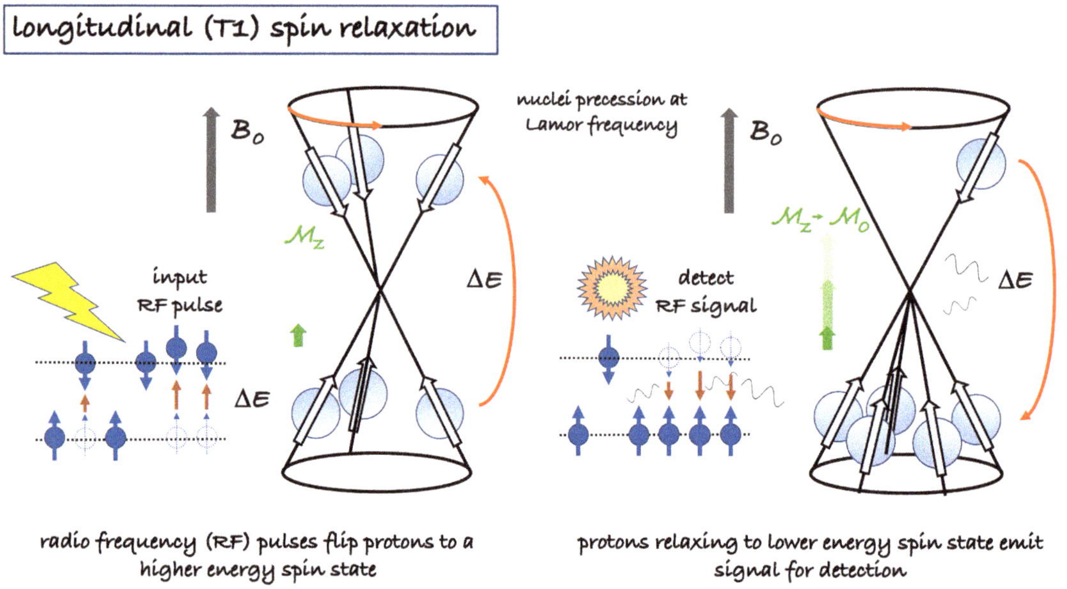

Figure 7.42 NMR – Longitudinal (T1) spin relaxation. The nuclear spins undergo a precession movement at the Lamor frequency around the externally applied static magnetic field. A radio frequency (RF) pulse flips many nuclei's spins from the lower to the higher energy spin state, resulting in an increased polarization in the direction of the magnetic field. Once the nuclei are allowed to relax, they will return to the base level of spin magnetization. This is known as longitudinal spin relaxation or as T1 relaxation.

The exact frequency for each nucleus depends on the electron cloud environment of the nucleus, which exert a "shielding" effect onto the nucleus. Hence, the frequency for resonance to occur will be determined by the electronic environment for each nucleus, a phenomenon also known as chemical shift. Chemical shift is a tiny fraction of the frequency and often expressed in parts per million (ppm). Chemical shift is an indicator of the local electron distribution around the nuclei, and thus characteristic shifts can be attributed to certain chemical functional groups. Integration

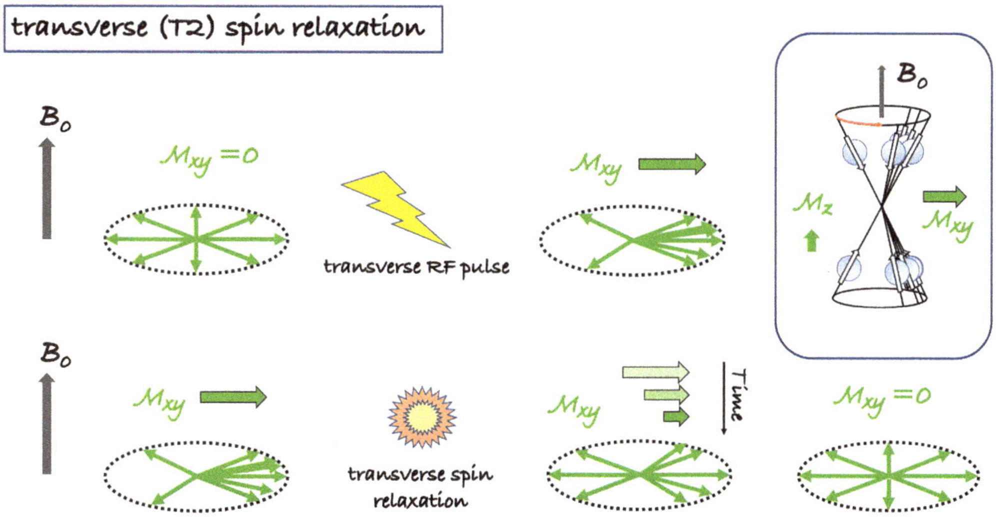

Figure 7.43 NMR – Transverse (T2) spin relaxation. Application of an appropriate RF pulse leads to nuclear spin magnetization from the longitudinal axis (M_z) to a transverse plane (M_{xy}) perpendicular to the constant magnetic field. The system is allowed to relax its transverse spin reducing the M_{xy} magnetization to zero. This is known as transverse spin relaxation or as T2 relaxation.

of the area under the peak gives an indication about the number of nuclei contributing to the respective peak.

However, the integrated peak intensity can be positively or negatively affected by the so-called Overhauser effect, which is closely related to the spin–lattice relaxation (with its time constant T1), where spins relax from their excited state back to a thermal equilibrium distribution.

In the Overhauser effect, nuclear spin polarization is transferred through space from one population of spin-active nuclei to another in close proximity. This phenomenon is known as cross-relaxation. The distances of two hydrogen atoms can be determined by the analysis of unambiguously assigned, well-resolved, high signal-to-noise cross-peaks in so-called Nuclear Overhauser Effect Spectroscopy (NOESY) spectra. NOESY provides key information about the close vicinity (<6 Å) to each nucleus in space (not through chemical bonds) and thus provides constraints for the 3D folding of the macromolecules.

Information about relative chemical bond lengths and angles can be determined from the so-called J-coupling (also known as spin–spin coupling or indirect dipole–dipole coupling), where electrons in the chemical bond affect the spins, which leads to sometimes complex splitting of resonance peaks in the NMR spectra.

The shielding effect also will depend on the orientation of the molecule with respect to the external field. However, in conventional solution NMR molecules adopt random orientations and therefore the chemical shift anisotropy averages out, leading to an average chemical shift. In solid-state NMR, this problem is solved by spinning the sample at a so-called "magic angle" with respect to the external field.

7.3.4 Instrumentation and Experimental Setup

The key component for NMR spectroscopy is the magnet to provide the stationary magnetic field B_0, with stronger magnets allowing a higher resonance frequency signal to be collected, which usually means higher resolution spectra. Magnets are often described by the frequency at which a hydrogen atom will show resonance. For example, a frequently used magnet would be a 900 MHz magnet, which corresponds to a magnetic field of 21 Tesla.

Inside the strong magnetic field of an NMR spectrometer reside a spinning sample holder, a RF pulse emitter and a radio-frequency antenna that receives the signal of the sample after perturbation of the stationary magnetic field by the RF pulse emitter. To ensure homogeneity of the magnetic field throughout the sample volume to a precision of parts per billion, one needs to resort to "shimming," which is the process of detection and compensation for magnetic field inhomogeneity, typically accomplished by an additional RF emitter.

As ordinary water (H_2O) predominantly consists of ^1H, and thus would contribute a large NMR signal, biological samples are usually studied in deuterated solvents, e.g., D_2O or deuterochloroform ($CDCl_3$), depending on the solubility requirements of the sample. The choice of solvent may affect chemical shifts, and thus calibration of the NMR experiments against a known proton peak standard is necessary.

7.3.5 Data Collection and Analysis

Upon perturbation of the magnetic field by a short RF pulse (in the μs range), the magnetic precession axis of the nuclei switches 90° from the longitudinal axis, which results in a signal that can be detected by the sensitive radio antenna. Over time (typically in the seconds range) the magnetic moment relaxes back to its longitudinal axis, which is known as free induction decay (FID), hence the NMR signal decays, a process that is also known as T2 relaxation (Figure 7.44). The FID signal is Fourier transformed, resulting in a resonance spectrum of the examined nuclei (e.g., ^{1}H). Since each FID signal has a low signal-to-noise ratio, the perturbation experiment is repeated many times until through averaging of the signal a high-quality NMR spectrum can be obtained. Depending on the nuclei under examination this process can take minutes or hours.

The resonance peaks tend to differ by parts per million from a reference peak (e.g., the ^{1}H peak of tetramethylsilane), which is knows a "chemical shift." Chemical shifts for protons are characteristic for the presence of certain electron density environments, which cause a shielding effect for the nuclear spin, which causes a shift in the resonance spectrum, hence from the chemical shift one can determine the presence of certain chemical functional groups, a process also known as assignment of the spectrum, and in the case of ^{1}H is carried out by analyzing the peaks' position and integrate the area under each peak (Figure 7.45). For more complicated NMR experiments, e.g., the study of ^{13}C NMR spectra, assignment can be more difficult.

J-Coupling

J-coupling (also known as scalar coupling) arises from the influence of a nuclide's spin from its neighboring atoms through the chemical bond that connects them, which results in the splitting of the respective NMR signal, thus given rise to complex spectra, particularly if two different types of nuclei are involved. Coupling combined with chemical shift analysis provides information about the

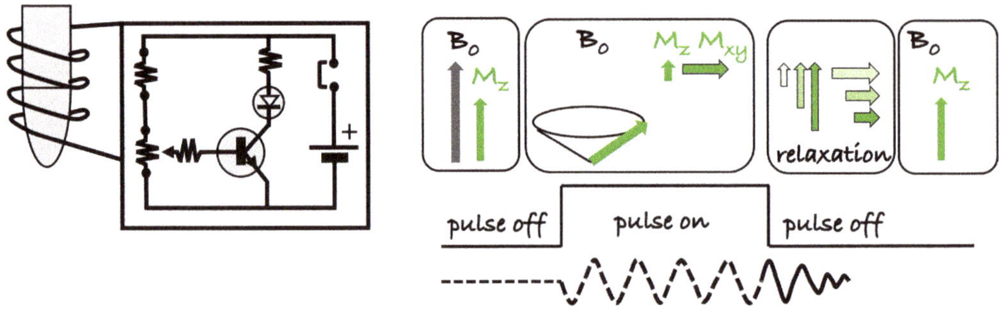

Figure 7.44 NMR – RF-pulse excitation and spin relaxation. In a constant strong magnetic field, most (but not all) nuclear spins align with the field, resulting in a large nuclear spin magnetization M_z along the magnetic field B_0. Upon excitation with an RF pulse, the M_z component decreases as the nuclear spin magnetization (M_{xy}) in the plane perpendicular to B_0 increases. After the RF pulse is switched off, the system undergoes transverse (T2) spin relaxation.

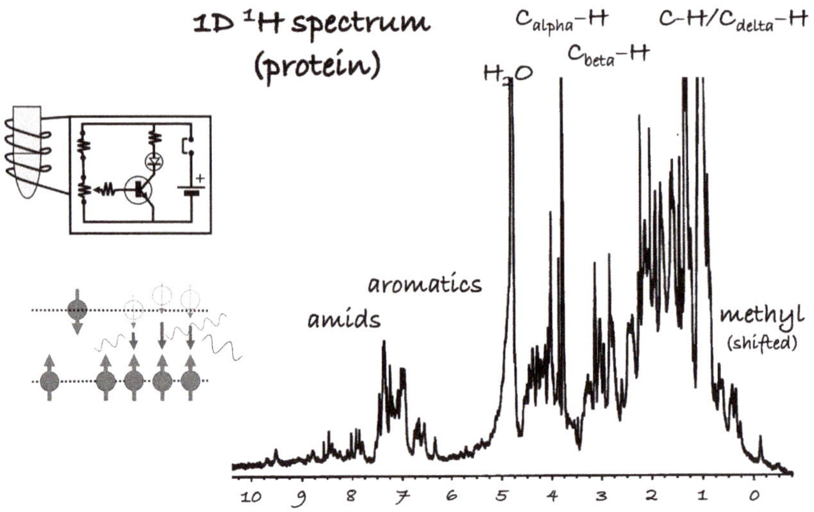

Figure 7.45 NMR – Chemical shift and peak assignment. The NMR signal detected during spin relaxation is typically plotted as signal strength as a function of parts per million (ppm) chemical shift (compared to the signal of a reference peak, such as tetramethyl-silane). There are characteristic fingerprints in the spectrum that can be assigned to certain chemical functional groups.

chemical environment the nuclei reside in, as well as information about neighboring NMR-active nuclei. Thus, coupling can be very valuable when attempting to distinguish different nuclei in complex spectra with multiple peaks at similar chemical shifts.

Nuclear Overhauser Effect (NOE)

The NOE describes the phenomenon of spin cross-relaxation, i.e., the transfer of nuclear spin polarization from one nuclei population to another one through space.

The NOE is important in the assignment of NMR resonance peaks, as this transfer, which leads to an enhancement or suppression of peak intensity, depends on the nuclei being spatially in close contact. Thus, NOESY experiments provide space constraints that help elucidate and confirm the 3D structure of biological macromolecules in solution. The NOE can be homonuclear (e.g., between ^{1}H and ^{1}H) or heteronuclear (e.g., between ^{1}H and ^{13}C), which can be exploited for correlation spectroscopy experiments (Figure 7.46).

Correlation Spectroscopy

2D-, 3D-, 4D-NMR are forms of correlation spectroscopy (also known as COSY experiments), where two, three, or four kinds of nuclides are probed for their signal, with each nuclide type (e.g., ^{1}H, ^{13}C, ^{15}N), requiring recording of different NMR spectra for each nuclide.

In 2D correlation methods the sample (and thus their nuclide spins) are subjected to a sequence of RF-pulses, rather than single pulses as is typical for 1D NMR experiments. Introducing the second frequency dimension leads to a higher-resolution spectral information and to information about which nuclei have contact with one another in form of a 2D correlation spectrum. Such correlation methods are key for the structure determination of biological macromolecules. The COSY-NMR experiment has four distinct periods, namely first the preparation period, where the equilibrium of the nuclear spin is distorted by one or several pulses. Second, in the evolution period, this non-equilibrium is allowed to evolve for some time, before in the third period, the mixing period, another set of pulses are applied. The last period is the detection period, where the NMR signal is recorded as a function of time, before another experimental cycle with these four distinct periods is started. A FT of the signal recorded during the detection period in combination with the length of the evolution period result in a 2D frequency spectrum.

NMR spectroscopy is the method of choice for small organic molecules, as it provides identification of their chemical structure. It is also powerful for the structure determination of biologically relevant macromolecules such as small to intermediate-sized proteins (<35 kDa) through the application of multidimensional NMR data collection of ^{13}C and ^{15}N derivatized samples. More recently, new data acquisition schemes, such as transverse relaxation optimized spectroscopy (TROSY) have been able to extend NMR spectroscopy to larger macromolecular assemblies.

Solid-state NMR spectroscopy (in combination with magic angle spinning of the sample) has also been used for structure determination of membrane proteins and proteins that form fibers.

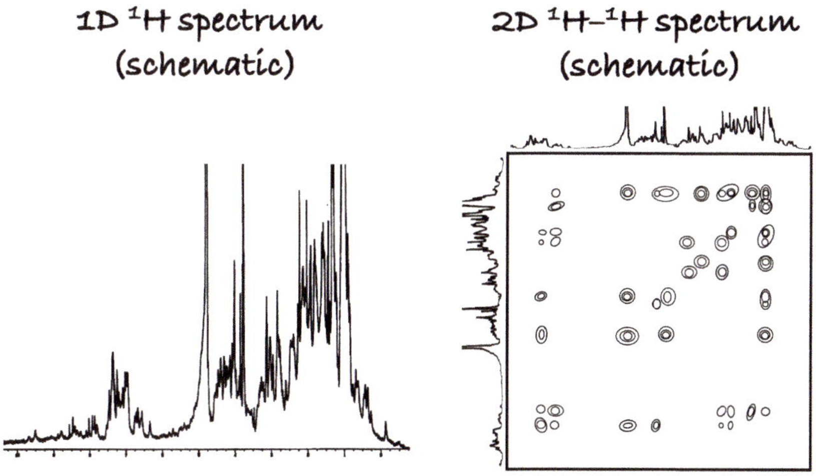

Figure 7.46 2D NMR spectroscopy. Compared to one-dimensional NMR spectroscopy, 2D NMR is defined by two frequency axes, each representing a chemical shift, rather than just one. Typical for 2D NMR is that there are pulses sequences with delay periods in between them, with timing, frequencies, and intensity being varied. One frequency axis refers to the length of the evolution time, the other one to the detection time. Fourier transform converts such time series to frequency series. The 2D spectra are plots of intensity value (contour line) for each pair of frequency variables. COSY and NOESY are examples of 2D NMR methods. 1D NMR spectra are often too complex and crowded to allow structure determination, thus further dimensions are added.

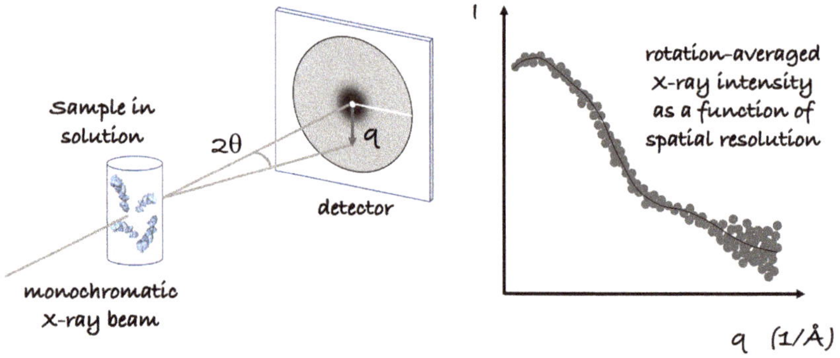

Figure 7.47 Small angle X-ray scattering. In small angle X-ray scattering (SAXS), X-rays are elastically scattered (at low angles) by macromolecules in solution. The scattering curve obtained depends on the size and shape of the macromolecule, and thus with a suitable macromolecular model in hand, one can compare the calculated scattering curve with the experimentally determined curve and thus distinguish between different conformational models. Note that the scattering curve is typically less well defined at higher spatial resolution. There is usually not enough information in the scattering curve to allow an ab-initio structure determination at high resolution, but it is an excellent tool to provide a low-resolution envelope and thus an overall shape of a macromolecule.

Despite the smaller percentage of hydrogen atoms in nucleic acids compared to proteins, the structural study of nucleic acids by NMR is feasible. However, structure determination by NMR spectroscopy is most powerful for RNA oligonucleotides, which tend to adopt complex 3D structures, whereas in the case of DNA double helices only local structural constraints are detectable, as unlike protein amino acid chains, DNA double helices do not fold back on themselves, thus long-range correlations of distant parts of the DNA do not occur. Use of NMR spectroscopy on carbohydrates is challenging as there are only very few functional groups, resulting in poor spectral dispersion.

7.4 Small Angle Scattering – SAXS and SANS

7.4.1 Small-Angle X-Ray Scattering (SAXS)

Small-angle X-ray scattering (SAXS) is an elastic X-ray scattering technique at low angles (0.1°–10°) that allows the determination of the size and shape of nanoparticles. It uses a collimated, monochromatic X-ray beam at a wavelength of 0.07 nm (0.7 Å) to 0.2 nm (2 Å) and depending on the angular range recorded, it can provide information about particles between 1 and 100 nm in diameter. One of its advantages is that unlike in X-ray crystallography, SAXS does not require the protein to be in a crystalline state. It is often used for determining conformational changes that occur in solution, e.g., by binding to a small molecule or another protein.

A scattering curve is recorded, with the signal from the unscattered beam being blocked. Point-collimation instruments have a centrosymmetric distribution as samples are randomly oriented in solution; hence the analysis of a single cross-sectional line is sufficient for analysis. Iterative rounds of model building of the macromolecule, calculation of its SAXS profile and comparison with the real measurement, can lead to a refined model that is consistent with the data. SAXS is well suited to discriminate between different confirmations of a protein, but the amount of data contained in a scattering curve does not warrant an ab-initio atomic structure determination at high-resolution (Figure 7.47).

7.4.2 Small-Angle Neutron Scattering (SANS)

Small-angle neutron scattering (SANS) is similar to SAXS but uses neutrons for structural investigation of particles of 1–100 nm in size. Unlike SAXS, where X-rays interact with the electron cloud, SANS employs neutrons that interact with the nucleus of an atom (Figure 7.48).

SANS is an imaging technique that is particularly well suited for light elements such as deuterium, and offers the possibility of isotope labeling, as the scattering behavior of hydrogen is very distinct from that of deuterium. Also, neutrons are strongly scattered when interacting with the magnetic momentum of unpaired electrons (Table 7.4). Macromolecules often adopt a very different neutron scattering signal when dissolved in water versus in deuteriated

Table 7.4 Nobel Prize involving neutron scattering.

Year	Laureate	Prize category	
1994	Bertram Brockhouse Clifford G. Shull	Physics	For pioneering contributions to the development of neutron scattering techniques for studies of condensed matter

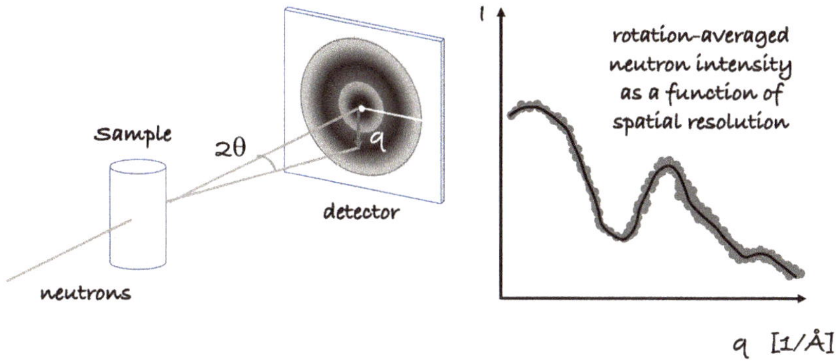

Figure 7.48 Small-angle neutron scattering (SANS). In small angle neutron scattering (SANS) one exploits the ability of light elements (such as hydrogen or deuterium) to scatter accelerated neutron beams through the direct interaction of the neutrons with the atom's nuclei. The result is a scattering curve that shows the scattering intensity as a function of spatial resolution. One of the major applications is to distinguish between protonated and deuterated portions of a macromolecule, as hydrogen and deuterium adopt very different scattering behavior resulting in high contrast.

water, with hydrogen atoms exchanging easily with deuterium atoms. Such differences in scattering can be exploited for contrast variation, including contrast matching where a mixture of hydrogen and deuterium can be used. To use contrast variation, different component must scatter differently: thus, some components are deuterated, whereas others are protonated. It should be noted that SANS instrumentation is typically only available at neutron facilities such as research reactors or at dedicated spallation sources.

7.5 Atomic Force Microscopy (AFM)

AFM is a type of scanning probe microscopy, that can resolve the topography of a biological sample at ~1 nm resolution under ideal conditions. Unlike other types of microscopies, AFM does not employ electromagnetic or particle radiation (and thus is not diffraction-limited), but instead brings the sharp tip of the AFM (the probe) in close contact with the sample, and upon raster scanning across the sample surface keeps a constant distance (probe-sample force) to the sample, therefore moving the AFM tip up and down via a Piezo feedback loop. In the process AFM provides topographical information about the sample, with the position of the tip being attached to the cantilever whose position can be read out by a laser (i.e., by interferometry), thus the surface is monitored via "touch," not unlike a needle of a vinyl record turntable player (Figure 7.49).

The precursor to the AFM, the scanning tunneling microscope, was invented in the early 1980s by Gerd Binnig and Heinrich Rohrer, which earned them the 1986 Nobel Prize for Physics (Table 7.5). Commercial AFMs were introduced in 1989. The AFM also plays a role in near field scanning optical microscope (SNOM/NSOM).

Among the demonstrated applications in molecular biology has been the structural conformational changes in the purple membrane protein bacteriorhodopsin and the study of microtubules including the measurement of their stiffness.

An AFM probe typically consist of a sharp tip (in the nanometer diameter range), attached to a cantilever (in the micrometer size range) protruding from a holder (in the millimeter size range). The back of the cantilever may be gold-coated to increase its reflectance and thus improve the deflection signal readout. There are several forces between the tip and the sample that need to be considered, including Coulomb forces, double layer forces, van der Waals forces, hydrophobic forces, as well as hydration and solvation forces. The forces also depend on the tip geometry. Also of interest are the water meniscus forces, when operating the AFM in air, as the moisture in the air leads to a thin layer of water forming between the tip and the sample.

AFMs can be operated in one of three modes, namely (1) (static) contact mode, (2) (dynamic) tapping mode, and (3) (dynamic) vibrating mode.

In contact mode, the tip is moved across the sample in firm contact with the solid surface (the overall force is repulsive), with a readout of cantilever deflection or – more commonly – readout of the feedback signal required to keep the cantilever in a constant position. One of the challenges in contact mode are the strong capillary forces,

Table 7.5 Nobel Prize involving atomic force microscopy.

Year	Laureate	Prize category	
1986	Gerd Binnig Heinrich Rohrer	Physics	For their design of the scanning tunneling microscope

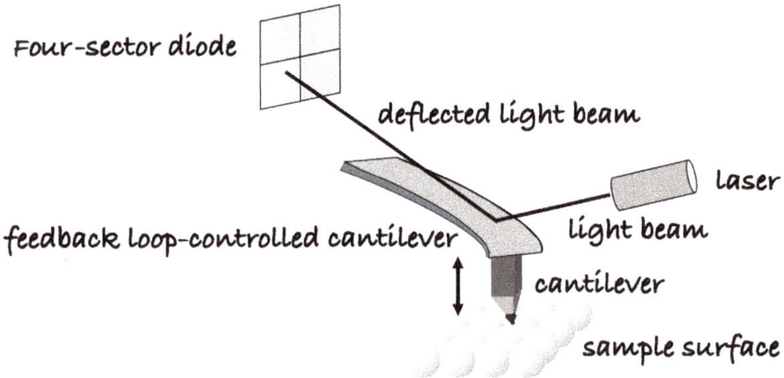

Figure 7.49 Atomic force microscopy. An atomic force microscopy (AFM) probe consists of a holder, a cantilever and a nanoscopic tip that scans the topographic surface of a biological sample, e.g., via a Piezo-driven feedback loop. The movement of the tip is monitored by a laser beam and a four-sector diode light detector. The AFM can be operated in contact mode, tapping mode as well as vibrating mode.

arising from the water film forming between the tip and sample surface, which can lead to sample damage. This problem can be overcome by dynamic imaging modes such as the tapping mode.

The key objective in tapping mode with its tip oscillation is to prevent the tip from being stuck to the surface. Tapping mode is the most frequently used mode in AFM, particularly when operating in ambient air conditions or liquids. In tapping mode, the force interactions (van-der-Waals, dipole–dipole and electrostatic forces) decrease the amplitude of the cantilever oscillation. Tapping mode, being an intermittent contact regime, is often found to cause less damage to the sample compared to contact mode.

In the (non-contact) vibration mode, the tip is also oscillated like in the tapping mode, but the probe never makes direct contact with the sample surface. Using van-der-Waals forces and the resulting decrease in resonant frequency, combined with the feedback loop system, the tip-to-sample distance can be measured, resulting in a topographic image of the sample surface. When operated in amplitude modulation mode, changes in oscillation amplitude or phase can provide the feedback signal used for imaging of the sample surface. Either the *Z*-position of the probe is read out (e.g., by using a negative feedback loop mechanism to keep the exact same distance) or one detects changes in the frequency shift in constant height images where the probe stays exactly at the same height, but the distance to the sample surface slightly varies.

Cantilever height can been read out by the beam-deflection method (sometimes referred to as the optical lever method), where a solid-state diode laser is reflected off the back of the cantilever and hits closely spaced

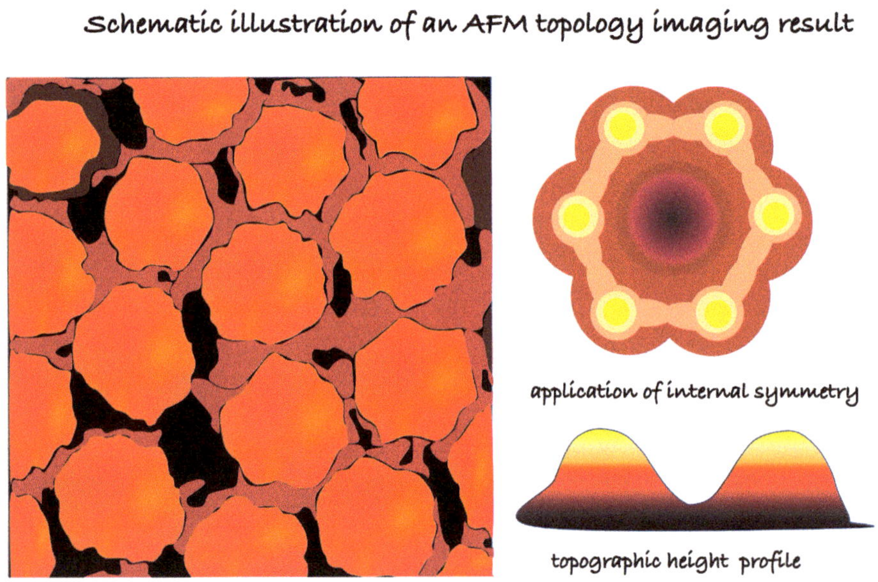

Figure 7.50 Atomic force microscopy – Schematic imaging result. Atomic force microscopy yields a topographic *Z*-height as a function of *X* and *Y* raster positions of the probe. Topographic *Z*-height changes may indicate conformational changes of the macromolecule, and like in electron crystallography, external (2D crystal symmetry) as well as internal symmetry (e.g., threefold or sixfold symmetry) can be exploited to get to a *Z*-height average.

photodiodes of a position-sensitive detector. The amount of light detected by each photodiode indicates the amount of deflection and thus the height-position of the cantilever. Its advantage over other deflection measurement methods (such as piezoelectric detection, piezoresistive detection, laser Doppler vibrometry, optical interferometry or capacitive detection) is its high sensitivity and simplicity.

AFM has been shown to have the potential for high resolution topographic information of samples in a vacuum, air, or liquid, with the sample size being ~150 nm by ~150 nm (Figure 7.50).

However, scan speed of an AFM is rather low (thus vulnerable to thermal drift artifacts), and only topographic (surface) information can be obtained. Also, the topographic information can be compromised due to the combination of tip geometry and sample properties, such as steep changes in height or overhangs. Furthermore, operating the cantilever submerged in liquid as is often the case for biological systems, can be problematic in terms of temporal and spatial resolution due to the damping effect of the water's viscosity. Encased cantilevers operating under water in an air bubble (scuba-design) combined with spiral scan algorithms can overcome such limitations. It can also be combined with a variety of optical and spectroscopic imaging technique to enable scanning near field optical microscopy and nano-FTIR.

In addition to imaging, AFM can also be used for force measurements and to mechanically manipulate (i.e., poke) cells. Also, Chemical Force Microscopy can be carried out with an AFM whose probe has been derivatized with a functional group to detect specific sample interactions, but its use is very limited.

8

Techniques – Cell and Tissue Architectural Imaging

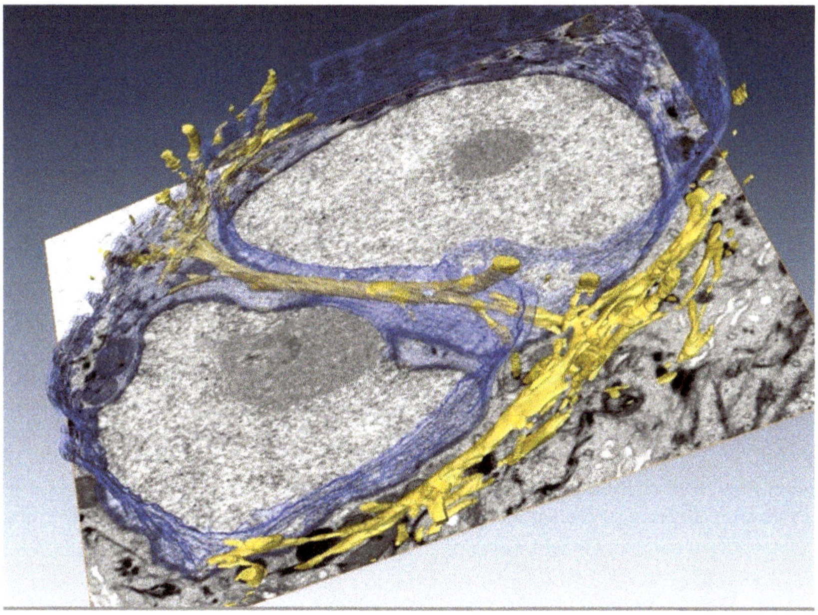

Cytoskeletal filaments tunneling through the cell nucleus in human HMT-3522 S1 cell acini are connected to the nuclear membrane (blue), thus showing a mechanical connectivity between the nucleus and the cell's microenvironment.

Techniques Discussed:

- Transmission Electron Microscopy (TEM)
  - Cryo-/Resin-Section 2D TEM
  - (Cryo-) Electron Tomography (3D)
- Scanning Electron Microscopy (SEM)
  - Whole-Mount 2D SEM
  - Array Tomography/Automated Tape-Collecting Ultramicrotome (ATUM) SEM
  - Serial Block Face (SBF) 3D SEM
  - Focused Ion Beam 3D SEM
- Helium Ion Microscopy (HeIM)
- X-ray Microscopy Tomography (XRMT)
  - Hard X-ray Microscopy
  - Soft X-ray Cryo-Microscopy

8.1 Overview

The previous chapter deals with various approaches to determine the 3D structure of macromolecules, macromolecular complexes, and supramolecular assemblies, ideally at the level of atomic details. There, the biological samples have been directly isolated and purified to homogeneity or reconstituted in-vitro from purified components. The main goal of structure determination at atomic resolution is to mechanistically understand enzymatic mechanisms or details of interaction between macromolecules that form an assembly. In-vitro re-assembly of purified components is often necessary so that we deal with a homogenous system, meaning that the components can be assumed to

Introduction to Biological Imaging, First Edition. Manfred Auer.

adopt a unique state/conformation or at least a relatively small number of defined states/conformations, which then can be sorted in a set of unique categories. One of the advantages of the in-vitro study of proteins and macromolecular complexes is that the experimenter has full control over all parameter, including pH, ionic strength but most importantly composition. Its disadvantage is that life does not happen in isolation, and that proteins and protein complexes function in the context of cells (and tissues).

This chapter aims to address the question of how individual components, whose structure may or may not be known at high resolution, associate into larger supramolecular assemblies. 3D architectural organization needs to be understood at the level of subcellular volumes, the level of organelles, entire cells and possibly even at the level of organoids or small portions of a tissue.

The cytoskeleton and the cell–cell or cell–matrix adhesion complexes it interacts with may serve as an example. The mere study of the 3D structure of actin-monomers and their assembly into filaments, albeit important, allows only limited insight into how their supramolecular assembly into actin stress fibers alters the properties of cells. Likewise, determining the atomic 3D structure of individual cytokeratins does not reveal how they form a dense network of intermediate filaments that distributes mechanical forces across the entire cellular volume, and how changes in organization of such networks may alter cellular behavior, and maybe even lead a cell from senescence to malignancy, proliferation, and invasive migration.

One could argue that the atomic 3D-structure of a cytoskeletal protein is not necessary to understand high-order function, and in many cases, it may well be sufficient to assume cytoskeletal filaments as a set of flexible ropes that may be assembled in thicker ropes or into a net. Such higher-level organization provides information about their respective mechanical properties. In other words, there is information in the 3D architecture that is relevant and independent of the exact shape and atomic-level structure of the underlying components. One likely feature of such higher-level organization is heterogeneity, as no cell can be expected to be built exactly like any other one. Still, there are likely to be many similarities in terms of ultrastructure, as the ultrastructural architecture likely reflects the functional needs of a cell. An analogy can be drawn to the discipline of civil engineering and building architecture, where houses or office buildings will share certain characteristics with respect to type of floor plan, number of windows and doors, one may say that in cellular biology form also follows function, and there must be 3D cellular architectural signatures that reflect the functional state of the cell in its specific spatial and temporal context. Let us take epithelial cells as an example. Independent of the organ they reside in, they all display apical-basolateral polarity with a distinct distribution of cell-adhesion complexes and comparable cytoskeletal organization. They are clearly distinguished in their ultrastructure from cells of the nervous system, muscle tissue or connective tissue. Hence despite all the possible heterogeneity of the exact ultrastructure, one can postulate an ultrastructural 3D architectural fingerprint that identifies a cell as an epithelial cell. Hence, the exact shape of a particular ultrastructural features may be less important than the ability to clearly categories the observed feature into one of the many categories, and only then to determine quantifiable volumetric properties. Such properties could be the size of the various cell–cell adhesion sites, which in first approximation may provide information about the strength of cell–cell adhesion between adjacent cells, or the abundance and distribution of mitochondria, which may provide information about the overall and cell-regional energy needs.

When asking questions of this sort, it is not necessary (nor particularly useful) to reach near-atomic resolution. However, it may be much more important to cover a large volume, ideally multiple cells to get a sense of abundance, size, shape, distribution, and 3D organization of such organelles or supramolecular assemblies. While we may call this approach Structural Cell Biology, the goal of architectural imaging at the subcellular, cellular and tissue level is fundamentally different from the classical goal of structural biology.

A variety of technologies can help to determine such 3D architectural organization and determine ultrastructural signatures, including three-dimensional transmission electron microscopy (TEM), including electron tomography, and three-dimensional scanning electron microscopy (SEM), also known as volume-EM (vEM), as well as hard and soft (cryo-) XRMT (Figure 8.1).

The border between ultrastructural imaging techniques and (superresolution) fluorescence localization microscopy is blurry, as macromolecules of the cytoskeleton, adhesion complexes or mitochondria (to name a few) can be specifically targeted with a fluorophore and hence fluorescence imaging also will provide information about their spatial distribution. However, to truly establish ultrastructural 3D cellular signatures one needs the ability to image at high resolution many structures simultaneously, which is limited by the availability of non-overlapping fluorophores. Also, in fluorescence imaging one can only see what has been labeled, hence the architectural imaging may be limited to very few target molecules at any given time. Optical techniques, including fluorescence localization microscopy, will be discussed in more detail in Chapter 9.

This chapter will address the differences in specimen properties (e.g., sample dimensions/specimen thickness), specimen preparation requirements, field-of-view/volume-of-interest imaging, as well as in types of information that each technique can provide.

subcellular, cellular, and tissue 3D architecture

key objective: to identify features of interest and determine their spatial relationships

	cryo-XRMT	cryo-ET	cryo-FIB-SEM	micro-CT XRMT	vEM: serial section TEM	vEM: array tomography	vEM: SBF-SEM	vEM: FIB-SEM
sample preparation	vitreous: unstained, frozen-hydrated			stained	heavy metal stained, dehydrated, and resin-embedded			
sample type	cells in capillary	Sections lamella	cells lamella	tissues organs	cells, tissue sections	tissue/organ/ animal	tissue/organ/ animal	tissue/organ/ animal
sample thickness	< 15 μm	<1 μm	<200 μm	>10 mm ~65 μm	>1 mm	~1 mm	~1 mm	~1 mm
data volume	15x15x15 μm³	4x4x0.5 μm³	10x10x10 μm³	5x5x1 mm³	200x200x20 μm³	4x4x1 mm³	50x50x50 μm³	50x50x50 μm³
resolution (x,y)	30–50 nm	2–5 nm	7–10 nm	~600 nm 30–50 nm	1–3 nm	7–10 nm	7–10 nm	7–10 nm
resolution (z)	30–50 nm	6–15 nm	7–10 nm	~600 nm 30–50 nm	70 nm	30–50 nm	20–30 nm	7–10 nm
acquisition speed	fast	fast	slow	fast	slow	Slow/medium	medium	slow

Figure 8.1 Cell and tissue architecture imaging. The key objective of subcellular, cellular, and tissue 3D architectural is to determine the spatial relationship of macromolecular machines, supramolecular assemblies, organelles, and other cellular features in the cell and tissue context. Cryo-electron tomography (cryo-ET) and cryogenic soft-X-ray microscopy tomography (cryo-XRMT) image samples in an unstained, frozen-hydrated near-native state, with a sample thickness of less than 1 and 15 μm, respectively. Hard-X-ray microscopy (XRMT), serial section transmission electron microcopy (ssTEM), array tomography/automated tape-collecting ultramicrotome (ATUM) scanning electron microscopy (AT-SEM/ATUM-SEM), serial block face scanning electron microscopy (SBF-SEM) and focused ion beam scanning electron microscopy (FIB-SEM) all rely on heavy-metal staining for contrast generation. If the samples need to be imaged in a vacuum, as is the case for volume-EM (vEM), samples are typically resin-embedded. Note that sample thickness is limited to 1 mm for conventional diffusion-based chemical imaging and staining and to 200 μm when high-pressure freezing cryogenic sample preparation is used. Data volumes are rough estimates as they also depend on detector properties, the use of stitching/montaging software as well as scanning size and image storage limitations. In ATUM/array tomography large volumes require the use of multibeam (e.g., 91 beam) SEM setup. Note that resolution limits for SEM are ~1 nm at 15 kev and ~1.5 nm at 1 keV. Resolution estimates given here are based on the Nyquist sampling theorem and thus typically given as 2–3 times the pixel size used for imaging. As always, larger areas can be imaged if the pixel resolution is lowered.

8.2 Historical Perspective/Milestones

In the late 1920s and early 1930s Ernst Ruska and Max Knoll conceived and constructed the first transmission microscope (TEM), soon followed by Manfred von Ardenne in 1939 who developed the scanning electron microscope (SEM), which used electron beams not in a transmission mode but in a reflected mode. Ruska and von Ardenne could not possibly know at that time how their newly created instruments would ultimately transform our understanding of biology and help us explain the inner workings of life as manifested in the ultrastructural organization of cells and tissues. Ernst Ruska shared the 1986 Nobel Prize in Physics for the design of the first electron microscope.

The first TEM images of cells were taken in the late 1930s by Helmut Ruska, the brother of Ernst Ruska, which showed some badly preserved viruses and bacteria. The first electron micrographs of eukaryotic cells were published by Keith Porter and colleagues in 1945 and depicted the thin edge of cells cultured directly on the EM support grid, as the center of the cell was too thick to be penetrated by the electron beam. In the 1950s, new data on the ultrastructure of cells was starting to pour in, with many new discoveries by Palade, Porter, and others such as the endoplasmic reticulum, the inner membrane configuration of mitochondria, ribosomes, chemical synapses, details on the Golgi complex, the centriole as well as cell–cell adhesion complexes, such as gap junctions, tight junctions, and desmosomes. Huxley used TEM in the 1950s to verify the sliding filament theory of muscle contraction. In the 1960s and 1970s, every self-respecting cell biologist had undergone some training in electron microscopy, and optical microscopy seemed outdated, reduced to a steppingstone to identify the region of interest for EM. Palade went on to share the 1974 Nobel Prize in Physiology or Medicine for his discoveries regarding the structural organization of the cell, while Porter despite his many important contributions never did (Table 8.1). Figure 8.2 shows muscle tissue in cross-sectional and longitudinal view. Note that there is organization at different levels of magnification, and thus

Table 8.1 Nobel Prizes involving cell and tissue architecture.

Year	Laureate	Prize category	
1906	Camillo Golgi Santiago Ramón y Cayal	Physiology/ Medicine	In recognition of their work on the structure of nervous system
1953	Frits Zernicke	Physics	For his demonstration of the phase-contrast method, especially for this invention of the phase contrast microscope
1974	Albert Claude Christian de Duve George E. Palade	Physiology/ Medicine	For their discoveries concerning the structural and functional organization of the cell

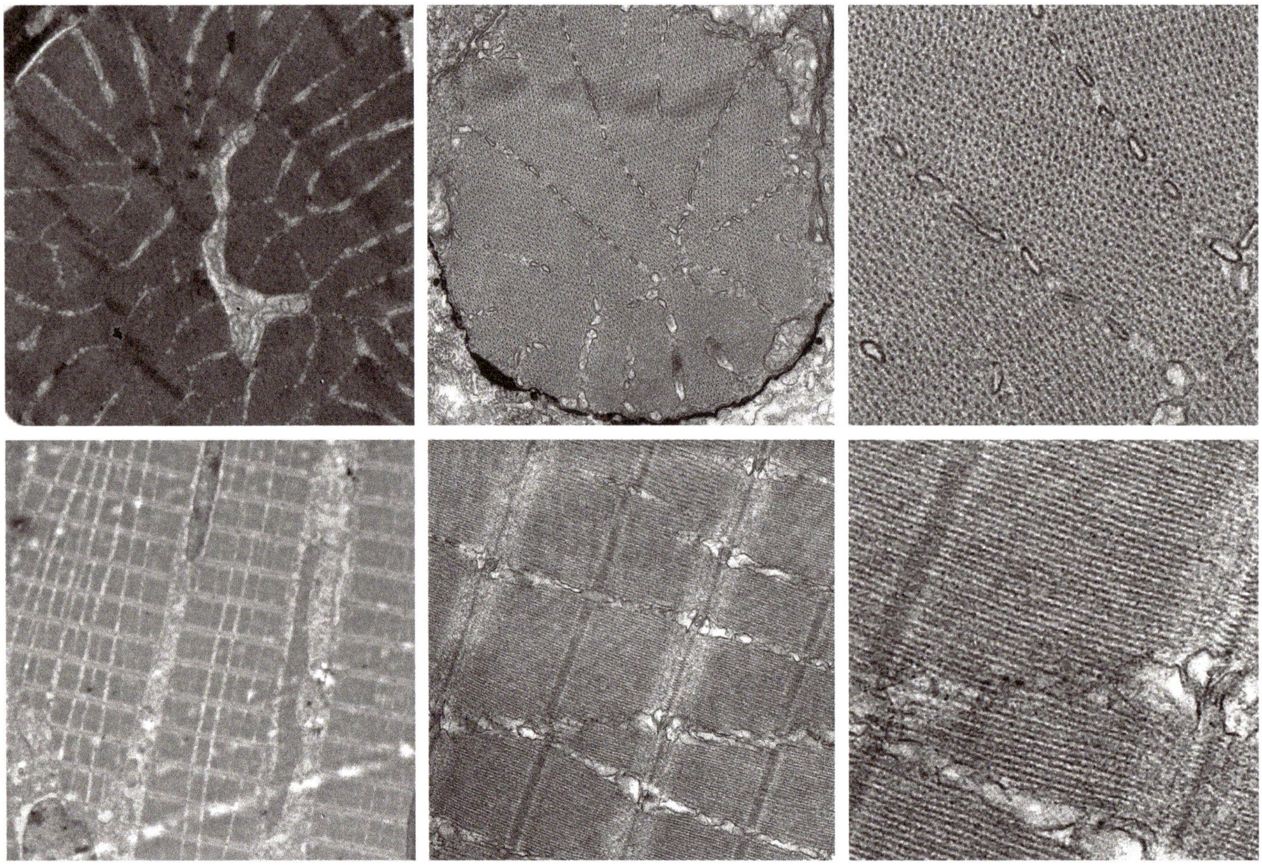

Figure 8.2 Ultrastructure of muscle tissue. These images show at different scale and resolution skeletal muscle tissue from 5-day post fertilization zebrafish larvae as imaged by TEM of 70 nm ultrathin resin-sections. Top row shows muscle tissue in cross-sectional orientation at increasing magnification, whereas the bottom row shows the muscle tissue in longitudinal orientation. A closer inspection of the higher magnification view reveals the actin and myosin filaments that make up the muscle tissue. Note that there is organization at all three different scales shown.

to gain a comprehensive insight into muscle function, muscle tissue needs to be studied at different magnification and thus levels of detail.

Since the early days of electron microscopy, it was clear that for electrons to penetrate thicker samples the acceleration voltage needed to increase from 50–100 kV to 200 kV, 300 kV or even 1,000,000 V. Such high voltage transmission electron microscopes became available in the late 1970s, and allowed the study of thicker samples (e.g., whole mount cells), however, it became soon apparent that the projecting a thicker sample on a 2D plane wasn't really the answer to the study of the three-dimensional organization of cells, and that with thick samples cellular structures were simply superimposed onto one another in projection. Even when retrieving information along the *Z*-axis, e.g., by electron tomography (ET), thinner samples are preferred.

To accomplish the same 3D resolution as for thin samples, the tilt angle increments would need to become smaller for thicker sample, and thus the number of images that need to be collected would significantly increase. However, this would lead to much higher electron dose and exceed an acceptable dose limit.

As TEM imaging required thin samples that could withstand the vacuum of the electron microscope, new sample preparation techniques needed to be developed. Thus, not too surprisingly, given the critical role of sample preparation in TEM (and SEM) imaging, the history of EM to a large extend is also the history of sample preparation, both of whole-mount samples and sections.

One easy solution is to simply lyse the cells and study the cell fragments. Cell lysis which can naturally occur in osmotically shocked cells, leads to thin, yet extracted whole-mount cells or cell debris. This approach could be combined with negative staining, which allowed certain cellular constituents such as ribosomes, microtubules (which are hollow rods), intermediate filaments or actin filaments (then still called microfilaments) to be studied in situ or in in vitro. However, it was clear that such macromolecular complexes or supramolecular assemblies experience different conditions in lysed, enriched, or purified samples compared to when they reside in their intact cellular environment. Hence, soon it became apparent that this approach was going to be limited in its usefulness for cell biology.

Other ways had to be found to limit sample thickness and deal with the microscope's vacuum, and the answer for the longest time would lie in resin-embedding followed by the cutting of ultrathin sections. However, acrylic resins are not water miscible, hence a dehydration-step was needed, typically in the form of a graded ethanol series, sometimes with an additional acetone step before resin-infiltration could occur. To improve sample preservation and to ensure that the biological system would not respond to the insult of the organic solvent replacing cellular water, chemical fixation (typically in form of a paraformaldehyde and/or glutaraldehyde aqueous solution) preceded the dehydration step and infiltration step. In addition, since acrylic resin material are carbon- and oxygen-based and thus in composition very similar to biological samples, contrast for imaging needed to be created via exposing the biological material to heavy metal ions, such as osmium, iron (ferrocyanide), or chromium, all of which bind to biological material and ensure high contrast upon electron microscopy imaging. Heavy metal staining also helped with radiation damage as the stained material was more electron radiation-resistant, an approach not unlike that of positive or negative staining used in early days of macromolecular EM imaging. The hydrophobic resin monomers took up the space occupied by the organic solvent (which during dehydration had replaced cellular water molecules) and were polymerized by radical-chemistry, and with the help of heat.

The harsh chemical treatment of biological systems frequently resulted in aggregation artifacts of cellular ultrastructure, and to some degree also in the extraction of cellular volumes, and thus in the alteration of cellular ultrastructure. Systematic studies on what effect the temperature has on sample preservation showed that at temperatures lower than −35 °C, the sample seemed to be protected from aggregation artifacts. This led to the so-called progressive lowering of temperature (PLT) dehydration approach for chemically fixed samples, and to freeze-substitution for samples that had been either plunge-flash frozen, slam-frozen, or high-pressure frozen (cryo-immobilized). Plunge-freezing into a liquid ethane (kept at liquid nitrogen temperature) works best for specimen less than 1 μm in thickness, slam-freezing will work for a region ~5–15 μm deep into a tissue, with the first ~5 μm possibly being destroyed due to the impact of the sample when slamming into a copper block (which had been cooled to liquid nitrogen temperature). High pressure freezing on the other hand works well for tissues up to 200–300 μm thickness. However, one should also be aware that in many cases some form of cryo-protectants is used to reduce ice crystal formation.

Cryogenic sample preparation such as high pressure freezing followed by cryo-sectioning or frozen-hydrated lamella-preparation via cryo-focused ion beam milling is widely considered the gold standard in faithful sample preservation, particularly when followed by cryo-imaging of the thin cryo-section/cryo-lamella in its unstained, frozen-hydrated state. However, excellent results are also obtained by high-pressure freezing, freeze-substitution, where the cellular water is replaced by an organic solvent at −90 °C (e.g., by acetone) and subsequent resin-embedding, particularly if the goal of visualization is to assess higher level 3D organization of cells and tissues, and not the exact (high-resolution) shape of each protein or macromolecular complex. Figure 8.3 shows the ultrastructure of a 70 nm thin section of an frog inner ear sensory epithelial hair cell with its characteristic apical hair bundle, the actin meshwork-rich cuticular plate, its vesicle- and membrane-tube-rich cytoplasm, and the darkly stained mitochondria. Note the richness of ultrastructural features and the good preservation, e.g., of the cell-cell adhesion complexes with their extracellular filaments connecting adjacent cells.

Sample preparation for SEM for many biological samples such as cells and soft tissues overlaps greatly with that of TEM sample preparation. The main difference is that a specimen needs to be "dry" for its surface to be studied

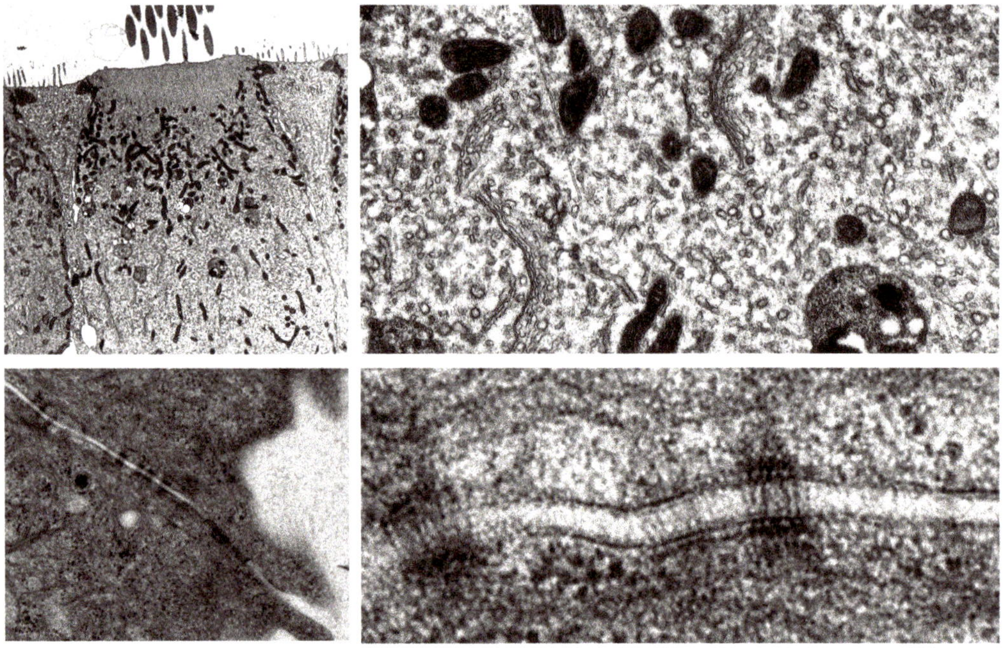

Figure 8.3 Cellular ultrastructure – Organelles and supramolecular assemblies. Ultrastructural organization of inner ear sensory epithelia hair cells as shown by TEM imaging of ultrathin sections: Top row: Cytoplasm with mitochondria, cytoplasmic membrane systems and vesicles, as well as microtubules; Bottom row: Cell–cell adhesion complexes such as tight junctions and desmosomes. Note the fine details visible in a close-up view of desmosome complexes revealing the filamentous nature of cell–cell connections.

by SEM. This is not a problem for hard dry biological material such as wood, bone, feathers, dried insects, or shells, but for soft, hydrated samples, the water needs to be removed.

This is done by replacement of the water with an organic solvent, followed by replacement of the organic solvent with liquid carbon dioxide in a process called critical point drying. Raising the sample temperature and pressure to 31 °C and 7.4 MPa/1,073 psi, one reaches the critical point of carbon dioxide, where carbon dioxide is in a supercritical state, where there is no gas–liquid interface. This means that there is no meniscus or other capillary forces that would alter delicate ultracellular structure as carbon dioxide transitions from a liquid immersed state to a dry gaseous state. Lowering the pressure at constant temperature returns the CO_2 to a gaseous state without ever crossing the liquid-gaseous boundary.

Such dried samples are then typically mounted on a SEM specimen stub via a glue or electrically conductive double-sided adhesive tape, and sputter-coated with a thin heavy metal (e.g., gold, palladium, platin) and/or graphite carbon layer to enhance conductivity and thus reduce charging upon SEM imaging. This step of metal or graphite carbon coating is not needed for HeIM imaging, where charging either is no issue or can be dealt with by irradiation with an electron beam.

Alternatively, if the SEM is equipped with a cold stage, low-temperature SEM can be performed. Impressive results have been obtained from cryo-samples that have been freeze-fractured (with fracture planes typically occurring through biological membranes or at water–fat interfaces). Also, freeze-etching has been used to study cytoskeletal supramolecular assemblies inside cells, but both freeze-fracturing and freeze-etching can now be considered a "lost art," with few people still knowing this delicate art and craft of low-temperature sample preparation for cryo-SEM.

Environmental SEM (ESEM) was commercially introduced in the late 1980s, which uses differential pumping and pressure-limiting apertures to separate the vacuum of the gun and lenses from the specimen chamber. Also, a secondary electron (SE) detector was developed that can operate in the presence of water vapor. While the sample chamber is evacuated for air as is typical for SEM imaging a relatively high water-vapor pressure surrounds the sample keeping the sample near 100% relative humidity. However, in the process of specimen transfer, the sample is not kept fully hydrated all the time, which may be one of the reasons why to this day ESEM did not get much traction for cellular imaging. Another reason may be that without introducing heavy metals, the sample contrast is very low. Also, another issue is that the electron bombardment of the sample in the microscope prevents imaging of living samples anyway, which is an issue independent of the challenge of imaging in a vacuum and thus the drying of the sample in this process.

While SEM is best known for imaging of (critical point-) dried samples, more recently, SEM imaging of the surface of resin-blocks or vitreous ice-embedded samples hold great promise for the future of bioimaging by SEM. In this approach the sample is prepared identically as for TEM imaging (typically though with more heavy metal staining), but instead of thin sectioning or cryo-ion beam thin lamella preparation, the block surface is imaged at low voltage by SEM. Note the wealth of information gained by the ability to image the interior of the samples instead just imaging the sample from the outside. Figure 8.4 shows a comparison of images obtained by conventional SEM off critical-point-dried *Myxococcus xanthus* bacterial biofilm and a eukaryotic cancer cell adhered to a 2D surface, with their corresponding resin-embedded samples, with thin slices of the 3D volume recorded by electron tomography or focused ion beam SEM, respectively.

Resin-blocks samples are also the preferred specimen for hard XRMT, whereas soft X-ray cryo-microscopy tomography/cryogenic soft-X-ray microscopy tomography (cryo-XRMT) typically relies on unstained, frozen-hydrated vitreous ice-embedded sample. While cryo-XRMT has the advantage of imaging samples in their frozen-hydrated state, the sample size limitation for cryo-imaging in the X-ray water window of ~15 μm diameter means that microbes, and individual eukaryotic cells can be studied, whereas multicellular organoid cell culture systems or tissues are too thick for soft X-ray cryo-microscopy tomography.

8.2.1 Transmission Electron Microscopy (TEM) Imaging

Traditional 2D TEM imaging has been very straightforward. Due to heavy metal staining, amplitude contrast is the main mechanism for image generation. TEM imaging predominantly images the heavy metal stain distribution, with the implied assumption that wherever the electron beam is strongly scattered (elastically and inelastically), there must be the location of the heavy metal stain and thus of the stained biological material. One way to obtain a 3D volume

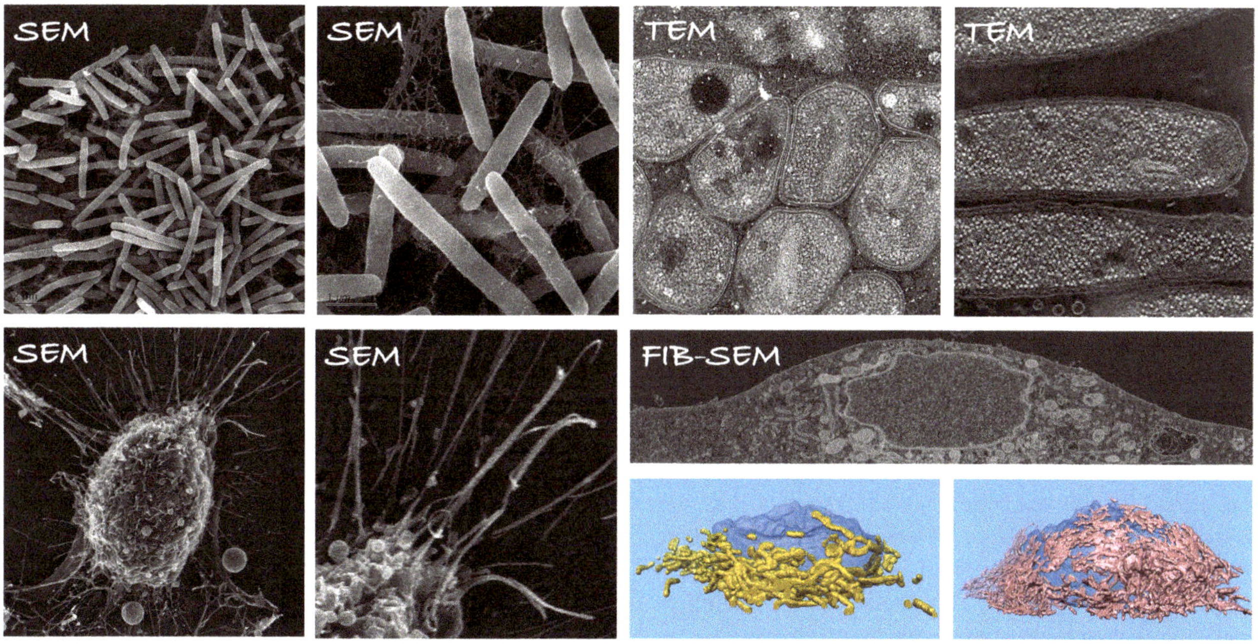

Figure 8.4 Conventional SEM, TEM electron tomography and Focused Ion Beam SEM. The traditional type of samples for SEM imaging are whole-mount samples that have been chemically fixed, heavy-metal-stained, dehydrated, and critical point dried before being heavy-metal (and sometimes also carbon-coated), such as the *Myxococcus xanthus* bacterial community (top left: overview and close-up view) and a cancer cell (bottom left: overview and close-up view). Note that only the outside of the sample can be seen, whereas internal structures are not visible. For TEM imaging, samples are typically chemically or cryo-fixed, heavy-metal-stained, dehydrated, resin-infiltrated and resin-embedded, before the resin is being hardened by polymerization. Samples embedded in such hard resin-blocks can be sectioned, and such ultrathin resin-sectioned can be subjected to conventional 2D TEM imaging or 3D TEM tomography imaging (top right), which reveals internal structures of the *Myxococcus xanthus* bacterial community. However, the structures imaged are limited to the thickness of the ultrathin section. Larger volumes can be obtained by serial section TEM imaging. More powerful however for large volume imaging is Focused Ion Beam SEM (FIBSEM; also known as dual beam SEM) imaging, which can build up 3D volumes of entire cells at 5–10 nm isotropic resolution, as is shown on the bottom right for a cell adhering to a surface. Upon segmentation and surface rendering, internal structures such as the cell nucleus (shown in dark blue), mitochondria (shown in golden/yellow) and the endoplasmic reticulum (shown in salmon/red) can be visualized.

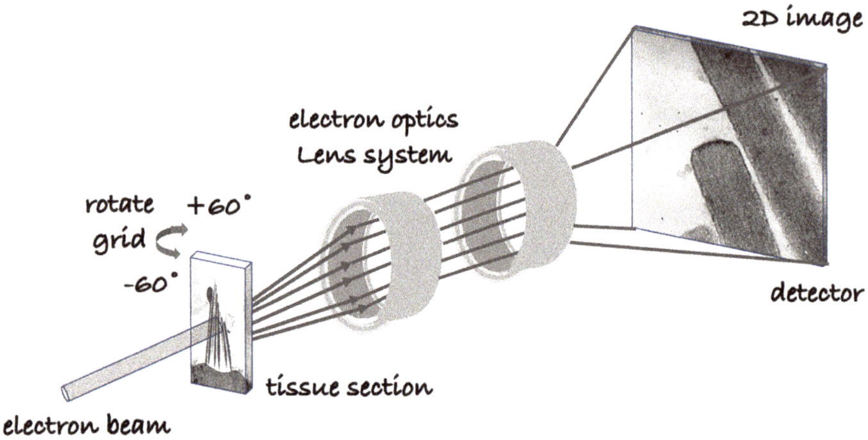

Figure 8.5 Transmission electron microscopy (TEM) imaging. In TEM imaging, an ultrathin sample (typically 70–150 nm in thickness) is irradiated by an electron beam, which – upon refocusing by an electromagnetic lens system – results in 2D images at the detector level. For 3D imaging, the sample is rotated typically up to ±60–70°, resulting in a tilt series that after alignment can be reconstructed into a 3D volume.

by TEM imaging is electron tomography, where the samples is tilted along one axis or two perpendicular axes. A 3D volume is reconstructed by combining the aligned projection views of the tilt series (Figure 8.5).

Alternatively, a 3D volume can be reconstructed by combining the projection views from serial sections and by interpolation of the density along the *z*-axis. Serial section TEM is considered one approach for volume-EM imaging with an excellent *x*,*y*-resolution, but its poor *z*-axis resolution and the high probability for sectioning artifacts makes this approach less attractive, particularly for large volumes.

Cryo-imaging on the other hand implies that most of the contrast is due to phase contrast, which means that the mainly elastically scattered electrons will be phase-shifted to the unscattered electrons, and hence scattering center positions will be revealed as locations of interference. Also note, that the observed contrast will be modulated by the contrast-transfer function, which is a defocus-dependent microscope property, and for an underfocus setting typically results in a negative CTF value in the low-resolution shell, and thus to contrast inversion.

8.2.2 Scanning Electron Microscopy (SEM) Imaging

While traditional SEM imaging has been very successful for imaging of whole-mount, bacteria, cultured cells or epithelial tissues such as inner ear sensory epithelia with its impressive hair bundles, the number of samples is limited where it is useful to use traditional SEM as a visualization of the specimen from the "outside," and therefore, after the initial euphoria of the 1960s and 1970s, the interest in traditional SEM imaging of biological samples has somewhat declined. In classical 2D SEM, both back-scattered electrons as well as secondary electrons are used for detection and generation of an image. The image depends both on the chemical composition (stained versus non-stained region) as well as specimen topography (Figure 8.6).

However, within the last decade, renewed interest in SEM has emerged due to advances in volume-EM (vEM), which includes (serial section) array tomography SEM (also known as automated tape-collecting ultramicrotome SEM; ATUM-SEM), Serial Block Face (SBF) SEM and Focused Ion Beam (FIB) SEM (also known as dual beam SEM). What makes these techniques so attractive (particularly in the last few years) is the possibility to image large volumes of biological cells and tissues at macromolecular (5–10 nm) resolution. Unlike in ET (which achieves a comparable resolution), the volumes that can be imaged are gigantic, and comprise of entire individual cells and groups of cells and small regions of tissue. These technologies have been introduced in the context of "brain connectomics" and they allow EM reconstruction of very large volumes (albeit at coarser voxel size). Large volume SEM imaging has the potential to be a game changer for cell biological imaging as the resolution is sufficient to detect, identify and quantify supramolecular assemblies such as the cytoskeleton, cell adhesion complexes and ribosomes, and all organelle-like features in a cell, yet at the same time very large volumes can be imaged.

8.2.3 Helium Ion Microscopy Imaging

HeIM is the "new kid on the block" and has the advantage over SEM that specimen charging can be easily dealt with. Therefore, samples do not need to be metal sputter coated,

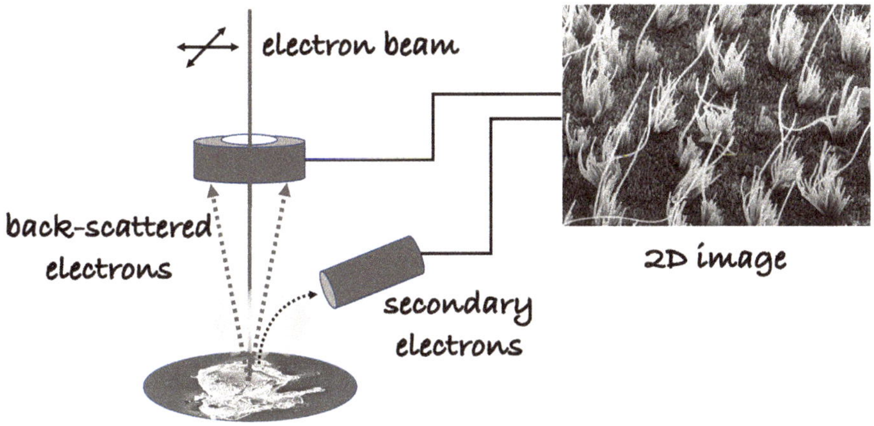

Figure 8.6 Scanning electron microscopy (SEM). Upon irradiation of the surface of a resin-block or whole-mount sample, electrons of the primary beams are either back-scattered or lead to the emission of secondary electrons, each of which are detected independently. To form a 2D image, the primary electron beam raster-imaged across the sample.

allowing the fine delicate structures of extracellular filaments to be detected without the thick heavy metal layer that obscures all details. HeIM is based on the emission (and detection) of secondary electrons upon interaction of the helium ion beam with the sample (Figure 8.7). The resulting positive charging can be compensated with an electron beam.

Helium ions can be focused into an even smaller beam size, which means higher resolution imaging is possible. Furthermore, HeIM has an even larger depth of focus as SEM, which means the entire field of view is in focus.

The usefulness of HeIM for block face imaging on the other hand is not as clear, as for block face imaging, helium ion beam bombardment of the block surface only results in SE formation, whereas the backscattered electron (BSE) signal, essential for contrast generation in block surface SEM imaging, is missing. As a result, the contrast of block surface images is very low in HeIM.

8.2.4 X-Ray Microscopy Tomography Imaging

For the longest time, imaging in the hard X-ray window of the electromagnetic spectrum was the domain of medical imaging, including chest and bone X-rays as well as computed (axial) tomography (CAT/CT). Micro-CT builds on the same principle by using X-rays to cast a shadow of

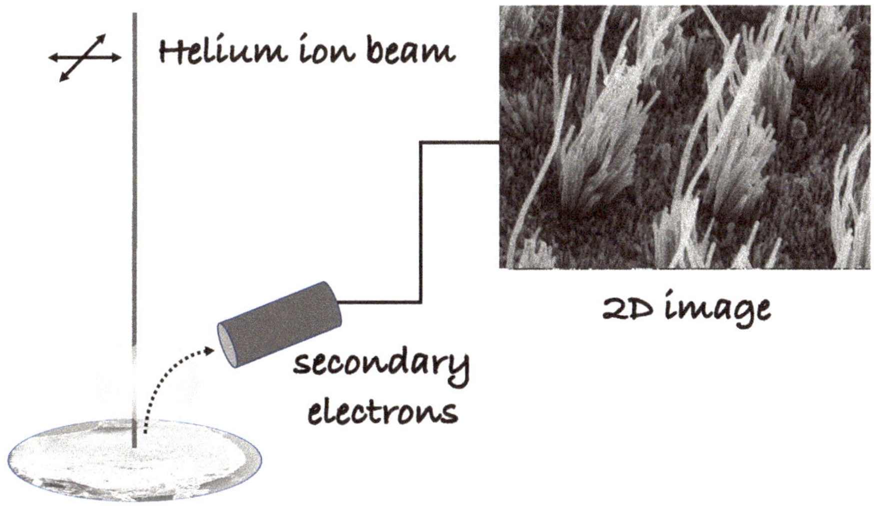

Figure 8.7 Helium ion microscopy (HeIM). Helium ion microscopy (HeIM) is like scanning electron microscopy, except that a helium ion beam instead of an electron beam irradiates the sample. For this reason, there are no back-scattered electrons, instead contrast is accomplished by the detection of secondary electrons. Advantages of HeIM over SEM is the lack of sample charging and the large focus depth. 2D images are recorded by raster-imaging of the sample.

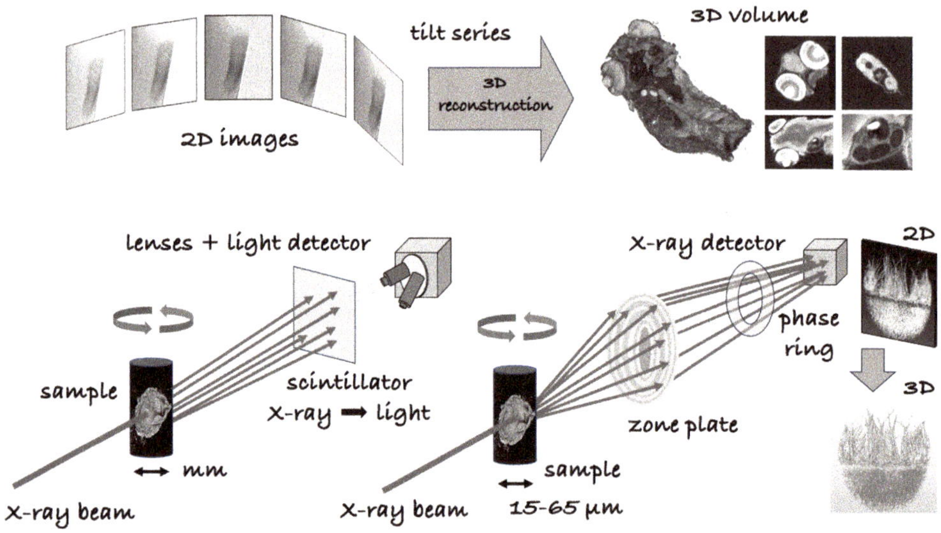

Figure 8.8 X-ray microscopy tomography (XRMT). In X-ray microscopy tomography, a sample is rotated 180° through an X-ray beam, which results in a tilt series of 2D images, which upon back-projection can be reconstructed into a 3D volume with isotropic resolution. There are two different ways to create images: The first approach, omits refocusing of the scattered X-rays, and uses a scintillator to convert the X-ray photons into visible light photons with the image being magnified and detected by an optical microscope. The second approach uses zone plates (in combination with a phase ring) to refocus the scattered X-rays back and to generate contrast using an X-ray area detector (CCD or CMOS). Note the size limitations for each approach. While XRMT with scintillator and optical light detection can handle specimens of several millimeter in size (and larger), XRMT using phase plate is limited to ~65 µm for heavy-metal stained, resin-embedded samples or ~15 µm for cryogenically preserved unstained samples, which are imaged by cryo-XRMT.

objects of higher density (such as bones) onto a flat panel detector without any attempt to refocus the X-rays behind the specimen (Figure 8.8). X-ray Microscopy Tomography (XRMT) comes in two variations. The first setup is not unlike the one found in micro-CT but with a more condensed beam penetrating the sample before hitting a scintillator-material of a screen, which results in a fluorescence image. This fluorescence image can be imaged using optical low-power and high-power lenses, which results in an overview image and a zoom-in image of the sample (Figure 8.8). Besides the geometric magnification that depends on the distance of the source and detector to the sample, there is also an explicit optical magnification. The second setup uses Fresnel zone plates, which act like lenses to re-focus the X-ray beam. XRMT is a relatively recent technology, which may explain why it is not used very much in cellular and tissue imaging, despite its huge potential. By using hard X-rays and heavy metal-stained samples, one can examine entire (small) organisms like zebrafish larvae or organs like mouse cochlea, and one can readily determine the cell and tissue organization. In some cases, even prominent organelles can be identified, such as hair bundles emerging from the sensory epithelial apical hair cell surface.

Samples can be imaged at a resolution of ~500–600 nm (with voxel sizes of 50 µm), which is comparable to that of optical microscopy. Hence, XRMT in its own rights is an excellent tool for studying organ and tissue organization in whole animals or for studying cell and tissue organization in isolated organs of small animals such as mouse. Given that samples can be optically opaque (black) and millimeter-sized, hard X-ray XRMT is also ideally suited as a bridging technology between fluorescence microscopy and electron microscopy, as it can pin-point with cellular precision to a region of interest identified by fluorescence imaging. This region can then be prepared for subsequent much higher resolution imaging, e.g., by FIBSEM. Also, like it is the case for cryo soft XRMT, a resolution of ~50 nm (at 16 nm voxel size) can be accomplished by hard XRMT of resin-embedded heavy-metal-stained samples, however, imaging at such high resolution requires the samples to be physically trimmed to ~65 µm diameter.

Imaging by Cryo Soft X-ray Microscope Tomography has the advantage that the sample is not stained (heavy metal-contrasted) but only frozen, with imaging occurring in the soft X-ray water window (X-ray wavelength between 2.2 and 4.4 nm), where oxygen and thus water does not absorb X-rays, whereas carbon (and thus biological material) does. This creates maximal contrast between the organic molecules that cells are made of and its surrounding water. Since biological material is radiation sensitive, XMRT is carried out with frozen-hydrated samples kept frozen at liquid nitrogen temperature where the effects of radiation damage are being kept minimal.

Among its advantages is that the sample can be rotated a full 180° (or 360°), hence the resulting resolution is isotropic in *X*, *Y*, and *Z*, and that sample preparation is fast, allowing high throughput imaging, e.g., by translating the specimen along its axis, thus exposing a new volume for imaging without the need to mount another sample.

However, like with any techniques there are some caveats for cryo-XRMT: The need for the high beam brightness that a synchrotron radiation facility can offer also means that only few such facilities are available for data collection, and hence it remains uncertain, how widely adopted this technology for bioimaging of cellular samples will become in the cell biology community. Its most significant drawback is the size limitation (diameter) of the sample, which is currently ~15 μm, and hence about the size of a single eukaryotic cell. At this point in time, soft-X-ray XRMT is not suited to study tissues, which means that its applicability is limited, also in the light of the somewhat limited resolution of ~50 nm (Figure 8.8).

8.2.5 Optical/Fluorescence Light Microscopy Imaging

Since its inception, optical microscopy offered insight into architectural organization, first through inherent optical absorption contrast (e.g., the dark green color of chloroplasts in plant cells) or through phase contrast. Using stains, large organelles such as mitochondria and cell nucleus/chromosomes, could be revealed. Ultimately, using synthetic or genetically encoded fluorescence markers, the location of certain targeted cellular components could be determined. As an example, fluorescent phalloidin-derivatives could reveal the location and thus organization of filamentous actin, whereas antibodies to tubulin could reveal the localization and thus the cytoarchitectural organization of microtubules. Fluorescent proteins genetically fused to a protein that is known to target to mitochondria then reveal position, size and shape of mitochondria. Yet another protein may be a component of an adhesion complex, thus by genetic engineering fusion proteins can be generated to visualize adhesion complexes. Yet another form of targeting are fluorophore-conjugated antibodies. Fluorescence based on targeted fusion protein, synthetic fluorophores conjugated to molecules with a natural affinity to cellular components or antibody-conjugated fluorophores yield information about the 3D distribution of such selected fluorophores and thus specific proteins and/or supramolecular complexes inside cells, whereas ultrastructural imaging by electron microscopy yields an account of all cellular ultrastructure (Figure 8.9).

The border between localization and architectural imaging is somewhat blurry, even more so, since superresolution fluorescence light microscopy attains a resolution not too far from what the classical approach for ultrastructural imaging, namely the TEM, can offer. And while the electron microscope cannot help but see all the existing ultrastructure, an approach based on high-resolution fluorescence optical imaging can select for only few components of the ultrastructure, which can be a blessing (as one reduces complexity) and a curse (as one can only observe what has been labeled).

Historically, there has been a back and forth between optical and electron microscopy imaging. While optical imaging has taken a back seat in the 1970, when ultrastructure was all the rage, it made a formidable comeback in the 1980s, outpacing EM in the three decades since, due to its new capabilities to study the dynamic of biological processes in cells whereas EM could only provide a static view or a time series at best. By the end of the 20th century, it seemed that we had a basic understanding of the cell's ultrastructural inventory, and now the time had come to study its dynamic behavior rather than its static ultrastructure. Hence, many asked the question whether cellular EM was dead and as a result most electron microscopists took to macromolecular imaging, which looked increasingly intriguing as discussed in the previous chapter.

The pendulum swung back in the first decade of the 21st century as cell biologist realized that the fluorescence microscopy signals, even those that transcended the diffraction limit of visible light, needed to be grounded in some ultrastructural reality/context, and thus two methods learned to co-exist, with neither one claiming anymore the other no longer to be relevant. As will be discussed in the end of this book, the information that both techniques can provide are sufficiently different from one another, yet also relatable to one another, that it may be wise to combine the information both approaches provide, a goal that can be accomplished in a correlative bioimaging or an integrated bioimaging approach.

8.3 Theoretical Background

8.3.1 Contrast Generation in Transmission Electron Microscopy

Contrast in TEM can stem from both amplitude and phase contrast, with amplitude contrast being caused by the removal of electrons (due to absorption, or high-angle-scattered electrons which are then blocked by the objective aperture), whereas phase contrast relies on the interference of the electron wave front scattered with the unscattered electron wave front.

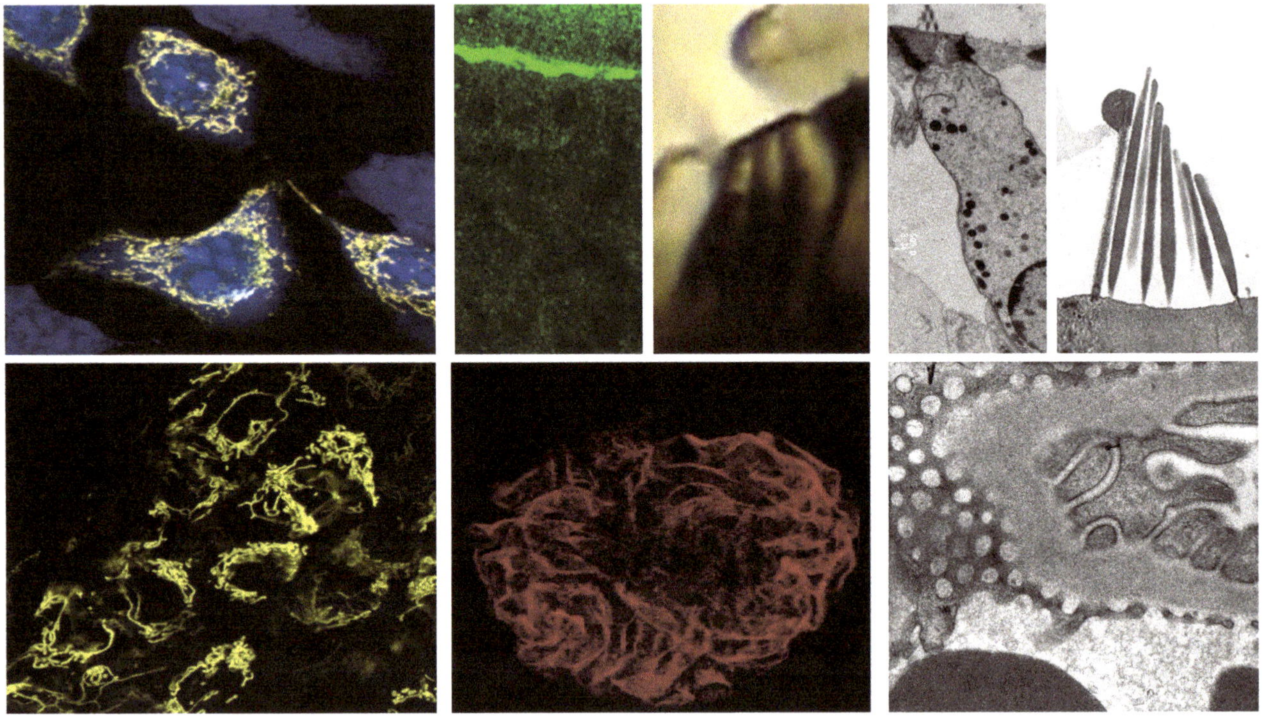

Figure 8.9 Fluorescence, optical, and electron microscopy – Examples. Left column: HeLa cells (top) and zebrafish larvae (bottom) expressing YFP genetically fused to a mitochondria-specific protein. HeLa cells are counterstained with DAPI to show location of cell nuclei. Top row (middle and right side) shows hair cells residing in inner ear sensory epithelia. From left to right: antibody labeling of a hair bundle protein, light microscopy image of a thick section of mouse cochlear samples, displaying three layers of outer hair cells and one layer of inner hair cells. Electron micrograph montage of an ultrathin section of an outer hair cell. Electron micrograph of a bullfrog sacculus hair bundle, protruding from the apical surface of the hair cell; bottom middle, immunolabeling of kidney glomeruli with a podocyte-specific protein antibody. Bottom right: close-up view of kidney podocyte foot processes with slit diaphragm and glomerular basement membrane.

Traditionally, for cellular TEM imaging amplitude contrast has been a major mode for contrast generation, particularly for samples that have been heavy-atom-stained. Amplitude contrast can be either due to high atomic mass or due to sample thickness (e.g., by multiple inelastic scattering). It constitutes the main contrast mechanism for low magnification TEM imaging, even for unstained specimen that are imaged in phase contrast at higher magnification. Phase contrast in TEM imaging has been extensively discussed in the context of macromolecular imaging (Figure 8.10).

8.3.2 Contrast Generation in Scanning Electron Microscopy (SEM)

The main signal types in SEM for structural information stem from either the scattering of electrons upon collisions with atoms backscattered electrons (BSE) or the electron beam-stimulated emission of secondary electrons (SE). BSE come from deeper regions of the sample, whereas SE originate from the first few nanometers of the surface. The SE signal provides more detail information about the specimen surface and is useful for determining sample surface topography.

Depending on the primary electron beam energy, the atomic composition and density of the sample, electrons can penetrate the sample up to 5 μm in the so-called interaction volume, that typically adopts the shape of a teardrop. In this interaction volume, high energy electrons are scattered both elastically (sometimes multiple times) and inelastically. BSE and SE carry different types of information, with BSE images showing high sensitivity to differences in atomic number. The higher atomic number the material the stronger it scatters electrons, and thus the brighter the image appears.

The bombardment of the specimen surface with high energy electrons can also lead to the emission of X-rays and light through a process known as cathodoluminescence, which can be used for determining the elemental composition of the specimen. Furthermore, one can measure the absorbed (specimen) current as well as the transmitted electron signal.

BSE have a much higher energy than SE, typically in the keV-range for BSE and ~50 eV for SE, which means that SE are highly localized and can only escape from the top few nanometers of the sample, whereas BSE emerge from deeper

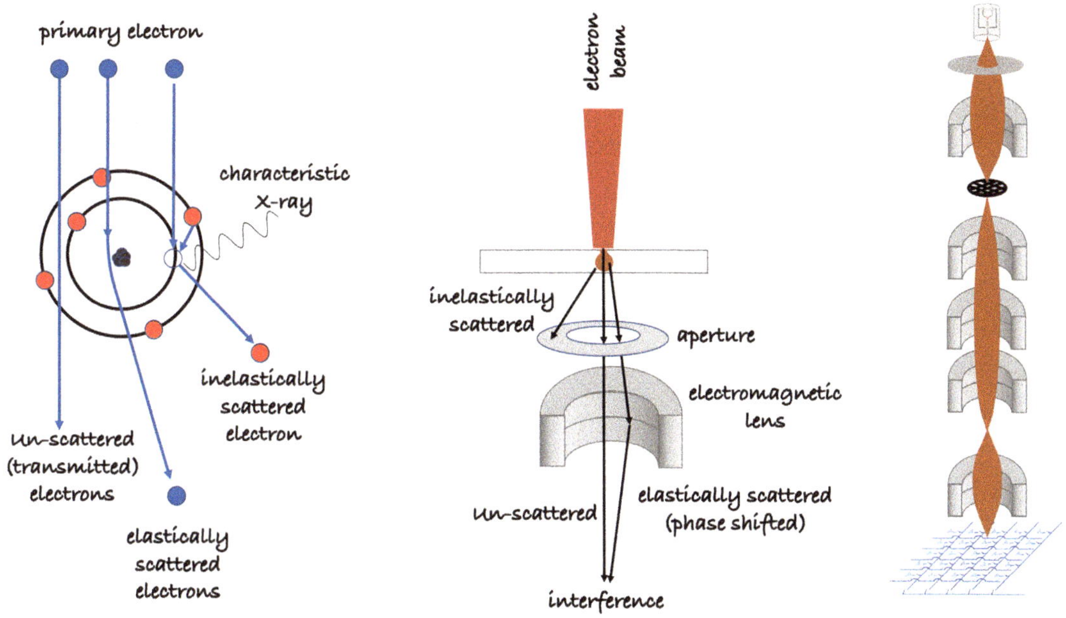

Figure 8.10 TEM contrast generation in heavy-metal stained samples. Unlike phase contrast that relies on the interference of unscattered and elastically scattered electron wavefronts, contrast generation in heavy-atom-stained samples are the result of inelastic scattering that typically results in the emission of electrons at angles high enough that they are filtered out by the microscope's objective aperture.

regions within the specimen. Thus, the BSE signal is less localized, hence the resolution of the BSE signal will be lower.

Since the BSE signal also depends on the atomic number (Z) of the backscattering element, BSE is often used for elemental mapping in combination with the X-ray signal that results from an ejection of an inner shell electron and the re-filling of the shell from an outer electron shell. Note that while the BSE signal is stronger with heavy elements, and thus appears brighter, the BSE signal alone cannot provide the atomic identity of the sample. It is the wavelength (energy) of the X-rays emitted that is detected in wavelength-dispersive X-ray spectroscopy (WDS) or Energy-Dispersive X-ray Spectroscopy (EDS) and which allow elemental mapping (Figure 8.11).

8.3.3 Contrast Generation in Helium Ion Microscopy (HeIM)

The contrast in HeIM derives predominantly from SE emitted from near the surface of the sample. Since the beam is more highly collimated to begin with, and given that the interaction volume is much smaller, the SE signal in HeIM is much more localized, thus resulting in higher (lateral) resolution images in HeIM compared to SEM. A lateral resolution of 0.24 nm (2.4 Å) has been demonstrated. Furthermore, the SE signal yield in general is much higher upon helium ion bombardment than it is for electrons (but also varies considerable for different materials). The SE have a low energy (e.g., ~15 eV) as only a small fraction of the helium ions' energy (~25 keV) is being transferred, resulting in a strong edge and topography contrast (Figure 8.12).

In addition to SE emission, HeIM has another unique contrast mechanism, known as Rutherford Backscattering Imaging (RBI): when helium ions collide with heavier ions, they transfer some of their momentum to the heavier atom. The remaining energy of the backscattered helium ions is determined by both the atomic mass of the target atom and the angle of scattering, with heavier target nuclei producing higher energy backscattered helium ions. Hence, while backscattered helium ions are not as abundant as SE, they do provide a unique contrast mechanism that allows quantitative discrimination between different material at sub-micron spatial resolution.

8.3.4 Contrast Generation in X-Ray Microscopy Tomography (XRMT)

Like in TEM, X-ray imaging uses either amplitude contrast or phase contrast. Amplitude contrast in hard XRMT arises from heavy metal-stained samples, whereas cryo-soft XRMT predominantly relies on phase contrast imaging of fully hydrated, unstained samples in the ~2.3 to ~4.4 nm X-ray wavelength water window, where water interacts very weakly with X-rays. X-rays passing through electron cloud that surrounds each nucleus are either unscattered,

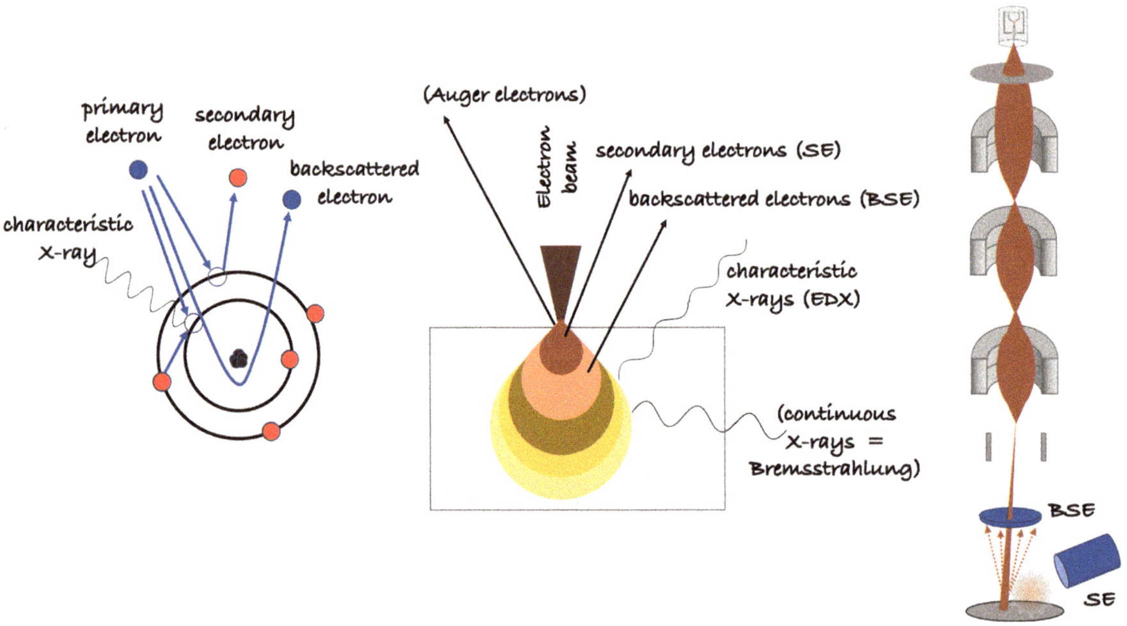

Figure 8.11 Contrast generation in the SEM. The main mechanisms of contrast generation in the SEM are the emission of backscattered electrons (BSE) as well as secondary electrons (SE). BSE typically arise from deeper in the interaction volume and have high energy, whereas SE originate from the surface of the interaction volume and have comparably very low energy. BSE and SE are detected by two different types of detectors and provide different information about the sample. BSE is sensitive to the atomic number and thus discriminates the heavy atoms of the stain, whereas SE provide topographic information of the sample.

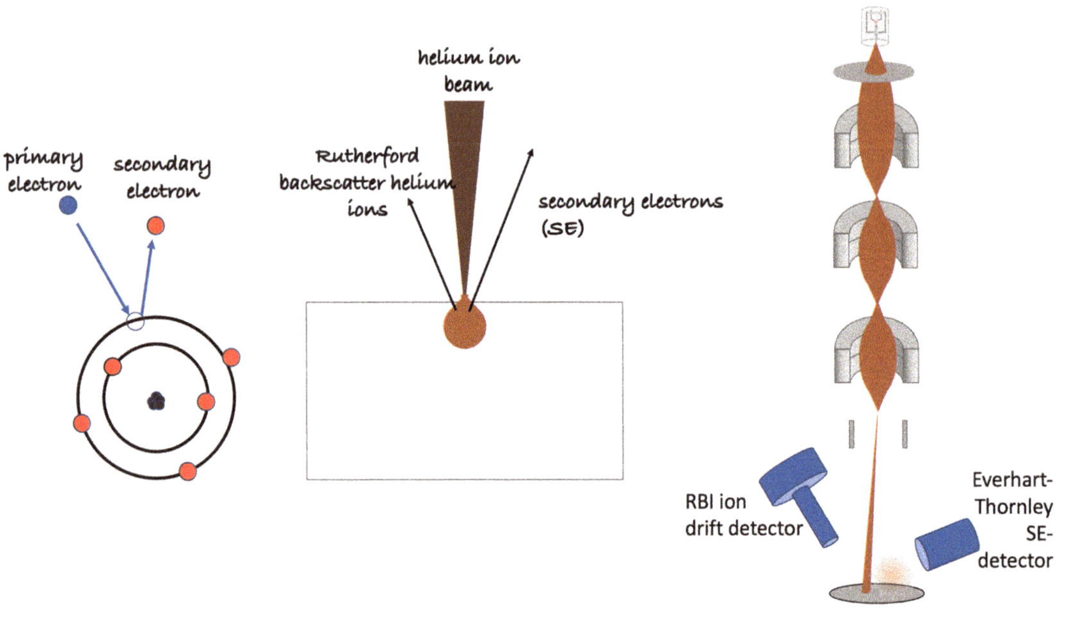

Figure 8.12 Contrast generation in the helium ion microscope (HeIM). The main mode of contrast generation in the HeIM is the emission of secondary electrons (SE) from the surface of a small interaction volume (both axial and lateral), resulting in much sharper features with strong edge and topography contrast. In addition to SE, there is Rutherford backscatter contrast with helium ions colliding with heavier atoms' nuclei. Upon collision, some of the energy is transferred to the heavier atom, and thus analysis of the energy and the angle of the Rutherford backscattered helium ion (RBI) leads to a discrimination between different elements at high resolution.

elastically scattered or inelastically (Compton) scattered. With the help of a Fresnel zone plate and a phase ring, elastically scattered X-rays interfere with unscattered X-rays, resulting in phase contrast in cryo-XRMT, whereas hard-X-ray microscopy tomography typically relies on amplitude contrast, with a loss of X-rays scattered at high angles and/or inelastically (Figure 8.13). Classical micro-CT (micro-computed tomography) X-ray techniques rely solely on amplitude contrast with no refocusing of scattered X-rays. As discussed above, detection of X-rays in micro-CT occurs via X-ray flat panel detectors solely relying on geometric magnification. In commercially available conventional XRMT instruments, the X-rays are detected as fluorescence signal on a scintillator screen, with the signal being read out by a lens-based optical microscope, where an overview picture can be obtained by using a low-powered lens, whereas higher resolution data to about 500–600 nm can be collected with a higher-powered lens. However the trade off for higher resolution is a much more limited field of view. Higher-resolution XRMT, where resolution data of much better than 100 nm can be collected, requires Fresnel zone plates and phase rings for refocusing X-rays and higher contrast, respectively. Fresnel zone plates act as lenses and consist of radially symmetric rings, which alternate between being opaque and transparent for X-ray photons, which leads to constructive interference of diffracted X-rays at the focal point. The spacing of the rings, which gets progressively smaller toward the edge, ultimately limits the achievable resolution to ~25–50 nm. While higher resolution (~15 nm) seems possible, there is a tradeoff between spatial resolution and field of depth. As X-rays pass through a Zernike phase ring, additional phase contrast emphasizing edge information is produced (not unlike it is the case in optical phase contrast microscopy).

An additional contrast mechanism is the so-called linear absorption coefficient (LAC), which describes the fact that different material absorbs X-rays differently. For example, lipid droplets have a higher LAC value than vacuoles that have a higher water content. For cell-biological samples this means that mitochondria, nucleus, nucleolus, vacuoles and lysosomes have characteristic LAC values, which can be used for automated segmentation and annotation.

8.3.5 3D Reconstructions of Pleiomorphic Objects

As discussed extensively in the chapter of macromolecular (cryo-) electron microscopy imaging, 3D objects with no symmetry (pleiomorphic objects) can be calculated from 2D projection images of the objects by tilting (rotating) the 3D object and recording a tilt series (a series of projection images at different angles, e.g., in 1° increments). Unlike it is the case in single particle analysis, where single images of identical particles in random orientation can be combined and averaged, cellular sceneries require a tilt series of the exact same object rotated around one of two axes for 3D reconstruction (Figure 8.14). Images of the tilt series are first aligned (registered), often with the help of fiducial

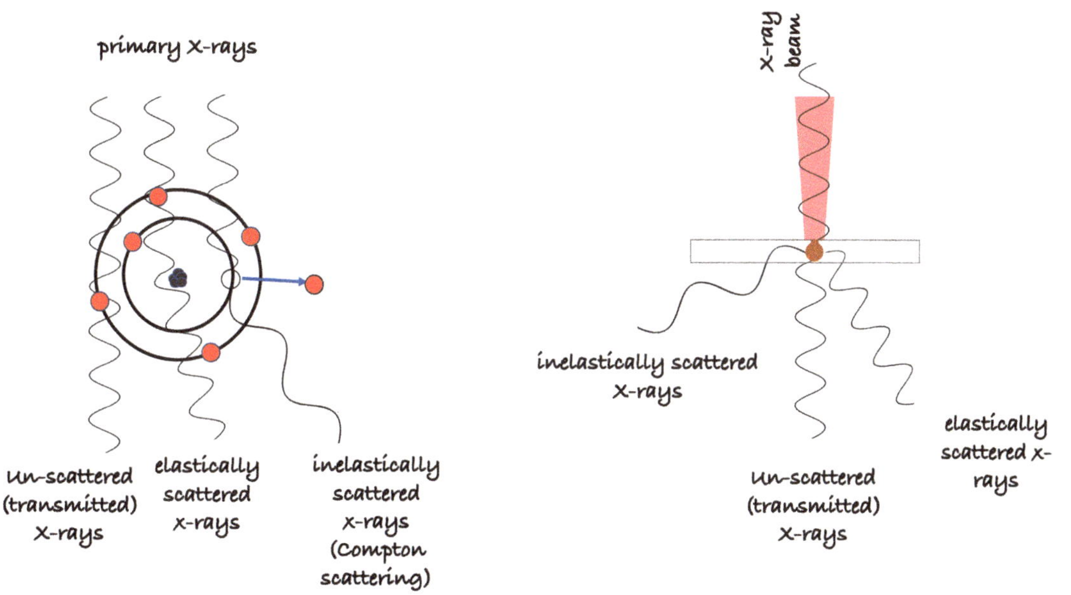

Figure 8.13 Contrast generation in X-ray microscopy tomography (XRMT). As X-rays interact with the electron cloud surrounding each nucleus, X-rays may pass as unscattered, elastically scattered or inelastically scattered photons (Compton scattering). Elastic scattered X-rays interfere with unscattered transmitted X-rays to yield phase contrast, whereas inelastically scattered X-rays, which are typically scattered at high angles are lost, which results in amplitude contrast.

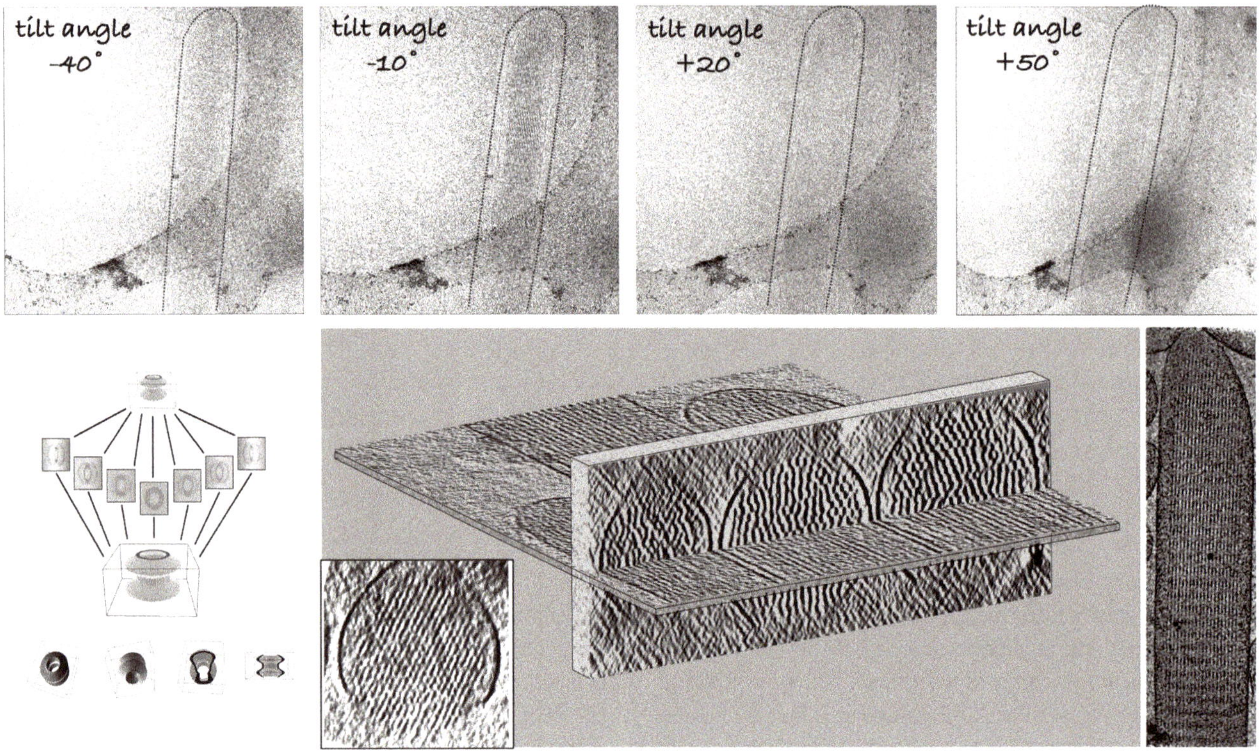

Figure 8.14 3D reconstruction from tilt series – Tomographic imaging. Shown here is an example of inner ear hair cell stereocilia attached to a holey carbon support film that were obtained by blotting hair cell stereocilia directly from the hair bundles of the apical surface of sensory epithelia onto an electron microscopy grid. Four representative images of the tilt series are shown in the top row, at −40°, −10°, +20°, and +50°. As the contrast is very low due to low-dose imaging and vitreous ice-embedding, the outline of the stereocilia is indicated by a dotted line. Upon alignment of the tilt series 2D projection images, a 3D tomographic volume is reconstruction by weighted back-projection. The insert shows a 15-slice average of the stereocilia with its hexagonally packed actin bundle. On the right, a 15 nm thin slice in longitudinal direction shows high regularity of the actin filament network.

markers or by cross-correlation approaches, and the 3D volume is reconstructed, e.g., by weighted back projection (WBP) algorithms, the algebraic reconstruction technique (ART) or by the simultaneous iterative reconstruction technique (SIRT), to name a few.

Among the challenges is the fact that in TEM imaging, the sample cannot be tilted for more than 120° (±60°) or 140° (±70°), which means that for a single-axis tilt series, a missing wedge of information exists that compromises the resolution in the direction of the electron beam. Dual (orthogonal) axis data collection schemes reduce the missing information to a pyramid instead of a wedge but cannot fully overcome this problem of resolution anisotropy due to limitations in data collection geometry. In yet another data collection scheme, called conical tomography, the specimen is first tilted to a certain angle and then imaged with the sample holder and its EM grid being rotated, however this data collection approach is rarely used in ET. It is conceivable that in the future focused ion beam milling would be used to create pillar-shaped specimen that would allow a full 180° data collection.

Another challenge is the high dose needed to collect a complete tilt series. Low-dose imaging and dose fractionation demands that the total allowable dose is spread over the entire tilt series, which results in individual tilt series images with very high noise (and therefore a high-noise 3D reconstruction).

Once 3D volumes are obtained and certain macro-/supramolecular complexes have been identified, approaches like the ones used in macromolecular imaging techniques (i.e., single particle cryo-EM) can be employed to enhance signal-to-noise and improve resolution. This approach is also known as subvolume or subtomogram averaging.

Based on geometrical considerations alone, the theoretical resolution can be calculated as a function of sample thickness "*D*" and number of different views "*m*" being taken in a tilt series. Assuming the ideal case that images are spaced evenly throughout 180° (which we know is not correct) the resolution limit (*d*) is approximately given by $d = \pi D/m$, which means that for a 100 nm thin section and 140 images recorded at 1° increments the best-case resolution is ~2.3 nm, whereas for a 200 nm section, it is closer to

5 nm. Likewise, one can use the formula $m = \pi D/d$ to estimate the minimum number of views (m) needed for any object of a diameter of D at a desired resolution d. This formula is also known as the Crowther criterion.

The actual quality and fidelity of the reconstructed volume will also depend on the noise level, any alterations that may have occurred during sample preparation, the amount of radiation damage suffered during data collection, and reconstruction artifacts that arise from imperfections of image frame alignment and the interpolation algorithms used for 3D reconstruction. However, averaging techniques – as discussed in the previous chapter – can be used to go beyond the initial resolution seen in the raw tomogram.

An impressive example is the microtubule doublet, whose 3D structure could be determined to 2.9 nm (29 Å) resolution, using cryo-tomograms as a starting point and followed by a customized helical averaging approach that took into consideration the oval (and thus non-perfect circular) shape of the microtubule doublet. This structure allowed the known tubulin atomic 3D structure to be docked into the resulting density map and predicted additional proteins that were needed in the microtubule doublet formation (see Figure 7.36 in the previous chapter).

8.4 Sample Preparation

Sample preparation is arguably the most crucial of all steps toward faithful imaging of the cellular macromolecular inventory and its respective 3D architecture, and despite its importance it is rarely discussed. This section will aim to address the various choices one has for sample preparation and explain the rationale behind the various protocols.

8.4.1 Electron Microcopy

The need for extensive sample preparation for TEM is the result of the strong interaction of electrons with matter, which limits the sample thickness that can be penetrated by an electron beam. This strong interaction requires the sample to be imaged in a vacuum as a few millimeters of air would completely stop an electron beam. Inelastic scattering is the underlying reason for radiation damage, as inelastically scattered electrons deposit energy into the biological specimen, which leads to chemical bond breakage and formation of radicals. This ultimately destroys the structural integrity of the biological sample.

8.4.2 Need for Thin Samples

Due to the limitations in specimen thickness, only bacteria, viruses, organelles, or the very edge of flat eukaryotic cells can be imaged as whole mounts. They can be either examined in their unstained, frozen-hydrated state using cryo-EM low-dose imaging or as positively or negatively heavy metal-stained samples by exposing the sample to diluted uranium, osmium, lead, or other heavy metal salt solutions. Heavy metal-stained biological samples show a higher tolerance to the electron dose and display amplitude contrast, which facilitates visualization. However, heavy metal staining bears the potential of structural reorganization of the macromolecules as well as the danger of uneven or preferential staining, which may alter the appearance of the structure of interest (as mainly the stain distribution is imaged as a proxy for the underlying biological structure).

All samples thicker than ~500–1,000 nm need to be thinned, ideally to a thickness of ~100–150 nm, with thinner samples being preferential for 2D and 3D imaging. For samples significantly thicker than 100 nm (which approximately translates into up to 20 layers of small proteins of ~5 nm thickness, note also that microtubules have a diameter of ~25 nm), the chance of overlap of cellular features increases, which can result in confusing 2D projection images. Features along the electron beam path be resolved by electron tomographic imaging, however, thicker samples mean an inherently lower resolution of the 3D reconstruction, if the total electron dose cannot be increased.

8.4.3 Conventional TEM Sample Preparation

The conventional solution to (ultra-) thin sectioning has been the embedding of the (heavy metal-stained) biological specimen in a liquid epoxy-resin (or other "plastic" resin) liquid, which is then hardened by addition of a radical starter solution and heating for hours in an oven at an elevated temperature of 60–70 °C. Prior to embedding, the biological samples need to be infiltrated with the resin-monomer solution. Since epoxy resins are not water-but organic solvent-miscible, the original cellular water needs to be replaced by an organic solvent, most frequently by a graded (30%, 50%, 70%, 100%, 100%, 100%) ethanol series, and/or acetone. This step of dehydration, i.e., the replacement of cellular water by an organic solvent, appears to be the most detrimental of all sample preparation steps, and if not done at temperatures below −35 °C often results in aggregation artifacts due to conformational changes of proteins upon removal of their hydration shell, which in turn exposes hydrophobic regions of the protein's sequence, leading to protein aggregation.

To reduce the effect of the solvent exchange, biological samples are typically exposed to primary fixatives, typically glutaraldehyde, and to secondary fixatives (heavy metals) such as osmium tetroxide and uranyl acetate prior to dehydration. The idea is that the fixatives will physically connect the network of macromolecules into a giant gel-like structure, which in turn should resist aggregation during dehydration. These chemicals penetrate the sample by diffusion, which results in rapid fixation for objects thinner than a few micrometers in the shortest dimension but may take several hours or even much longer for larger pieces of tissues or organisms due to natural diffusion barriers such as animal exocytoskeletons, protective layers around embryos, or plant cell walls. These barriers may lead to slow cell death and sometimes to gross alterations of cell architecture, such as autolysis or membrane blebbing. Aldehyde-fixation will only cross-link certain protein residues, but not nucleic acids, carbohydrate, or lipids, hence extended exposure to solvents in the dehydration, especially when performed at room temperature, and resin-infiltration process can lead to extraction of unfixed macromolecular components, often generating the impression of sparse protein distribution within cells. In reality however, proteins are so densely packed that they literally touch each other. This is known as macromolecular crowding. In a way, good sample preservation can be inferred from cell and tissue samples that appear very dense with proteins and macromolecular complexes literally touching one another.

The relocation of proteins within the cells, their extraction and vastly altered membrane structures (blebbing, which is most likely due to a cellular stress response of dying cells), have given conventional EM sample preparation a bad reputation. Fortunately, there exist sophisticated methods that can overcome most if not all these artifacts., such as ultrarapid freezing. Also, the use of low-power microwave irradiation can help in speeding up chemical fixation and heavy metal staining, which also results in better ultrastructure. Interestingly, there are still some investigators that prefer the artifacts associated with conventional protocols over the more densely populated, complex, as contrast of features of interest inside the cell maybe be lower in images that result from cryogenic faithful cell and tissue preservation, due to the dense packing of surrounding macromolecules.

8.4.4 Cryogenic EM Sample Preparation

Cryogenic sample preparation approaches including plunge freezing and high-pressure freezing immobilizes all cellular molecules within milliseconds, therefore "fixing" molecules in their respective position and avoiding any fixation artifacts. From such cryo-immobilized samples, TEM data such as cryo-tomograms can be collected directly if sample thickness if below 300–500 nm. For sample much thicker than 1 μm, cryo-sections can be cut by cryo-ultramicrotomy. Alternatively, samples can be thinned using ion beam milling to create thin frozen-hydrated cryo-lamella that can be imaged by cryo-tomography or frozen lamella can be produced by cryo-focused ion beam milling, which are then lifted out (cryo-FIB liftout), placed on a EM grid with a support film and then imaged in their unstained, frozen-hydrated state by cryo-electron tomography (Figure 8.15).

Alternatively frozen samples are subjected to a process called freeze-substitution that is designed to minimize dehydration artifacts. Dehydration of frozen-hydrated specimen occurs over the course of several days or according to more recent protocols over the course of a few hours at dry-ice temperature, using either liquid acetone (or methanol) as the organic solvent. While the detailed mechanism remains unclear, it was empirically found that at such low temperature the macromolecules are shielded from the effect of changes in their hydration state. It is presumed that at a temperature of less than −35 °C macromolecules have a limited ability to undergo drastic conformational changes in response to the changes of the solvent, therefore avoiding protein denaturation and subsequent aggregation. Once the solvent is exchanged, macromolecules seem stable in the new solvent environment: they can be warmed up to room temperature and resin-infiltrated without apparent changes to the ultrastructure. Typically, fixatives, such as glutaraldehyde and osmium tetroxide or uranyl acetate, are dissolved in the organic solvent, but it is assumed that they chemically fix the samples only after the solvent exchange has taken place and when the sample is being slowly warmed up, with glutaraldehyde and osmium tetroxide beginning to be chemically reactive at about −50 °C and about −30 °C, respectively. Therefore, at the temperature that macromolecules can undergo conformational changes the cells are already fixed.

Freeze-substituted samples can be warmed up to room temperature and subsequently infiltrated with commercially available epoxy-araldite or LR White resins (for morphological or immunolabeling studies) and polymerized at elevated temperature (~60–70 °C). Alternatively, cells can be infiltrated with methacrylate resins (such as Lowicryl HM20 or K4M) and polymerized by UV irradiation at −25 to −70 °C. Infiltration at room temperature can be accelerated by using a suitable specialized microwave oven. One of the caveats of freeze-substitution is that membranes often appear less pronounced and often missing. Such short-comings can be avoided by deliberately retaining trace amounts of water (up to 5%) throughout sample preparation or by adding tannic acid to the freeze-substitution. Both approaches for EM sample preparation, i.e. conventional protocols (also known as bench top processing) and high-pressure freezing, freeze substitution, are widely in use, and end in the infiltration and embedding of the sample in a resin, that can be hardened through

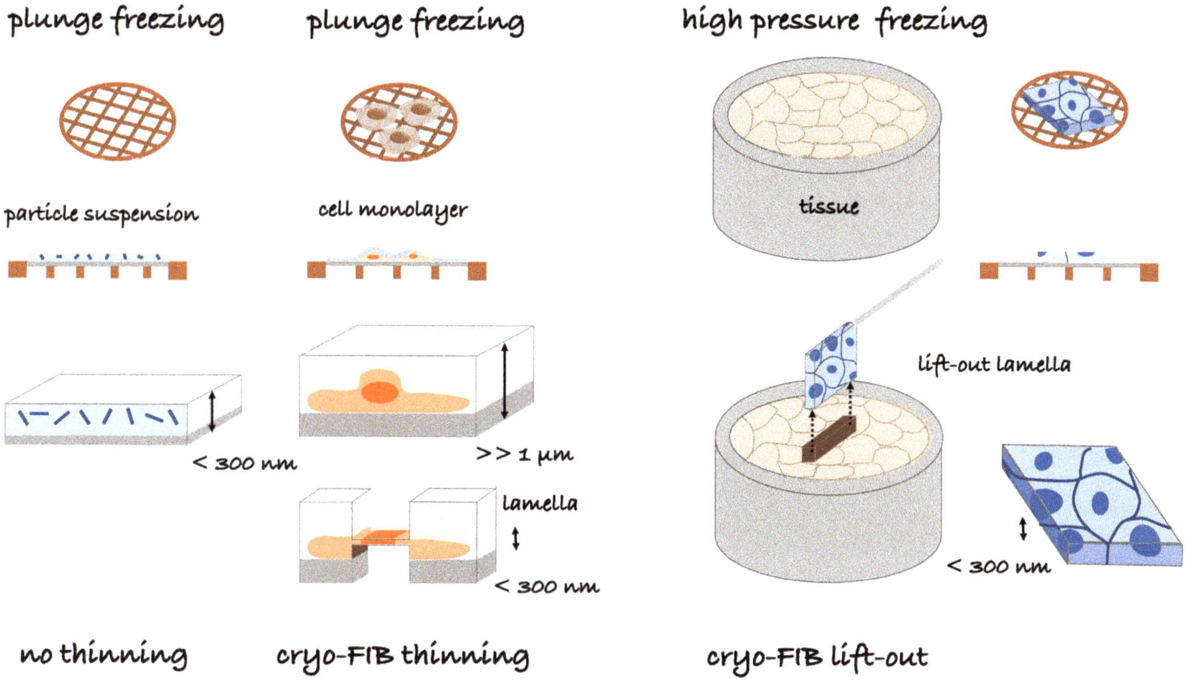

Figure 8.15 Cryogenic sample preparation for TEM – Thinning. Biological samples up to ~300–500 nm can be imaged as whole-mounts without thinning (e.g., organelles and particle suspensions). Any samples thicker need to be thinned, either by using cryo-focused ion beam milling (removing layers that are not relevant for imaging) or by trenching of a larger cell/tissue sample, so that a frozen-hydrated cryo-lamella can be lifted out of the tissue and placed onto an electron microscopy grid for cryo-imaging. Note that samples up to several micrometers thickness can be vitrified by plunge freezing into liquid ethane held at liquid nitrogen temperature, whereas larger cells and tissues need to be ultra-rapidly frozen, typically at high pressure and in the presence of cryo-protectants.

polymerization by a radical chemical, heat, or UV-radiation. The resulting resin blocks that can be imaged directly by block surface SEM or sectioned and imaged by TEM (Figure 8.16).

The main objective of successful rapid freezing is the "vitrification" of the biological specimen, meaning here the avoidance of ice crystal formation, which threatens to damage the cell's ultrastructure. Therefore, the heat needs to be conducted away rapidly from the specimen. For very thin objects, less than about 1 µm in thickness, vitrification can be accomplished by plunge freezing into liquid ethane. Thicker samples including tissues are best cryogenically preserved by high-pressure freezing, where millisecond freezing of the sample under high pressure discourages ice-crystal growth due to the density differences of water and ice. The addition of cryo-protectants further helps in controlling ice crystal formation but can provoke an unexpected biological response and can be a challenge for osmotically sensitive systems. It should be noted that when a live sample is subjected to high pressure freezing it may take a minute or more before the sample is prepared for high pressure freezing. During that time the sample is out of its tissue environment or culturing conditions, and often exposed to a cryo-protectant prior to high-pressure freezing, which could lead to an osmotic stress for the sample. Hence, while it may seem counterintuitive, an argument can be made (and experience shows) that excellent preservation of biological samples can also be accomplished by fast chemical fixation with glutaraldehyde over the course of tens of seconds to one minute by using a gentle dose of microwave radiation at room temperature or on ice, before proceeding to high-pressure freezing and freeze-substitution. The advantage of this approach is that the biological processes are swiftly stopped, which means all one needs to worry during sample processing is about the chemistry of the system and not any biological response to a change of the microenvironment. One could even consider carrying out a microwave-assisted rapid chemical fixation, followed by a heavy metal staining step and only then high pressure freeze the sample. In our experience, this approach has led to exquisite preservation and excellent contrast of the cellular ultrastructure, including of internal membranes.

Cryogenic approaches should always be considered when preparing biological samples. While the introduction of heavy metals bears the risk of changing cellular

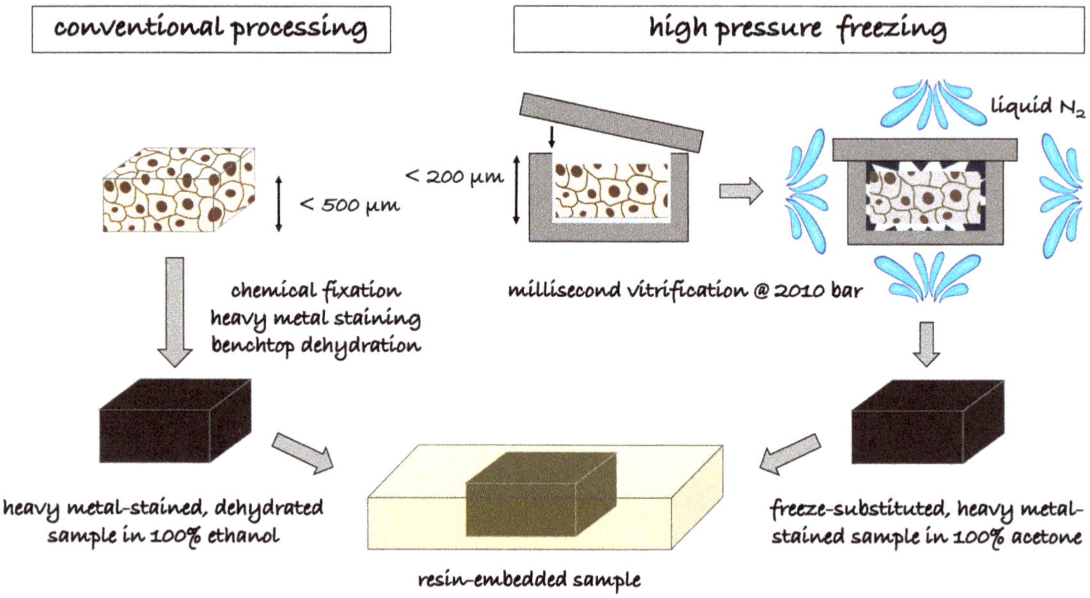

Figure 8.16 Sample preparation for TEM – Conventional processing versus high pressure freezing and freeze-substitution (HPF/FS). Conventional processing protocols rely on room temperature or on-ice chemical fixation by glutaraldehyde over the time course of hours or days. Samples are subjected to heavy-metal salt staining, benchtop dehydration (typically in a graded ethanol series), before being infiltrated, embedded in an organic solvent-miscible resin, and heat polymerized for hardening of the resin-block (with the embedded sample) to allow ultrathin sectioning. In high-pressure freezing, samples are ultra-rapidly frozen, resulting in cryo-preservation of the sample, followed by freeze-substitution to allow resin infiltration, embedding, and polymerization for subsequent block surface SEM images or TEM imaging of ultrathin block sections.

ultrastructure and can be avoided for thin or thinned specimen that can be subjected to cryo-ET, it may be necessary to create sufficient contrast for imaging, such as is the case for large-volume SEM and HeIM imaging, as well as for hard-X-ray Microscopy Tomography. We should however remind ourselves that large volume SEM imaging is not operating at the resolution level of individual proteins. Instead, it aims to determine the overall cellular architecture and the underlying 3D spatial relationship between various distinguishable subcellular components, such as organelles or supramolecular complexes. For such applications, the introduction of stain seems acceptable, if during the dehydration step the denaturation of proteins and thus aggregation is avoided (as is typically the case for high pressure freezing/freeze substitution approaches).

8.4.5 Sample Preparation for cryo-XRMT

Soft X-Ray Cryo-Microscopy Tomography (cryo-XRMT) in the X-ray water window is typically done on unstained samples and exploits differences in X-ray absorption for various cellular components (e.g., DNA versus protein or lipids). However, sample thickness is typically restricted to 15 µm and thus to about the diameter of a single eukaryotic cell. Larger samples, such as tissues or organs as well as millimeter-sized whole animals such as zebrafish larvae, are typically imaged by room temperature hard X-ray Microscope Tomography (XRMT) and typically rely on heavy metal staining.

8.5 Instrumentation

Each of the microscopy approaches (i.e., TEM and SEM, HeIM, and XRMT) requires a radiation-source, an optical system to focus the radiation, a specimen-holder and one or several detectors (Figure 8.17).

Both electron microscopy and HeIM require the sample to be imaged in a high vacuum, whereas X-ray imaging can be done under ambient atmosphere conditions, which significantly simplifies instrumentation requirements.

However, all techniques have in common that the specimen is bombarded with high energy radiation, which means that samples have been either radiation-hardened by heavy metal staining (or coating) prior to imaging, or that they need to be imaged in their frozen-hydrated state at liquid nitrogen temperature to mitigate and locally confine the effects of radiation damage. For the latter approach, the microscope also needs to be equipped with a cryo-stage suitable for low-temperature imaging.

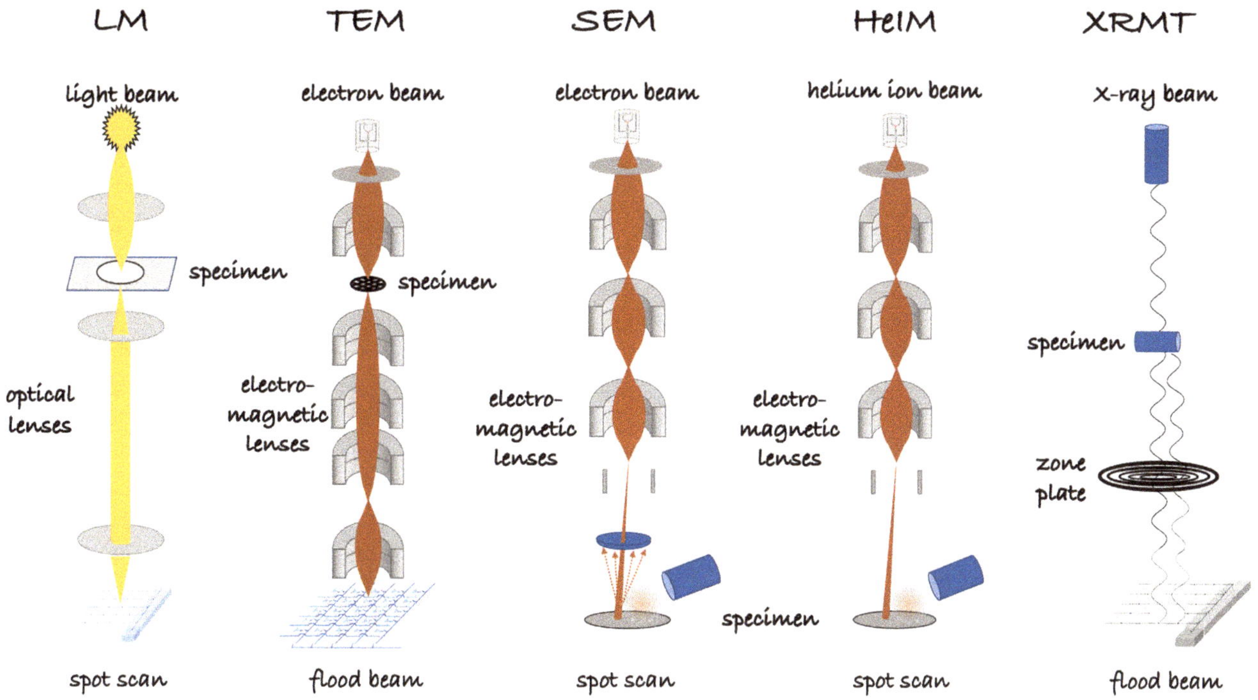

Figure 8.17 Instrumentation: Optical microscopy, transmission and scanning electron microscopy, helium ion microscopy, and X-ray microscopy tomography. All of these imaging techniques require a radiation source, an optical system to focus the radiation, a specimen holder, as well as one or more detectors. (Note: Rutherford backscattered ion detection is not shown here.)

If 3D imaging is the goal, the stage needs to be either tiltable or rotatable to record tilt series 2D images that can then be reconstructed into a 3D volume. Alternatively, as is the case for block face SEM, an entirely different approach to building up a 3D volume is to repeat a cycle of imaging of the block-surface and removal of a thin layer, which for each cycle exposes a new block surface for subsequent imaging. The removal of a thin layer can be accomplished by either using an ultramicrotome (which is built into the SEM) or a focused ion beam for milling.

Additional analytical instruments (detectors) may be present that can probe for the distribution of the elemental and/or molecular composition.

8.5.1 Radiation Source

Both TEM and SEM use as thermionic electron emission source either a tungsten hairpin filament or a lanthanum hexaborite (LaB_6) single crystal cathode. For hairpin filaments tungsten is the preferred metal as it has the highest melting point and lowest vapor pressure of all metals. The LaB_6 source has a low work function and is ideally suited for thermionic electron emission as free electrons emerge from a small volume at the tip of the crystal, thus exhibiting excellent spatial coherence of the electron beam. The state-of-the-art technology is field electron emission, where free electrons are not produced by heating but by high-intensity electric field extraction at the filament tip from a tungsten filament. There are cold cathode-type field emission guns (FEG) that use tungsten single crystal emitters or the thermally-assisted (heated) Schottky type FEG, that uses tungsten single crystals coated with zirconium oxide. FEG technology provides bright electron beams with excellent spatial and chromatic (energy) coherence.

The free electrons reside inside a Wehnelt cylinder, whose purpose is to focus the emitted electrons into a beam. The electrons are accelerated by a high voltage (typically at 100–300 kV for TEM, and at 15–20 kV in regular SEM mode or at 0.4–4 kV in low voltage SEM mode) and pass through an aperture before encountering the field of the electromagnetic lenses of the EM optics system.

In HeIM a cryogenically cooled, sharp tip resides in an ultra-high vacuum to which small amounts of helium gas are admitted in a controlled way. A large electric field is formed at the sharpest corner of the tip, which ionizes neutral gas atoms within a few Å (0.1 nm), resulting in a very narrow (~0.5 nm) helium ion beam. The narrow beam size contributes to the higher resolution that can be accomplished by HeIM.

For XRMT, conventional X-ray sources (such as rotating anodes which were discussed on the context of X-ray crystallography) can be used and are commercially available as single laboratory-scale stand-alone machines. However, synchrotron radiation with its high beam intensity and coherent, highly collimated beam is the preferred source for soft X-ray Microscopy Tomography, however access to soft X-rays in the water window is limited to few facilities.

8.5.2 Electron/Ion/X-Ray Optical System

In light microscopy, photons passing through different materials display a different velocity (refraction), a phenomenon that can be used to focus light using appropriate lens materials and shapes, which in turn allows an object to be magnified, e.g., in a compound optical microscope. There is no simple equivalent of a optical lens for electrons and other charged particles like helium ions or for X-rays, hence other ways of focusing the radiation are needed.

Electromagnetic lenses and electrostatic plates (surfaces) are ideally suited to alter the trajectory of charged particles and thus to guide (bundle and deflect) the electron or ion beam, simply by changing the electromagnetic and/or electrostatic field strength. Therefore, electromagnetic lenses and electrostatic plates in combination with appropriate apertures constitute the core of electron and ion microscope optics.

Electromagnetic lenses are made of solenoid coils surrounded by ferromagnetic materials. Application of an electric current to a lens forces the charged particles entering the electromagnetic field inside the hollow lens cylinder onto a spiraling trajectory around the curved magnetic field lines. This focuses the particle beam, with a lens' focusing power being dependent on the magnitude of the lens current. Optical lenses are superior to electromagnetic lenses in many properties, such as aberrations and other imperfections. However, one big advantage of electromagnetic lenses over optical lenses is that the same lens configuration can be used for different magnifications, simply by changing the lens currents (with the caveat that lens hysteresis limits the speed by which such switching can be accomplished). Furthermore, electromagnetic lenses typically need to be water-cooled to prevent overheating.

Deflectors and stigmators are small electromagnets that allow deflection of the beam and compensation for asymmetrical beam distortions due to differences in lens focal strength in different directions (astigmatism). High-end electron microscopes offer customs lens configurations that are corrected for spherical aberration, and energy filtering can be used to correct for electron chromatic aberration.

Apertures, which are circular holes in a metal strip, allow the removal of electrons or ions that do not follow the desired electron/ion-optical path or that would pass through the peripheral parts of the magnetic lenses, where aberrations are large. They also play a role in preserving the vacuum in the different parts of the microscope.

Transmission electron microscopes employ a condenser lens system that is responsible for primary beam formation, focusing the electron beam to a chosen size and at a particular location on the specimen. The objective lens system focuses the radiation that comes through the sample to form an image in the back-focal plane. Finally, an intermediate/projector lens system is then used to magnify the image onto the surface of an image recording device (the detector). Magnification can range from 100× to 1,000,000×, but most typically magnifications ~1,400× to ~20,000× are used for low-resolution overview as well as high-resolution close-up images, respectively. Below ~1,400×, image quality is often poor, whereas magnifying the image above 20,000×–40,000× is often unnecessary and only results in oversampling with no real benefit in terms of resolution (depending on the exact pixel-size of the detector).

In a scanning electron microscope (SEM), the magnification of an object can range from 10× to 800,000×, but biological samples are typically imaged at a magnification of 3,000× – 20,000×. In SEM, magnification is not defined by the power of the objective lens, but by the beam focus size and the incremental distance by which each pixel of the image is being imaged. The role of the lens system in the SEM is to focus the electron beam. When the sample has been hit by the electron beam, the entire signal that the specimen produces at this pixel location is being collected.

In an X-ray microscope (XRM), there are two principles used for the focusing of X-rays, namely (poly-) capillary wave guides and Fresnel zone plates. Capillary wave guides are an array of small hollow glass tubes that are tapered at one end and reflect X-rays at shallow angles by a mechanism known as total external reflection (which is related to total internal reflection used in fluorescence light optical microscopy). Since poly-capillary optics are achromatic, they can be utilized over a broad X-ray spectrum. X-rays passing through poly-capillary optics end up in a single point, which is why poly-capillary optics are often being used as a condenser lens to provide even illumination upon the sample.

Fresnel zone plates are composed of radially symmetric rings (also known as Fresnel zones), with adjacent zones either absorbing or phase-shifting X-rays. The larger the rings/zones' radius (the closer to the edge) the narrower is their widths. Zone plates focus X-rays through constructive interference. Zone plates are frequently used as an objective lens to focus the transmitted X-rays. Unlike poly-capillary optics, zone plates are highly chromatic, which means that they are typically designed for a narrow

X-ray bandwidth. Hence for high resolution imaging, monochromatic X-rays are highly desirable. X-rays may also pass through a Zernike phase ring, which results in an edge-enhancing phase contrast effect, not unlike phase contrast imaging in optical microscopy. Further magnification can be accomplished in XRMT by producing an X-ray-generated optical image with the help of a scintillator that is then optically magnified before reaching the charge-coupled device (CCD) detector.

8.5.3 Detectors

Given the different types of radiation employed in TEM, SEM, HeIM, and XRMT and the fact that two types of illumination and imaging modes (flood beam or raster scanning) are employed, it should not be surprising that different types of detectors are needed to capture the different radiation signals and create an image.

Key concepts such as detective quantum efficiency (DQE), point spread function (PSF), modulation transfer function (MTF), contrast transfer function (CTF), pixel and array size, noise, data readout speed, sensitivity, radiation hardness, as well as modes of detection of different types of radiation have been extensively discussed in the chapter on detectors and elsewhere in this book. Here we only provide a short summary of the detector technology that is being employed, and only as it is relevant understanding image formation for these four techniques.

Transmission electron microscopes (TEM) traditionally used X-ray films for data collection, particularly when high-resolution information was the goal of imaging. However, in any TEM session only a limited number of images could be obtained, and since film plates first needed to be photographically developed, results could not be viewed in real time. In the late 1990s, CCD cameras became the method of choice for recording the light signal created by electrons hitting a scintillator layer, but CCDs have slow read-out times and require an intermediary scintillator step to convert the high energy electron signal into a light signal. Complementary metal-oxide semiconductor (CMOS) detectors are more resistant to radiation damage than CCDs and have been introduced by 2005 to TEMs, where they are known as direct detectors, since they no longer need a scintillator intermediary, and thus can detect incoming electrons directly. Further development of the CMOS technology in the early 2010s allowed the detection of single electrons, and thus CMOS cameras could be run in electron counting mode, which had a huge impact on macromolecular structure determination by cryo-EM single particle analysis. Given their advantages over CCD cameras, CMOS detectors are likely to have a similar impact on cellular cryo-EM imaging, in particular cryo-ET.

Scanning electron microscopes (SEM) employ separate detectors for BSE and SE. BSE detectors are either scintillator- or p–n junction-based solid-state detectors that are based on the inner photoelectric effect, where the number of electron–hole pairs created (and thus the electrical current generated) depends on the quantity and energy of the BSE. The doughnut-shaped BSE detector with its hole in the middle is placed above the sample and allows the primary beam to reach the sample, while maximizing the collection of BSE. The BSE detector has four quadrants that can be read out independently. Reading out all quadrants allows elemental identification (atomic numbers), whereas differences in the quadrant signal read out provides topographical information about the object.

The most commonly used SE detector is the Everhart–Thornley detector, which is a positively charged Faraday cage, typically positioned to one side of the specimen. Low energy SE are attracted by the positive charge and hit a scintillator material, which converts the SE's energy into visible light before reaching a photomultiplier (Figure 8.18).

X-rays produced by cathodoluminescence in a SEM are detected by Silicon Drift Detectors (SDD), which can measure at high-count rate the energy of the incoming X-ray photon through the amount of ionization it produces in the detector. This type of detector, with its transversal field generated by several ring electrodes, which causes electrons to drift to a small collection electrode, is used for EDS, which allows elemental mapping.

HeIM produces a high amount of SE for image formation, which can be readily detected by the SE-based Everhart–Thornley detector. Helium ion Rutherford backscattering can be measured via a Silicon Surface Barrier Detector (Silicon Charged Particle Radiation Detector), which function by electron–hole pair creation, like the BSE detector described above but with the detector being optimized for helium ions instead of electrons.

X-rays in XRMT can be detected either directly by semiconductor detectors (e.g., CMOS) via electron–hole pair formation (inner photoelectric effect) or indirectly by a CCD camera via a scintillator-mediated conversion of the X-ray photons to visible light photons. For micro-CT imaging of larger specimen, X-rays hit a scintillator, and the signal is read out with an optical microscope set-up featuring two different lenses which results in two different magnification settings of the image.

8.5.4 Specimen Stage

Not surprisingly, sample/specimen stages for TEM, SEM/HeIM, and XRMT are very different, owing to the different specimen types (e.g., ultrathin sections or macroscopic whole-mounts) and states (stained or metal coated for radiation

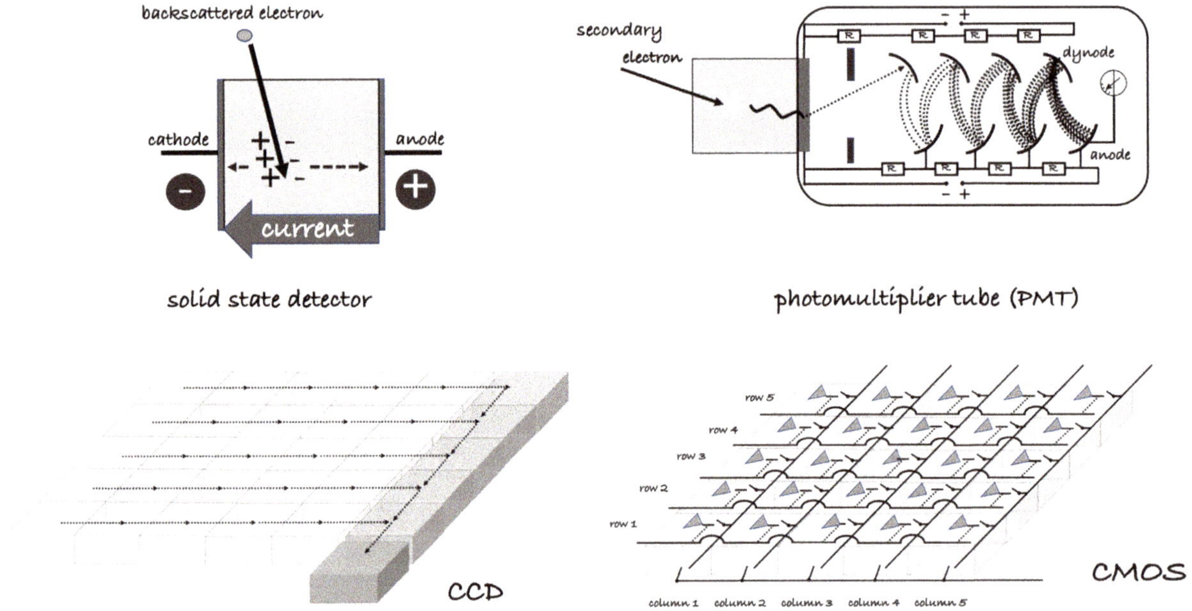

Figure 8.18 Detectors used in TEM, SEM, HeIM, and XRMT. CCD and CMOS detectors are commonly used in TEM, whereas solid state detectors and photomultiplier tubes are used for electron detection in SEM. Note that the Everhart–Thornley detector used for detection of secondary electrons in both SEM and HeIM is a combination of a Faraday cage collecting secondary electrons and a photomultiplier tube with a scintillator in between to convert the electron signal to an optical signal. XRMT employs either CMOS detectors or are scintillator/CCD-based.

hardening or unstained frozen-hydrated), penetration depths of the radiation, type of specimen preparation and modes of image formation (e.g., transmission or reflection).

In TEM, due to their size and delicate nature (e.g., ultrathin sections) samples are typically supported by a metal grid 3.05 mm in diameter with grid bars spaced every ~50–100 μm, coated with an ultrathin carbon, Formvar (a polyvinyl alcohol/formaldehyde copolymer) or a variety of commercially available support films. The support film can be continuous, have holes of predictable positions and size, a random number and size of holes as in holey carbon film or look more like a meshwork as is the case for lacey carbon. The grid with its support film is then inserted into a sample holder, which can be either a single-axis or a dual axis tilt holder. Side entry holders, which are inserted through an airlock into the microscope (ideally with the vacuum being maintained during specimen transfer), have one end of the holder remaining outside the microscope (Figure 8.19). Top entry holders typically detach a cartridge or the tip of the sample holder inside the microscope. Side-entry holders, suitable for cryo-electron microscopy, have a bulky liquid nitrogen-filled Dewar sticking out of the airlock, which is less than optimal with respect to specimen vibration as well as mechanical or thermal specimen drift. Hence for high-resolution cryo-EM data collection, top entry stages are preferable. State-of-the-art sample holders typically store multiple grid holders in the vacuum of the microscope and allow a fast change of multiple specimens for efficient data collection. The stages with the sample holder in it are usually motorized and allow coarse and fine *X*, *Y*-translation to find the grid region of interest, as well as eucentric *Z*-height adjustment. Typically, the entire stage is being tilted for tilt series data collection, which for side entry holders with liquid-nitrogen-filled Dewars can lead to bubbling of liquid nitrogen upon rotation, and thus holder vibrations during data collection.

For SEM and HeIM, the design of the sample holder and the transfer of the sample into the microscope is much simpler but requires air-venting the microscope chamber prior to specimen insertion. For room temperature SEM and HeIM imaging, the specimen is typically fixated onto a metal plate sample holder with an electrically conductive glue material. After insertion of the specimen, the sample chamber is gas-evacuated before imaging.

For XRMT, samples do not need to reside in a vacuum but can be in air or in a liquid or frozen-hydrated state (Figure 8.20). Cryo soft X-ray microscopy can penetrate ~15 μm, hence the biological samples (typically individual cells) are placed in a capillary before being ultrarapidly frozen and imaged in its unstained, frozen-hydrated state. Cryogenic preservation also helps to reduce the effects of radiation damage by the X-ray beam (Figure 8.20).

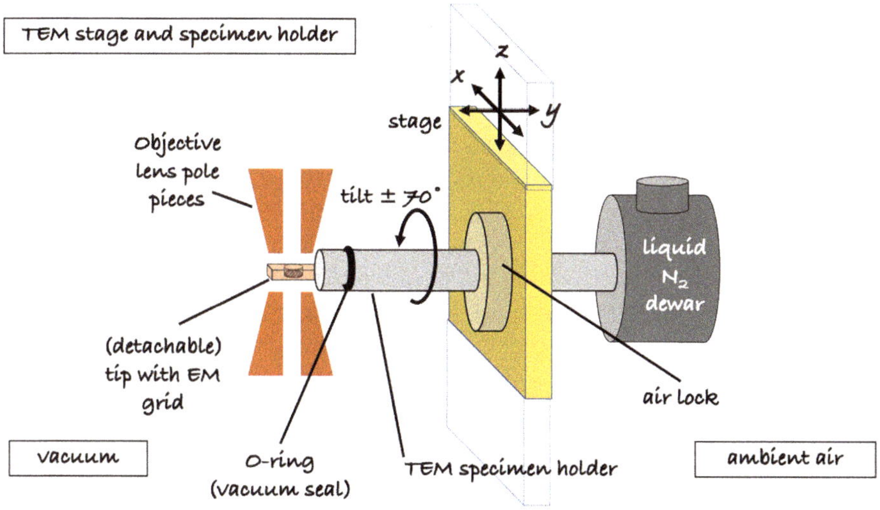

Figure 8.19 Specimen stage: Side entry grid holder for TEM. Side entry sample (grid) holders for TEM imaging consist of a long rod with a tip that places an EM grid between the objective lens pole pieces. On the other end of the long rod is a liquid nitrogen Dewar outside the microscope's vacuum that keeps the EM grid at liquid nitrogen temperature. An O-ring on the rod and an airlock ensure that the microscope vacuum remains intact during the insertion of the holder. The entire stage including the specimen holder are typically adjustable in *X*, *Y*, and *Z*-direction.

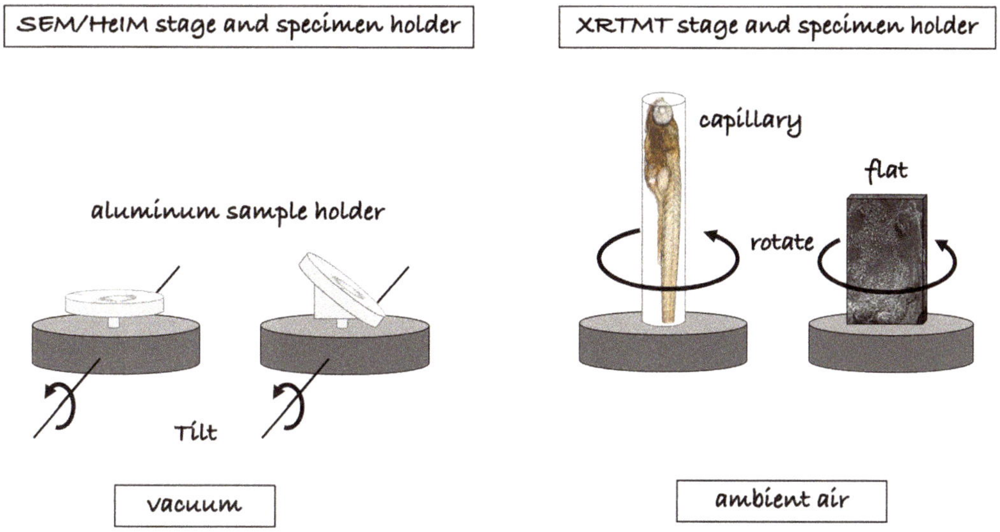

Figure 8.20 Specimen stage: Sample holder for SEM/HeIM, and XRMT. Compared to TEM cryo-sample holders, sample holders for SEM are relatively simple. In the simplest case it just a metal stub (flat or tilted at ~45°) onto which the sample is glued. This stub resides typically on a motorized stage that can be adjusted in *X*, *Y*, and *Z* and that can be tilted. For XRMT, typically a capillary containing the sample or a sample slab is mounted on a stage that can be rotated for tomographic data collection.

8.5.5 Vacuum System

TEM, SEM, and HeIM require the entire electron/ion-optical path including the sample to reside in a vacuum to increase the mean free path of the electrons/ions. Microscopes typically have several vacuum pumping systems and airlocks, as well as pressure-limiting apertures. Field emission technology has higher vacuum demands than LaB_6 crystal or thermionic tungsten filament sources. A high vacuum is not only needed for field emission to work properly, but also helps to avoid the generation of an arc when applying a high voltage in the electron/ion gun to accelerate the charged particles. Furthermore, the higher the vacuum the lower is the probability of contamination of frozen-hydrated samples held at liquid nitrogen temperature.

High vacuum values are achieved in multiple steps. An initial low (roughing) vacuum is produced by a rotary vane pump or a diaphragm pump, which is then needed for the turbo-molecular/diffusion pump to create a higher vacuum. The highest vacuum exists in the electron gun courtesy of ion getter pumps which adsorb and chemically bind gas molecules to the getter material. With all these three vacuum systems the pressure in the electron gun can be reduced to 10^{-6} Pa, which is ~11 orders of magnitude below ambient atmospheric pressure.

8.6 Data Collection and 3D Reconstruction

2D projection data collection is straightforward for TEM, SEM, HeIM, and XRMT and involves finding the region of interest (typically at low magnification) and after adjusting appropriate illumination and finding focus, the simple recording of an image.

For TEM imaging of unstained samples (as a weak phase object) at high resolution, where contrast solely relies on phase contrast, images are taken with a small amount of underfocus to gain additional contrast, while keeping the modulation of the contrast by the CTF in an acceptable and more importantly predictable range. The concept of the CTF has been discussed in detail in the chapter on macromolecular electron microscopy imaging. Also, for unstained, frozen-hydrated samples, a low-dose imaging data collection scheme is advised, where the predominant fraction of the total dose is used for data collection, whereas positional adjustments of the region of interest are carried out at low magnification and focusing does not occur in the region of interest, but at a deliberately chosen adjacent area of the specimen.

For 3D (volume) imaging in TEM, ET and XRMT, samples are tilted or rotated, respectively, to obtain a series of projection 2D images, from which upon X, Y alignment (often with the help of fiducial markers or by simple cross-correlation) a 3D volume can be calculated through some 3D reconstruction algorithms, such as weighted back-projection or algebraic reconstruction technique (Figure 8.21). Given that in ET the tomographic data collection is limited to a tilt angle of up to ±60–70°, the resolution of the reconstructed 3D volume is anisotropic. XRMT on the other hand allows 180° rotation of the sample and thus the resulting 3D volume displays isotropic resolution.

8.6.1 Serial Section TEM

Serial section TEM is based on the physical sectioning of a sample embedded in a resin block. With ultrathin sections cut at ~50–100 nm thickness, one can collect serial sections and 2D image them one after the other one (Figure 8.22). The images – once taken – are then aligned with one another, ranging ideally in a X,Y-resolution of 1–5 nm (depending on magnification and detector pixel size), whereas the axial resolution cannot be better than the ~50–100 nm thickness of the section. However, there are a variety of problems associated with serial sections. It is very challenging to cut more than a few consecutive sections and transfer them to an EM grid support film without the section being physically altered, displaying compression or wrinkling artifacts. This only becomes obvious in the final serial reconstructions if one tries to align the images of the consecutively cut sections. Another challenge arises from repeatedly trying

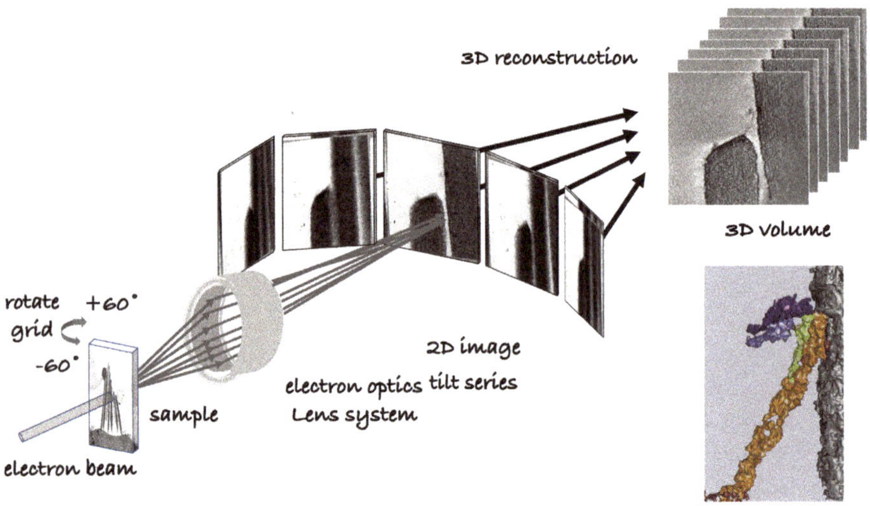

Figure 8.21 TEM tomography – 3D reconstruction from tilt series. In electron tomography (ET) a sample (e.g., a section) is tilted in electron microscope up to an angle of ±60–70°, resulting in a tilt series that upon alignment can be reconstructed into a 3D volume by weighted back projection or other iterative 3D reconstruction algorithms. After segmentation, macromolecular details such as the 3D organization of tip link, a protein central in the process of mechanoelectrical transduction, can be visualized.

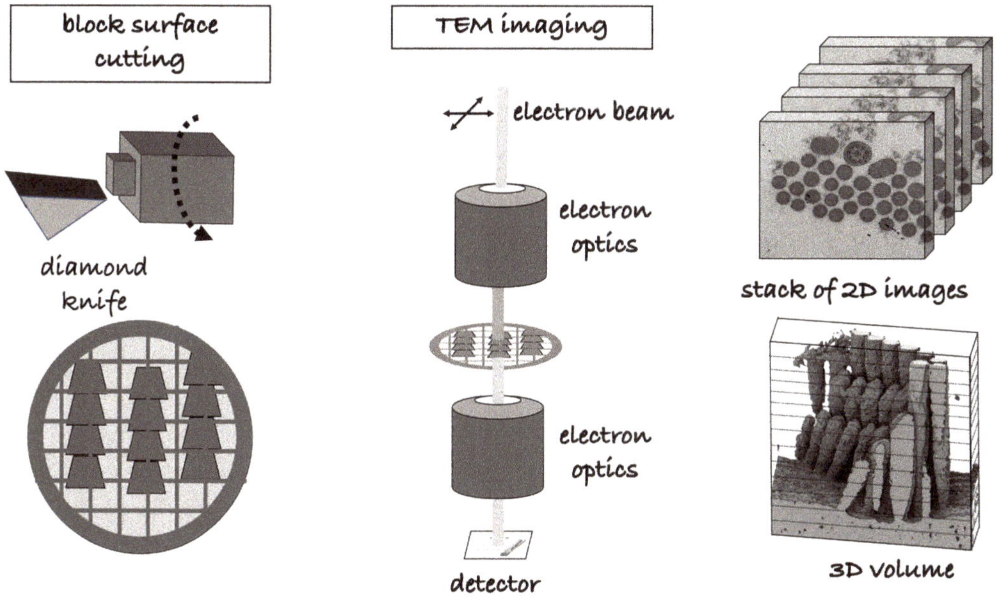

Figure 8.22 Serial section TEM. In serial section TEM, the resin block (with the embedded sample) is sectioned repeatedly using a diamond knife, and ribbons of the sections are collected from the knife boat's water surface with a TEM grid. 2D projection images of the ~50–100 nm thick sections are aligned with one another and stacked into a 3D volume with significant anisotropic resolution.

to find and image a very small region of interest (a few microns at best) within the entire section which could be hundreds of microns and even millimeters in diameter. Furthermore, due to compression of the block hitting the ultramicrotome's knife, it is possible that some sections are unintentionally thinner or thicker than others, or some may be missing altogether. For all these reasons, serial sectioning is rarely performed these days.

8.6.2 Serial Section SEM

A related but slightly different approach is taken in Array Tomography and Automated Tape-Collecting UltraMicrotome (ATUM) microscopy, where serial sections (at ~50–100 nm thickness) are collected by a tape right after ultramicrotome sectioning. Note that ultramicrotome sectioning is carried out outside the SEM at ambient pressure. The tapes containing the sections are placed onto silicon wafers, which in turn are then glued onto SEM sample holder stubs before the section ribbons are being imaged by SEM (Figure 8.23). ATUM has the advantage over serial section TEM that the sections are fully supported by the tape and thus manual handling is easier and gentler and thus the danger of mechanical damage is somewhat less of a concern. However, this approach has similar caveats as serial section TEM, such as resolution anisotropy. Yet this approach has been routinely and successfully been used in the context of "brain connectomics".

8.6.3 Serial Block Face SEM

In the case of SBF SEM imaging, the ultramicrotome is placed inside the microscope and operates under vacuum conditions. Instead of collecting the serial sections, the microtome is only there to reveal a new block surface by shaving off resin material, which is discarded. The new block surface is then imaged by the SEM, followed by another round of ultramicrotome sectioning. This repeated approach allows the buildup of the 3D volume slice by slice. Since the section is discarded and does not need to be collected for imaging, the sectioning allows a step-size of ~30 nm (or even less). The alignment of the images usually is straightforward as the block surface (given the massive size of the block) does not experience compression artifacts, unlike it is the case for ultrathin sections (Figure 8.24).

8.6.4 Focused Ion Beam (Dual Beam) SEM

A repeated cycle of block surface imaging and block surface material removal/block surface renewal also lies at the heart of focused ion beam (dual beam) SEM. In this approach the block is exposed to a focused ion beam, which ablates the resin material and thus creates a new block surface with an ~3.5–5 nm increment/step size. Often only the region of interested is ion-milled, resulting in trenches that are imaged by SEM at comparably low voltage (typically at ~1 keV). A stack of serial 2D images of the

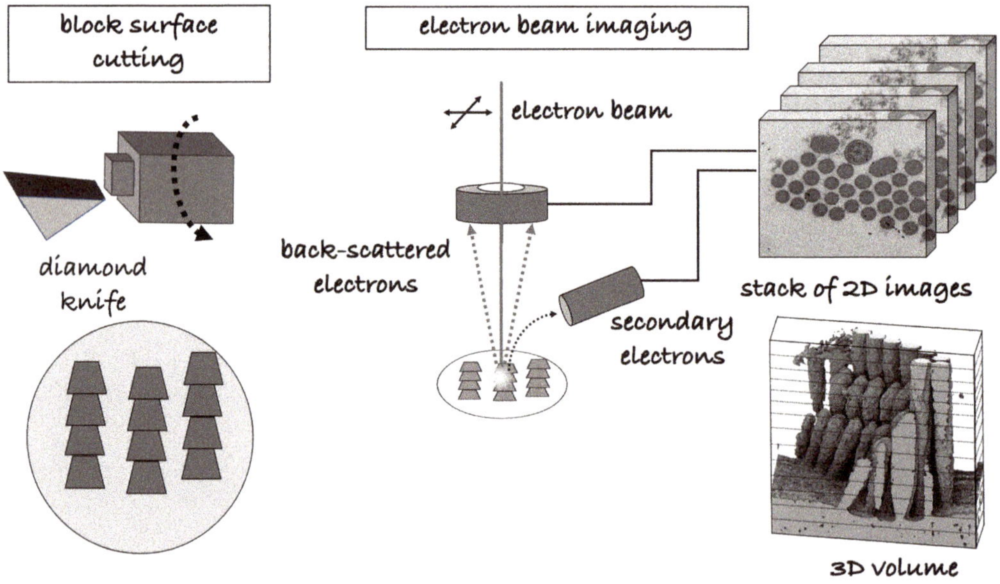

Figure 8.23 Array tomography/Automated Tape-collecting UltraMicrotome (ATUM) – Serial section SEM. In ATUM-SEM, serial sections are cut with a diamond knife from a resin block surface, collected by a tape running at constant speed. The tape pieces with the serial sections are placed on a silicon wafer which is glued to a SEM stub and imaged in 2D. The stack of images is aligned, and a 3D volume can be built up from the serial sections.

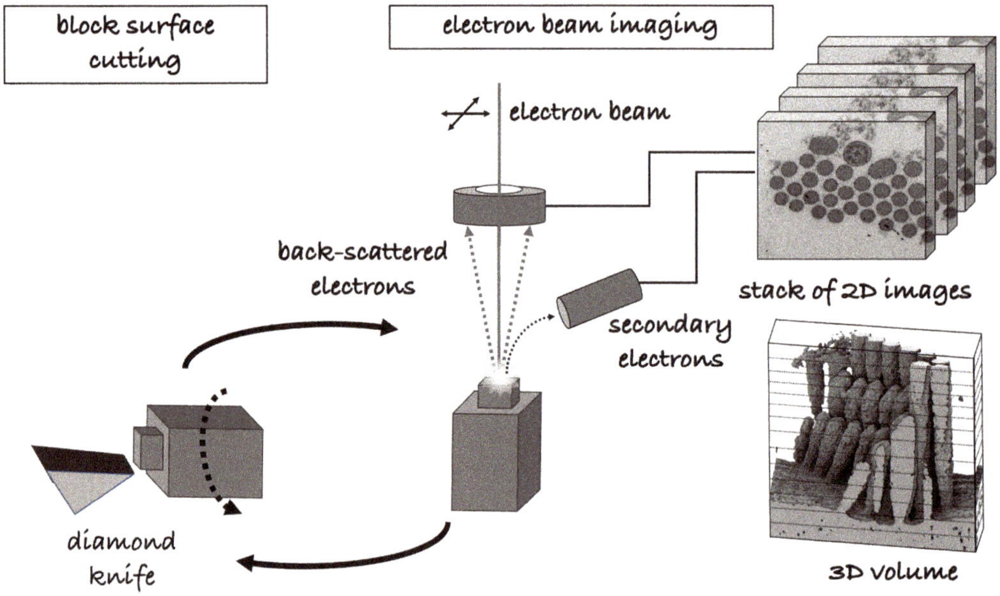

Figure 8.24 Serial Block Face SEM. For Serial Block Face SEM a diamond knife ultramicrotome is used to cut a 30 nm ultrathin section off the block surface. The section is being discarded, as it is the newly revealed block surface that is imaged by SEM. Low voltage imaging (at ~1 keV) results in a 2D image of the block surface with a small penetration depth of only a few nanometers. The images typically align very well with one another, and a 3D volume can be built easily.

block surface directly builds up the 3D volume (Figure 8.25). Some challenges arise from the fact that trenches can only be of a certain depth for imaging, and hence other approaches are currently in development to gain better access to the region of interest.

8.6.5 X-Ray Microscopy Tomography

In X-ray microscopy, the sample (either stained or frozen) is irradiated by an X-ray beam, and the scattered X-rays can be refocused by zone plates to generate 2D images. The sample is rotated at ambient pressure and a 2D tilt series is

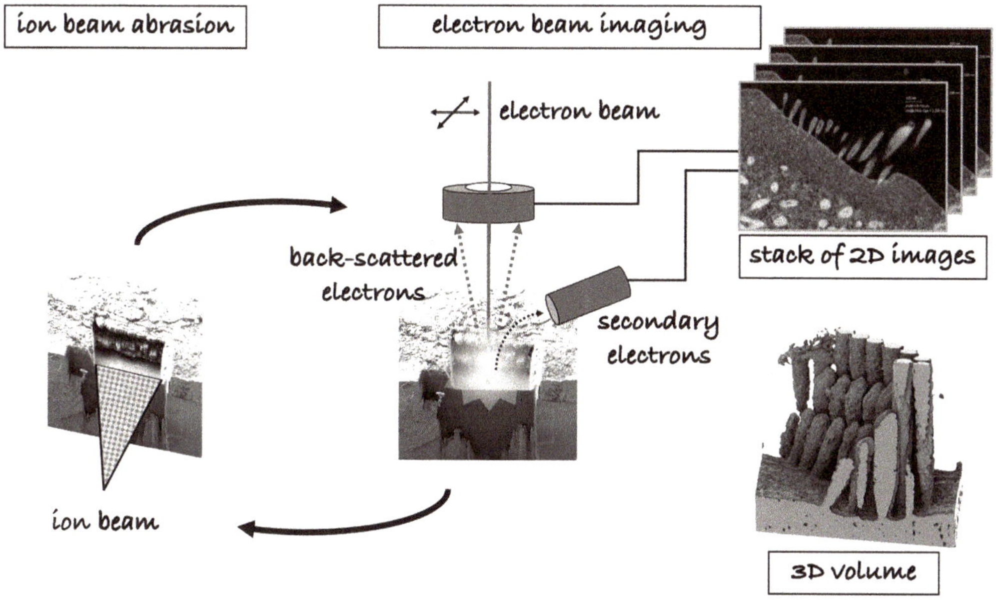

Figure 8.25 Focused Ion Beam (dual beam) SEM. In Focused Ion Beam (FIB) SEM (also known as dual beam SEM), an ion beam is used to mill away resin material to expose a new resin block surface for SEM imaging, typically at a step size of up to ~3.5 to ~5 nm. Often only the region of interest is ion beam-milled to save milling time, leading to trenches into the resin block from where 2D SEM image stacks are recorded. Given the small step size, serial block face images typically align very easily to generate a 3D volume such as the hair bundle shown.

obtained which can be reconstructed into a 3D volume using back projection methods (Figure 8.26).

Note: While the term "3D volume" is redundant (as a volume is always three-dimensional), it is chosen to make a clear distinction between individual images that are typically two-dimensional (2D) and the reconstructed 3D volume.

8.7 Data Visualization and Analysis

Independent on how the 3D volume information was obtained (i.e., ET/cryo-ET, serial section TEM, block-face SEM, FIBSEM/dual beam SEM or XRMT), it is just the beginning of a long and tedious process of visualization, feature extraction and analysis. In fact, it may take a few hours

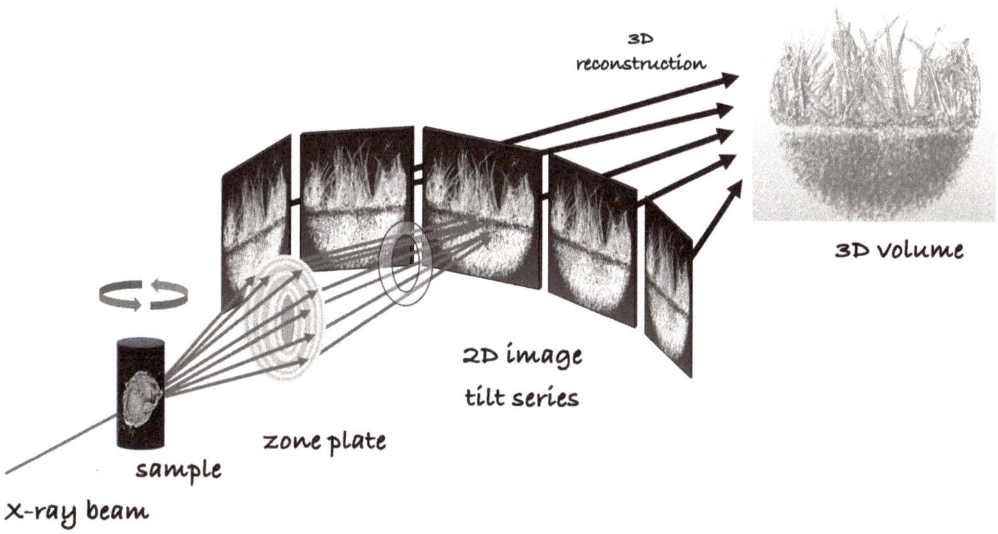

Figure 8.26 X-ray microscopy tomography. The samples in X-ray microscopy tomography are either heavy metal-stained or kept frozen in a vitrified state. Upon irradiation of a rotating specimen with an X-ray beam and refocusing of the scattered X-ray with the help of zone plates a 2D image tilt series can be recorded which is then reconstructed into a 3D volume.

(or days) to get the 3D data, and many months or possibly years to thoroughly analyze them and extract biological meaning from that large 3D arrays of voxels of intensity.

In other words, the visualization and analysis may well be the most time consuming and challenging aspect to ultrastructural imaging, and the one that may be the least developed in this pipeline of preparing the sample, 3D imaging and deriving meaning from the imaging data.

First, often there are some practical shortcomings to be dealt with, such as data anisotropy (a significantly worse resolution along in a direction versus perpendicular to the direction of the beam) due to the limited tilt range in ET or section thickness in serial TEM, serial SEM/ATUM, or Serial Block Surface SEM, as well as a high level of noise, courtesy of dose fractionation in cryo-ET and/or reconstruction artifacts, including shadowing artifacts of high contrast features.

However, by far one of the biggest challenges arises from the fact that the macromolecular composition is ill-defined, and hence assignment of macromolecular feature often is somewhat tentative and requires intensive prior knowledge about the biological system under investigation. This tedious process of deriving biological meaning is typically divided into four stages: (1) visualization of very dense and complex 3D data; (2) extraction of features of interest, also known as segmentation; (3) (quantitative) analysis of such extracted features; and (4) deriving some biological meaning from the 3D image data. The third point is often skipped, and the last point often requires a biological expert to look at the image data and interpret them in the context of current knowledge and uncertainties about the biological system.

8.7.1 Visualization of Cellular Sceneries

Visualization of cellular sceneries can be challenging to the fact that the macromolecular composition is not well established, but also because (sub)cellular volumes are often complex in their 3D organization. Furthermore, complex 3D volumes are plagued by high noise levels, which further obscure features of interest. Figure 8.27 shows an example where mouse inner ear hair cell stereocilia have been blotted onto an EM grid support film, and cryo-tomograms of such unstained, frozen-hydrated have been obtained. Such stereocilia contain a bundle of closely-spaced parallel actin filaments that are heavily

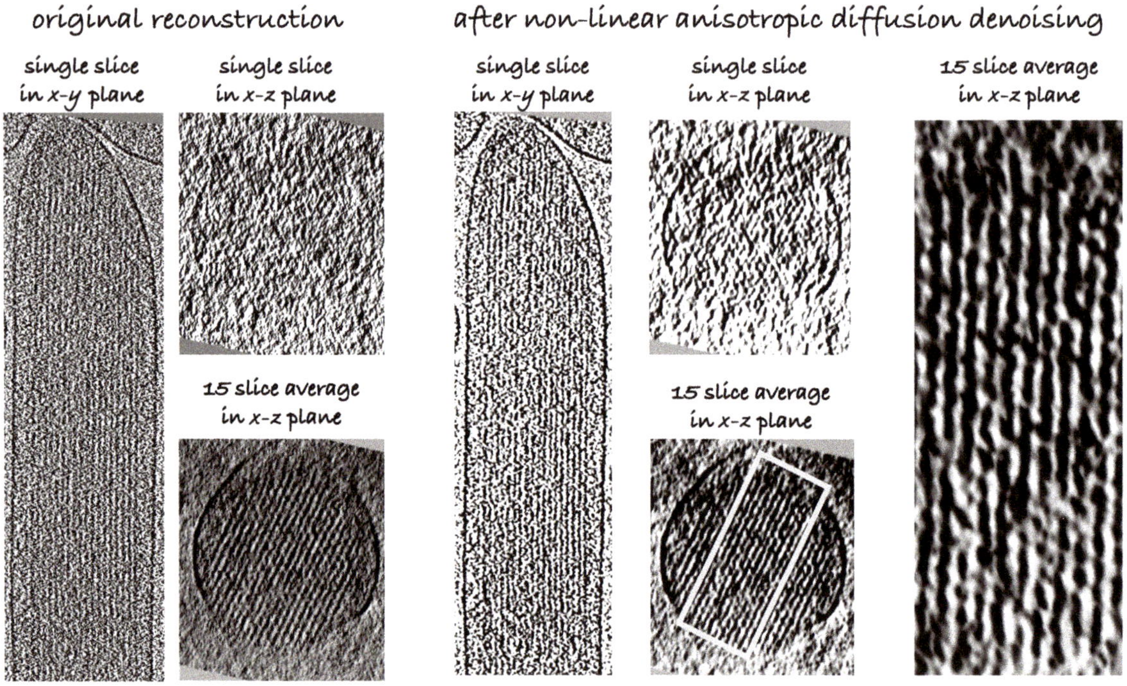

Figure 8.27 TEM tomography data visualization of original and denoised data. Reconstructed 3D volumes of electron tomography samples are characterized by a high noise level for single slices of the 3D reconstruction (left two columns). Averaging over 15 slices in the X,Z plane significantly improves the signal-to-noise ratio (note the difference to a single slice in the X,Z plane), and reveals a significant level of order present in the actin bundle of stereocilia. Denoising algorithms such as non-linear anisotropic diffusion, significantly suppresses noise, which results in better contrast between features and the background (right three columns). For denoised image datasets, even single slices reveal order in the actin bundle organization. However, also note that data anisotropy can make unambiguous assignment of filament organization rather challenging.

cross-linked. Noise-reduction algorithms such as non-linear anisotropic diffusion and/or averaging over several slices (in the correct orientation) are needed to distinguish thc pattern of actin filaments from the background. Note that macromolecules literally touch one another, a phenomenon known as macromolecular crowding. It is estimated that inside the cells cytoplasm the protein concentration may be as high as 100 mg/ml, which higher than what is often used for 3D crystallization for X-ray crystallography.

While some macromolecular complexes such as ribosomes, proteasomes, F-type ATPases as well as supramolecular assemblies such as microtubules, intermediate filaments or actin filaments can be recognized through their shape and/or subcellular localization, other macromolecular machines and individual proteins appear rather unremarkable, and at a resolution of ~3–5 nm not distinct enough for direct identification.

Subvolume/subtomogram averaging, which is increasingly being adopted in cryo-ET, can help increase the resolution of the 3D structure of macromolecular complexes in their native cellular environment. However, the determination of the exact shape/3D structure of macromolecular complexes is not always the goal in 3D cellular imaging. A very valuable goal instead may well be to determine the overall organization of organelles and supramolecular complexes like the cytoskeleton, cell–cell or cell–matrix adhesion complexes, without aiming for the exact details with respect to their precise shape and 3D structure.

It is not only that the organization of each object (macromolecular complex, supramolecular or organelle assembly) is complex and that the exact composition cannot be assumed with certainty, but also the very fact that all these components are tightly spaced, which makes visualization difficult, as objects in the front obscure other objects further behind, and thus the spatial relationship cannot easily be appreciated, even if it is possible to somewhat separate the objects from one another and annotate them.

Virtual Reality (VR) caves allow immersive exploration of 3D volumes, which means one can stand virtually in the middle of one's data and explore the data 'from the inside' instead 'from the outside', which can indeed be an intense experience. However, not only are there limits set on the size of the data set that can be rendered in a stereoview headset, but also, VR approaches suffer from the same problems that are outlined above, such as macromolecular crowding and the lack of clear spaces in between different macromolecular components, a somewhat undefined set of possible macromolecular constituents. Comparably low resolution does not allow unambiguous annotation of each feature, and one can be easily overwhelmed by the high density of components.

To reduce complexity, it may still be valuable (and probably it is still the most common way to interact with the 3D volume) is to visualize the 3D volume as consecutive 2D slices that build up the 3D volume, often in form of a looped movie that allows the brain to capture the features of interest and develop an intuitive understanding of the cellular scenery, which then later helps in segmentation. Often segmentation is done slice-by-slice, or at least a feature of interest is identified in a 2D slice of the 3D volume, which serves as a start for semi-automated 3D volume segmentation algorithms (Figure 8.28).

8.7.2 Segmentation/Feature Extraction

After an initial visualization, individual features of interest need to be distinguished from the background and from one another. This is more complicated than it may seem, as proteins and protein complexes literally touch one another due to macromolecular crowding. Hence, there are often no obvious empty gaps between the different objects in a cell. The lack of clear boundaries is further complicated by the noise inherent the datasets. Resolution anisotropy and the general lack of high-resolution data further contributes to the problem of fuzzy boundaries between different macromolecular components in the 3D volume. Also, one often approaches the segmentation of such volumes with preconceived ideas of what shapes one may find, and which shape or arrangement a certain object may adopt, which makes visualization and manual feature extraction somewhat biased from the very start. More objective approaches, such as template matching may not only be computationally very demanding, particularly for large volumes, but also fail altogether due to all the same problems discussed above.

For the time being, expert user knowledge is often still being required and advanced software packages allow a user to point and click on a few pixels of an object, and an algorithm typically based on partial differential equations, watershedding, level set methods, graph cuts or other segmentation approaches will identify the boundaries around the object, which then is either accepted as the segmented volume or further modified by the expert user, who may decide to further divide or merge regions.

More recently, through manual segmentation of parts of the volume that are considered as correctly segmented examples, ground truth is established that allows training of deep learning algorithms with their convolutional neural networks. Such neural networks, after an initial period of training, can find similarly looking objects in the remainder of the volume (Figure 8.29). However, ideally such supervised deep learning approaches rely on large training datasets as ground truth, which can be difficult in biological imaging. Hence unsupervised approaches that do not require

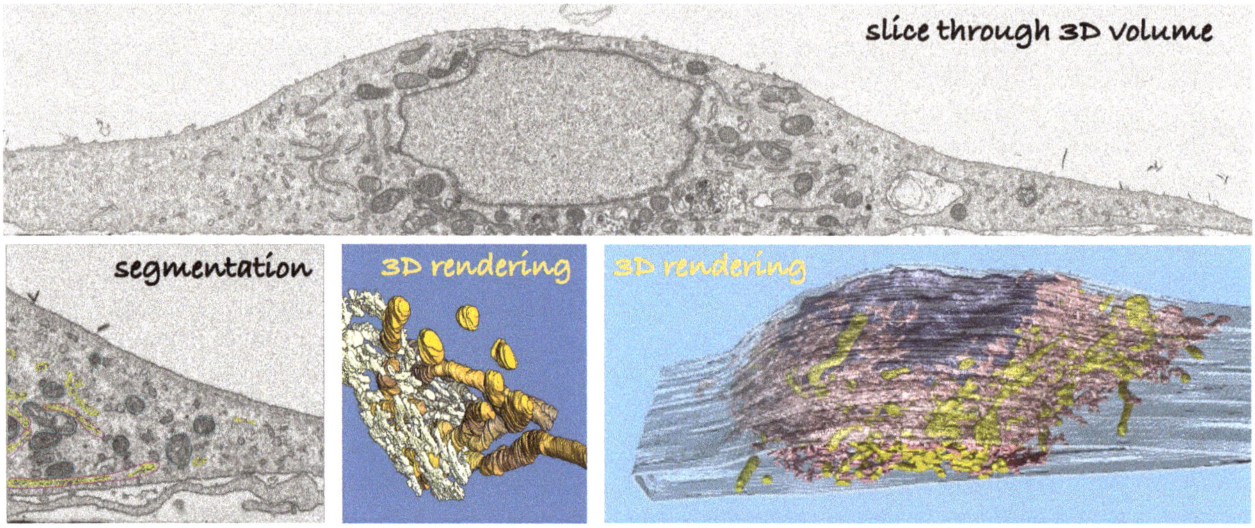

Figure 8.28 Visualization and manual segmentation of cells. Top: Single slice of a 3D FIBSEM dataset of one half of a fibrosarcoma cell cultured on a coverslip. Note that cells can adopt the shape reminiscent of a fried egg, typically for many cells cultured in the absence of an extracellular matrix on hard surfaces. Bottom left: Manual segmentation of mitochondria and the endoplasmic reticulum (ER). Bottom, middle: 3D rendering of the small region depicted at the bottom left with mitochondria rendered in golden and the ER in yellow color. Bottom right: 3D rendering of the entire FIBSEM volume with nuclear membrane being shown in navy-blue, mitochondria in yellow, the ER in salmon and the plasma membrane in a highly transparent white. Note that the high complexity and the network-like appearance of the ER and the mitochondria can only be appreciated after 3D rendering of segmented volumes.

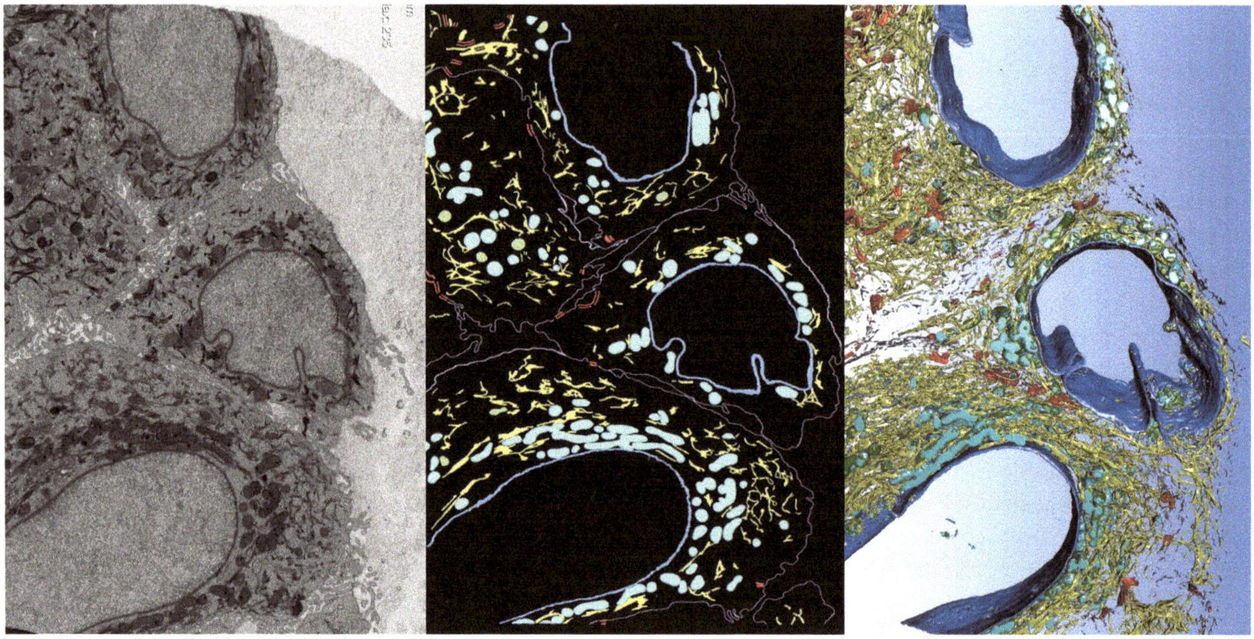

Figure 8.29 Segmentation (feature extraction) of large cellular volumes by Deep Learning. Left: Single slice through large volume 3D reconstruction of HMT-3522 S1 cell acini, cultured in a collagen-rich 3D matrix showing portions of four cells in their acinar context. Middle: Few individual sections with manual segmentation were provided as ground truth for training the U-Net CNN (convoluted neural network as part of the Deep Learning tools in the visualization package ORS Dragonfly. Right: Rendering of 3D volume segmented by the Deep Learning tools in the visualization package ORS Dragonfly. Depicted in blue are the nuclear membranes, in cyan are the mitochondria, in yellow is the cytoskeleton, and in red are cell–cell adhesion complexes (desmosomes).

training are being developed. This area is a fast-progressing field, driven by the demand for automated approaches for the very large datasets that now can be routinely generated.

8.7.3 Model Building and (Quantitative) Analysis

Segmented volumes can be surface-rendered and color-coded, which for many people marks an endpoint of their analysis. Such renderings, when done in sophisticated software with ray tracing and surface texture mapping, can look very impressive, and are often presented in forms of (animated) movies, showing the features of interest from all perspectives, and possibly interacting with one another.

However, beyond the "pretty picture" and the "impressive movies" there exists another world, which is rarely explored, but maybe should be explored more. Images (and in extension 3D volumes) are not only pretty to look at but contain an enormous amount of geometric (= 2D)/volumetric (= 3D) information, including information about size (volume, surface, diameter, axes-ratio, etc.) of a feature of interest and its localization and/or distribution with respect to a cell-framework or with respect to other features of interest (Figure 8.30).

The key to quantifying cellular features may lie in the generation of resolution-faithful volumetric models, hence moving from the voxel space (segmented volumes) to the vector space, where features are approximated (depending on the resolution attainable) by volumetric models based on basic shapes such as ellipsoids, curved planes, tubes, etc. The segmented volumes serve as the starting point for such automated model building, but it is the volumetric models that will be retained for the quantitative analysis, whereas the segmented volumes (in voxel space) will be stored away but for the analysis are no longer needed. Going from voxel space to geometric vector space can also help compress data by a factor of ~10,000, hence this approach may also be useful for displaying larger volumes. Furthermore, each model can be switched on or off for visualization, which is very useful for an understanding of the 3D organization.

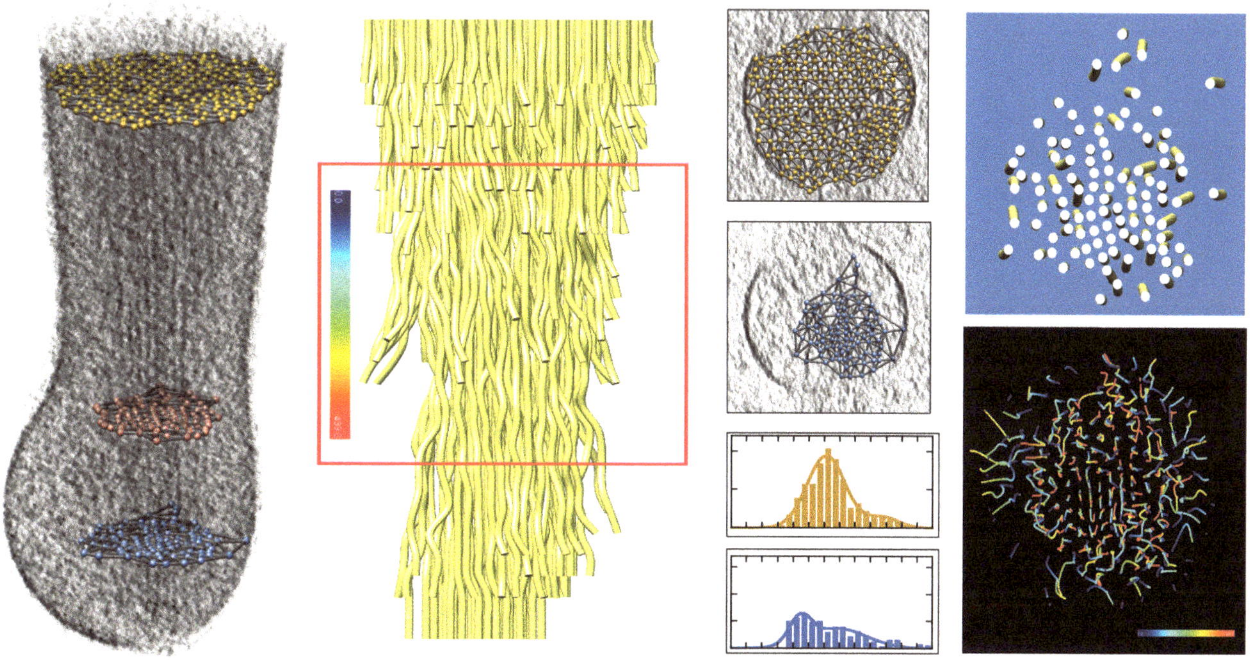

Figure 8.30 Volumetric model building and quantitative analysis. Segmented volumes can be replaced by volumetric models, as is the case here for the actin bundle of the taper and rootlet region of inner ear hair cell stereocilia. Simplified ball-and-stick volumetric models of actin filaments were directly placed into the density maps of the cryo-tomogram. Such model building allowed the tracing of individual filament density in this very complex region. At various positions along the actin filament core, distances between adjacent filaments were measured, which resulted in histograms of actin-actin distances. Interestingly, the histogram showed that in the rootlet, many of the actin filaments are closer spaced compared to the taper region (and also the stereocilia shaft region). This subtle change in spacing would have not been obvious from visualization and rendering of the segmented volumes alone. The path of individual filaments can be traced as individual rods (top right) or as skeletons (bottom right). In the case of skeletons, the filaments are color-coded from blue to red to reflect the different positions along the filament axis and thus a path of the individual filaments.

8.7.4 Deriving Biological Meaning Through Interpretation

The most difficult but possibly also the most rewarding aspect in the analysis of cellular ultrastructural data is to derive biological meaning from the imaging data. This requires an expectation of what to find in one's particular biological system. Some general cell biological knowledge helps to form an expectation of what the cellular ultrastructure should look like in terms of 3D organization and cellular distribution. For example, epithelial cells have a characteristic organization and distribution of actin filaments, apical-basal polarity and distinguished pattern of cell–cell and cell–matrix adhesion complexes, which is very different from mesenchymal and migratory cells. It is thus very likely that cellular function is reflected in the 3D organization. Distribution of mitochondria as the cell powerhouses may indicate where the highest energy needs are within the cell. The size and location of adhesion complexes gives an indication about a cell's neighborly potential and likely behavior. The cytoskeleton can generate force and also defines the mechanical properties of a cell, hence its organization is indicative for differentiation and/or migratory behavior. The shape of the nucleus and the plasma membrane, and the properties of other organelles such as the Golgi apparatus, the endoplasmic reticulum, peroxisomes may indicate whether a cell is in senescence, still has the potential to undergo cell division, or is in a pre-malignant or malignant state. However, sometimes the imaging result is rather surprising and completely unexpected, as was the case for a human breast cancer disease progression system we examined. Through volume-EM imaging of cells and acini, we discovered nuclear membrane-enclosed invaginations into and tunnels through the nucleus, with cytoskeletal filaments that are physically connected to the nuclear membrane and via the cytoplasmic cytoskeleton network and adhesion sites to the cell's microenvironment. These findings were confirmed by superresolution and confocal fluorescence light microscopy, using appropriate antibodies (Figure 8.31). Clearly, if it hadn't been for the volume-EM imaging data, we would have never suspected such ultrastructural features and would have never be able to show a strong candidate for how the cell detects tension changes in its

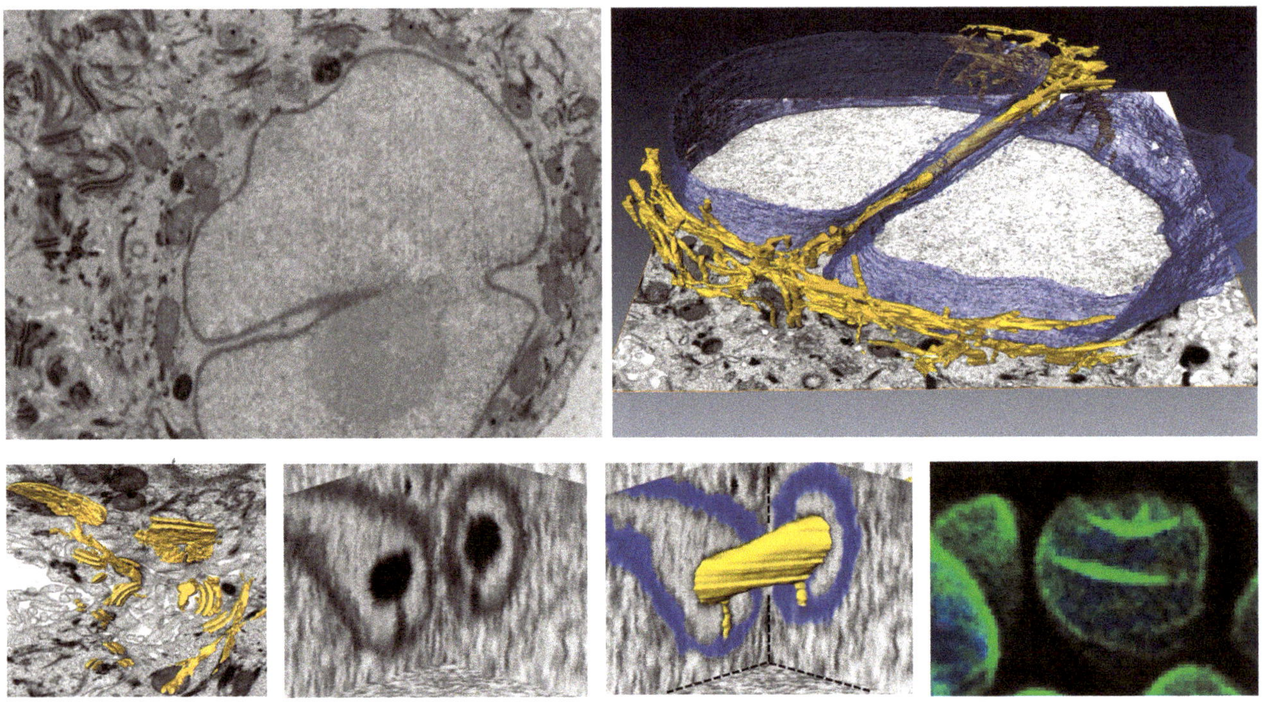

Figure 8.31 Deriving biological meaning from ultrastructural analysis. In the case of the HMT 3522 S1 acini, large volume FIBSEM imaging revealed the presence of deep invaginations into the nuclear membranes and existing tunnels through the cell's nucleus (with the cell being in the state of senescence). Inside such invaginations and tunnels, one finds cytoskeletal filaments (which by superresolution STORM fluorescence microscopy were identified as actin filaments and intermediate filaments) that are anchored to the nuclear membrane, thus mechanically connecting the nuclear membrane with cell–cell adhesion complexes. The sensing of the mechanical forces inside a cell and its mechanical connectivity to its microenvironment may turn out to be key in our understanding of cancer and malignancy. The results obtained in FIBSEM imaging were too obvious to be ignored, and the presence of such features for about half of the cells that were studied was confirmed by immunofluorescence microscopy, which is compatible with higher throughput imaging.

microenvironment, which may have fundamental implication for disease progression and malignancy. Or to put it in a different way: Not every discovery is hypothesis-driven, sometimes it just pays to look at it to paraphrase the famous physicist and Nobel Laureate Richard Feynman, who in 1959 declared in a lecture to the American Physical Society that it was "very easy to answer many fundamental biological questions. You just look at the thing", stating that structure is the key to understanding function.

One may even postulate distinct cellular ultrastructural signatures that reflect cellular function, and possibly even be indicators for cellular health or in pathogenesis. How strong such correlations are is the subject of ongoing research and will require quantitative analysis on larger sample sizes to get a sense of variability of the 3D organization and distribution, and thus of the cellular ultrastructural heterogeneity.

As ultrastructural analysis requires a broad expertise, from knowledge in the biological domain to knowledge in sample preparation, imaging, image analysis, and bioimage informatics, it is key to work in a team, and to automate and standardize as many aspects as possible.

9

Techniques – Cell and Tissue Characterization and Localization Imaging

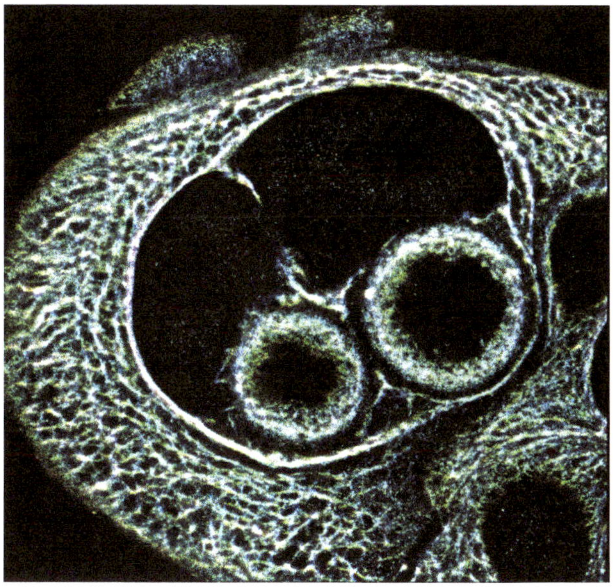

Superresolution STORM imaging of actin filaments in HMT 3522 S1 cells forming growth-arrested acini when cultured in a collagen-rich extracellular matrix. *Source:* With permission by Ke Xu, UC Berkeley.

Techniques discussed:

- White light microscopy
  - brightfield, darkfield, phase contrast, DIC, AVEC
- Fluorescence light microscopy
  - epifluorescence
  - deconvolution
  - confocal laser scanning, spinning disk, 4Pi, theta
  - two-photon
  - single plane illumination (light sheet)
  - total internal reflection (TIRF)
  - superresolution – single molecule localization: STORM, PALM
  - superresolution – patterned illumination: STED, SIM
  - superresolution – near-field microscopy
  - molecular dynamics: FRAP, FLIP, FSM, FRET, FLIM

9.1 Overview

The optical microscope is the oldest scientific instrument to visualize objects that cannot be seen with the unaided (naked) eye. It is one of the four major branches of microscopy, with the other three being electron microscopy, scanning probe microscopy, and X-ray microscopy. Optical microscopes have played an important role in biological imaging with several Nobel Prizes being awarded in the field of cell and tissue characterization and localization Imaging (Table 9.1). Optical microscopes utilize the visible light portion of the electromagnetic spectrum, and typically use lenses (and mirrors) to shine visible light onto or through a sample/object. The sample is either illuminated in flood light mode or raster-scanned across the sample by a small spot. The scattered light (either reflected from the surface or transmitted through the sample) is collected to create an image of the object. The resulting image was traditionally detected by the eye or photographic film, nowadays predominantly by some kind of digital detector. The most basic microscope possesses one lens, whereas the compound microscope uses two or more lenses, to obtain a magnified image of the sample. The design of the compound microscope, known as far back as at least 1621, is still the basis for modern-day microscopes.

The contrast in optical microscopy in bright-field mode arises from absorption (typically using contrasting agents/dyes), whereas in dark-field mode contrast stems from light scattered by the object. (Cross-)polarization microscopy is enabled by a rotation of the polarization plane of the light by the sample. In phase-contrast microscopy contrast arises from the interference of unscattered light with scattered light.

Contrast of a different kind is obtained in fluorescence microscopy, which is based on the emission of fluorescence light by a reporter fluorophore, which got activated by a shorter-wavelength illumination. Emission of the light (and thus a signal) only occurs in region where the fluorophore was illuminated.

Introduction to Biological Imaging, First Edition. Manfred Auer.

Table 9.1 Nobel Prizes involving cell and tissue characterization and localization imaging.

Year	Laureate	Prize category	
1906	Camillo Golgi Ramón y Cajal	Physiology and Medicine	For their work elucidating the structure of the nervous system
1953	Frederik Zernike	Physics	For his demonstration of the phase contrast method, especially for his invention of the phase contrast microscope.
2008	Osamu Shimomura Martin Chalfie Roger Tsien	Chemistry	For the discovery and development of the green fluorescent protein (GFP)
2014	Eric Betzig Stefan W. Hell William E. Moerner	Chemistry	For the development of super-resolved fluorescence microscopy
2023	Moungi Bawendi Louis Brus Aleksey Yekimov	Chemistry	For the discovery and synthesis of quantum dots

Due to the phenomenon of diffraction in optical systems, any point source will be imaged as a so-called Airy disk (a fuzzy central disk with a central maximum that becomes weaker until it reaches the first minimum, surrounded by rings of diminishing intensity). An object is considered resolved if the two point-sources are separated by the radius of the first minimum of the Airy disk, in other words when the maximum of one Airy disk is positioned at the first minimum of its neighboring Airy disk. The resolving power of the microscope depends on the wavelength of the light being emitted, and the numerical aperture (NA) of the objective lens. Putting all other imperfections (such as aberrations) aside, the diffraction limit is set at about half the wavelength, hence for fluorescence microscopy about 220–300 nm.

For diffraction-limited optical imaging, any object spaced closer than 220–300 nm will not be distinguishable as two separate objects. It should be noted however that a single point source can be located with much higher accuracy as the center of its Airy disk can be determined in the order of a few nanometers. This is one of the ways that the Abbe's proclaimed resolution limit can be overcome.

Several super-resolution fluorescence imaging techniques, including photoactivated localization microscopy (PALM) and stochastic optical reconstruction microscopy (STORM) build up an image sequentially from many diffraction-limited images, each of which with a sparse distribution of individual Airy disks. For each of these diffraction-limited images only a small number of fluorophores are activated, resulting in a small number of clearly separated Airy disks, whose center can be determined with high accuracy. The final image is then calculated by adding up all determined Airy disk center positions.

Stimulated emission depletion (STED) microscopy works on an entirely different principle, by minimizing the area of illumination at the focal point, by using an additional high intensity (high photon-flux) laser to suppress excitation fluorophores that are not exactly in the center of illumination.

Near-field scanning optical microscopy (NSOM) uses a scanning probe (e.g., an atomic force microscope (AFM)) to deliver the light to the immediate surrounding of the scanning probe, and thus fluorescence becomes a highly localized phenomenon.

Structured illumination microscopy (SIM) is built on an interference pattern of two lasers, which alters the point-spread function (PSF) of the illumination, resulting in higher-resolution information to be collected.

Apart from efforts to improve resolution, one key agenda of cell biology experimentalists has been to reduce phototoxicity. One solution has been to use two-photon microscopy, which uses a pair of longer-wavelength (lower-energy and thus lower phototoxicity) photons to activate a fluorophore, and at the same time reduces illumination to the focal point where photon density is high enough to support two-photon adsorption. Other efforts, such as Total Internal Reflection Fluorescence (TIRF) imaging, have concentrated on reducing illumination volume, which also improves contrast as background signals are minimized/eliminated. There are a variety of techniques that have been successful in minimizing photobleaching and/or phototoxicity, including single-plane illumination microscopy (SPIM).

There are a whole range of related techniques that allow the visualization of dynamic processes of molecules in cells, and/or probe the close spatial proximity of two reporter-tag fusion-proteins in vivo (Figure 9.1).

9.2 Historical Perspective/Milestones

9.2.1 What Is Light?

Early on, light was known to propagate in straight lines and could be thought of as rays, a concept that has survived to this day and forms the basis of ray tracing and thus geometric optics. A basic knowledge of the concept of refraction and of lenses already existed in the early civilizations in Mesopotamia, Egypt, and Crete/Greece. Independently, early theories about light were put forward by the philosophical schools of Samkhya and Vaisheshika in ancient India, as well as by Mo Zi in ancient China. Thus, early concepts of geometrical optics go back to and possibly even precede Euclid in the 3rd century BCE.

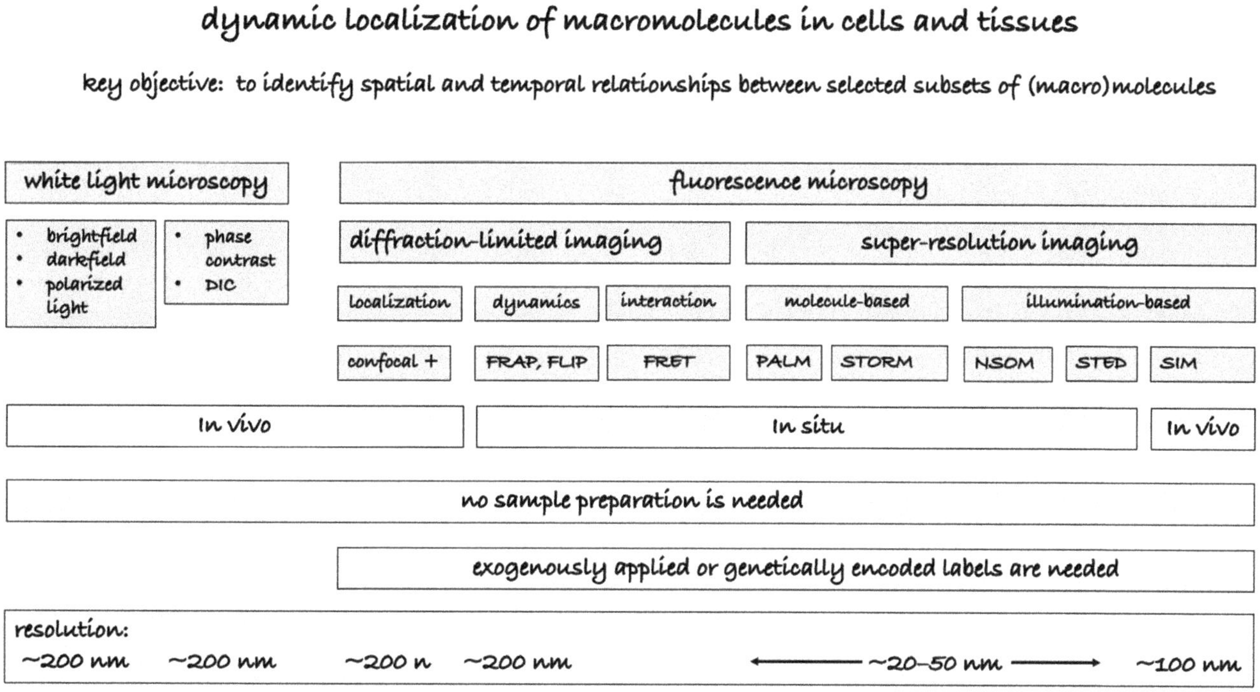

Figure 9.1 Cell and tissue characterization and dynamic localization of macromolecules – Overview. Optical light microscopy is well suited to image biological objects in a field of view of tens to hundreds of micron in diameter, such as cells and small tissue regions, using either white light to monitor live cell behavior or using fluorescence to identify spatial and temporal relationships between selected subsets of macromolecules. White light imaging employs brightfield and darkfield imaging, polarized light imaging as well as phase contrast and differential interference contrast (DIC) imaging. Apart from localization, molecular dynamics and interaction partners can be monitored. All white light imaging is diffraction limited. Fluorescence imaging is divided into diffraction limited and superresolution imaging, with superresolution imaging techniques such as PALM, STORM, STED, NSOM, and SIM using a variety of different tricks to overcome Abbe's diffraction limit. Note that for a variety of reasons including but not limited to phototoxicity, not all samples can be imaged in vivo. Most imaging techniques do not require specific sample preparation, except for the labeling with a fluorophore or the genetic expression of tags to which fluorophores will bind or fluorescent proteins that are genetically encoded proteins, fused with a target protein.

Al-Kindi, an Arab Muslim philosopher, mathematician, physician, and music theorist, who lived in the 9th century, stated in his work known as "De radiis stellarum" that "everything in the world... emits rays in every direction, which fill the whole world." This theory had an important influence on later scholars like Ibn al-Haytham (also known in Western Europe as Alhazen). In the late 10th century, the Persian Islamic mathematician Ibn Sahl worked on how curved mirrors and lenses bend and focus light, resulting in a law of refraction that is similar to Snell's law, postulated much later in 1621.

The Arab mathematician, astronomer, and physicist Alhazen is considered by many to be the father of modern optics. He is credited to produce a comprehensive and systematic analysis of Greek optical theories and to further explore concepts in optics, including geometrical optics in his six volumes of the "Book of optics", published between 1011 and 1021 CE. Against the opinion of the influential philosopher Ptolemy, Alhazen insisted that light rays were reflected off objects before they reach the eye, instead of originating from the eyes.

In terms of optical theory, Isaac Newton, building on earlier ideas by René Decartes, proposed in 1704 in his book "Opticks" a corpuscle theory of light, where he stated that white light was a mix of colors (which he thought of as different corpuscle sizes) that can be separated with the help of a glass prism. Newton's corpuscle theory of light was in contrast to Huygens' wave theory of light published 1690 in his book Traité de la Lumière (Treatise on Light), which Huygens had developed based on earlier ideas by Robert Hooke. Huygens' wave theory, states that each point on a wave front can generate a secondary spherical wavefront. Francesco Grimaldi is widely credited to have coined the term diffraction, which literally means for light to break into pieces. His careful observations regarding light diffraction were published in 1665 after his death.

While the Newtonian corpuscle theory of light could not explain refraction, diffraction, interference, and polarization tied to birefringence of calcite, it was favored until the early 19th century when Thomas Young and Augustin-Jean Fresnel carried out experiments, including the famous single-slit and double-slit experiments, that could not be explained by Newton's corpuscle light theory and thus established the wave nature of light. Their work also paved the way to understand refraction (and thus dispersion) as a frequency-dependent change of the speed of light in medium other than vacuum, with the refractive index of a material being the ratio of the speed of light in vacuum and its speed in a medium. Furthermore, the wave-like behavior of light could explain diffraction as differences in light path, and thus shifts in the phase of sinusoidal waves which leads to either constructive or destructive interference.

James Clerk Maxwell in the 1860s formulated a set of partial differential equations that (together with the Lorentz force law) laid the foundation of classical electromagnetism, and essentially postulate the following: (1) Static electric fields are generated by charges, (2) Magnetic force lines form closed circles, (3) A changing magnetic field generates an electric field, and (4) Electric current and changing electric field generate a magnetic field. Light was now understood as a propagating wave with both an electric and an orthogonal magnetic field, which could be described by the direction of propagation, its wavelength (or frequency), its amplitude, its phase shift, as well as the directions of electromagnetic field within a plane perpendicular to the direction of propagation direction.

Building on his study of black-body radiation, Max Planck around the year 1900 discovered that light could only be emitted in quantized form, and that its energy was proportional to its frequency. He was awarded the Nobel Prize in Physics in 1918 "in recognition of the services he rendered to the advancement of Physics by his discovery of energy quanta," and he is considered the founding father of quantum mechanics.

At the beginning of the 20th century Albert Einstein postulated the photon as a particle-like entity to explain the photoelectric effect, which needed to possess a certain amount of energy (thus frequency) to be able to free an electron from the surface of a metal. He was awarded the 1921 Nobel Prize in Physics "for his services to Theoretical Physics, and especially for his discovery of the law of the photoelectric effect." Niels Bohr's model of atoms with its discrete orbits/shells provided an explanation for the discrete amount of energy being absorbed or emitted in the form of photons when electrons move to a different shell. Niels Bohr was the recipient of the 1922 Nobel Prize in Physics for "his services in the investigation of the structure of atoms and of the radiation emanating from them."

The conceptional conflict whether light should be thought of as either made of particle or considered as electromagnetic waves was laid to rest by Louis de Broglie, who stated in his doctoral thesis in 1924 the hypothesis that electrons have both particle-like and wave-like properties, which is a central point in the theory of quantum mechanics. After the Davisson–Germer experiment in 1927, which demonstrated diffraction of electrons by a nickel crystal, Louis de Broglie was awarded the 1929 Nobel Prize in Physics "for his discovery of the wave nature of electrons." De Broglie's wave-particle-duality hypothesis could be applied to photons, as well as to a large range of particles including protons, neutrons, or electrons. If only a few photons are detected, light appears particle-like with individual photons that can be detected one by one, whereas in the case of a larger number of photons, photons are better described in statistical terms, as they exhibit wave-like properties.

The science of the interaction of photons with atoms and molecules, including the study of the particle-like properties of photons became known as quantum optics, which led to such important discoveries such as microwave amplification by stimulated emission of radiation (maser) in 1953 and its optical equivalent, the light amplification by stimulated emission of radiation (laser) in 1960.

9.2.2 Optical Instruments and Microscopy

The origins of lens making are thought to date back more than two and a half thousand years to the Old Kingdom of Egypt, and first written accounts of lenses as magnifying glasses date back to the reign of the Roman Emperor Nero in the 1st century.

Roger Bacon's writings on optics at the end of the 13th century, which were based on earlier works of Arab writers, described corrective lenses for vision. However, it would take until the early 17th century until lenses were used to build telescopes and compound microscopes.

Antoine van Leeuwenhoek in the 17th century built his own simple single-lens microscope to make many observations of the microscopic world including the discovery of protozoa and bacteria. While being simple, van Leeuwenhoek's instrument had a small, but strong lens. The compound microscope was invented at the end of the 16th century and further refined in the 17th century (as was the refracting telescope). Its principle is still the foundation of modern-day optical microscopy. However, it took the compound microscope 150 years of further developments before it could match the image quality of van Leeuwenhoek's instrument.

By the mid 19th century, optical microscope performance had improved significantly by a combination of craftmanship and manufacturing tradition (Carl Zeiss), physics (Ernst Abbe), advanced glass making (Otto Schott), and high-resolution test gratings (Friedrich Norbert). Around the same time, the first usable binocular microscope became available. In 1893 August Köhler developed the so-called Köhler illumination, which illuminated the sample evenly and no longer left the light bulb filament visible in the image of the sample.

Another important milestone was the development of phase contrast microscopy, for which the Dutch physicist Frits Zernicke was awarded the 1953 Nobel Prize in Physics.

In this technique, unstained samples can be imaged, with contrast being based on interference rather than absorption of light by the sample stain. In 1955, the Polish Physicist Georges Nomarski laid the foundation for DIC microscopy.

In the early 1900s, fluorophores started to be used for staining biological samples, which led to the development of fluorescence microscopes by the optical factories of Karl Reichert and of Carl Zeiss. Antibody-targeted fluorescence labeling was demonstrated in the early 1940s and remained for several decades a major avenue for visualization of (macro-)molecular targets of interest. Figure 9.2 shows a selection of microscope designs of the last few centuries. Antibody-labeling typically required chemical fixation and permeabilization of the samples, which also meant that cells and tissues could not be studied alive.

This all changed with the discovery and cloning of green fluorescent protein (GFP) from the jellyfish (*Aequorea victoria*). The demonstration of GFP as a genetically encoded tag (in form of a GFP-target fusion protein) and the development of spectral variants that would have different excitation and emission spectra, and thus different colors, revolutionized cell biology in the 1990s. It was now possible to study the dynamic aspects of living biological systems without the need for antibody labeling sample preparation and its associated artifacts. GFP-tagged fusion proteins allowed the direct visual assessment of protein expression levels as well as subcellular localization in living cells. For this reason, the 2008 Nobel Prize in Chemistry was awarded to Osamu Shimomura, Martin Chalfie, and Roger Y. Tsien "for the discovery and development of green fluorescent protein, GFP."

Another milestone in advanced optical imaging was the development of the confocal microscope, which due to its simplicity in operation became the work horse of cell biological imaging, as it allowed 3D volumes of fluorescence to be collected. The beginnings of confocal optical systems go back to 1940, when the ophthalmologist Hans Goldmann developed a slit lamp for eye examinations. Zyun Koana in 1943 and his colleague Horoto Naora in 1951 published designs for a confocal microscope, but it wasn't until 1955,

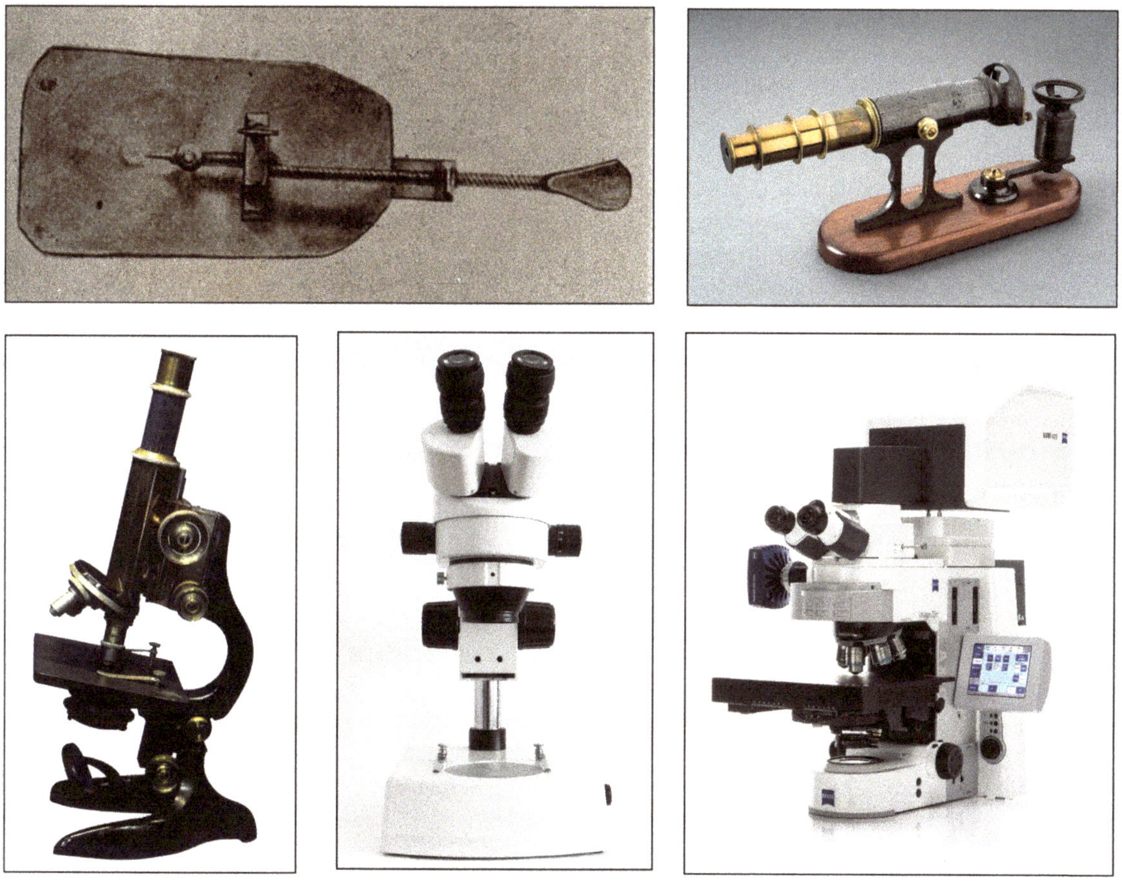

Figure 9.2 Microscope design over the last few centuries. A selection of microscope designs over the last few centuries. *Source:* Wellcome Collection / Wikimedia Commons / CC BY 4.0, Rama / Wikimedia Commons / CC BY-SA 3.0 FR, Pawel Czerwinski / Unsplash.com / Public Domain, ZEISS Microscopy / Flickr / CC BY 2.0. Top left: Single lens microscope design as used by Leeuwenhoek; Top right: Early compound microscope design. Bottom left: Compound microscope design in the early 20th century; Bottom middle: Current day stereomicroscope; Bottom right: Up-right epifluorescence microscope.

when Marvin Minsky built the first confocal scanning microscope, which was then patented in 1957. Prior to confocal microscopy, epifluorescence imaging was the main fluorescence imaging mode. However, epifluorescence suffers from the fact that all molecules in the path of the light (z-direction) are excited and thus emit a fluorescence signal, which means that there is little to no resolution in the z-direction, and there is significant out-of-focus contribution that degrades image quality. In the early 1960s, Minski added pinholes in front of the light source and in front of the detector, which blocks the light that comes from regions outside of the focal plane, resulting in images with higher resolution, greater contrast, and less out-of-focus noise. He patented the so-called "double focusing system," which became the basis for modern confocal microscopes.

In a laser scanning confocal microscope (LSCM), the pinhole in front of the light source is unnecessary since a sharply focused laser beam is used for illumination of the sample. Images are then recorded one pixel at a time by raster-scanning the laser beam across the sample, which can be a time-consuming process. An alternative to LSCM is spinning disk confocal microscopy, which has hundreds of pinholes (arranged in spirals) that rotate at high speed and thus build up (row by row) an image in a much faster way than LSCM. Also, since only a small part of the sample at any given time is illuminated, photo damage is considerably reduced. The precursor to modern day spinning disk confocal microscope was built and a patent was filed in the 1960s by Mojmir Petran. The first laser scanning microscope emerged in 1969 from the work of M. David Egger and Paul Davidovits, using a 5 mW Helium–Neon laser with light at 633 nm being reflected by a semi-transparent mirror and an objective lens onto the sample. The light from the object was focused by a lens onto a photomultiplier tube (PMT), before being displayed via cathode-ray tube of an oscilloscope, which moved simultaneously with the objective lens. In the mid 1980s Brad Amos and John Graham White built the first confocal beam scanning microscope (with the beam moving not the sample), which initially wasn't met with much interest by established microscope manufacturers, but later became the blueprint for commercially successful laser scanning confocal microscopes.

Other technologies to improve z-resolution were 4π (4Pi) microscopy and two-photon microscopy, with 4Pi relying on an orthogonal geometry of illumination and detection, and two-photon relying on the simultaneous absorption of two longer-wave photons. Two-photon microscopy requires the high-photon density only found in the focal spot of the microscope.

While all these techniques were largely used for the localization of candidate proteins in form of fluorescence-tagged fusion protein, several related techniques were invented to address the molecular dynamics aspect as well as the co-localization aspect of proteins inside cells. These techniques include Fluorescence Recovery after Photobleaching (FRAP), Fluorescence Loss in Photobleaching (FLIP), Fluorescence Lifetime Imaging Microscopy (FLIM), Photoactivation (PA) microscopy, Fluorescence Correlation Spectroscopy (FCS), and Förster Resonance Energy Transfer (FRET) microscopy.

All the previously discussed techniques are diffraction limited. Hence the achievable resolution is on the order of half the wavelength of the light used in each experiment. A variety of very different approaches have overcome Ernst Abbe's diffraction limit barrier, including SIM, STED, PALM, STORM, as well as NSOM/scanning near-field optical microscopy (SNOM). Many of these techniques surpassed Abbe's postulated diffraction limit by a factor of 10–20, which is why Eric Betzig, William Moerner, and Stefan Hell were awarded the 2014 Nobel Prize in Chemistry for the development of super-resolved fluorescence microscopy.

Apart from improving resolution, one goal in cell biology has been to make optical imaging less harmful for biological samples. Two-photon microscopy uses two longer-wavelength (thus lower energy photons) to activate a fluorophore at half the wavelength, which results in substantially lower phototoxicity. Another approach taken was to restrict the volume that is illuminated to only the region that is meant to be imaged. Light sheet and the related lattice light sheet fluorescence imaging significantly reduce the illumination volume and thus phototoxicity.

9.2.3 Application of Microscopy to Biological Samples

Having built his own compound microscope, the English physicist Robert Hooke studied a sample of cork, and in 1665 described the regular compartments as "cells", because they reminded him of monks' living quarters. The name stuck, and soon after cells of all sorts have been the favorite topic for optical microscopy.

Soon after, Antoine van Leeuwenhoek, a businessman and self-taught scientist used a one-lens high power magnifying instrument to study household objects including red blood cells, protozoa, and sperm. His most famous discovery (in 1683) were bacteria, which was heavily disputed at the time. While individual cells could clearly be observed without staining, they were not detectable when in a tissue context. Hence in the 18th century cells were not yet considered as the basic units of living organisms.

By the mid 19th century, however, the idea that all organisms were made up of cells was widely accepted, in part due to microscopic work by Theodor Schwann and Matthias Jakob Schleiden. The last hold-out was the study of the brain, until the Czech anatomist Jan Evangelista

Purkinje (Purkyně) was able to describe what amounted to very large cells with unusual features such as long protrusions and large amount of branching. It was the combination of using a metal stain (potassium bichromate), an organic solvent (glacial acetic acid) and a resin (Canada balsam; balsam of fir) that after infiltration would harden, which would allow Purkinje to cut very thin slices by using a microtome, and to examine these sections under a light microscope with good contrast.

The Italian physician Camillo Golgi (1843–1926) further refined the metal staining process adding silver nitrate after potassium bichromate staining (now known as the Golgi stain), which led to a dramatic improvement of contrast. The recipe was further refined by the Spanish physician Santiago Ramón y Cajal (1852–1934), who used higher concentrations of the chemicals as had been prescribed by Golgi and added a methylene blue staining step. Not only was Ramón y Cajal able to find differences between the staining behavior of bird versus mammalian brains, but also between embryonic and adult brain. Most importantly he was able to settle the controversy that existed at the time to whether the brain was a large continuum (reticular theory) or was made of discrete cells. Ramón y Cajal's microscopic discoveries of the plasticity of axons strongly supported the theory that the nervous tissue consisted of discrete cells (neurons), which then could form structures that looked like a reticulum, due to the formation of dendrites, which Ramón y Cajal referred to protoplasmic branches (and thus constitute extensions of the nerve cell bodies). Cajal and Golgi shared the 1906 Nobel Prize in Physiology and Medicine for their work elucidating the structure of the nervous system. It should be noted that both Golgi and Ramón y Cajal made drawings of what they saw, as cameras recording an image were not available at the time (Figure 9.3).

The cell biologists and embryologists Margaret Reed Lewis and Warren Lewis published in 1915 a time lapse study of mitochondrial dynamics in living cells. Polarization microscopy was applied since the 1930s to birefringent supramolecular structures such as protein crystals, muscle cell fibril, microtubule bundles and the myelin sheath of nerve fibers. White light and fluorescence microscopy are currently widely used in biological imaging, studying organ, tissue and cell organization as well as protein localization in live and chemically fixed animals, tissues and individual cells (Figure 9.4).

9.2.4 Fluorescence Microscopy

The discovery of fluorescence is credited to Frederick W. Herschel in 1845, who observed that a quinine solution (tonic water) emits blue light when excited by UV light. Sir George G. Stokes was the first to realize that the emitted fluorescence light was red shifted with respect to the incident light that causes the excitation in the first place. In the early 1900s fluorophores were used in biology to stain

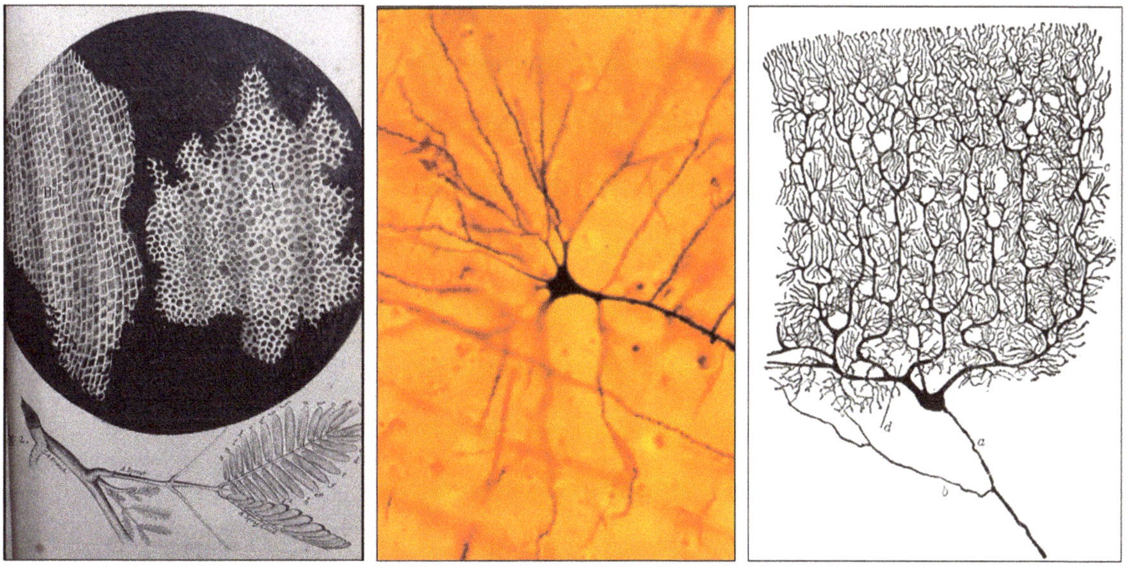

Figure 9.3 Applications of microscopy to biological samples. *Source:* Robert Hooke / Wikimedia Commons / Public Domain, Bob Jacobs / Wikimedia Commons / CC BY-SA 3.0. In 1665 in his book Micrographia, Robert Hooke used an early version of the compound microscope to study the living plant tissue cork. He coined the word cell, as the regular compartments (surrounded by the plant cell wall) he observed reminded him of the living quarters of monks. By using and sectioning of hard resins, Jan Evangelista Purkinje discovered the unusual structure of neurons with their axon and dendrites. Building on this work and further refining heavy metal staining techniques, Camillo Golgi, and Ramón y Cajal revealed the complexity of the nervous system, which earned them the 1906 Nobel Prize in Physiology and Medicine.

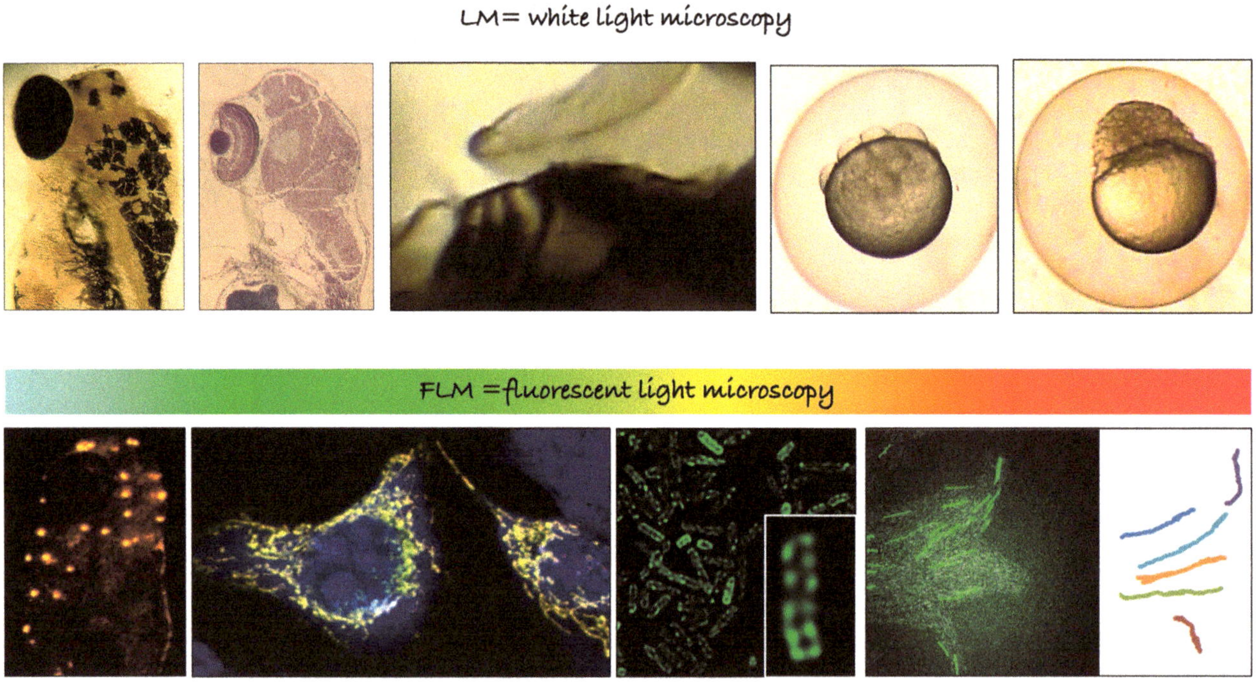

Figure 9.4 Examples of white light and fluorescence microscopy applications. Applications of white light and fluorescence microscopy to biological samples. Top row, from left to right: Light micrograph of a high-pressure frozen, freeze-substituted zebrafish larvae head whole-mount, embedded in an Epon resin block. Light micrograph of a ~500 nm thin section through the resin-embedded head, counterstained by Toluene Blue. Light micrograph of a ~1 μm cross-section of guinea pig cochlea's organ of Corti, showing three rows of outer hair cells and one row of inner hair cells. Brightfield images of an early and later stage of zebrafish egg development. Bottom row, from left to right: Neuromast labeling by DiAsp fluorescent reagent of live zebrafish larvae head region. YFP-fusion protein labeling of a mitochondria-specific target protein. SNAP-tag labeling of an anaerobic bacterium *Desulfovibrio vulgaris* expressing MinE protein. Tracking *Myxococcus xanthus* swarming behavior by using a mixture of fluorescent protein expressing and wildtype cells.

tissues as well as microbes. Fluorescence microscopes were developed by Carl Zeiss and Carl Reichert. Protocols for fluorescence labeling were developed in the 1940s. However, it wasn't until the early 1990s when jellyfish GFP and its spectral derivatives became widely available. The ability of genetic engineering to create fusion proteins of a GFP-tag with the target protein revolutionized cell biology, as it was now possible to study the in vivo subcellular localization and dynamic properties of the target protein, courtesy to its endogenous fluorescent tag that could be imaged with high contrast and specificity. "The discovery and development of the green fluorescent protein, GFP," was recognized by the 2008 Nobel Prize in Chemistry, awarded to Osamu Shimomura, Martin Chalfie, and Roger Tsien. Since then, a large variety of fluorescence imaging techniques have evolved (Figure 9.5), the most spectacular ones are the various superresolution fluorescence microscopy techniques, which are able to overcome the diffraction limit of light, first postulated by Ernst Abbe in 1873. Superresolution fluorescence light microscopy had a profound impact on cell biology, a fact recognized by the 2014 Nobel Prize in Chemistry, awarded to Eric Betzig, Stefan Hell, and William E. Moerner.

9.3 Theoretical Background

The theory of how light interacts with matter goes back centuries in physics both at a macroscopic level as well as an atomic level and constitutes a large portion of modern physics. The Snell's laws of refraction describe the behavior of light rays when they enter an optical medium with an altered speed. The law of reflection, which says that the angle between the incident light ray and the surface normal is the same as the angle of the reflected ray with the normal, can be logically derived from Snell's law, but was postulated nearly 2,000 years earlier. The practical application of Snell's law is the design of lenses, with convex lenses bundling (converging) light rays, whereas concave lenses diverge light rays. For each medium the speed of light (the phase velocity) depends on its frequency/wavelength, with the refractive index being different for

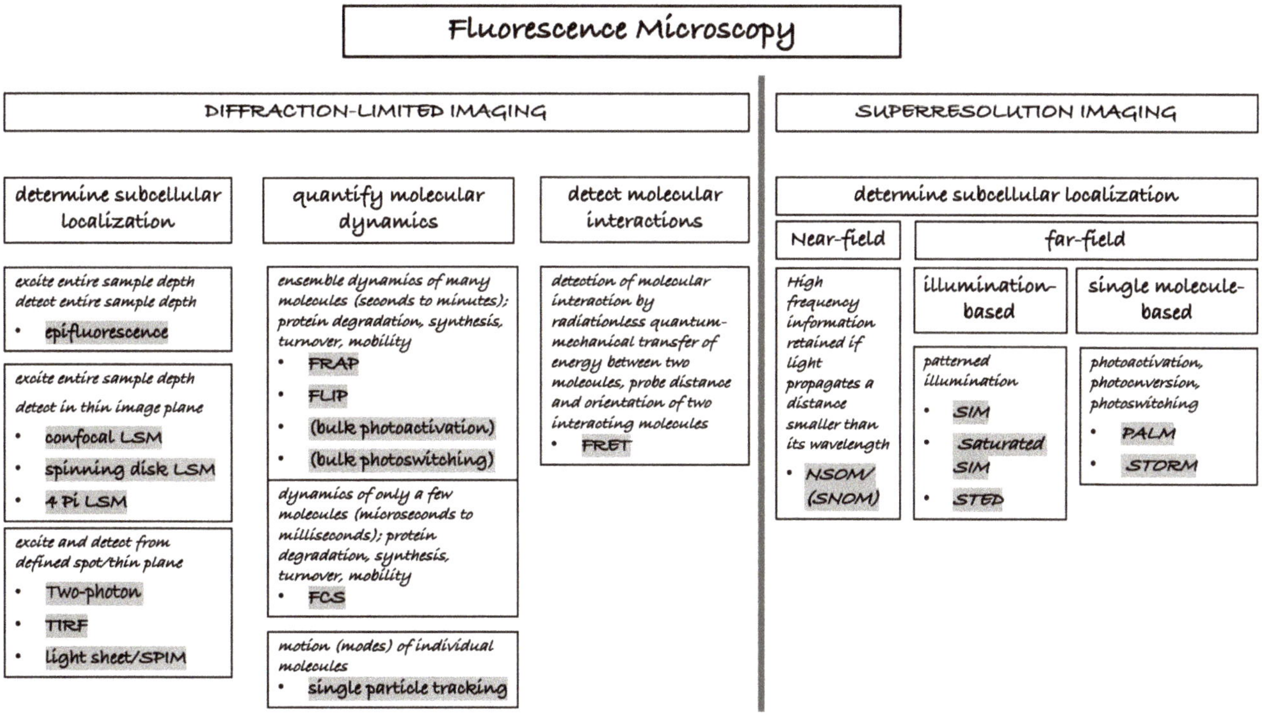

Figure 9.5 Fluorescence light microscopy – Overview. In fluorescence microscopy one distinguishes diffraction-limited imaging from superresolution imaging that – in terms of resolution – goes beyond Abbe's diffraction limit all optical microscopy is subjected to. For diffraction limited imaging, there are three very different goals for imaging, such as determination of subcellular localization, quantification of molecular dynamics and detection of molecular interaction. With respect to diffraction-limited subcellular localization, some techniques such as epifluorescence excite and detect a signal from the entire field of view, independent of the axial position of the fluorophore with respect to the focus. Confocal laser, spinning disk and 4π laser scanning microscopy excite a fair amount of the sample depth, but detect in a rather thin focal imaging plane. Out-of-focus contributions are filtered out by pinholes. On the other hand, two-photon, total internal reflection, and light sheet/single plane illumination microscopy all excite and thus detect from a small spot or thin plane, which results in the least phototoxicity, as unnecessary irradiation is avoided. When it comes to quantification of molecular dynamics, one can study the ensemble dynamics of macromolecules in the seconds to minutes range, using fluorescence recovery after photobleaching (FRAP), fluorescence loss in photobleaching (FLIP), bulk photoactivation and photoswitching, or the dynamics of only a few molecules in the microseconds to millisecond range using fluorescence correlation spectroscopy imaging (FCS), as well as track the motion of individual molecules. Close molecular interactions are detected by Förster-resonance energy transfer (FRET) imaging. The goal in superresolution imaging is typically the determination of subcellular localization. One distinguishes near-field scanning optical imaging (NSOM) from far-field approaches such as structured illumination (SIM), stimulated emission depletion (STED), stochastic optical reconstruction (STORM), and photoactivation localization (PALM) microscopy.

different wavelengths. Prisms can disperse light and thus split white light into its spectral components displaying a continuous spectrum of the light. The presence of certain emission lines or dark bands in an absorption spectrum (e.g., sunlight), can then be indicative for the presence of certain elements or molecules.

As light interacts with matter, it gets scattered, with each scattering center being the origin for a new light wave. Scattering can be elastic (e.g., Raleigh scattering) or inelastic (e.g., Compton scattering), meaning that after scattering has occurred the wave has either the same or a different (lower) frequency, respectively.

Such new light waves, each emitted from a scattering center, will interfere with one another, which means that they can reinforce one another (constructive interference) or cancel each other out (destructive interference), depending on the relative phase shift of the waves at any given point in space. If there are many scattering centers that are periodically arranged (like in a crystal lattice), there will be predictable positions where scattered waves will interfere constructively. Such reflections, also known as diffraction spots, are central to X-ray crystallography and electron crystallography, and thus key to the structure determination of macromolecules such as proteins and/or nucleic acids (as was discussed in Chapter 7).

Double-slit experiments have demonstrated the wave-like properties of light, where each of the two slits can be considered as the origin of spherical waves which will undergo interference and thus create periodic patterns with minima and maxima. This result could only be understood with a

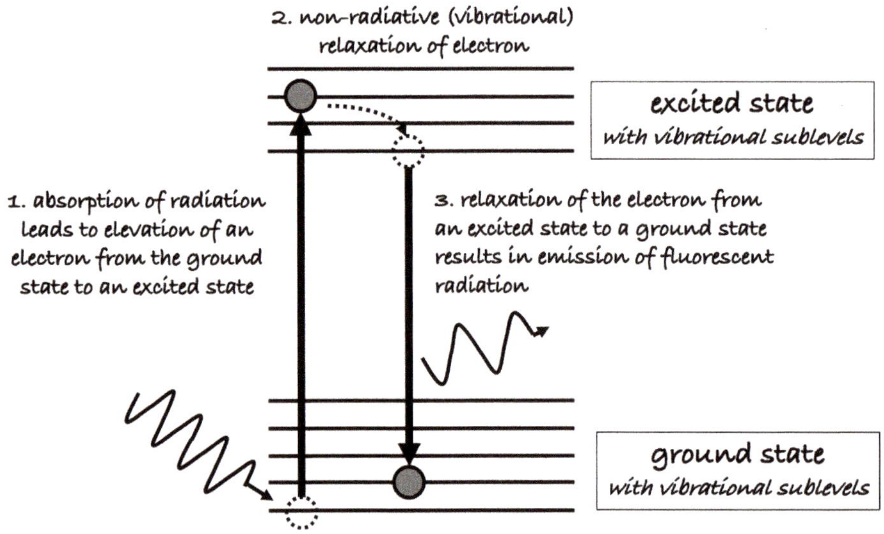

Figure 9.6 Theoretical background of fluorescence. For fluorescence to occur, electrons in a molecule have to absorb a photon (typically in the visible light radiation range) with a certain energy to lift them from a ground state to an excited state. Such excited electronic states will have several vibrational sublevels. The electron will relax to the lowest vibrational sublevel of the excited state in a non-radiative manner, from where it will relax back to the ground state. In this process of relaxation of the electron to any of the vibrational sublevels of the ground state, the electron will emit a photon, whose wavelength will be longer (hence its energy will be lower) than the photon that was absorbed for excitation.

classical view on wave mechanics, and called into question the long-held idea that light has only corpuscle/particle-like properties.

However, the photoelectric effect, where photons with a sufficient energy can knock out electrons from atoms is a clear indication that indeed light has corpuscle-like properties. This apparent contradiction was solved when it was acknowledged that light has both wave-like and corpuscle-like properties, which is known as the wave-particle duality of photons. The concept of wave-particle duality also applies to electrons, protons, neutrons, and ions, all of which are subject to the laws of quantum mechanics.

The atomic model and the molecule model of matter, with their discrete energy orbital spaces where electrons are likely to reside, are the key for understanding electron valency as well as vibrational and rotational states. Changes in electron valency is the foundation for understanding fluorescence, where a shorter-wavelength photon is absorbed by the molecule, exciting it to one of several excited states, from which the electron in a non-radiative way relaxes to a slightly lower excited state, before it relaxes back to its ground state, emitting a longer-wavelength photon in the process (Figure 9.6).

The emitted photon is always lower in energy (hence longer in terms of wavelength), except when two photons of much lower energy (higher wavelength) are absorbed at the same time and their energy is combined, hence the wavelength is half of each photon's wavelength. This is the foundation of two-photon microscopy, which, despite the high intensity lasers, does not only lead to less photobleaching and/or phototoxicity, but also reduced the interaction volume of light with matter, thus suppressing out-of-focus signals, and therefore improving image quality and resolution.

Reducing the volume that is irradiated to only the region from which images are recorded, and thus to reduce phototoxicity and bleaching is a common goal for a variety of imaging techniques, such as single-plane illumination, light sheet and lattice-light sheet imaging, as well as TIRF imaging.

Optical systems in general only allow diffraction-limited imaging at a resolution about half the wavelength of the light being administered. This is called the useful (or beneficial) magnification. While additional magnification is possible, such magnification is "empty" magnification, as no additional detail is revealed at this point.

A variety of efforts have been dedicated to breaking Abbe's postulated diffraction barrier, to achieve superresolution. In STED microscopy and reversible saturable optical fluorescence transitions (RESOLFT), the region just outside the very center of the illumination spot is depleted of a fluorescence signal by using a second, barrel-shaped laser illumination.

Another approach is to localize single molecules by repeatedly inducing the fluorescence of only a small subset of all the molecules present and determining the center of each of their Airy disks. Using this strategy, a final super-resolved image can be obtained, based on the accumulation of enough sequential localizations of Airy disks. Stochastic Optical Reconstruction Microscopy (STORM), Photo-activated Localization Microscopy (PALM), and Point Accumulation for Imaging in Nanoscale Topography (PAINT) are all based on this principle but employ different types of fluorophores to accomplish single molecule localization. STORM typically uses organic fluorescent dyes such as cyanines and rhodamines together with a specific imaging buffer to allow blinking of the fluorescent molecules, whereas PALM employs photo-activatable, photo-switchable, or photo-convertible tag fusion proteins, such as, e.g., PA-GFP, PA-mCherry, mEOS, mMAPLE. PAINT uses reversibly binding fluorescent probes such as Nile Red.

Yet another approach is to reduce the PSF (and thus size of Airy disk) by about a factor of two, by discarding traditional uniform Köhler illumination, and replacing it by illumination with spatially modulated (patterned) light, with periodically spaced bright and dark regions (Structured Illumination Microscopy, SIM). As a result, one can image a sample with a lateral (*X*, *Y*) resolution of ~100 nm, and axial (*Z*) resolution of ~300 nm. Saturated Structured Illumination can extend the resolution further to ~50 nm.

4π/4Pi microscopy also relies on the constructive interference of two wave fronts, resulting in a nearly isotropic (spherical) PSF, and thus increased axial resolution. It should be noted however that structured illumination (superresolution) microscopy is very complex and computationally intensive, and a full understanding of its theoretical basis requires a strong foundation in the underlying mathematics and physics.

Yet another, completely different approach to breach the resolution barrier is used by near-field scanning probe microscopy (also known as NSOM or SNOM), which does not use (diffraction-limited) apertures and lenses in the classical sense, but instead a laser is guided to the tip of a scanning probe (e.g., an AFM), with the result that fluorophores from only a small immediate region around the atomically-sized/nanometer-sized tip are excited, and hence will give off a fluorescence signal in close proximity of the scanning probe tip.

As may be obvious by now, different imaging techniques rely on different types and geometries of illumination, different optical light paths (including filters, apertures, lenses, beam splitters) as well as different type of detectors and modes of signal detection and data collection. This will be discussed in more detail in Section 9.4.

Limitations in optical/fluorescence microscopy are the total light dose fluorophores can accept before they bleach (thus stop to fluoresce) and the risk of phototoxicity (the production of highly reactive small molecule species), which makes long-term live imaging of complex biological systems such as organoids, tissues, and organs a challenge. Solutions can be to employ more robust fluorophores, use longer wavelength illumination, keep illumination to a minimum and/or use scavenger chemicals that react with the highly reactive small molecules and thus have a photoprotective effect. A more general limitation of fluorescence microscopy (of any flavor) is that one only sees what is labeled, hence, the cellular context of the fluorophore can be difficult to determine. Also, there are only a few colors that can be used for each experiment, hence only a small number of different molecules or cellular structures can be detected simultaneously.

9.4 Instrumentation/Experimental Setup

The optical microscope, also known as light microscope, uses the visible light portion of the electromagnetic spectrum in combination with a system of apertures and lenses to record magnified images of (biological) samples that are too small to be seen by the naked eye. The basic design of the compound microscope is simple and has not changed all that much since its invention in the 17th century, however design complexity is added to improve sample contrast and/or resolution.

There are a large variety of optical microscopy techniques, each with their own instrumental requirements and setup. However, they all share basic components, such as an *X*, *Y*, and *Z*-adjustable stage (coarse and fine) with sample holder to move the specimen into focus, an illumination source, optical light path components, including apertures, filters, condenser, lenses (often arranged into an objective turret or revolver), possibly (dichroic) mirrors and (dichroic) beam splitters, as well as a detector (and/or eye pieces).

9.4.1 Frame, Stage, and Sample Holders

Regarding the frame, stage, and sample holders, commercial microscopes are either regular upright microscopes or inverted microscopes.

Upright microscopes are used for samples that can be squeezed between a glass slide and a coverslip. White light trans-illumination of the sample occurs from the bottom of the stage via a condenser lens, and the transmitted light is detected from the top. The objective lens in upright microscopes either operates in air near the coverslip or in a drop of water or immersion oil that bridges the gap between the objective lens and the coverslip.

Inverted microscopes are particularly well suited for live cell imaging (e.g., cell cultures), where white light trans-illumination comes from the top and detection of the transmitted light happens below the sample. The advantage of an inverted microscope is that in a cell culture dish, with a coverslip at the bottom, the objective lens resides just below the coverslip of the dish, typically with immersion oil. Also, the dish can be environment-controlled with respect to temperature and ambient gases (as CO_2 is often needed for cell culture). If cells adhere to the coverslip, this microscope configuration ensures that all cells are in focus. There is no need to squeeze a coverslip onto the sample. The cells in the culture dish are readily accessible to micropipettes and there is no direct physical contact (and thus no source of contamination) between the cells and the microscope equipment (Figure 9.7).

Fluorescence microscopy can be used either in an upright or an inverted configuration, but most frequently it is used in epi-illumination mode in combination with cell culture dishes with a coverslip-bottom, and thus with an inverted microscope. However, epi-illumination implies that excitation and detection of the emitted photons occurs from the same side (from the bottom). In such a configuration, a dichroic mirror will only allow the emitted light to reach the detector, whereas the excitation wavelength is rejected (Figure 9.8).

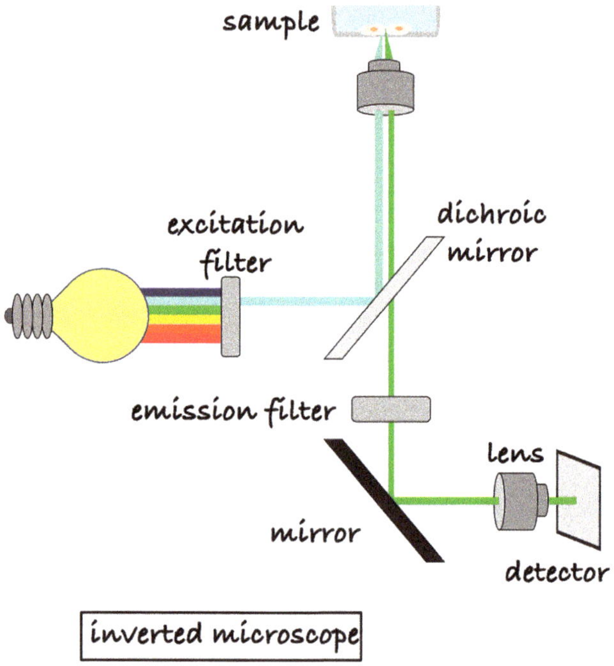

Figure 9.8 Fluorescent light microscopy in epi-illumination. A typical setup for fluorescence microscopy consists of a strong light source, a set of excitation and emission filters as well as a dichroic mirror, and a detector. Note that the fluorescence signal is typically collected in epi-illumination mode, and thus from the same side of the specimen as the excitation illumination.

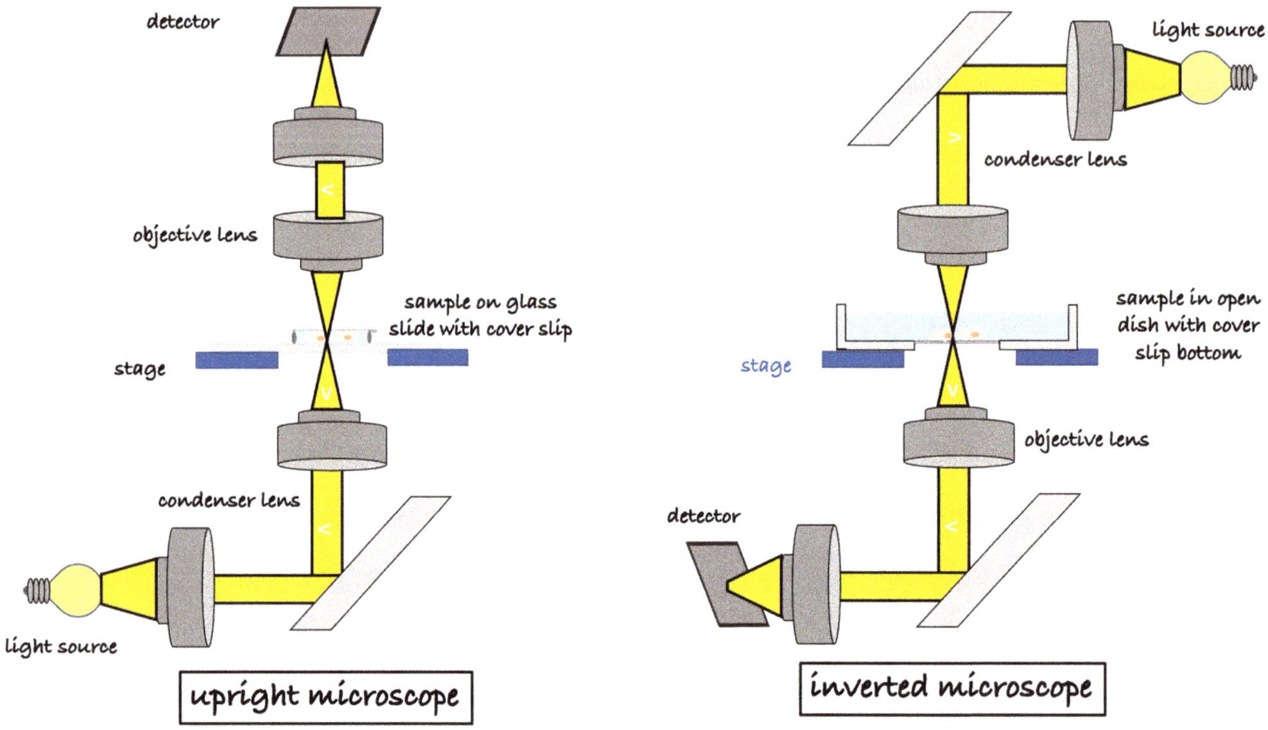

Figure 9.7 Upright versus inverted microscope for trans-illumination. For white light imaging both upright and inverted microscopes use trans-illumination, which means that light is transmitted through the specimen. In the case of an upright microscope, illumination occurs from the bottom and detection from the top, whereas in the case of an inverted microscope, illumination originates from the top and detection occurs at the bottom. Inverted microscopes are well suited for liquid filled, open cell culture dishes with a coverslip at the bottom, whereas upright microscope usually require a sample to be mounted (squeezed) between a glass-slide and a coverslip.

9.4.2 Light Source and Illumination

There are a variety of light sources suitable for microscopic imaging, including halogen lamp glowing light, xenon- or mercury arc lamps, metal halide lamps, light emitting diodes (LED) or lasers. Halogen lamps are often not bright enough for fluorescence microscopy, hence xenon-arc lamps or mercury-vapor lamps are common light sources for epifluorescence microscopy. However, arc-lamps are increasingly replaced by high-power LEDs, since arc-lamps need to be replaced frequently, and are sometimes hard to align. Also, in the case of the mercury arc lamp, a broken arc-lamp can be highly toxic. LED on the other hand can be turned on and off very fast, and do not become hot. For high-end configurations, solid-state lasers are the preferred source of illumination, due to their high intensity and coherence. Figure 9.9 shows the emission spectra of tungsten-halogen incandescent lamps, mercury and xenon arc lamps, as well as krypton and argon lasers. Note that lasers only deliver specific wavelength, whereas incandescent and arc lamps offer a more or less continuous spectrum.

There are different ways for illumination depending on what type of microscopy is being performed, e.g., brightfield or darkfield microscopy. In the so-called Köhler illumination which is used in most optical microscopes these days, the condenser lens will focus the light of a radiating point source onto the specimen in an even, uniform manner.

There are some specialized applications that require different types of illumination and or additional equipment as part of the illumination. For example, structured illumination is one form of superresolution imaging technique and surpasses the diffraction limit by about a factor of two. Polarization microscopy is useful, e.g., for the optical study of protein crystals and other biological objects that may alter the polarization of light waves. In phase contrast imaging, ring-like illumination is accomplished by a condenser annulus to allow constructive and destructive interference mechanisms to provide specimen contrast. Near-field illumination is based on entirely different principles, and does not require lenses in a classical sense, but just the guidance of highly focused laser light very close to the sample surface.

For epifluorescence microscopy, there are dichroic beam splitter cubes, which contain an excitation filter, a dichroic mirror, and an emission filter, designed to match spectral excitation and emission characteristics of each fluorophore. Each dichroic beam splitter filter has a specific combination of excitation and emission filters suitable for certain fluorophores. If one wants to record multiple fluorophore signals, one must exchange the filter cubes for

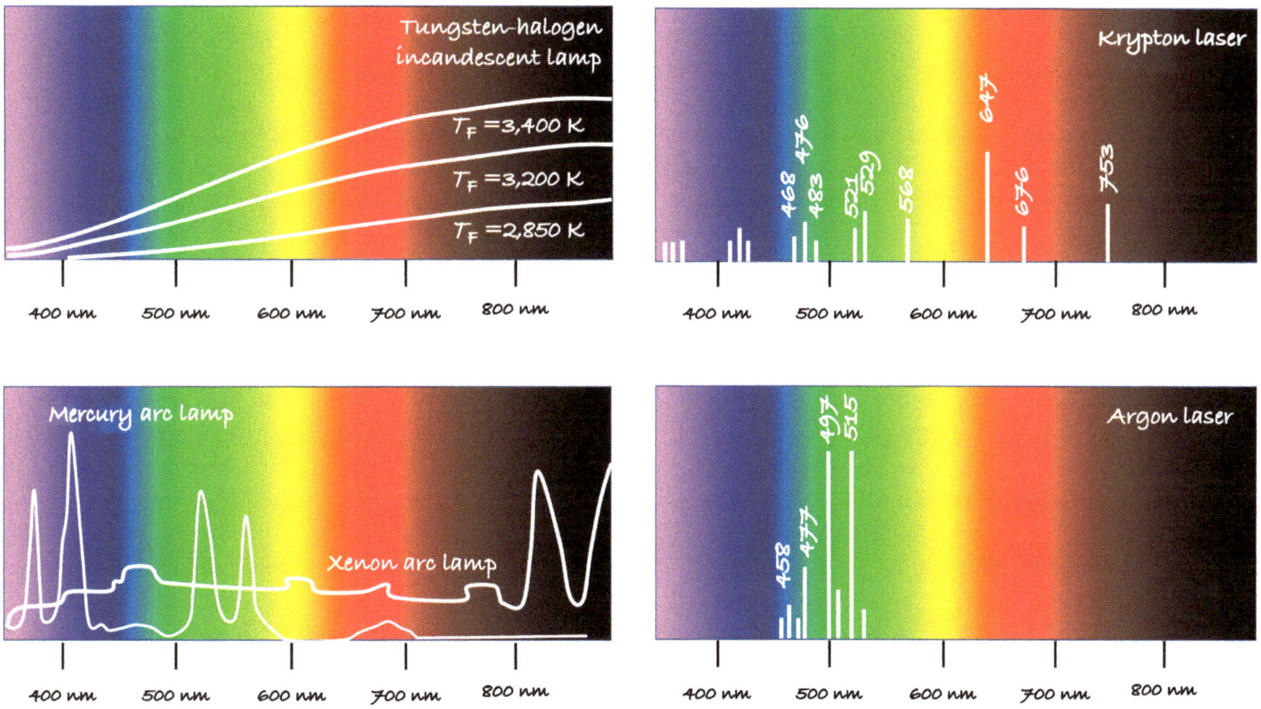

Figure 9.9 Emission spectrum of different types of light sources. Different types of light sources have very different light emission spectra that can be used for excitation of fluorophores, with the spectra of tungsten halogen incandescent lamps (at different temperatures) showing a broad range of light emission. Lasers on the other hand have a very sharp distribution and hence fluorophore and laser need to be compatible and optimized with one another. Arc lamps are in between with some portions of the spectrum yielding a strong signal, whereas in other regions of the spectrum the emission may be weak.

each fluorophore. The use of dichroic beam splitter cubes will result in a dark (black) background and thus optimal fluorescence contrast.

9.4.3 Optical Path

In terms of the optical path, the simplest microscopes involve a single lens, which simply magnifies an object not unlike a magnifying class. This concept is still in use for some cheap commercial digital microscopes. However, most microscopes used for research are compound microscopes. Compound microscopes are based on at least two lenses, one lens to create a virtual image, which is then further enlarged by a second lens to provide a much higher magnification. Stereomicroscopes are typically low-powered microscopes that allow stereoscopic viewing of the sample, e.g., for dissection of organs and tissues. Stereomicroscopes keep the optical paths (including objective lens and eyepieces) of the right eye and left eye separate, resulting in two slightly different viewing angles for each eye, which results in a 3D impression of the object.

Due to the diffraction limit of light in optical microscopy, the maximum magnification power is limited to ~1,000×, with an eye-piece magnification of 10× and an objective lens magnification of about 100×. A typical compound microscope has several different lenses for lower and higher magnification. These lenses are typically arranged in an objective lens turret (revolver) to allow switching between different magnifications, with the sample and thus the field of view remaining in place.

Microscope objective lenses are typically described by two parameters, namely magnification (typically ranging from 5× to 100×) and a numerical aperture (NA) that typically ranges from 0.14 to 0.7 in air, and up to ~1.5 in immersion oil.

The NA is the product of the refraction index n times the sine function of the maximal angle at which light originating from a point source enters the lens. This is also known as the acceptance cone of an objective and defines its light-gathering ability and its resolving power. Since high-NA lenses collect a broader light cone, they are brighter and contain higher resolution details compared to low-NA lenses. With the refractive index being $n = 1.0$ for air, $n = 1.33$ for water, and $n = 1.52$ for immersion oil, high-NA lenses must be used in either water or immersion oil. The maximum NA for oil immersion is 1.5 ($n = 1.52$) and for water 1.27 ($n = 1.33$). Because of the acceptance cone, high-NA lenses have a short working distance, whereas low-NA lenses have a longer working distance.

While the Raleigh criterion of lateral resolution is somewhat arbitrary it is a useful way to characterize the resolving power of a microscope. When two Airy disks are spaced apart that their respective maxima coincide in the first minimum of its neighboring Airy disk, the intensity between the two overlapping Airy disks drops by 26%, and we call the two points (that are at the center of such two Airy disks) as resolved.

The resolution is dependent on the wavelength (lambda) and the NA and is 0.61 × lambda/NA, and thus in the best-case scenario 0.48 × lambda in water and 0.4 × lambda in immersion oil, or roughly half the wavelength. Apart from the NA, and the wavelength at which one images, correct sampling is key for success, with sampling according to Nyquist's law (or Nyquist–Shannon sample theorem) must be at least twice as fine as the detector pixel spacing, but ideally is 2.5×–3× as fine. Fine sampling will reduce aliasing, the discrete (pixel-by-pixel) sampling of a continuous object brightness function.

The useful magnification of a microscope system is considered ~500×–1,000× times, but sample, illumination, optical path (aberrations) and detector properties as well as adequate sampling spacing further complicate the matter. At magnification exceeding the value of 1,000× one speaks of empty resolution, as no new details are being revealed, the image instead is just further magnified.

Since optical systems are never perfect, a variety of aberrations are known, and in high-end microscope, much effort has been undertaken to correct for these aberrations. It is not uncommon for objective lenses to contain up to 17 independent lenses and a high-end objective lens may cost as much as the entire rest of the microscope. Furthermore, there can be additional components in the light path, including filters, apertures, mirrors, interferometers, electronic light amplifiers, and spectrometers.

There are a variety of aberrations, among which the most serious issue is spherical aberration. Spherical aberration results in the blurring of an image near the edge as the result of an uneven focus of monochromatic light due to the curvature of lenses. Likewise, regions deep inside the specimen can come to focus on a different point than regions at the surface of the specimen, which is another source of spherical aberrations. In addition, there can be (axial) chromatic aberration, which is an uneven focus for each wavelength in polychromatic light due to dispersion, the wavelength-dependent propagation of light in an optical material. As a result, red, green, and blue light come to focus on different points on the Z-axis. Axial chromatic aberration is usually corrected for by using chromatic doublet lens groups that contain a mixture of convex and concave lenses with slightly different properties. In practical terms, axial chromatic aberration can also be the result of the objective lens not being properly matched with its immersion oil (Figure 9.10).

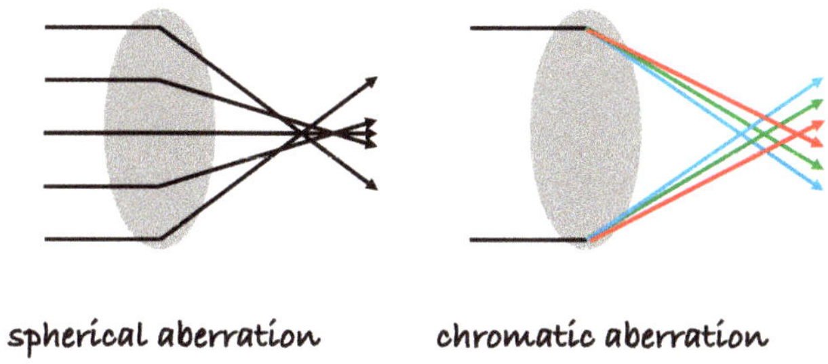

Figure 9.10 Spherical and chromatic aberrations. Among the various aberrations, spherical and chromatic aberrations are the most important ones for optical imaging. With respect to spherical aberrations, an uneven focus of monochromatic light leads to image blurring near the edges, whereas for chromatic aberrations different spectral parts of polychromatic light come to focus on different points on the *X*-axis.

Petzval field curvature can also be considered an aberration and results from the fact that not all parts of the specimen (e.g., center versus periphery) come to focus on the same plane (e.g., on a detector plane) as they would on a curved detector such as the retina in our eyeballs. Solutions to this issue can be to use an aperture to restrict the field of view to the central portion of the image (which however reduces the light collection power of the lens), or to use a curved detector design (as is the case for the Kepler Space Observatory).

Astigmatism leads to blurring of a point from a circle to an ellipse, with the directionality changing at focus. Astigmatism can be due to asymmetric lens manufacturing or misalignment.

Coma is often caused by misalignment and is characterized by point sources appearing as a streak of light widening at the periphery (due to uneven focus of light that passes through the center versus light that passes through the periphery of the lens). Coma is due to off-axis illumination, and thus different from spherical aberration, which is an on-axis illumination phenomenon.

9.4.4 Detector

Digital detection of visible light is largely based on the photoelectric effect (e.g., in PMTs) or the inner photoelectric effect (e.g., in semiconductors). Older technologies were photographic film and phosphorescent image plates. Charge-coupled device (CCD) technology has dominated the field for the last two decades, but increasingly direct detectors are becoming the detector of choice also for optical microscopy. One distinguishes between single point detectors and "multi-point"/area detectors, which are arrays of photosensitive elements, and are also described as cameras. For each detector type, the photons impacting the detector result in electrons being created, and the resulting voltage/current is recorded as a digital number.

Singe point detectors, such as PMTs are very linear, have a very high gain, and a fast response rate, however, their quantum efficiency is typically only 25%, which means that on average it takes four photons to produce one electron. PMTs can be run in photon-counting mode, with a near-zero background, but detection by PMT is typically a very slow process. In linear mode, current is being measured, which can be a fast but noisy process. Another type of a single-point detector is a so-called avalanche photodiode, that is semiconductor-based, not unlike a CCD. Avalanche photodiodes can be operated in photon-counting mode with a high quantum efficiency of ~90%, but if they are run too fast, they can overheat.

Current-day area detectors/cameras are semiconductor-based and rely on the inner photoelectric effect to form electrons, which are accumulated in a potential well, and read out afterwards. The two architectures are complementary metal-oxide semiconductor (CMOS) and CCD technologies, with CMOS technology featuring a charge-to-voltage converter for every pixel in the chip, whereas in CCD there is a single read-out amplifier. CMOS technology has the advantage of being much faster than CCDs, but until recently CMOS was considered noisy and thus less precise than CCDs. For a long time, CCD was preferred due to its precision, but CMOS technology has significantly improved since, and is now the preferred choice for detectors as the new CMOS camera generation (unlike CCD cameras) is characterized by a high quantum efficiency.

The read-out of the CCD is frequently compared to a "bucket-brigade," where the charge in each pixel is transferred to the neighboring pixel and then to the final "bucket," where the charge is then read-out. This process is inherently slow, but very precise. Speeding up of the read-out process leads to lower precision. Also, care must be taken that an individual pixel with its potential well does not receive too many photons during light exposure as it otherwise "overflows," which then leads to "blooming" artifacts.

There are three different designs of CCD architecture, namely full frame, frame transfer and interline transfer CCD (Figure 9.11). Full frame CCD are rarely used anymore, frame transfer CCD are used nowadays in most electron-multiplying charge-coupled devices (EMCCDs), along with interline transfer CCD, which is a commonly used design for CCD detectors. Full frame architecture has a regular serial register read-out with no additional storage area. The frame transfer uses an aluminum-shielded duplicate CCD array at the bottom of the camera, that serves as a storage area. Charges from the image section are serially shifted to the store section, from where they can be read out, while the light-sensitive top part of the CCD camera can be used again for acquiring an image. In the case of an

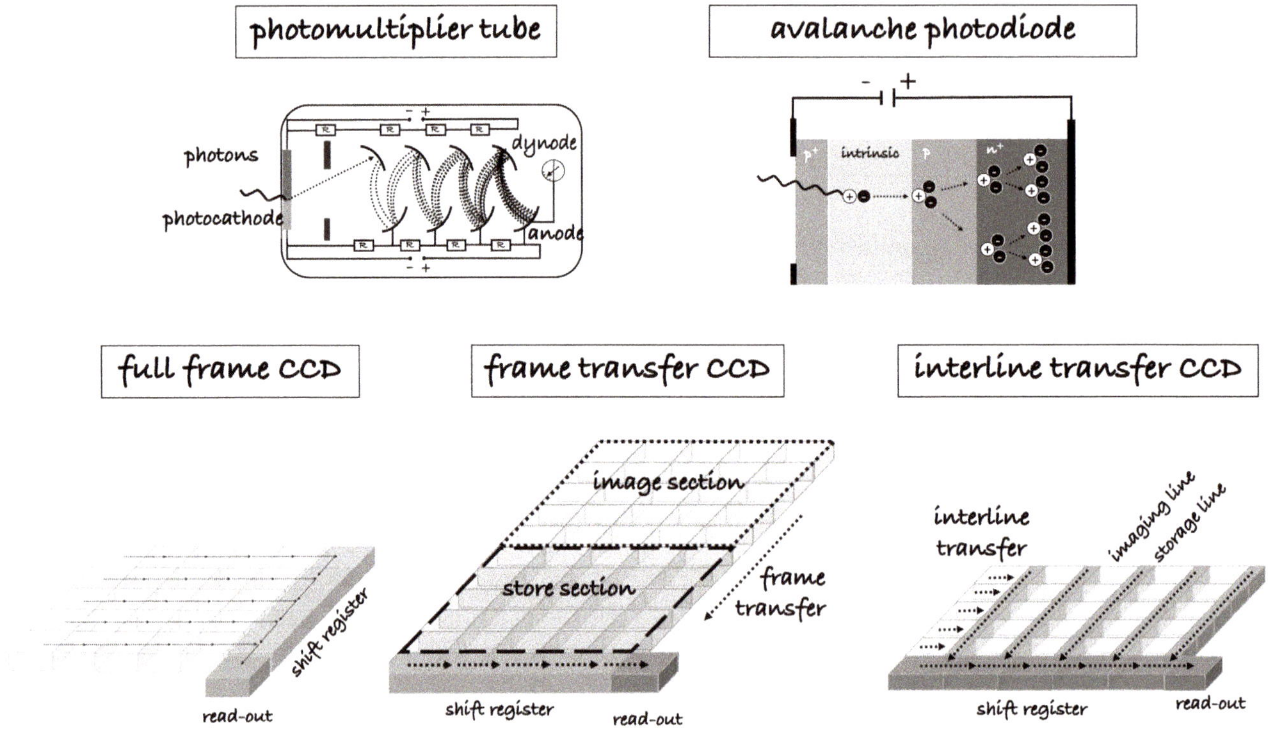

Figure 9.11 Optical/fluorescence microscopy detectors. The most prominently used point detectors are photomultiplier tubes and avalanche photodiodes, where CCD technology is frequently used either in form of full-frame CCD, frame-transfer CCD or interline CCD. However, the most recent development are CMOS detectors (not shown), with each pixel having its own amplifier. CMOS detectors are preferred in high-end applications for their fast frame rates, high sensitivity, high dynamic range, and low noise.

interline transfer there exists a row of light-sensitive pixels next to an aluminum-shielded row, to which the charge can be transferred, and from where the charge can be read out, while the light sensitive row is available again for light exposure.

EMCCDs contain an on-chip multiplication (amplification) that renders EMCCD cameras able to be ultra-sensitive and able to detect single photon events. Clock-induced charges occur and lead to charge amplification through a process known as impact ionization, where a charge has sufficient energy to create another electron–hole pair. Cooling the camera further increases the probability of charge multiplication and thus the gain of the camera. By amplifying the signal prior to the read-out (charge to voltage conversion), read-out noise become negligible, however the high gain of EMCCD can affect the dynamic range of the camera. For low signal intensity, with less than one photon per pixel per frame, EMCCDs can be used for single photon counting.

There are different sources of noise that affect data collection: photon shot noise, readout noise, fixed pattern noise and dark current noise. Photon shot noise is due to the stochastic nature of photons hitting the detector, with the signal-to-noise (S/N) ratio and scales with the square root of the number of photons. Longer exposure times will improve image statistics. Also, 2×2 binning (integrating the signal of four pixels into one pixel) doubles the S/N but also increases the pixel size and thus halves the resolution. Readout noise is independent of the number of photons reaching the detector and is inherent in the CCD readout design. The magnitude of readout noise depends on the bandwidth of the charge amplifier, which is low in slow-scan CCD cameras but gets higher (and thus noisier) with fast readout. Fixed pattern noise reflects the fact that not all pixels respond equally to photons. This type of noise scales linearly with the signal and can be adjusted for by flat-field correction. Dark current noise stems from the thermal accumulation of electrons, that were not the result of light exposure. It can be overcome by cooling the camera.

Color CCDs as frequently used in consumer electronics are not used in scientific CCD cameras, as every pixel in color CCDs just consists of four monochromatic detector elements, two with a green, one with a red and one with blue color filter. Hence, color CCDs "waste" photons, whereas in fluorescence microscopy one would like to catch every photon.

CCD cameras can be either front-illuminated or back-illuminated, with back-illuminated cameras achieving a much higher quantum efficiency and thus being the preferred choice. Care must be taken, that camera pixel size and attainable resolution are matched according to the criteria laid out by the Nyquist–Shannon sampling theorem, that recommends at least 2-fold (better is 2.5–3-fold) oversampling. Also, when choosing a camera, one should consider the speed, the quantum efficiency, gain, as well as the dynamic range as well as cost of the respective camera choice.

9.5 Data Collection

There are different types of optical microscopy, ranging from the conventional use of white light to study a biological sample in real time with low phototoxicity to the use of fluorescence to only look at small region of the electromagnetic spectrum for subcellular localization of a small subset of molecules.

9.5.1 Choosing the Right Microscopy Technique

Given the large variety of optical imaging techniques, choosing the right approach can be daunting. One fundamental decision is whether one wants to use transmitted light or fluorescent light for imaging.

Transmitted white light is good for measuring cell behavior, requires no genetic encoding or labeling with a fluorophore, and compared to fluorescence imaging is in general less damaging to the biological sample. Examples of transmitted white light imaging are brightfield differential interference contrast (DIC) microscopy, also known as Nomarski phase contrast microscopy, phase contrast microscopy of cells and cell cultures/organoids, or darkfield microscopy of microtubules and other supramolecular complexes.

Fluorescence light imaging usually measures the behavior of molecules in vitro or inside cells. Which of the many fluorescence imaging technique is best suited depends on the thickness of the specimen. Also, the choice will be affected by the choice of sample (alive or in a fixed state), the rate of data acquisition needed, and the system's tolerance to photodamage.

The advantage of epifluorescence microscopy is the low cost and ease of use. No expensive lasers or complex microscopy optics are required; however, the out-of-focus fluorescence contributions lead to a lower S/N ratio and more damage to the sample.

Deconvolution microscopy requires extensive computational processing of a Z-stack of images to sharpen the in-focus light but is easy to implement on an epifluorescence microscope as it only needs a motorized *Z*-axis stepper and appropriate software for deconvolution microscopy.

The choice of the right laser-scanning optical sectioning microscopy depends on whether the object is close (within ~50–200 nm) to the coverslip surface, in which case TIRF microscopy is an excellent choice. For cells and tissues up to ~100 μm in thickness, pinhole microscopy such as regular laser point-scanning, laser line-scanning, or spinning disk confocal microscopy are the imaging methods of choice. Laser point-scanning and laser line-scanning confocal microscopy are good for fixed specimen of less than 100 μm in thickness, where photodamage is less of a concern.

Spinning disk confocal microscopy is ideal for live cell samples, ideally less than 30 μm in thickness, where fast data acquisition is the prime goal. For thicker samples (~100–500 μm), two photon microscopy is best, for even thicker samples, array tomography, meaning physical sectioning instead of optical sectioning, followed by epifluorescence imaging of consecutive thin sections is considered a suitable alternative. Light sheet (selected plane imaging) microscopy excels for rather thick live samples, such as zebrafish or mouse embryos, given its low phototoxicity and fast data acquisition.

While all the approaches discussed so far are diffraction limited, superresolution imaging approaches exist and in terms of resolution go beyond the diffraction limit by about a factor of 10. However, given that superresolution imaging is technically more complex, one should ask oneself whether one would truly benefit from the high resolution these techniques offer. Or to put it in other words, what exactly would I learn at ~20 nm resolution that I cannot learn at ~200 nm. Conventional (diffraction-limited) imaging can achieve a resolution of 200–250 nm at best, whereas structured illumination can yield ~100 nm for live samples and STORM/PALM and STED super-resolution offer up to 20–50 nm resolution. Also, one should distinguish between resolution (the distance of two objects that can still be distinguished) and the precision to which the center of an Airy disk of a single fluorophore or a group of fluorophores (or transmitted light pattern for that matter) can be determined.

Also, as biology is becoming increasingly quantitative, one may want to ask oneself what kind of image analysis will follow the actual image data acquisition, i.e., whether one wants to track molecules, measure their velocities, or quantify their abundance and distribution in cells and tissues.

Ultimately, however, it may be wise to approach this question from a more practical point of view: one needs to answer the question of what one hopes to learn from the imaging experiment, whether one aims to quantify imaging data, and in practical terms what kind of imaging is readily available (Figure 9.12).

9.5.2 White Light Imaging

Bright field microscopy is the most basic technique, where white light illuminates the sample and is transmitted through the specimen before being observed (Figure 9.13). This form of microscopy is often used for samples that have

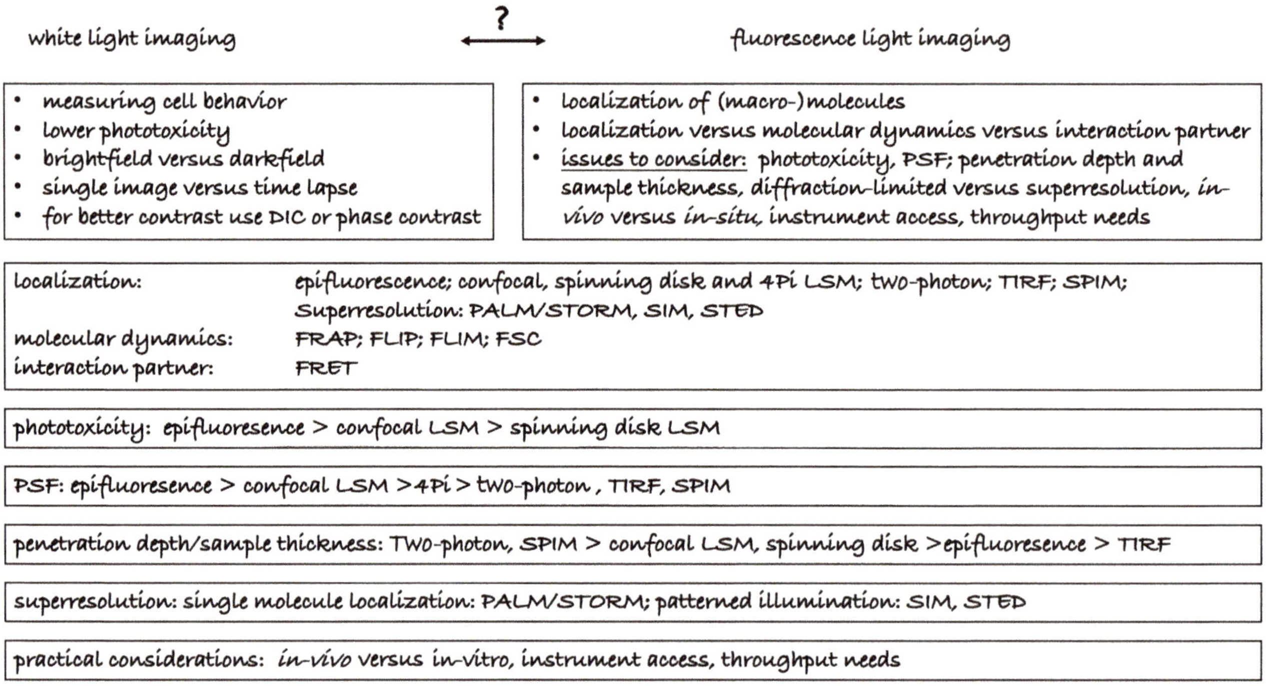

Figure 9.12 How to choose the right kind of microscopy. The best choice for light imaging depends on the goal of imaging, e.g., whether one is interested in monitoring and/or measuring quantitatively cell behavior, whether localization of a small subset of macromolecules is what drives the imaging. Alternative goals may also be to determine the dynamic behavior of molecules or to establish close interaction partners. Among the issues to consider are phototoxicity, whether the sample will be imaged in-vivo or in-situ, the sample thickness and penetration depth, the shape of the point-spread-function, and whether more is learned by superresolution imaging compared to diffraction-limited imaging, in addition to the more mundane questions of instrument access and throughput needs.

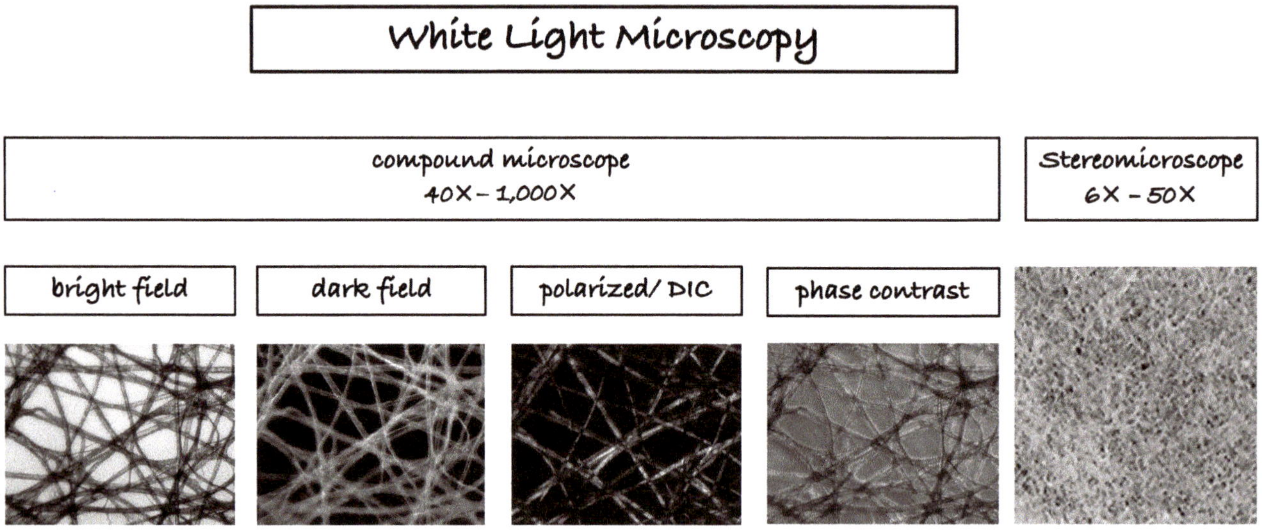

Figure 9.13 White light imaging of tissue paper. *Source:* Zephyris / Wikipedia Commons / CC BY-SA 3.0. Tissue paper consists of a network of fibers, which has a very different appearance when visualized by a compound microscope using brightfield, darkfield, polarized/DIC, or phase contrast imaging. For comparison an image obtained by a stereomicroscope at lower magnification is also shown.

been stained to distinguish organelles, cells or even tissues from their surroundings. If all objects of interest in the sample reside in a single focal plane, such as for individual cells in cell culture or thin tissue sections, out-of-focus contributions is not a problem, however, for more complex structures such as clumps of cells, organoids and/or tissues, blurring can severely degrade image quality and make the images difficult to interpret. In such cases oblique illumination (i.e., illumination from the side) can be advantageous, as the combination of light and shadows provides a three-dimensional-like appearance. Hoffmann's modulation contrast microscopy is based on the same principle and is often used in cell-culture experiments.

Dark field microscopy uses an illumination technique, where a darkfield condenser directs the light away from the objective lens. As a result, the non-scattered light will not be collected, and therefore any area where there is no scattering object (i.e., the background) will be dark. Only the light scattered by the sample is being collected, which will appear as bright objects against a nearly black background.

Phase contrast microscopy, originally developed by the Dutch physicist Frits Zernike in the 1930s, relies on differences in refractive index of biological structures, such as the cell's nucleus against the surrounding cytoplasm, and is used for thin samples. In phase contrast microscopy, a circular annulus in the condenser produces cone-shaped illumination, which is then collected by a similarly sized ring in the objective lens. This leads to an overall reduction in direct light intensity and most importantly to a quarter-wavelength phase shift of the non-diffracted light. Interference of the non-diffracted light with the light diffracted by the sample generates contrast which can be maximized by adjusting the phase ring setting, but also leads to the formation of a halo-light ring that can obscure details. Phase contrast microscopy is different from DIC microscopy and does not utilize polarized light.

DIC microscopy, also known as Nomarski microscopy, was invented by Georges Nomarski in 1952 and uses the principles of interferometry to enhance contrast in transparent, unstained samples. DIC images appear similar to phase contrast microscopy (black to white on a gray background) but lack the halo-light rings, typical for objects imaged by phase-contrast microscopy. In DIC, unpolarized light is polarized by a polarizer at an 45° angle of the polarization plane before split by a special prism (Wollaston prism or Nomarski prism) in the condenser into an ordinary beam that has a 0° polarization plane angle and an extraordinary beam that has a 90° polarization plane angle, with a small spatial difference (of ~200 nm) between the two beams. The Nomarski prism is a modification of the previously used Wollaston prism and consists of two wedges of birefringent quartz or calcite crystals, glued together by Canada balm resin. Upon entering the sample, light is 90° phase-shifted, but the polarization angle remains the same. A second Wollaston/Nomarski prism in the objective lens light path recombines the two beams with their perpendicular polarization planes into one beam that has a 135° polarization plane angle. The phase shift of the light that passed through the sample causes a change in amplitude. A second polarizing filter set at 135° just in front of the detector removes directly transmitted light. If the sample is homogenous with respect to refractive index, the image is uniform, however, at refractive boundaries (such as the nucleus/cytoplasm boundary) there will be contrast generated, appearing as a 3D relief in the image that emphasizes lines and edges. Contrast is direction-dependent, being maximal in one direction and minimal in the orthogonal direction. In the direction of maximal contrast, one edge often appears brighter than the background, whereas the other one being darker (depending on the off-set chosen in the "de Sénarmont" compensator).

(Allen) Video-enhanced contrast (AVEC) microscopy, developed by Robert Day Allen and Nina Stromgreen Allen in the early 1980s, is built on earlier work by Shinya Inoué in the 1950s. It uses DIC imaging and the power of frame-by-frame background subtraction (e.g., a slightly defocused brightfield image) to further enhance cellular features (particularly linear elements) that would have not been easily visible without the background subtraction, such as microtubules, intermediate filaments and actin filament bundles, however these structures are blurry due to diffraction limited imaging.

9.5.3 Fluorescence Microscopy

Fluorescence microscopy can yield highly specific, high-contrast, and quantitative information about (macro-) molecules of interest and can be compatible will live-cell imaging. As is best shown in a Jablonski diagram, light is absorbed by the fluorophore and an electron will move from one the ground states to one of the excited states. The electron will transition to the lowest of the respective excited states via non-radiative internal conversion (with the energy being dissipated into heat), from which the electron will relax back to a ground state. The time it takes for the electron to go back to the ground state is also known as the lifetime of the fluorophore. The brightness of the fluorophore depends on the likelihood of absorption (absorption coefficient) and the likelihood that an absorbed electron will lead to the emission of a fluorescent photon.

The PSF, and thus the data anisotropy, can be very different depending on the type of fluorescence microscopy employed. In all cases, except for two-photon microscopy,

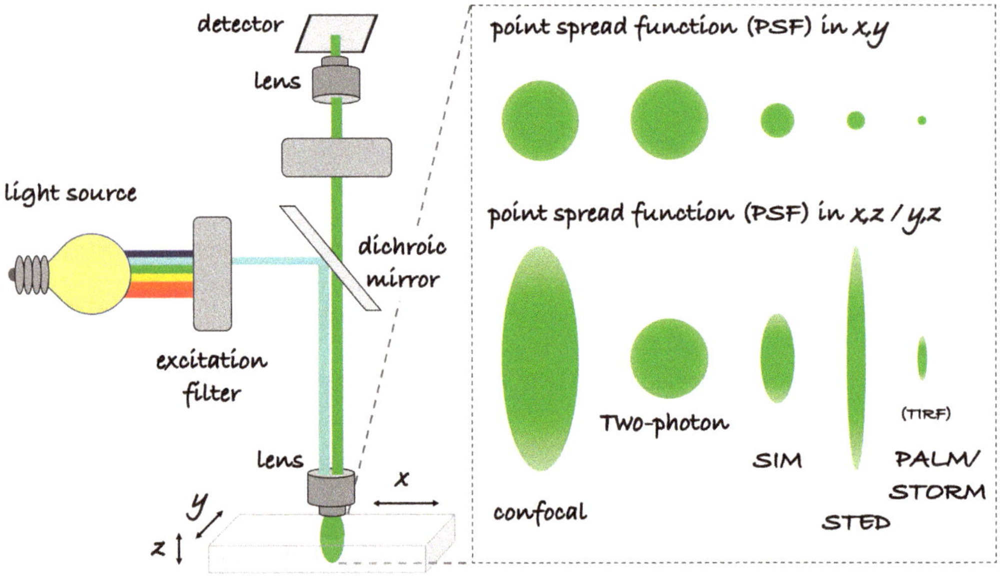

Figure 9.14 Point spread function for fluorescence microscopy. In fluorescence microscopy, the point spread function (PSF) is different for the different types of microscopies. Starting with a highly anisotropic PSF for confocal microscopy, one can obtain an isotropic PSF with two-photon microscopy. While all superresolution techniques such as SIM, STED, PALM, and STORM suffer from PSF anisotropy, the PSF in *X,Y* is significantly improved over the diffraction-limited confocal fluorescence light microcopy. The PSF in the *Z*-direction is also improved for SIM, PALM, STORM but not for STED.

the PSF is worse in the *Z*-direction (*X,Z*- or *Y,Z*-plane) compared to the *X,Y* plane. The PSF for superresolution techniques in *X,Y* is up to a factor of 10 better compared to diffraction-limited imaging but varies in terms of *Z*-resolution. The most extreme with respect to is STED, with a 10-fold improvement in lateral resolution but no improvement in axial resolution (Figure 9.14).

9.6 Fluorophore Considerations

It can be advantageous in biological imaging to reduce complexity, and instead of seeing the entire biological sample in all its complexity, one can focus on a few target molecules, e.g., by using a labeling strategy that will render the target macromolecule of interest fluorescent. Hence, fluorescence imaging will selectively report on the macromolecular target, while ignoring everything that is not fluorescent.

The detection of the fluorescence signal in diffraction-limited microscopes is limited by the number of photons that can be captured from a fluorophore before it photobleaches. Typically, ~1,000 photons are needed to determine the center of an Airy disk (which typically is ~450 nm in diameter for a point source). The more photons can be collected the more precise is the determination of the Airy disk center, hence brighter and more photostable fluorophores are desirable.

There are four types of fluorophores, such as synthetic small organic molecule fluorophores, semiconductor-based quantum dots, genetically encoded fluorescent fusion proteins, or small organic dye molecules covalently linked to a genetically encoded tag which is fused to the target protein of interest (Figure 9.15).

9.6.1 Synthetic Organic Dyes

Synthetic small organic molecule-based fluorophores have been used for a long time in biological fluorescence imaging. Fluorescein was first synthesized by Adolph von Bayer in 1871 and represents an example of an aromatic conjugated π-electron system.

The advantage of using them is that they are typically bright and photostable, and thus ideally suited for fluorescence imaging. Some of the more commonly used molecules are fluorescein and its derivatives (e.g., FTIC), coumarins, rhodamines, Texas Red, Alexa Fluors, cyanine dyes (e.g., Cy3, Cy5), as well as DyLight Fluor (Figure 9.16).

The cyanine Cy3/Cy5 dye pair was the original dye used in STORM imaging, as the probe can be switched reversibly for up to 1,000 times before it photobleaches. However, such molecules need to be somehow attached to the target macromolecule of interest, either by (immuno-)affinity (e.g., antibodies) or via genetically encoded tags (e.g., SNAP tag and others) that specifically bind a small molecule to which the synthetic dye is covalently linked to.

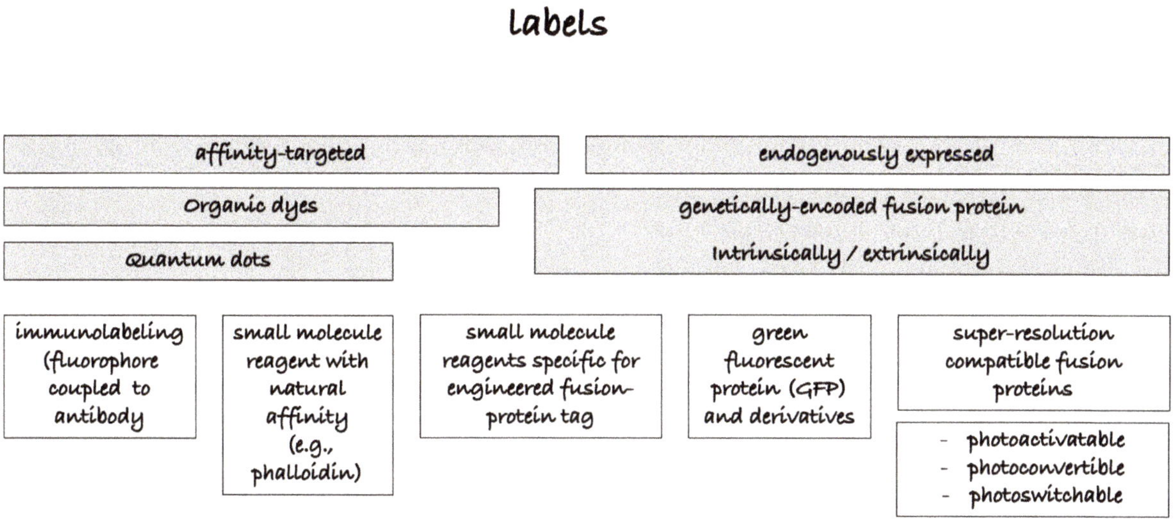

Figure 9.15 Fluorophore considerations – Overview. Labels are typically divided into affinity-targeted or endogenously expressed fluorescent labels. Furthermore, fluorophores can be of synthetic origins such as organic dyes or semiconductor nanocrystals (quantum dots), or they are genetically encoded proteins that are genetically engineered as fusion proteins with the target protein of interest. Genetically encoded fluorophores are either intrinsically fluorescent (such as GFP and its derivatives) or they are extrinsically fluorescent, which means that they constitute a non-fluorescent tag (such as a SNAP tag) to which a small molecule with a fluorophore binds with high specificity and affinity (sometimes covalently and thus irreversibly).

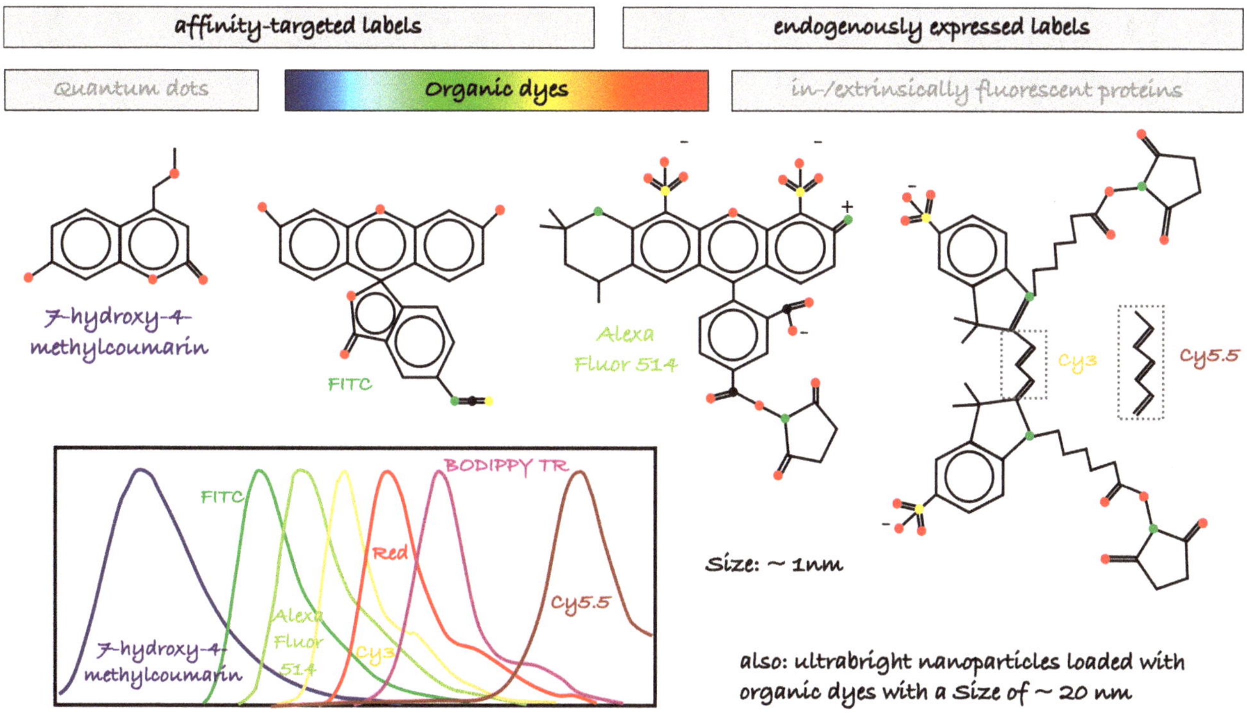

Figure 9.16 Synthetic organic fluorescent dyes. Organic fluorescent dyes are typically derivatives of conjugated π-systems, with different dyes having specific absorption and emission spectra. They typically are individual small organic molecules typically ~1 nm in size but can also be packed in high concentration into ~20 nm-sized ultrabright nanoparticles.

9.6.2 Quantum Dots

Quantum dots contain a core of certain semiconductor elements (CdSe-ZnS) surrounded by a biocompatible coating such as lipids or poly-ethylene-glycol (PEG), which can make them very large (Figure 9.17).

In terms of size, they are in the 3–10 nm range not unlike proteins (with their size being correlated to their emission wavelength). Their much higher brightness, broad (and thus overlapping) excitation spectra, narrow emission spectra, and high resistance to photobleaching make them ideally suited for fluorescence imaging, however, their size, their inability to cross biological membranes and the specific targeting constitute a challenge for experimenters. Also, they tend to blink which makes them non-ideal probes for single molecule-tracking. The significance and importance of quantum dots in chemistry has been recognized by the 2023 Nobel Prize in Chemistry, awarded to Moungi Bawendi, Louis Brus and Aleksey Yekimov for the discovery and synthesis of quantum dots.

9.6.3 Immuno-Affinity-Based Labeling

Still a widely used targeting approach is based on the affinity and specificity of primary antibodies, which are then detected by a fluorophore-conjugated secondary antibody. Also, certain molecules have a natural affinity to certain macromolecules such as phalloidin to filamentous actin or as DAPI to DNA.

Among the challenges with antibody-based fluorophore-labeling is antibody cross-reactivity, which results in high background and thus false-positive signals. But there are also false-negative signals, meaning there is no signal where there should be a signal. False negatives could be due to limited accessibility of the antibody to its epitope. This could be due to a barrier such as biological membranes that prevent the antibody ever getting close to its epitope or steric hindrance due to macromolecular crowding in a living cell. For these reasons, biological samples are frequently chemically fixed and detergent-treated, which also results in the loss of much of the cytoplasmic material, and thus also deals with macromolecular crowding. However, such protocols may not only alter the cellular ultrastructure but also interfere with the epitope's integrity, which means that the epitope, while present and sterically available, is no longer recognized by the antibody. It has been estimated that even under ideal conditions only ~30% of all epitopes are recognized by antibodies, and that in the case of immuno-electron microscopy with its extensive sample preparation protocols only 1–5% of all epitopes are recognized at all. False-positive and false-negative signals can lead to incorrect conclusions, and this problem is typically dealt with by including a variety of control samples that are aimed at getting an estimate of possible false-negative or false-positive results.

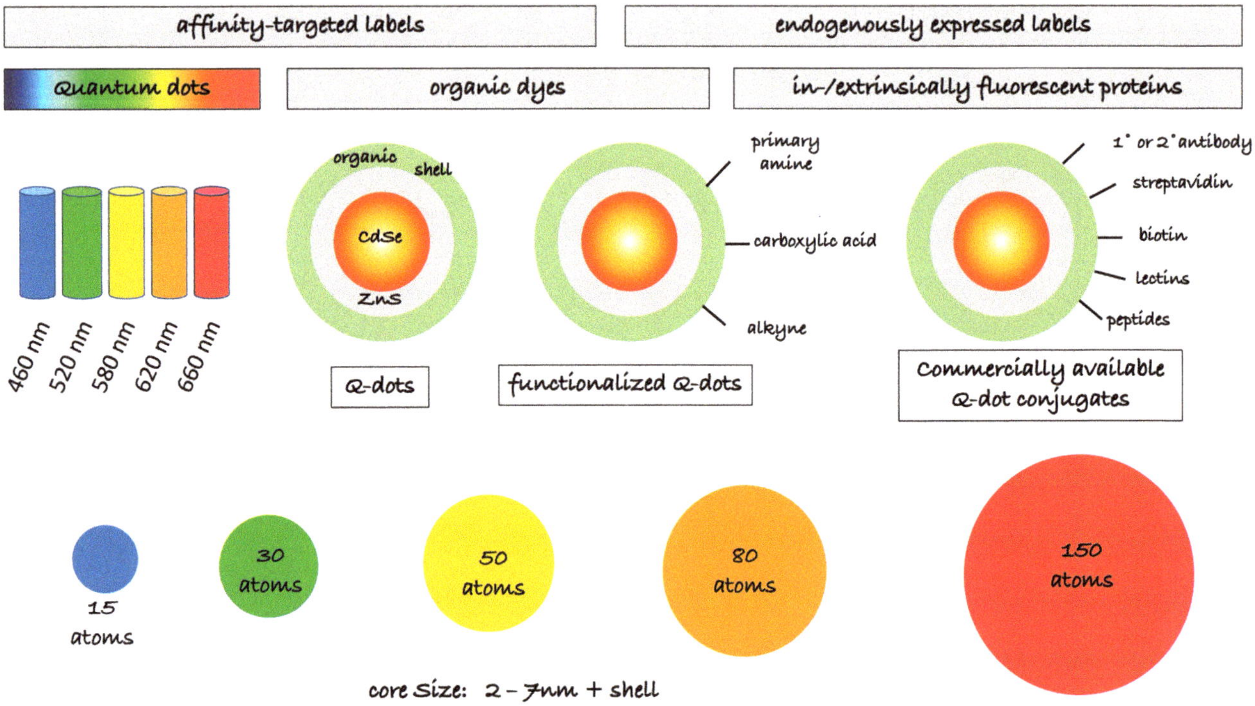

Figure 9.17 Quantum dots (Q-dots) fluorophores. Quantum dots are made of a core of the semiconductor elements cadmium and selenium, surrounded by a shell of zinc sulfide, around which there is another organic molecule coating (e.g., lipids, polyethylene glycol) that renders quantum dots biocompatible. Quantum dots are typically between 3 and 10 nm in diameter and require specific targeting. Q-dots are very bright, show high resistance to photobleaching, with a broad (overlapping) excitation spectrum and narrow emission spectra.

Apart from antibodies, affinity-based small molecules approaches continue to have their place in fluorescence imaging, particularly for fixed samples. For example, DAPI as a nucleic acid stain specifically labels the cell's nuclear DNA and thus DAPI is widely used to allow imaging of the cell nucleus. Labeling efficiency of affinity-targeted fluorescence probes is much lower compared to fluorescent-fusion proteins, with a high potential for non-specific labeling and thus background signal.

The discovery of fluorescent proteins and their spectral derivatives have revolutionized cell biology, which is why the discovery and development of GFP was recognized by the 2008 Nobel Prize in Chemistry. Fluorescent fusion proteins, which are genetically encoded, have allowed live cell imaging with high specificity and high labeling efficiency. However, genetically encoded fluorescent proteins typically require an oxidative environment for activation and multicolor imaging remains to be a challenge.

9.7 Genetically Encoded Fluorescent Proteins

One distinguishes intrinsically fluorescent proteins, which become fluorescent upon folding (usually in the presence of oxygen), from extrinsically fluorescent proteins, which either bind an endogenous fluorophore (already present in the cell) or an exogenous synthetic fluorophore. For this category, the protein portion is often referred to as a tag, that is genetically fused to the target protein of interest.

9.7.1 Intrinsically Fluorescent Proteins

Genetic protein engineering allows for the genetic encoding of an endogenous fluorescent signal, without the need for any of the classical fluorescence label targeting approaches. The genetic construct is the genetic fusion of a fluorescent protein with target protein, via a short protein linker sequence. Such fluorescent proteins have not only been engineered for spectral properties (different colors), but also for size (to avoid/minimize interference with the localization and function of the target protein), oligomerization behavior (to avoid aggregation), brightness (the product of extinction coefficient and quantum yield) and photostability (robustness to photobleaching).

Certain fluorescent proteins, where the fluorescence properties can be changed upon exposure to light, are called photoactivatable, photoconvertible, or photoswitchable, which means they can be activated from a non-fluorescent to fluorescent state, they can change their emission spectrum (green to red) or they can be reversely switched on and off, respectively (Figure 9.18).

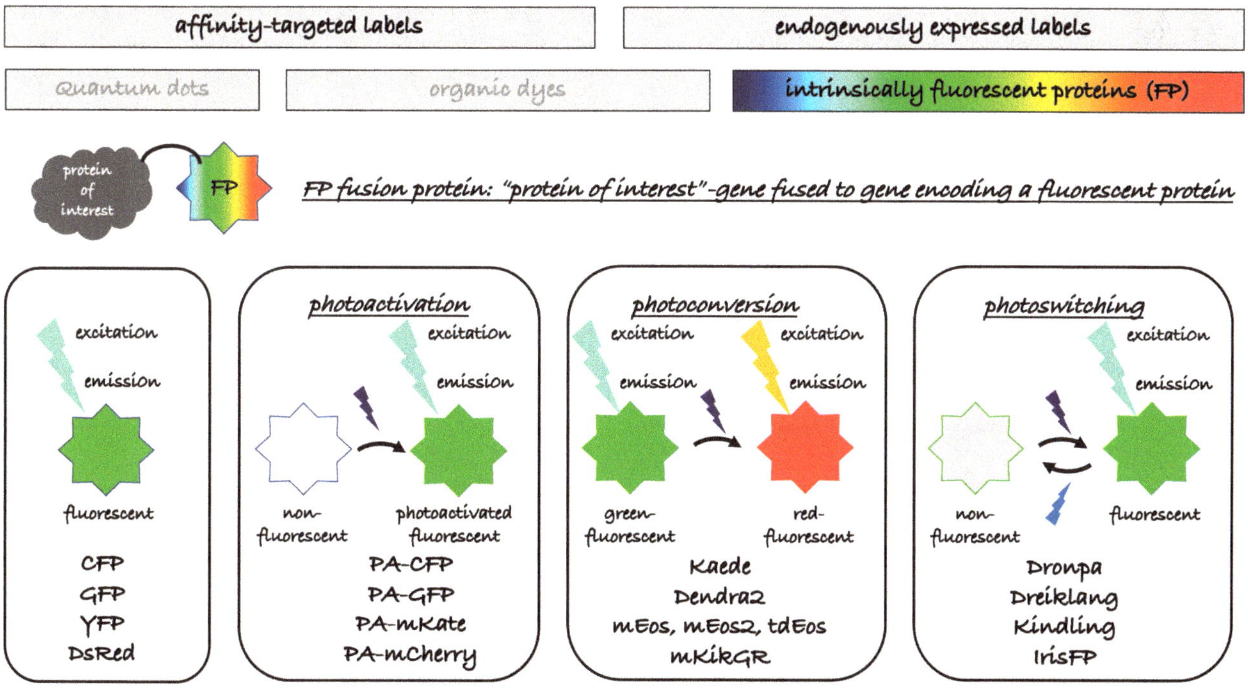

Figure 9.18 Intrinsically fluorescent proteins. Intrinsically fluorescent proteins (FP) are genetically expressed fluorophores, typically in form of a FP-target fusion protein. Among the intrinsically FP there are certain engineered versions that need to be photoactivated by a short pulse before fluorescent imaging, that can be photoconverted by a short pulse, switching from a green to red color, or that are photoswitchable, which means that one can alternate for many cycles between a non-fluorescent and a fluorescent state upon irradiation with the appropriate wavelengths.

9.7.2 Photoactivatable Fluorescent Proteins

Photoactivatable fluorescent proteins can be switched on by a short (<1 s) violet/blue light pulse, which means that the protein transitions from a low-fluorescent state to a high-fluorescent state (e.g., by a hundred-fold increase). In case of the PA-GFP, the underlying molecular process of photoactivation is the light-induced decarboxylation in one of the glutamate side chains. Photoactivatable fluorescent proteins are of particular interest for Photoactivated Localization Microscopy (PALM) superresolution imaging, but also for a variant of FRET imaging. Examples for photoactivatable fluorescent proteins are PA-GFP, PA-GFP/ECFP, PAmCherry, and PAmKate. It should be noted that photoactivatable fluorescent proteins are often less bright and less photostable than their non-activatable counterparts.

9.7.3 Photoconvertible Fluorescent Proteins

Photoconvertible fluorescent proteins were first discovered in stony corals. They irreversibly alter their emission spectra from green light to red (orange) light upon brief exposure to UV light. Examples of photoconvertible fluorescent proteins are Dendra2, Kaede, tdEosFP (dimeric), mEos and mEos2 (both monomeric) as well as mKikGR. The tags mKikGR, mEos2, and Dendra are frequently used in superresolution imaging such as PALM/STORM.

9.7.4 Photoswitchable Fluorescent Proteins

Photoswitchable fluorescent proteins, such as Dronpa, Dreiklang, Kindling FP, also alter their fluorescence emission states (non-fluorescent and fluorescent), but the conversion is reversible up to several hundred times without photobleaching. In the case of Dronpa, a light pulse at 405 nm will change Dronpa from a non-fluorescent to a fluorescent state, due to a trans–cis isomerization of a tyrosine side chain, which results in the protonation of the chromophore, whereas a light pulse at 488 nm will turn the fluorescence protein off.

IrisFP is a combination of photoconversion and photoswitching, whereas low-intensity 405 nm pulse turns the fluorophore from a dark state to a green-fluorescent stage (referred to as green IrisFP), and a 488 nm pulse switches it back to a dark state. A high-intensity 405 nm pulse turns green IrisFP dark state into red IrisFP dark state. A 440 nm laser pulse turns the red IrisFP on, whereas a 532 nm laser pulse turns the red-IrisFP from its fluorescent state back to its dark state.

Some fluorescent proteins act as reporters for pH, calcium, zinc, or chloride concentrations, phosphorylation, proteolysis (e.g., by cleaving the protein link between two fluorescent proteins, which leads to the loss of their ability for energy transfer from one fluorescent protein to the other, and thus a color change), or for the presence of certain lipids (e.g., by lipid-binding fluorescent protein fusion proteins). Also, there are commercially available organelle-specific probes (e.g., mitotracker, lysotracker) that are targeted by membrane potential.

9.7.5 Extrinsically Fluorescent Proteins

Extrinsically fluorescent proteins rely on the binding of an exogenous fluorophore and combine the advantages of specific labeling of the target protein (via genetic encoding of a tag fused to the target protein) with the advantages of synthetic fluorophores (such as brightness and photostability). The tags themselves are not fluorescent but covalently bind a label specific for the genetically encoded tag (Figure 9.19). Frequently one has a choice of labels linked with one of many different synthetic fluorophores, thus imaging experiments can be custom-tailored to experimental needs, using commercially available reagents with different colors or fluorophore properties. Simply by changing the label, while relying on the same protein tag, one can also carry out pulse-chase experiments.

Tags are often (but not always) smaller than intrinsically fluorescent proteins. The smallest example is the six-amino-acid long tetracysteine motif with a high affinity for arsenic-containing dyes such as FlAsH and ReAsH. SNAP and CLIP tags feature O^6-alkylguanine-DNA alkyltransferases that covalently bind benzylguanine and benzylcytosine derivatives, respectively. The Halo that is derived from haloalkane dehalogenase and reacts covalently with alkylhalides.

9.8 RNA/DNA – Fluorescent Probes

Also, tagged RNAs or RNA aptamers binding exogenous fluorophores exist as an alternative to fluorescent proteins. DNA Point Accumulation for Imaging in Nanoscale Topography (abbreviated as DNA-PAINT) uses fluorescent oligonucleotide DNA probes in combination with superresolution microscopy to map out DNA sequences on nuclear DNA. Fluorescence in situ hybridization (FISH) uses fluorescent probes attached to a nucleic acid sequence that is complimentary to the DNA target sequence of interest. It is often used for genotype- or species-identification (Figure 9.20).

While not much of an issue in regular fluorescence microscopy, the type of targeting of the fluorophore to the protein of interest becomes an important issue at high resolution. Synthetic dyes that are targeted to a macromolecule via a primary antibody, which are then recognized by

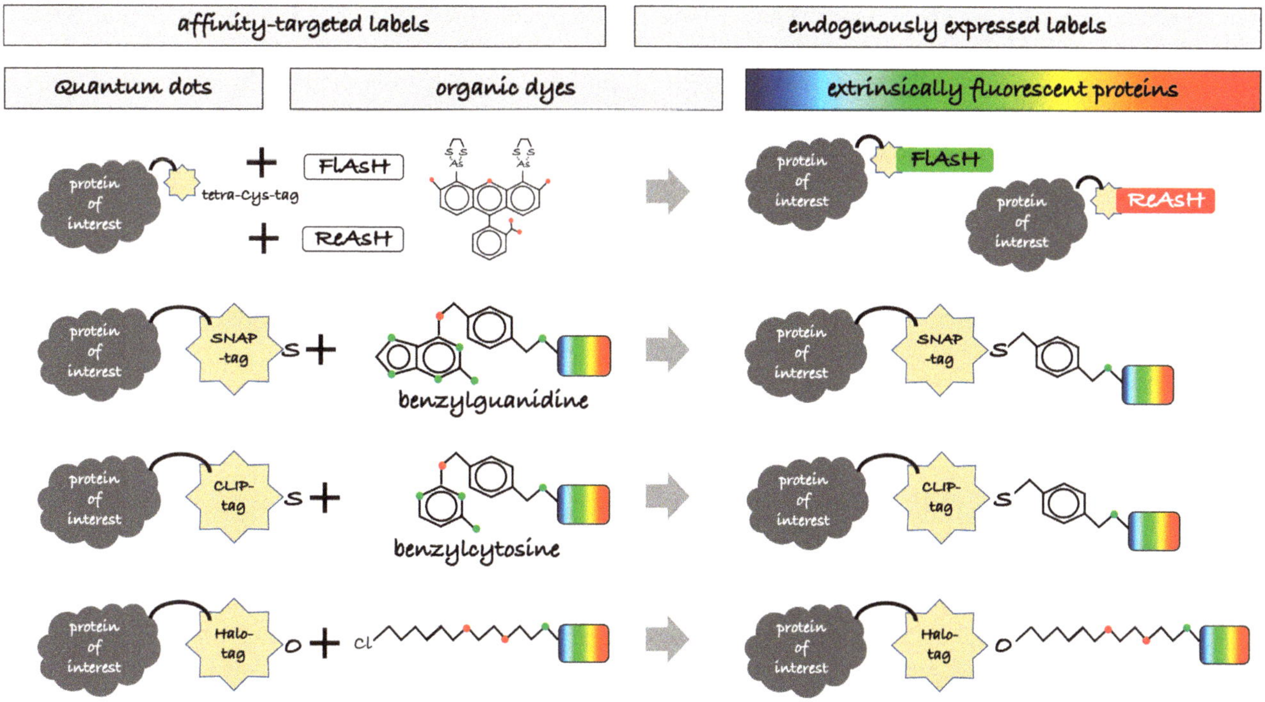

Figure 9.19 Extrinsically fluorescent proteins. Extrinsically fluorescent proteins are genetically encoded tags typically genetically engineered with a short linker to the target protein. The tags themselves are not fluorescent, but upon exposure to a label, which itself is conjugated to a fluorophore, the tags become fluorescent due to an irreversible covalent binding of the label (with its attached fluorophore). The most prominent tags are the tetracysteine tag (with the FlAsH or ReAsH label), the SNAP-tag (with the benzylguanidine label), the CLIP-tag (with the benzylcytosine label), and the Halo-tag binding alkylhalides.

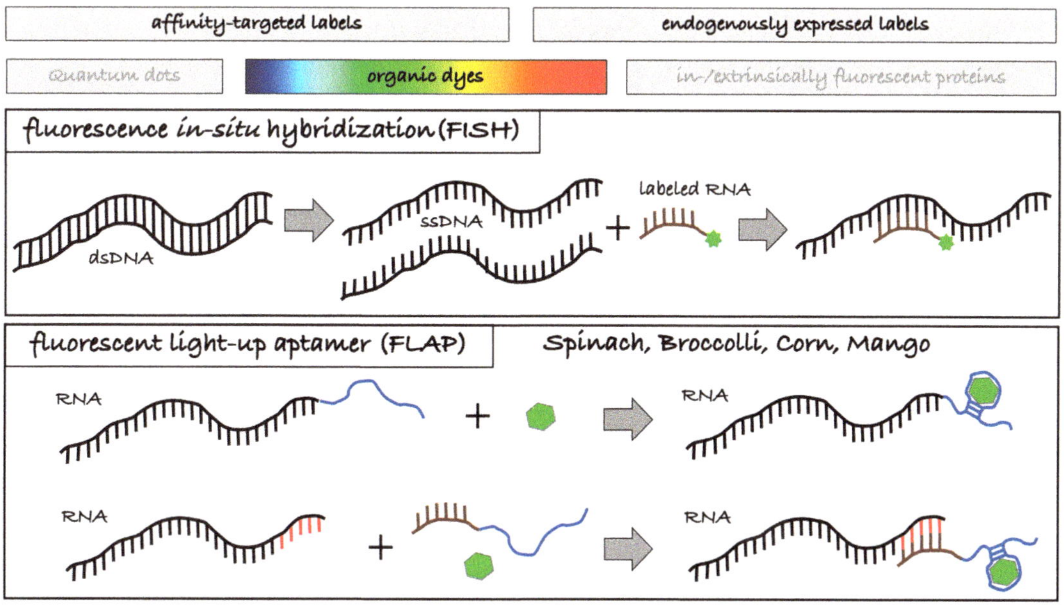

Figure 9.20 Fluorescent probes for DNA or RNA labeling. Fluorescence in-situ hybridization uses fluorophore-conjugated oligomeric nucleic sequences that are complementary and thus bind to their target sequences. Likewise, oligomeric DNA probes in combination with superresolution imaging can map out DNA sequences inside a cell's nucleus in a technique called DNA-PAINT. With respect to RNA, tagged RNA or RNA aptamers, also known as fluorescent light-up aptamers (FLAP), which include Spinach, Broccoli, Corn or Mango, can bind to single stranded RNA and then interact with a fluorophore upon refolding of the RNA sequence.

a fluorophore-conjugated secondary antibody have a high uncertainty of localization as the distance of the fluorophore to the target protein can be more than 20 nm, whereas in the case of fluorescent protein fusion proteins the distance is only ~3 nm.

Photobleaching (bleaching of the fluorophore upon imaging) and photodamage (damage to cellular health due to the conversion of regular triplet molecular oxygens to highly reactive singlet oxygen) remain a challenge in fluorescent imaging and many imaging approaches have been developed with the aim of reducing both. Removing oxygen or scavenging radical oxygen species helps in reducing photodamage.

9.9 Fluorescent Imaging Types

There are a variety of fluorescence imaging approaches, each with their own fluorophore property requirements, illumination requirements, optical path requirements, sample preparation requirements, data collection requirements, detector requirements, as well as processing requirements, ranging from the very simple (such as epifluorescence microscopy) to the very sophisticated (super-resolution microscopy).

One fundamental limitation of fluorescence imaging is photobleaching, which means there is typically a finite number of photons that can be detected from a single fluorophore. This affects decisions that need to be taken with respect to the object size that needs to be imaged, the resolution one aims for, the brightness of the signal one wants to collect, as well as the time period over which the sample is imaged. Much effort has been spent on the side of fluorescent dyes to engineer fade-resistant dyes or to use anti-fade compounds in the experiment. Another remedy is to budget the total amount of photons one has available, e.g., by only exposing the sample to photons while collecting data and by minimizing the volume that is exposed to excitation light. This will avoid excitation of out-of-focus that will not contribute to image formation (and only adding to a background signal). Generally, it is advisable to minimize exposure time and excitation power (Figure 9.21).

9.10 Detangling the Many Fluorescence Imaging Approaches

There were a variety of developments in fluorescence microscopy, which have resulted in the large variety of fluorescence imaging approaches available nowadays. Some developments have aimed to improve axial resolution (confocal, 4Pi, deconvolution), some others to minimize unnecessary light exposure to reduce photobleaching and phototoxicity, and thus allow long-term microscopic observation of living systems (two-photon, single-plane illumination, light sheet imaging), whereas yet other have focused to improving the lateral resolution including surpassing Abbe's diffraction limit of optical microscopy (superresolution techniques including SIM, STED, PALM, STORM, near-field imaging).

In addition, other imaging specializations have aimed to assess the dynamic behavior of macromolecules in living cells and tissues (FRAP, FLIP, FLIM, FCS, FRET).

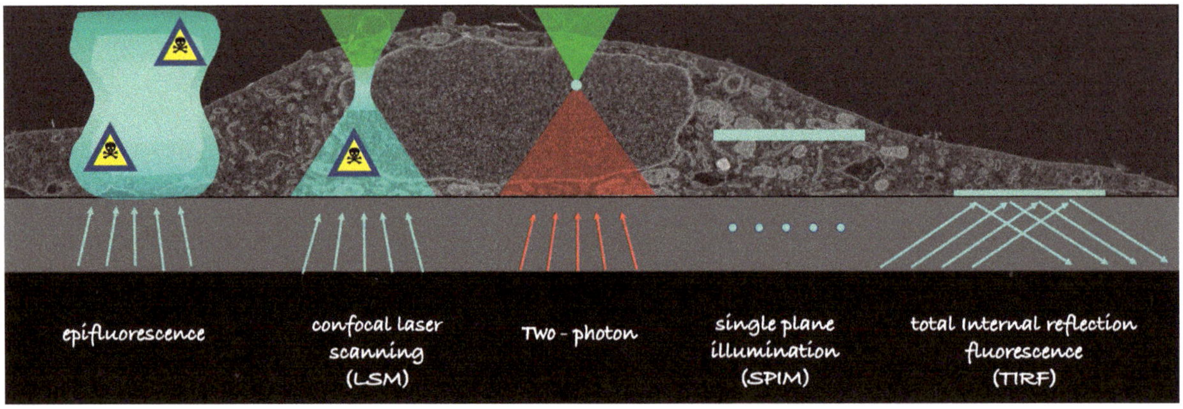

Figure 9.21 Different fluorescent imaging approaches: Epifluorescence, confocal, two-photon, single plane illumination, and total internal reflection fluorescence (TIRF) imaging. In epifluorescence, many out-of-focus fluorophores are unnecessarily excited and will contribute to a large background. Confocal laser scanning microscopy will reduce but not eliminate unnecessary irradiation. Two-photon overcomes unnecessary illumination, first by irradiating with photons twice the wavelength (which are much less damaging) and second by only exciting fluorophores in a small volume at the focus point where the photon density is high enough for two photons being absorbed simultaneously. Single plane illumination microscopy (SPIM) only excited a thin layer of the sample perpendicular to the imaging direction, from which an image is recorded. In total internal reflection fluorescence (TIRF) imaging, only a thin layer (the evanescent field) near the coverslip surface is being irradiated, hence the signal has very little background.

9.11 Improve Axial Resolution and Reduce Phototoxicity

Among the challenges of conventional epifluorescence microscopy is that all fluorophores that are irradiated give off fluorescence, whether they were in the focal plane or not. Out-of-focus fluorescence results in a large background signal, which degrades the images. Also, since the photons of the background signal do not contribute constructively to an image, they are wasted as the total dose a sample can tolerate is often limited due to phototoxicity and photobleaching. Thus, many photons may be unnecessarily excited without yielding any image information. Hence, there are two goals, namely to improve axial resolution and to minimize unnecessary irradiation.

9.11.1 Epifluorescence Microscopy

In epifluorescence microscopy, which is the most basic of all fluorescence microscopy techniques, illumination and detection occur from the same side of the sample (epi-illumination), with a light passing through a dichroic mirror cube with an excitation filter and the objective lens before illuminating the sample. The emitted fluorescence light is collected by the objective lens (ideally with a high-NA lens) from the same side as the illumination, and enters the dichroic mirror cube, where it is deflected (due to its altered wavelength) via an emission filter onto the detector.

9.11.2 Deconvolution Microscopy

Deconvolution microscopy is a strategy to mathematically deal with out-of-focus contributions from photons above and below the focal plane, which lead to blurring of the image features. Instead of simply rejecting such photons, which is the strategy of pinhole confocal microscopy, the contributions of the photons are "re-sorted to their respective image plane" by the process of deconvolution. In a deconvolution microscope one takes focus-series of the samples and mathematically treats the images knowing (or have an initial estimate of) what the PSF is. It is based on the idea that an object is convoluted with a microscope's PSF. Hence by collecting images at different focal planes, and having knowledge about the PSF, one can mathematically revert this process of convolution, hence the term deconvolution. This typically results in a much-sharpened depiction of the fluorescence signal. However, deconvolution bears the risk of artifacts and thus data from deconvolution microscopy must be interpreted with caution (Figure 9.22).

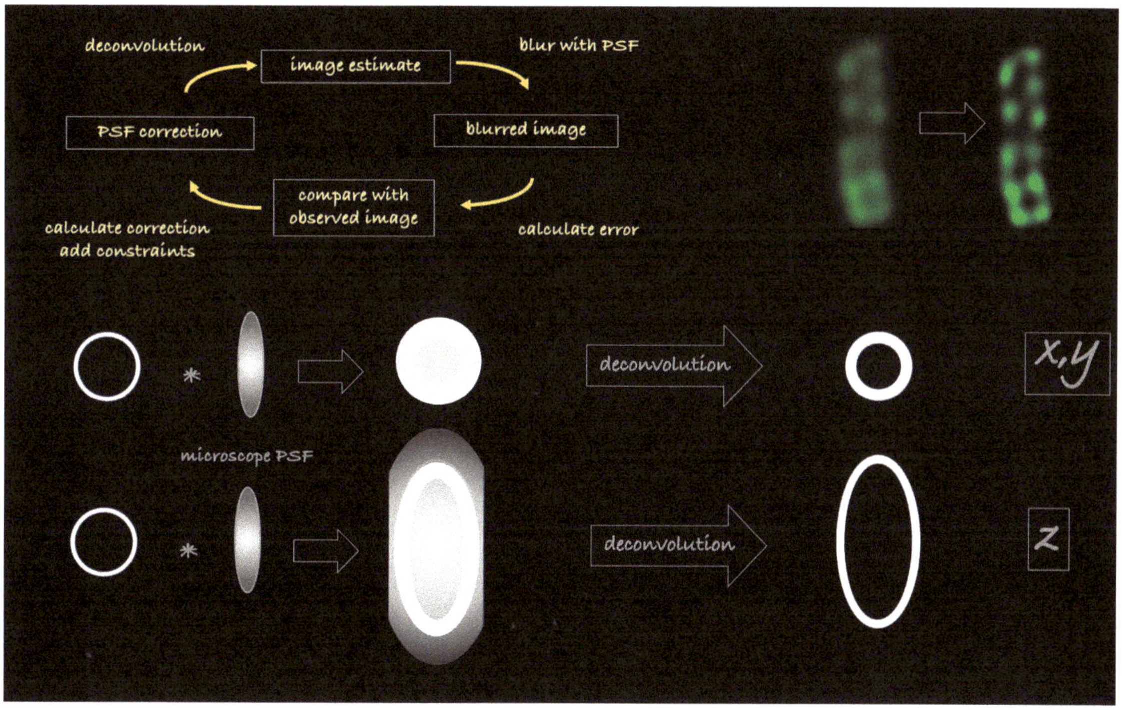

Figure 9.22 Deconvolution microscopy. Any point source in a microscope gets blurred by the microscope's point spread function (PSF). By using multiple images obtained at different focal planes, one can "re-sort" the contribution of out-of-focus photons to the image. Deconvolution is a rather complex mathematical process that uses information one has about the PSF to undo the blurring. To obtain best results, the parameters for deconvolution including assumptions about the PSF are iteratively refined. Deconvolution leads to much sharper images, but care must be taken not to introduce image artifacts.

9.11.3 Confocal Laser Scanning Microscopy

The experimental setup of a confocal laser scanning microscope (CLSM) differs from an epifluorescence microscope. A CLSM uses a laser for spot-scan illumination, a dichroic mirror and a pinhole aperture positioned near the detector. The emitted fluorescent light is being collected by the objective lens before it reaches a point detector (e.g., a PMT) via an aperture that rejects out-of-focus photons (Figure 9.23). However, while out-of-focus-light is rejected by the pinhole, fluorophores residing outside the focal plane were still excited and unnecessarily exposed to irradiation.

2D images are collected by moving either the stage with the sample or the beam (through the use of moving mirrors, which is faster and easier than moving the stage) laterally (in the *X*,*Y* directions). By moving the stage axially (in the *Z*-direction) through the focal point, one can build up a 3D volume, with a lateral resolution of ~200 nm and an axial resolution of ~500–800 nm, a process also known as optical sectioning.

9.11.4 Spinning Disk Confocal Microscope

Spinning disk confocal microscope is one form of confocal microscopy, which can scan multiple points simultaneously across the sample, instead of only one single point as regular CLSM do. This is accomplished by a set of pinholes in a disk that is rotating (Nipkow disk), eventually illuminating the entire sample (Figure 9.24). Microlens-enhanced or dual spinning disk confocal microscopes have a second disk spinning at the same speed that contains microlenses, which capture a broad band of light and focus it into the pinhole, thus increasing sensitivity.

The fluorescence signal is detected by a digital area-detector, typically an EMCCD or a CMOS detector, and a 2D image is formed by the fluorescent light detected at the respective spinning disk position. Among its advantages over conventional confocal laser scanning microscopes is that image acquisition is much faster. Also, phototoxicity and photobleaching are often reduced compared, making spinning disk confocal microscopes a preferred system for imaging live cells and organisms.

9.11.5 4Pi and Confocal Theta Microscopy

4Pi microscopy is an optical 3D imaging technique that improves axial resolution of a laser scanning microscope by a factor of ~3–5, and thus accomplishes a near spherical shape of the central portion of the PSF of ~100–150 nm, with an additional higher-order side lobe above and below. This accomplished by illuminating the sample with two opposing lenses of high NA, which leads to a coherent superposition of two focused wavefronts. The 4Pi microscope uses a beam splitter, two mirrors and objective lenses (one on each side of the specimen) to illuminate (and record fluorescence from) the common focal volume from both two sides (Figure 9.25).

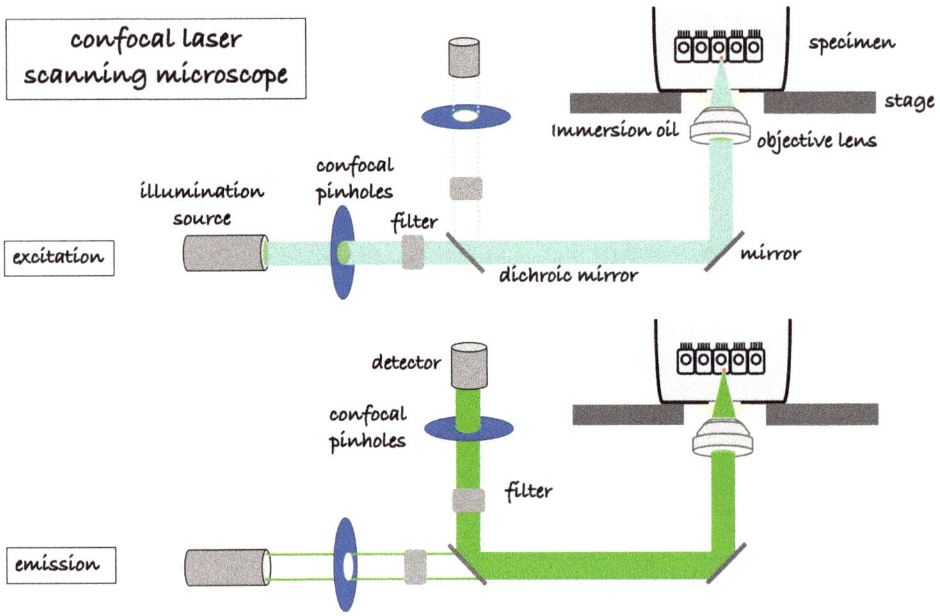

Figure 9.23 Confocal laser scanning microscopy. In a classical confocal microscope, two pinholes at equal focal length (hence the term confocal) are placed in the optical path to reject out-of-focus contributions from image planes above and below the focal plane. With the use of laser light for illumination, only one pinhole (in front of the detector) is needed. For data collection in confocal laser scanning microscopy (CLSM) the beam is typically scanned as a small spot over the sample with the help of two or more fast-moving mirrors, with the emitted fluorescence light reaching a point detector to build up the raster image point-by-point. To obtain Z-stacks, and thus 3D volumes, the stage is move via piezo motors through the focal plane.

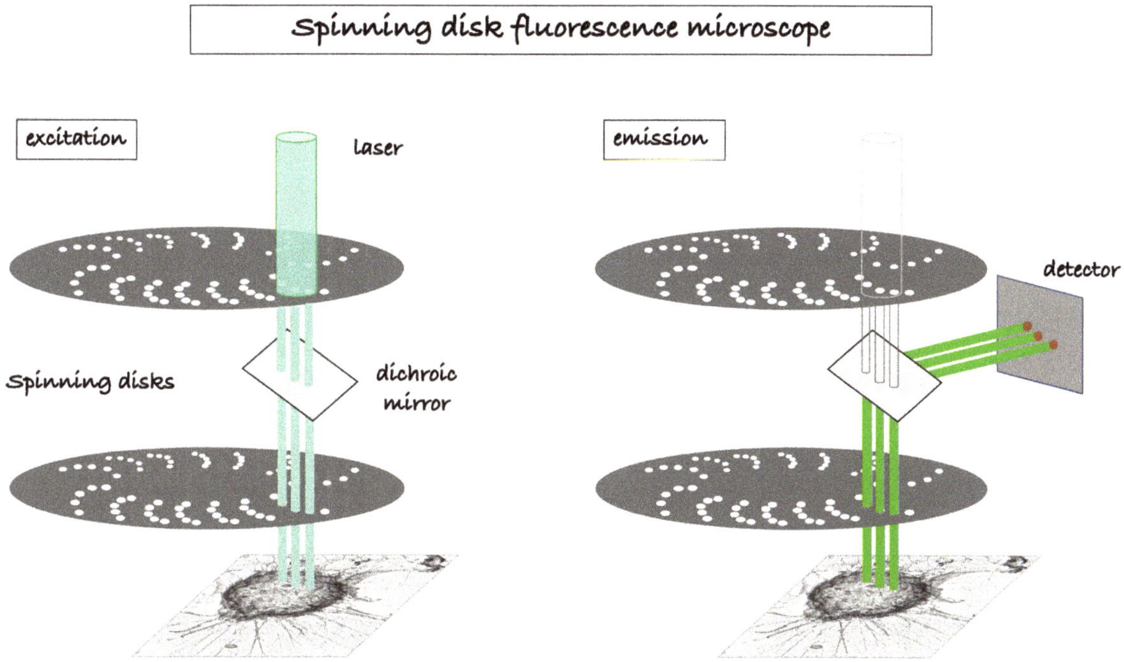

Figure 9.24 Dual spinning disk confocal microscopy. Spinning disk confocal microscopy scans multiple points across the sample simultaneously, courtesy of a set of pinholes in a rotating disk (Nipkow disk). In the case of (microlens-enhanced) dual spinning confocal microscope two disks are used that spin at the same speed, with microlenses (not shown here) focusing all incoming light into the pinholes of the second disk. The signal is read out by a digital area detector such as EMCCD or CMOS. Advantages of the dual spinning disk confocal microscope are the speed of data acquisition, the high sensitivity, low phototoxicity and photobleaching, which makes this approach ideal for imaging live cells and organisms.

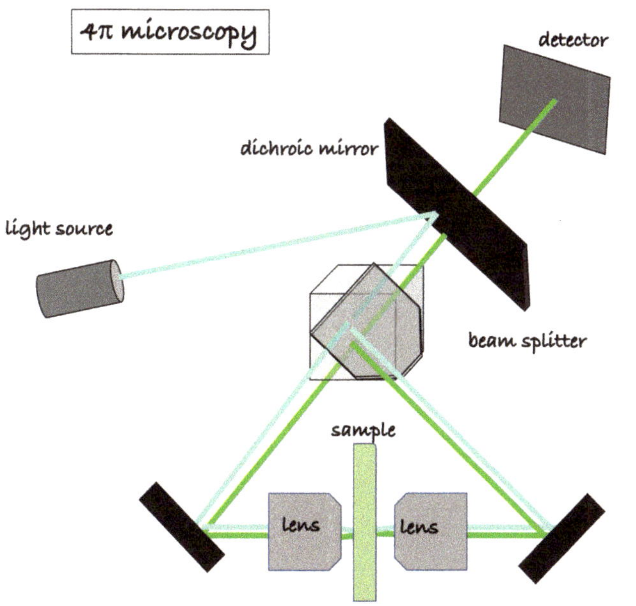

Figure 9.25 4Pi microscopy. In 4Pi microscopy, a sample is illuminated by a beam splitter, two mirrors and two opposing lenses of high numerical aperture, leading to a superposition of two wavefronts. This results in a central portion spherical PSF of ~100–150 nm, as well as a small higher-order lobe on both sides of the center, thus increasing axial resolution by a factor of 3–5. 4Pi illumination can also be combined with theta-microscopy, where the detection occurs at a 90° angle with respect to illumination axis.

Constructive interference will result in a spherical main maximum and two pronounced side lobes (one on either side). These higher-order side lobes are much lower in terms of intensity, and thus only contribute little to the overall image. Whereas the shape of the PSF of a conventional confocal microscope is highly elliptical (500–700 nm along the long axis), the PSF of a 4Pi microscope is nearly perfectly spherical. The combination of 4Pi microscopy with STED, e.g., in form of the RESOLFT microscopy with switchable proteins, allows imaging of living cells at low light levels with ~40 nm isotropic resolution.

Another way to increase axial resolution is confocal theta microscopy, where the sample is imaged with two or more objective lenses, positioned at an angle theta (ideal is 90° relative to the illumination axis). This approach also results in a near spherical observation volume and thus ~threefold smaller than in a conventional confocal microscope. Confocal theta microscopy can be combined with 4Pi illumination, further improving the resolution. Confocal theta microscopy paved the way for SPIM. Also, deconvolution can be employed to further improve contrast for both the in-plane and axial direction.

9.11.6 Two-Photon Microscopy

Two-Photon microscopy is an optical sectioning variant of confocal light microscopy and is best suited for thicker specimen, such as tissues of 200 µm to several mm of thickness. Two-photon microscopy is also particularly suitable for imaging cellular-level details in live samples, as for fixed samples there are alternative approaches such as physical sectioning or tissue clearing prior to imaging.

As absorption and scattering of shorter wavelength light limits tissue penetration depth, use of near IR radiation is the method of choice for deep tissue imaging, including for Cy7-dye imaging, commonly used for whole animal imaging. Alternatively, standard fluorescence dyes (e.g., Alexa dyes) with absorption and emission spectra in the visible light range can be used if two photons at the same frequency (wavelength) are absorbed simultaneously (within a femtosecond) by the fluorophore. Simultaneous two-photon absorption then result in the excitation of the molecule from a ground state to an excited state at an energy twice that of the original photons (Figure 9.26). Hence the molecules, by simultaneously absorbing two lower-energy photons, behaves as if it had absorbed a single photon at twice the frequency (half the wavelength). This requires a high-intensity laser, and since illumination is focused on a single point, photobleaching is reduced outside the focus, which is advantageous for imaging living samples. However, inside the focal volume, photon intensity is very high, and thus can be detrimental to the sample.

Pulsed infrared-lasers are used for excitation, with the photon intensity being only high enough in the focal point of the laser. Pulsed Ti:sapphire lasers are ideal (and thus have become popular workhorse lasers), as they are tunable between 700 and 1,000 nm, and attain a high peak power (~150,000 W) with an normal average power (1 W), due to the short laser pulse width (~80 fs) and a high repetition rate (80 MHz, 12.5 ns between pulses).

In two-photon microscopy, there is little to no out-of-focus fluorescence contribution, hence pinholes, as typically used in confocal microscopy, are not necessary. Ideal dyes have a broad excitation spectrum, so that a single laser can excite multiple dyes simultaneously, and multiple fluorescence emissions can be detected simultaneously, e.g., by using multiple dichroic mirrors that split the emitted light into the various color components. Longer-wavelength excitation means that incoming light is neither scattered nor absorbed before reaching the focal point. While shorter wavelength emitted fluorescence light may be scattered by the tissue, all light can be collected independent of its path and assigned to the focal volume, as this volume was the only volume that has been illuminated. Images are recorded by scanning a laser point-by-point over the sample and by recording all intensity at each spot, e.g., by a so-called "non-descanned" detector. Multiphoton imaging, i.e., excitation by three photons is only a marginal improvement; however, two-photon imaging is often referred to as multiphoton imaging as the more general term.

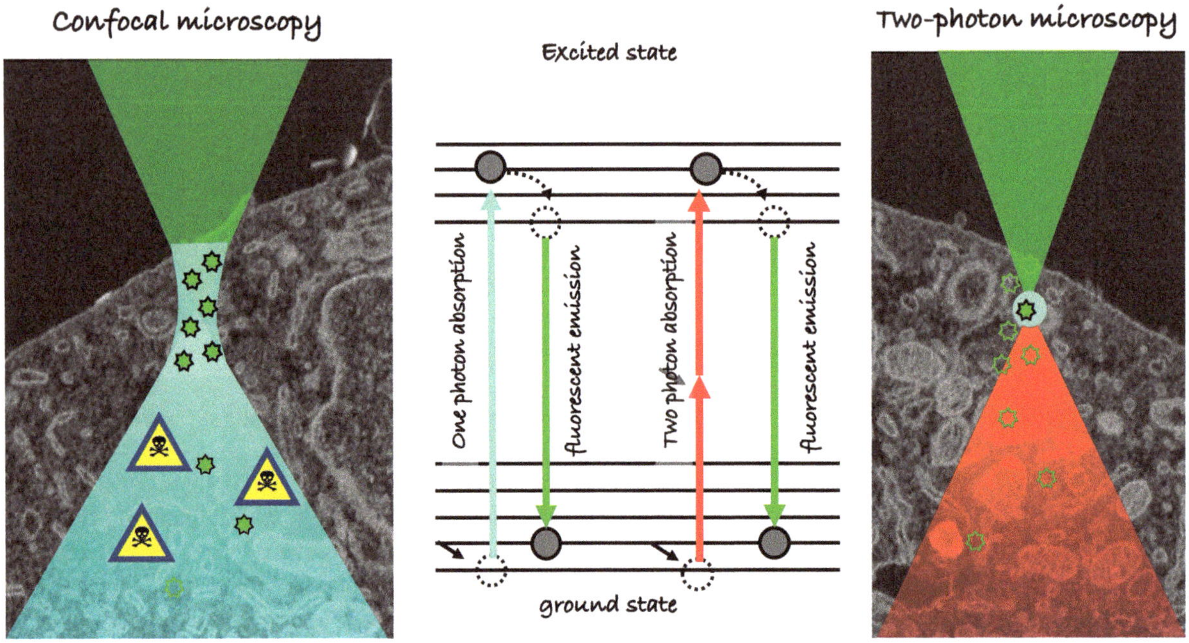

Figure 9.26 Two-photon microscopy. Two-photon microscopy uses a pulsed Ti:sapphire laser tunable to 700–1,000 nm for excitation of fluorophores in tissues thicker than 200 µm. In this spot-scan technique, fluorophore molecules absorb two photons (at double the wavelength) simultaneously, which only happens in the focal point where the photon density is high enough for simultaneous photon uptake to occur. This results in a very small volume from where emitted fluorescence can originate and thus high axial resolution can be achieved.

Second harmonic generation (SHG) microscopy is related to two-photon microscopy, with high-intensity laser light being absorbed in the near infrared and reemitted at double the frequency/half the wavelength of the incident light. It is a non-linear process, and thus brightness scales as the square of excitation light intensity, requiring bright-pulsed laser illumination. However, while two-photon microscopy is a fluorescence light technique, with dissipation of some energy in a non-radiative way, in SHG microscopy the emitted light is exactly half the wavelength of the incident light. SHG microscopy is ideal for visualization of certain anisotropic molecules such as collagen I and IV, cellulose and some amphiphilic or hydrophobic membrane dye molecules that can be aligned by the electric field present across cell membranes.

9.11.7 Single Plane Illumination Microscopy (SPIM)

Confocal microscopy with its confocal pinhole setup is in essence an out-of-focus light rejection technique, while still a substantial fraction of the sample is being illuminated, in other words, there is plenty of unnecessary light exposure, which leads to photobleaching and phototoxicity. SPIM, also referred to as light sheet microscopy, is one of the approaches that minimizes/avoids such unnecessary exposure. This makes SPIM the ideal tool in cell and developmental biology for long-term imaging studies of regions very deep inside a tissue with minimal detriment to the sample and retention of the imaging signal. Light sheet microscopy often penetrates even large specimen, and since it only illuminates a single plane, it results in several orders of magnitude lower energy compared to widefield or confocal microscopy, and thus less phototoxicity. Embryos, even if continuously imaged by light sheet microscopy, typically show no radiation stress and develop normally.

In SPIM, a defined homogeneous sheet of spatially constrained intense light illuminates the sample orthogonal to the imaging objective and stimulates fluorescence emission only within that volume. The fluorescence signal is collected by the objective lens which is orthogonal to the plane of propagation of the light sheet and reaches an area detector, such as a CCD or a CMOS detector. A 3D volume can be obtained in a similar way to regular confocal microscopy by moving the stage with the sample via Piezo actuators through the light sheet (Figure 9.27).

Creating thin light sheets can be difficult to accomplish, particularly for thick samples such as a mouse brain, whereas one can image a large specimen at low resolution or a smaller specimen at higher resolution. Another challenge for light sheet microscopy poses changes in the refractive index throughout the sample (e.g., air-filled compartments) as such changes will result in absorption and scattering of light. One solution may be to deploy multiple axially coincident light sheets from different angles (which can be experimentally difficult to attain) or to rotate the sample (e.g., mounted in agarose), if one wants to image live samples. Rotating the sample is much simpler than deploying multiple light sheets. 3D volumes are reconstructed from the multiple views of the rotating samples, to study the development of embryos (like zebrafish or *Drosophila melanogaster*). If the sample is chemically fixed, one can also carry out tissue clearing to improve light penetration.

Dual-View Inverted Selective Plane Illumination Microscopy (diSPIM) uses an inverted microscope setup with a sample stage that is accessible from the top to a pair of objective lenses, arranged at a 90° angle to one another,

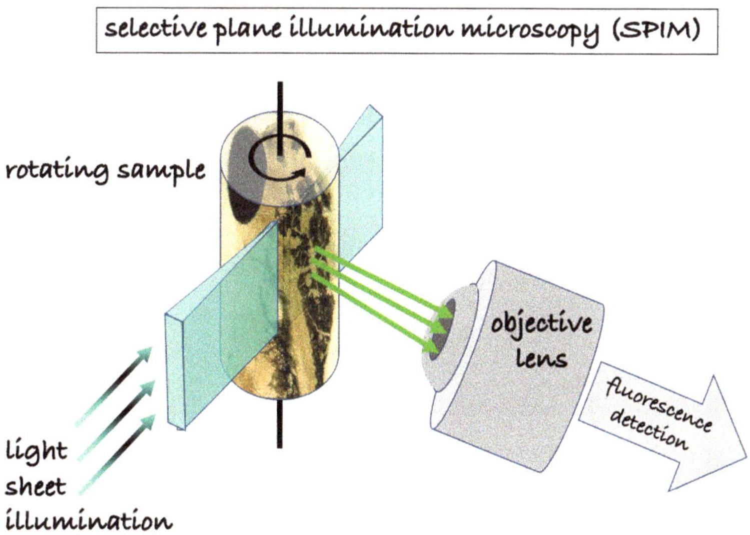

Figure 9.27 Single plane illumination microscopy. Single plane illumination microscopy (SPIM), also known as light sheet microscopy, illuminates a single plane of the sample and thus only excites fluorophores in that plane. Detection of the fluorescent signal is orthogonal to the light sheet by an area detector. SPIM avoids unnecessary irradiation, leading to less phototoxicity and thus is ideal for long-term studies in cell and developmental biology.

with both focusing on the sample using water-dipping lenses. Both lenses take turns to deliver a light sheet for excitation, while the other collects the fluorescence signal.

With this geometry, diSPIM overcomes one of the shortcomings of regular light sheet microscopy, namely the fluorescence signal anisotropy (three times better resolution in *X*,*Y* compared to *Z*), and produces images with isotropic high axial resolution details. By using very fast cameras and *Z*-axis control, collection of high-quality datasets is fast and non-detrimental to the development of *Caenorhabditis elegans* or *D. melanogaster*, however extensive post-processing of the raw image data is needed to obtain high-resolution data. There are commercial versions of the diSPIM microscope available.

Lattice light sheet microscopy uses spatially modulated light (and annular illumination) to create a defined Bessel beam profile being swept across a sample. While collecting the fluorescence signal from a very thin illumination layer orthogonal to the lattice light sheet is very simple, generating the Bessel beam can be extremely complex, however commercial solutions are available (although at a high price tag). Lattice light sheet microscopy displays high speed, high sensitivity and no apparent phototoxicity. A more cost-effective solution is the so-called "LITE" sheet approach that uses a barrel lens and an interference grating to generate a light sheet. Compared to lattice sheet microscopy, "LITE" sheet microscopy is also much simpler, not only for data collection but also for image reconstruction and post-processing. However, LITE sheet microscopy does not match the axial resolution of lattice sheet microscopy.

9.11.8 Total-Internal Reflection Fluorescence (TIRF) Microscopy

TIRF microscopy allows imaging of a sample very close (within ~100 nm) to the coverslip surface and thus greatly reduces the problem of background fluorescence. TIRF has been successfully applied to the field of single molecule (in-vitro) imaging and live cell culture (in-vivo) imaging. TIRF works by illuminating the sample (typically by a laser, but mercury arc lamps also work) at a very oblique angle close to the surface of a glass coverslip. As the light approaches at a large-enough angle the glass/water (buffer) interface, the beam is totally reflected (Figure 9.28).

However, there is a so-called evanescent (vanishing) field right beyond the glass-water interface, with a field strength decaying exponentially. Such oblique off-axis illumination is either accomplished by a trapezoid prism or a high-aperture condenser lens. The prism-less, objective based approach of TIRF imaging requires a lens with a NA being higher than the refractive medium, with the collimated (parallel) light being focused off-axis in the back focal plane. Among the useful features of TIRF is the very

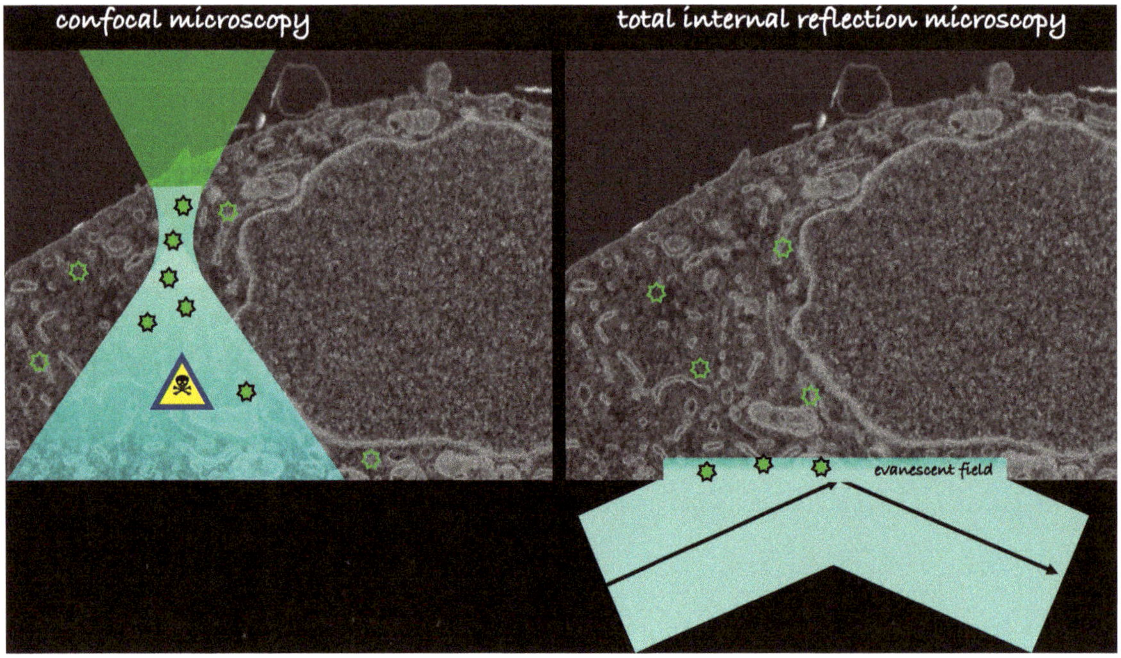

Figure 9.28 Total internal reflection fluorescence microscopy. In total internal reflection fluorescence (TIRF) microscopy, illumination at a high angle leads to internal reflection of the light at the coverslip-sample boundary. While the vast majority of the light is reflected, a very thin evanescent field enters the sample and falls off exponentially. This means that in the first 50–100 nm, there is sufficient light to excite fluorophores in that volume. Among its advantages TIRF shows no background fluorescent signal and shows no phototoxicity in the sample, but only a very thin region can be imaged.

low background in single molecule imaging and the very low phototoxicity for cell culture cells, as most parts of the cell are not illuminated by this technique.

9.12 Superresolution Imaging – Breaking the Resolution Barrier

Breaking Abbé's diffraction barrier of optical imaging has been a long-term objective in optical microscopy. Due to the diffraction-limit of optical microscopy, any point source of (fluorescent) light imaging is blurred into an Airy disk, which is equivalent to the point-spread-function. In practical terms that means that depending on the wavelength and lens' NA used, the maximum resolution in diffraction is between 200 and 250 nm (often set at ~220 nm).

While the center of such a single Airy disk can be determined with nanometer-scale precision, two overlapping Airy disks can only be distinguished as two separate Airy disks (each stemming from one of the two point sources of light), if the center of one Airy disk lies at least as far as the first minimum of its adjacent Airy disk. Any distance closer is considered not resolved.

At the center of most superresolution techniques are light-controllable (or photo-controllable) fluorescent proteins, whose fluorescent state can be regulated by irradiation with specific wavelengths. There are three categories, namely photoactivatable fluorescent proteins, photoconvertible fluorescent proteins, as well as reversibly photoswitchable fluorescent proteins.

9.12.1 Photoactivation

Photoactivation is a process by which a non-fluorescent version of a fluorescent protein undergoes an irreversible change that renders the genetically encoded fluorescent protein excitable and thus detectable upon emission of fluorescence, when excited by the correct wavelength. With only a small fraction of all fluorescent proteins being activated at a given time, only a small number of fluorescent proteins can be detected at any given time point. While the resulting images are still diffraction-limited, the sparse labeling leads to well-separated Airy disks whose center can be determined with high precision. Such centers are recorded for each image during data collection, resulting in a final fluorophore distribution upon superimposing all determined Airy-disk center positions (Figure 9.29).

9.12.2 Photoconversion

In the case of photoconversion, the distinguishing feature is not the transition of the reporter molecule from a non-fluorescent to a fluorescent state, but a change in the emission spectrum (and thus color) that similarly to photoactivation will only affect a small portion all available fluorophores. Hence, it is a small fraction of fluorophores

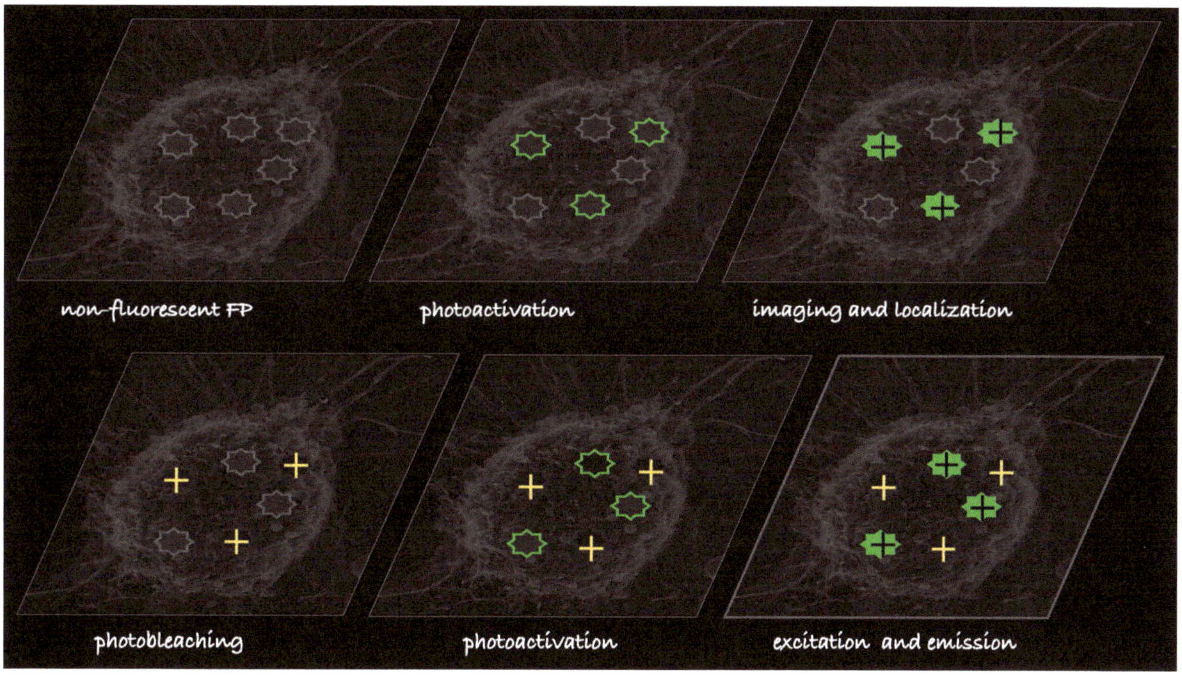

Figure 9.29 Photoactivation. In photoactivation, at any given time only a small fraction of all fluorescent proteins (FP) is activated and thus available for fluorescence imaging. After imaging, the activated FP are photobleached and a new round of photoactivation is initiated. For every image recorded only a small number of fluorophores and their Airy disks are detected. For every image, the center of each Airy disk can be established with high accuracy and will be stored to be displayed in the final image.

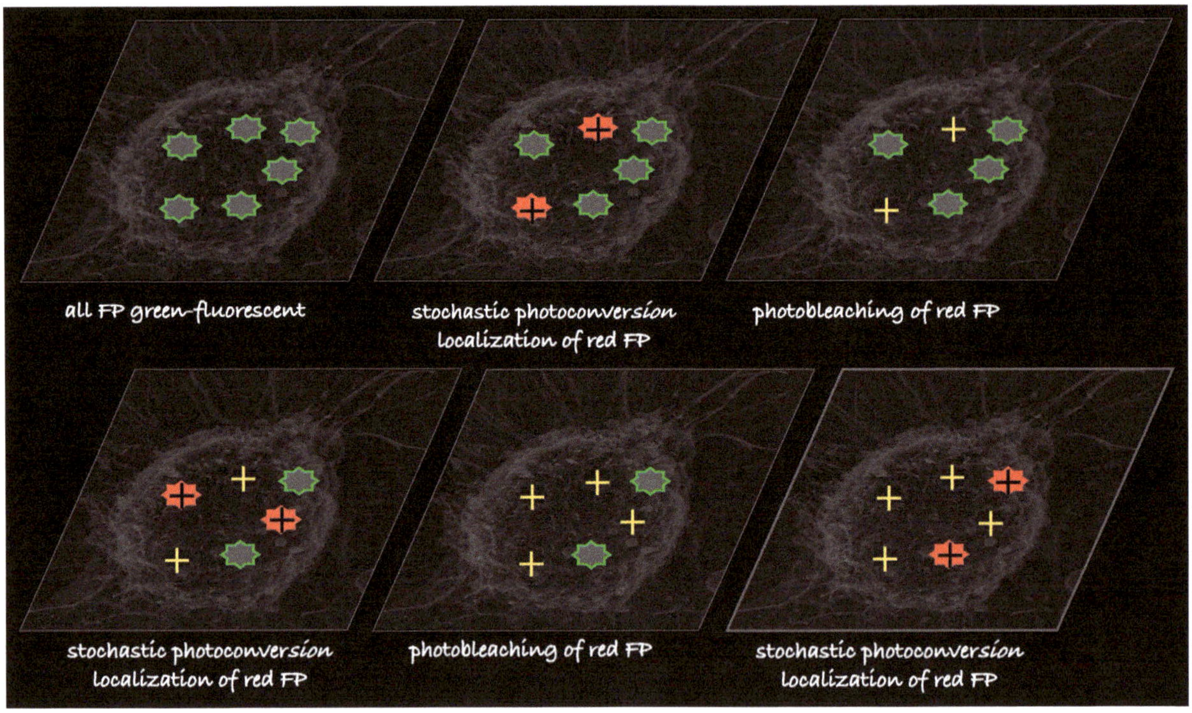

Figure 9.30 Photoconversion. Like in photoactivation, in photoconversion only a small portion of the fluorophores distinguish themselves in every round of photoconversion, changing their emission spectrum from green to red. Thus, the position of each Airy disk for all red signals can be determined with high precision, followed by photobleaching of the red fluorescent protein. The final image then lists all positions of all the Airy disks.

at any given time that had undergone such photoconversion from one emission spectrum (color) to another one. Likewise, its exact position can be determined (Figure 9.30).

9.12.3 Photoswitching

Photoswitchable fluorescent proteins can be switched between fluorescent and non-fluorescent (dark) states many times before they bleach, allowing the recording of a signal over many cycles of on- and off-switching (Figure 9.31).

9.13 Superresolution Imaging

To break the diffraction barrier of light there are two different approaches that are either based on (1) localization of single molecules or (2) on non-linear illumination approaches that reduce the size of an ensemble of fluorophores and thus sharpen its PSF. The second approach is sometimes also referred to as PSF engineering or patterned illumination approach.

9.13.1 Single-Molecule Localization Microscopy

In localization microscopy, only a small portion of all available fluorophores is photoactivated an any given time, resulting in a stochastic distribution of light emitting fluorophores. Hence, the Airy disks of single molecules emitting fluorescent photons can be imaged independently from one another as they on average are sufficiently spaced from one another. The sample is imaged repeatedly, with only a few fluorophores being activated stochastically at any given time. The light these individual fluorophores emit is collected and the activated fluorophores are eventually bleached (Figure 9.32).

STORM and photoactivated localization microscopy (PALM) are based on the principle that the center of each disk can be determined with high precision and thus its coordinates can be stored digitally. It should be noted however, that a sufficient number of photons is needed for an accurate estimate of the Airy disk center. In the case of sequential imaging of Airy disk centers, the final image is put together by recalling the coordinates from a long list of Airy disk center coordinates (Figure 9.32). However, the accuracy of determining the center also relies on the number of photons recorded, thus the experimentally measured localization precision is often worse than a theoretically possible value. The typical single-molecule density in biological samples ranges from 10^5 to 10^3 molecules per μm^2, allowing a lateral resolution of 6 to 48 nm, respectively. Also, PALM requires the recording of tens of thousands of images for a single superresolution image. Thus, PALM is a rather slow process, and often used for fixed samples rather than life sample, where the dynamics of the biological processes

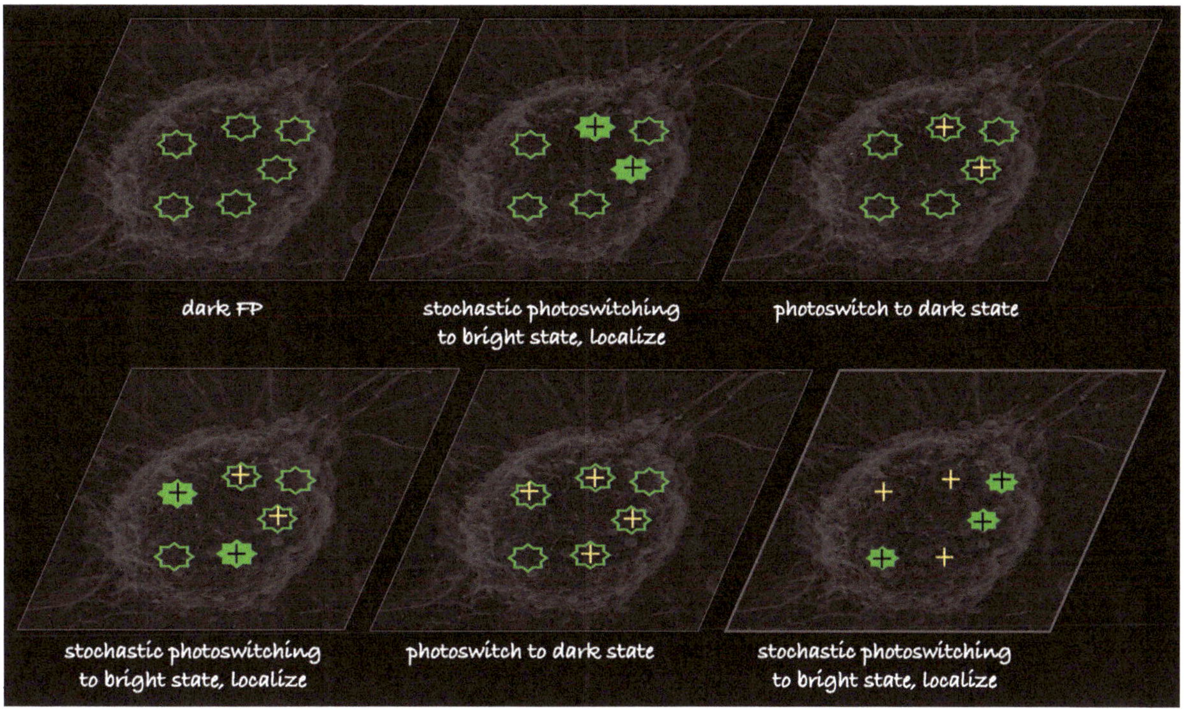

Figure 9.31 Photoswitching. In stochastic photoswitching, only a small fraction of fluorophores is switched at any given time between a bright fluorescent state and a non-fluorescent dark state. Like in photoactivation and photoconversion, the fluorophore's position is localized.

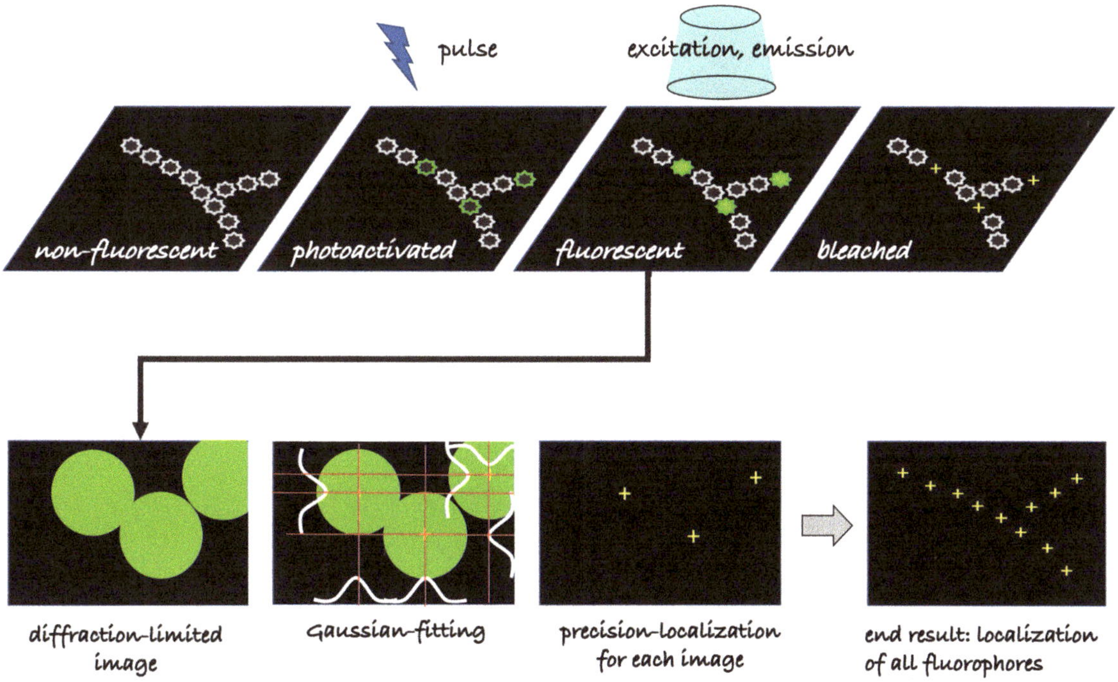

Figure 9.32 Single molecule localization microscopy – PALM. In single molecule localization microscopy, for every cycle only a small portion of all fluorophores is activated, and their Airy disks are detected. Gaussian fitting results in precision-localization of the center of the Airy disks. The final image is then a composition of all detected fluorophores.

have been fixed in place and time. More recently, variations on PALM relying in reversible switchable fluorescent proteins, such as PALM with independently running acquisition (PALMIRA), stroboscopic PALM (sPALM) or photochromic stochastic optical fluctuation imaging (pcSOFI) have been developed with the aim for faster data acquisition.

In comparison to patterned illumination approaches, the setup for PALM is easier, but data acquisition is more complicated and involves a significant amount of data processing. Localization microscopy is well suited for quantitative studies, as individual molecules can be counted, if blinking of fluorescent molecules can be accounted for. Multicolor imaging is also possible with PALM, courtesy to an ever-increasing number of suitable fluorescent proteins, many of which are photocontrollable.

Thick samples can be problematic for PALM as autofluorescence, absorption and scattering of the tissue result in a low S/N ratio. There is always a trade-off in superresolution imaging between spatial and temporal resolution, in part due to lengthy data acquisition time and/or photodamage.

9.13.2 Patterned Illumination Microscopy

The second approach uses non-linear optical approaches to reduce the spot size of an ensemble of fluorophores, which reduces the size of the PSF (Airy disk). This is the underlying principle of STED microscopy and all techniques that follow the RESOLFT concept, which is based on an optically driven saturable transition of reversibly photoswitchable fluorescent proteins between a fluorescent and a dark state. Apart from RESOLFT, patterned illumination approaches typically use permanently fluorescent proteins (Figure 9.33).

In STED imaging, a torus-shaped beam leads to STED at the periphery of the illuminated spot, whereas the center is allowed to emit a fluorescence signal. Hence the PSF is significantly narrowed. The high beam intensity needed for STED can be damaging to biological samples. Therefore, new approaches have been explored to reduce the required light intensities, e.g., by using ground-state depletion, where fluorophores are transiently driven to a metastable dark (triplet) state.

In RESOLFT, photocontrollable fluorescent proteins are used in combination with three light beams, namely the switching-on-laser, the excitation laser, and the switching-off laser, which when super-imposed, lead to a doughnut-shaped area with a bright center size of tens of nanometers and a surrounding dark region. Like in STED, the image in the RESOLFT mode is formed by scanning these beams pixel-by-pixel across the sample. As with other photocontrollable fluorescent proteins there is an increasing number of reversibly photowitchable fluorescent proteins available, enabling multicolor imaging. Among the challenges for reversibly photowitchable fluorescent proteins is that they need to withstand switching over 100 times for 2D imaging

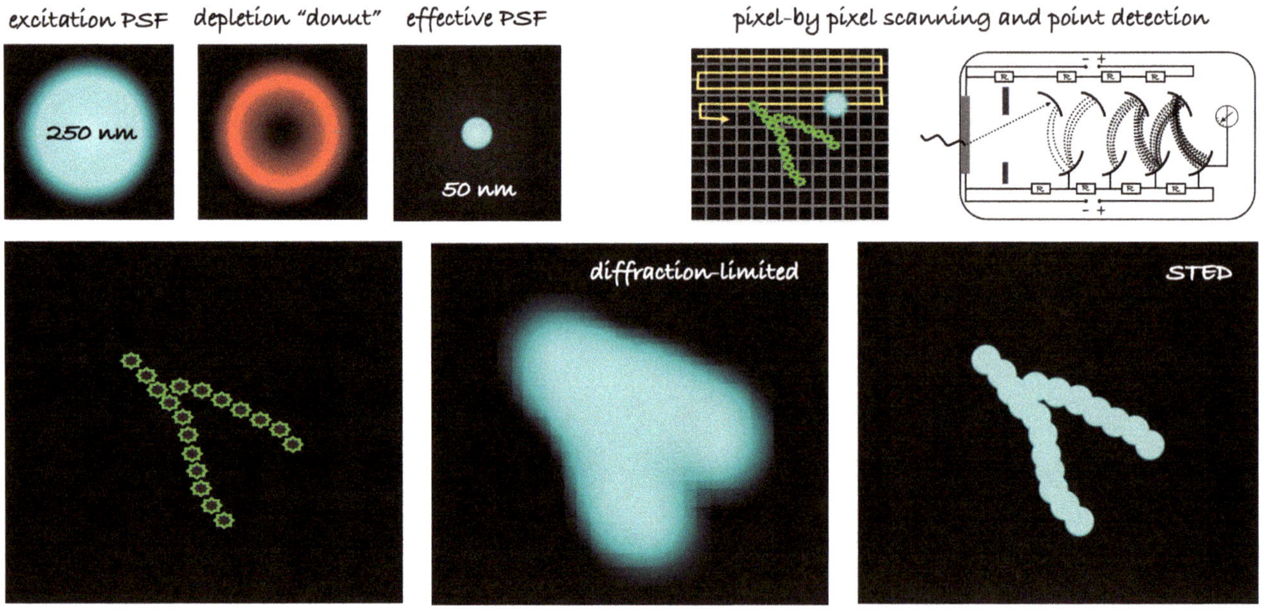

Figure 9.33 Patterned illumination microscopy – STED. Stimulated emission depletion (STED) is one form of patterned illumination microscopy, also referred to as point-spread-function engineering. By creating a depletion "donut" the effective point spread function (PSF) is reduced from ~250 nm to ~50 nm. With this smaller PSF, the sample is raster-scanned, resulting in a higher-resolution image compared to diffraction limited imaging.

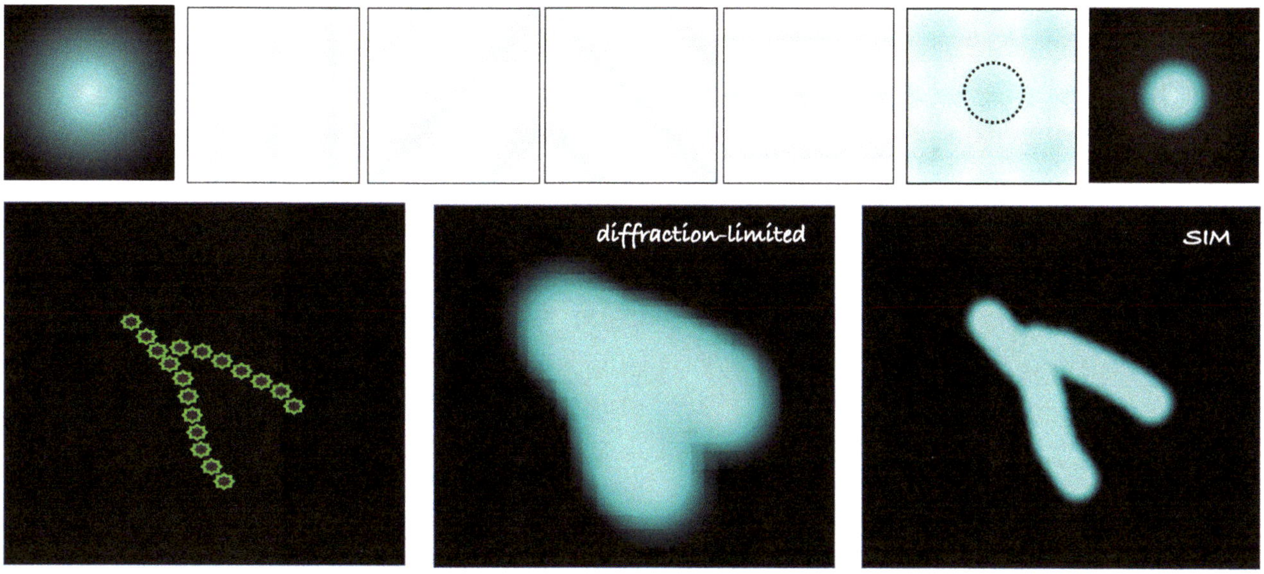

Figure 9.34 Patterned illumination microscopy – SIM. Structured illumination is another form of patterned illumination (point spread function engineering) and leads to the doubling of the resolution beyond the diffraction limit of light. It relies on the formation of Moiré patterns of structured light illumination. The images contain high-resolution information if appropriately analyzed in Fourier space as the convolution of the target structure with the illumination pattern.

and over 1,000 times for 3D imaging, with no loss of fluorescent signal.

Structured Illumination Microscopy (SIM) is another microscopy that uses PSF engineering. SIM is a method of superresolution imaging, developed at University of California at San Francisco by Matt Gustafsson in collaboration with David Agard. SIM relies on acquiring multiple images of the same sample, with sample illumination consisting of two patterns that are superposed, which gives rise to a Moiré pattern. This patterned illumination typically results in a twofold lateral improvement compared to diffraction-limited imaging (Figure 9.34). While the images at first appear coarser they contain high-resolution information, which is only appreciated in Fourier space. While the details of how it works are beyond the scope of this introduction, it may suffice to say that the image recorded is a convolution of the individual Fourier transform of the target structure with the illumination pattern. Hence, SIM requires significant computational analysis.

9.14 Near-Field Scanning Microscopy

Another way to overcome the diffraction-limit is NSOM or SNOM. NSOM/SNOM exploit the properties of evanescent waves that emerges from an aperture (or a tip) with a diameter that is smaller than the wavelength. In this near-field approach only fluorophores in the immediate vicinity of the scanning beam are excited, which can lead to an imaging of resolution of better than 10 nm.

9.15 Molecular Dynamics Study of Macromolecules

A variety of approaches have been developed that enable the visualization and analysis of complex dynamic cellular events. Fluorescence Recovery After Photobleaching (FRAP) and Fluorescence Loss In Photobleaching (FLIP) provide insights about the macromolecules' dynamics and diffusion potential in their native cellular environment, and to some degree so does Fluorescence-Lifetime Imaging Microscopy (FLIM), whereas Förster Resonance Energy Transfer (FRET) imaging allows the detection of direct protein–protein contacts if they are less than ~5 nm spaced apart and adopt a favorable orientation.

9.15.1 Fluorescence Recovery After Photobleaching (FRAP) Microscopy

In FRAP imaging, certain areas of the cell are bleached using point-scanning or line scanning illumination, which results in a dark area that over time recovers in fluorescence due to the dynamic behavior of the macromolecule of interest, i.e., the exchange of bleached and non-bleached fluorescent protein or protein-linked dye. The fluorescence recovery follows a typical saturation curve (Figure 9.35).

If after recovery there is a difference of fluorescence intensity in the saturated region from the original value one needs to assume an immobile fraction that can be either immobilized (e.g., cytoskeleton-associated), assembled (with another protein), confined, or shielded by other proteins.

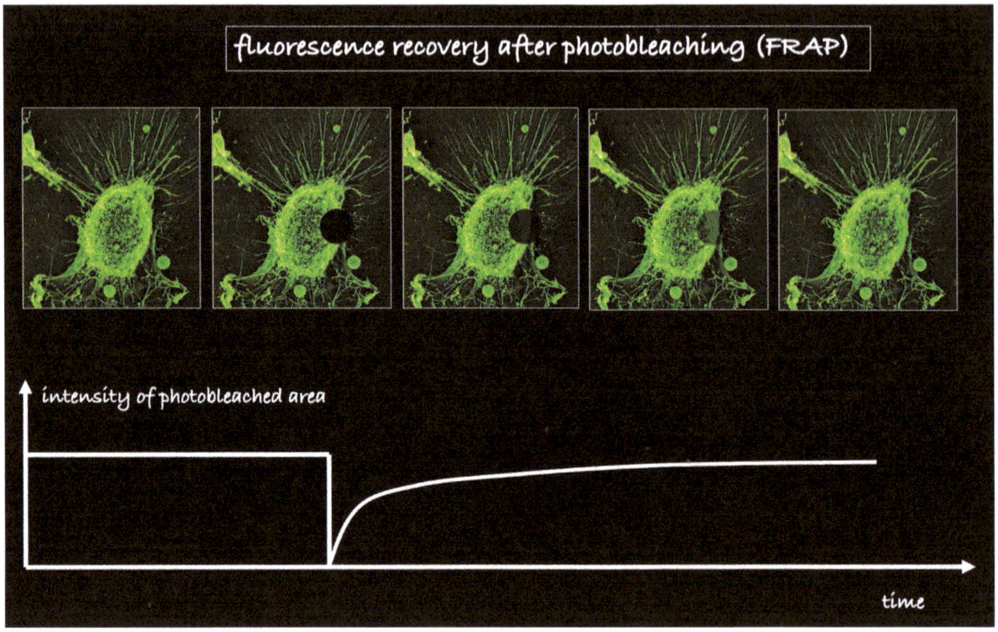

Figure 9.35 Fluorescence recovery after photobleaching microscopy. In fluorescence recovery after photobleaching (FRAP) microscopy, as the name implies, a region of the cell is photobleached and images are taken as a function of time to monitor the reappearance of a fluorescent signal, which provides information about the mobility of macromolecules in the vicinity of the photobleached region.

FRAP can provide insight about binding/release, transport by vesicles or diffusion through cytosol or within the membrane. Care must be taken to account for newly synthesized fluorescence protein.

9.15.2 Fluorescence Loss in Photobleaching (FLIP) Microscopy

An important difference of FLIP to FRAP is that the same area is repeatedly photobleached, which over time results in a reduction of fluorescence signal outside the photobleached area. While FRAP analyzes the signal recovery in the bleached area, FLIP images an area outside the repeatedly bleached area (Figure 9.36).

Both FRAP and FLIP provide information about the movement of macromolecules inside cells or cell membranes and are often used together to study the mobility of fluorescently tagged proteins. FLIP allows the study of molecular transfer between a range of regions in a cell, whereas FRAP is best suited for studying protein motility in the vicinity of the photobleached region. Like in FRAP, one must take into consideration the possibility of new fluorescent protein synthesis.

9.15.3 Fluorescence Speckle Microscopy (FSM)

Fluorescence Speckle Microscopy (FSM) allows determination of biochemical rate constants, such as binding to the cytoskeleton. FSM provides wide-field views and complements FRAP as it is capable of monitoring non-steady state dynamics and variations in molecular dynamics at high spatial and temporal resolution. FSM requires very sparse labeling (~0.1% to ~0.5%), with only 1–7 fluorophores representing one speckle. Among the advantages of FSM is that changes in the speckle pattern can be easily seen and quantitatively measured. A low background allows observation of thick specimen. The required hardware is relatively simple, and FSM is easily adapted to various modes of fluorescence microscopy. However, bright fluorophores that are immobilized are needed (as freely diffusing molecules are too fast to be detected adequately). Photobleaching needs to be prevented, e.g., by an illumination shutter or oxygen scavengers. Regarding hardware requirements, it is essential to be highly efficient in photon detection, hence simple light paths are preferred and DIC components should be removed. Focus should be highly stable, and a high magnification lens with an NA over 1.4 is required. As always microscope and detector should be resolution-matched, and the camera should be optimized for low noise, high dynamic range, and high quantum efficiency (Figure 9.37).

9.15.4 Förster Resonance Energy Transfer Microscopy

Förster Resonance Energy Transfer (FRET) microscopy allows the detection of direct protein–protein interaction, as in diffraction-limited imaging a mere co-localization by spatial coincidence is not conclusive. FRET from a donor

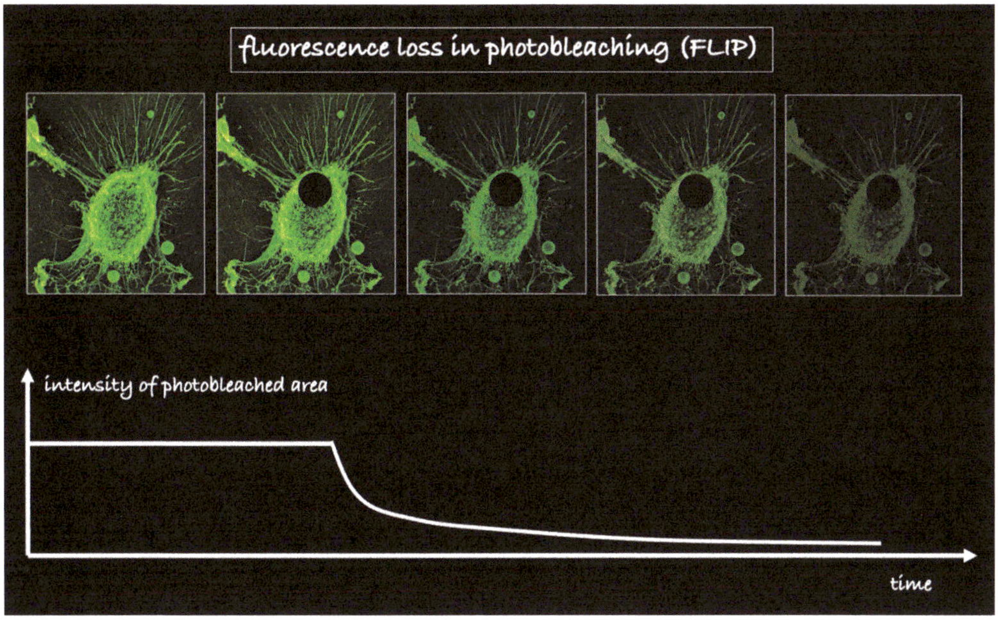

Figure 9.36 Fluorescence loss in photobleaching microscopy. In fluorescence loss in photobleaching (FLIP) microscopy, a cellular area is repeatedly photobleached. The monitored signal is the overall reduction in fluorescence outside the photobleached area. FLIP imaging allows the study of molecular transfer between different regions in a cell.

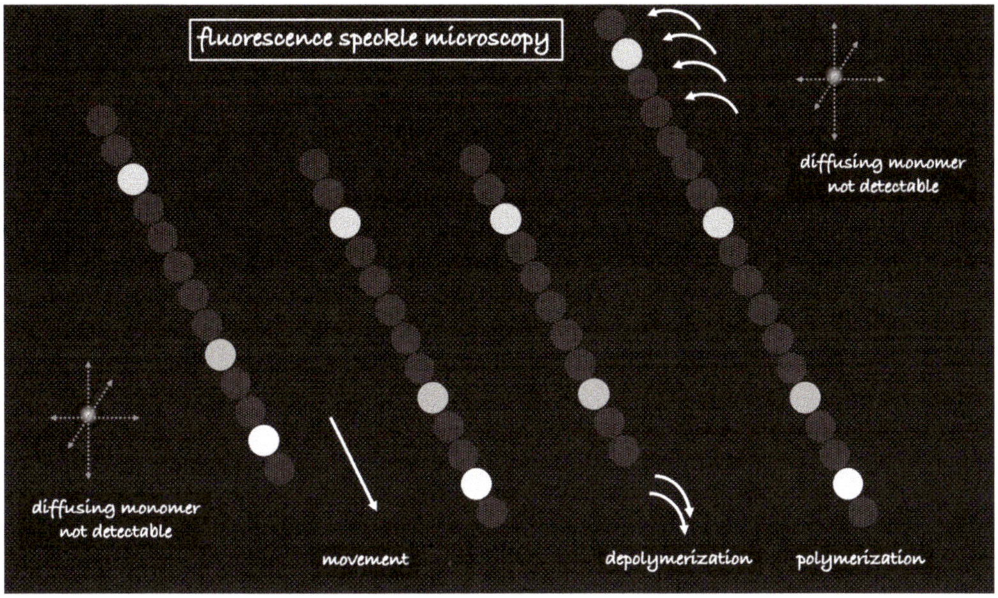

Figure 9.37 Fluorescence speckle microscopy. In fluorescence speckle microscopy (FSM), sparse labeling with a ratio of non-fluorescent target proteins to fluorescent target proteins of ~200–1,000, all of which need to be immobilized (part of a larger assembly), as free-diffusing molecules are too fast to be detected. If photobleaching can be prevented, one can follow frame by frame the pattern of fluorescent speckles and find out whether the assembly had moved, undergone polymerization, or undergone depolymerization.

molecule (e.g., cyan fluorescence protein, CFP or Cy-3) to an acceptor molecule (e.g., yellow fluorescent protein, YFP or Cy-5) scales with the inverse sixth-power distance between donor and acceptor. The Förster radius is the distance at which the transfer efficiency is 50% and is typically on the order of a few (1–10) nanometers. Förster transfer is a radiation-less energy transfer mechanism and usually only occurs when certain conditions are met: (1) the donor emission spectrum and acceptor absorption spectrum must overlap; (2) the proteins interact directly (are in very close contact) with one another; and (3) the chromophores' dipole moments show a favorable geometric alignment (Figure 9.38).

The FRET signal can be inferred from the dimming of the donor fluorescence, but the acceptor signal can also be

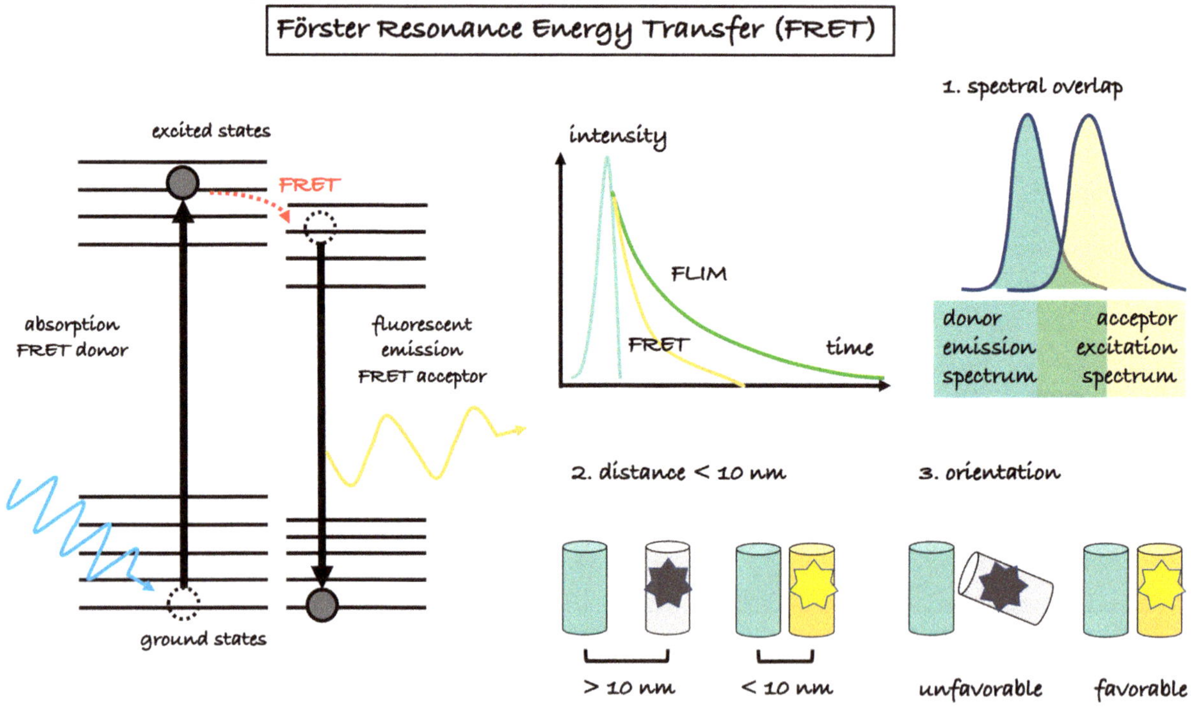

Figure 9.38 Förster resonance energy transfer microscopy. For Förster resonance energy transfer (FRET) to occur, there must be three conditions met: first, there must be spectral overlap between the donor emission spectrum and the acceptor excitation spectrum; second, the donor and acceptor molecules must be close to one another, i.e., within 5–10 nm; and third, the orientation of the chromophores must be geometrically favorable.

measured if bleed-through can be appropriately corrected for (e.g., by calibration). Also, CFP–YFP tandem-dimer tags linked by a protease cleavage sequence can be used a proteolysis assay. As is typical for single-molecule fluorescence detection, the detector needs to have high sensitivity and care must be taken to minimize (ideally eliminate) fluorescence background, e.g., by using total internal reflection illumination.

9.15.5 Fluorescence Lifetime Imaging Microscopy

FLIM is an imaging technique that measures differences in the exponential decay rate of fluorophore emission. Unlike a change of brightness, which could be due to photobleaching, scattering in thick layers, or illumination/background variation, the fluorescence lifetime depends only on the local microenvironment of the fluorophore (but not the concentration of the label). FLIM can be used for pH measurements inside cellular domains. Since FRET is another way the excited state lifetime of a donor could be reduced one should also examine the decay of the fluorescence lifetime, as faster than exponential decay indicates FRET. FLIM is often used in combination with FRET (FLIM–FRET) and allows fluorophore concentration-independent measurements and thus filter out potential artifacts in FRET.

9.16 Visualization

The visualization of white light and fluorescence light microscopy data is relatively straightforward, there are several visualization software packages that are often integrated with the data acquisition software and that make the inspection of 2D data straightforward and intuitive, including simple image restoration, denoising, segmentation, and quantitative analysis packages. Color image data is sometimes generated from grayscale image by reassigning the image data to either the red, green, or blue channel, which is also a favorite way to display multiple signals from different fluorophores by assigning them different colors.

As discussed earlier in Section 6.1.2 on image visualization, there are several non-commercial software packages including (ImageJ, Fiji, CellProfiler, VAAD, and others) that have capabilities like commercial packages, with ImageJ having been a long-standing visualization tool for which many plug-ins have been created by the image analysis community to address a large number of image analysis tasks. Some packages deal better with 3D data than others, some packages are more specialized for high-throughput imaging or deep-learning assisted classification.

It should be noted that for many fluorescence 3D datasets there is a significant resolution anisotropy, which can lead to substantial distortions in the *Z*-direction, which can render both visualization and quantitative analysis a frustrating endeavor.

9.17 Data Analysis

The analysis depends very much on the respective modes of imaging, white light imaging typically does not require much data analysis, according to the motto: what you see is what you get. The more advanced approaches such as the Allen Video Enhanced Microscopy have a real-time processing component that lies at the foundation of the respective technique, but the actual data that results from this real-time processing does not require any substantial further processing. Deconvolution microscopy heavily relies on the deconvolution of the image data with the microscope's PSF, and thus is computationally expensive, however, since deconvolution is often done by the acquisition software, it is typically carried out in the background, and thus the user typically sees the already deconvoluted images. There is substantial raw data processing to obtain precision measurements for the localization of single molecules (fluorophores) in techniques such as STORM or PALM, such as determining the center of each molecule's Airy disk. Extensive computation is also needed to extract the high-resolution information in SIM imaging.

As for all image data, one can aim to quantify the fluorescence signal, including the area, integrated fluorescence signal intensity or the amount of clustering. Those are data analysis steps that are not unique to optical microscopy data and aren't discussed in this context. All too often, images are used as "eye candy," with a selection of images being presented that support the overall biological conclusion. However, increasingly optical imaging data are being used to not just provide "pretty pictures" but as a mode of discovery and a source of information, including information about the heterogeneity of cellular responses, which in turn can reveal new aspects of a biological system.

Certain software packages are optimized for tracking of individual cells during organism/organ/tissue development or for tracking of individual molecule signal in a low background environment. However, those applications can be thought of as highly specialized and are therefore not discussed in detail in the context of a more general introduction to bioimaging.

Much effort has gone to high-throughput imaging, where the number of images that are recorded (often in an automated manner) is so large, that the image analysis can no longer be done manually, but also requires automated workflows (Figure 9.39). Systematic efforts

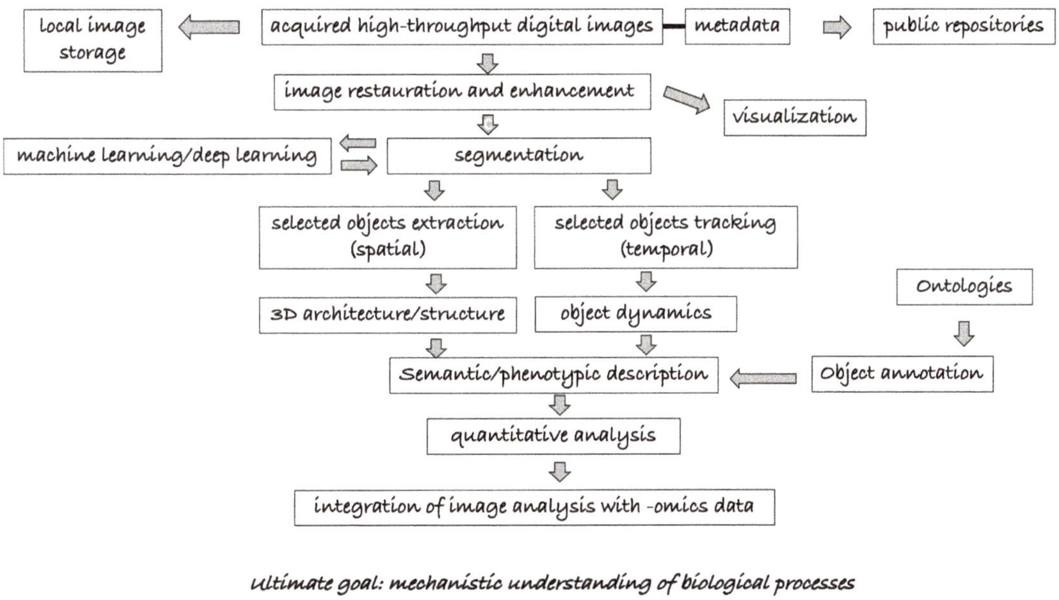

Figure 9.39 Data analysis of high-throughput imaging data. For high-throughput imaging data, it is often necessary to follow an extensive workflow to ensure a maximum amount of information from the collected images. Typically, the image data, along with the metadata are stored either locally on disks or in public repositories. After image restoration and enhancement, data is visualized, and segmented, ideally with the help of machine learning/deep learning. Selected objects of interest can then be extracted and/or tracked in time, resulting in information about the object 3D architecture and/or dynamics. With the help of ontologies and a controlled vocabulary, objects are annotated and phenotypically described. In some cases, the results are quantified and further integrated with knowledge from "omics data." The ultimate goal is a mechanistic understanding of biological processes.

for the characterization of cells with optical microscopy at their heart have emerged over the last decade, with one example being the Human Cell Atlas (HCA) initiative, which is supported by the Chan-Zuckerberg Foundation and other foundations. The HCA is designed to act as a cellular reference atlas for healthy and diseased human cells. Its aim is to catalog all cell types present in the human body, to map them to their respective tissue and organ location, and to study their architecture. Included in this rather ambitious goal is the identification of their developmental and cellular state (e.g., migration, proliferation, or senescence).

This is an early step in the right direction, arguably, as ultrastructural analysis should be included in such efforts and the approach shouwld be focused on tissues and organotypic 3D cell culture systems, as this is where ultimately health and disease of an individual plant, animal or human being is determined.

10

Techniques – Chemical Imaging at the Cell and Tissue Level

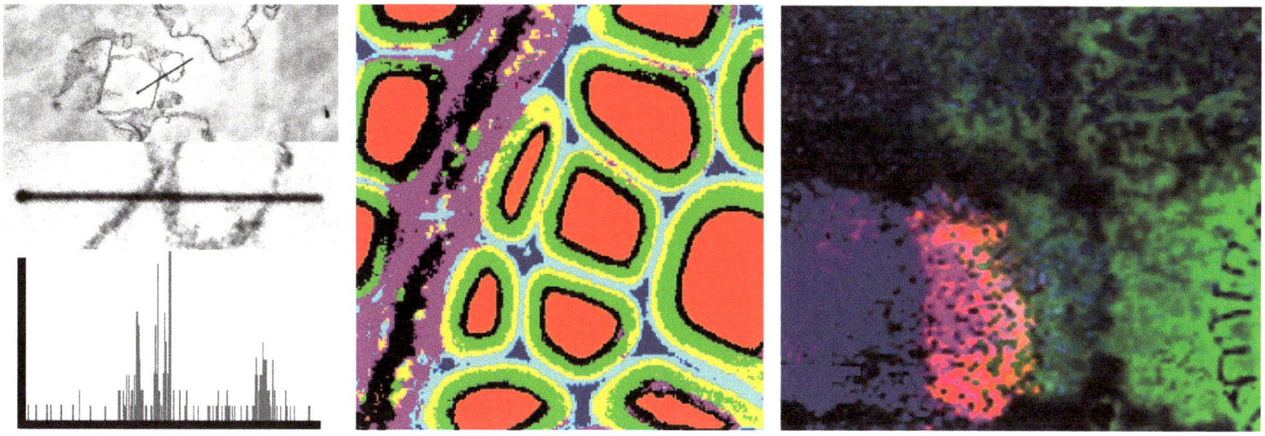

From left to right: X-ray microanalysis of extracellular metal deposits in *Desulfovibrio vulgaris* biofilms under electron-acceptor limiting conditions. Raman imaging of a thin section of plant tissue showing the self-similarity of the Raman signal for cell walls. Color-coded mass-spectrometry imaging of an interaction zone of *Myxococcus xanthus* and *Bacillus subtilis* colonies showing chemical warfare at the interface.

Techniques discussed

- X-ray Microanalysis
- Raman Imaging
- Fourier Transform InfraRed (FTIR)
- Mass Spectrometry

The goal in chemical imaging is to obtain spatially resolved compositional information about a specimen without the need for specific tags or other forms of specific targeting. Chemical imaging allows for the mapping of elemental, molecular or macromolecular constituents. Element identification relies on detection of X-rays with a specific energy/wavelength, which are emitted during the bombardment with electrons. Molecular and/or macromolecular identity can be deduced from changes in vibrational and/or rotational energy levels through the absorption of infrared radiation, through Raman scattering or by mass spectrometry imaging (MSI) (Figures 10.1 and 10.2). Due to the width of the spectral IR peaks, and the fact that only functional groups can be identified instead of the entire molecule, unambiguous identification can only be accomplished by MSI. MSI requires the ionization of the (macro-) molecules, followed by a separation and detection of the ions according to their mass-to-charge ratio (m/z). Such m/z peaks then can be compared to extensive databases for (macro-)molecular identification. Several Nobel Prizes have been associated with elemental and molecular identification and thus with chemical imaging (Table 10.1).

Spectral imaging combines spectral information with spatial information. The resulting data format is also known as a hypercube, with the X, Y coordinates representing the two-dimensional spatial dimension of the tissue slice, whereas the third dimension Z is typically given in units of wavelength and represents the spectrum. One speaks of hyperspectral imaging if continuous spectral bands are recorded. We speak of multiband imaging if the spectrum is divided into several discrete sections. Examples of hyperspectral imaging are NIR, mid-IR, and Raman imaging.

Introduction to Biological Imaging, First Edition. Manfred Auer.

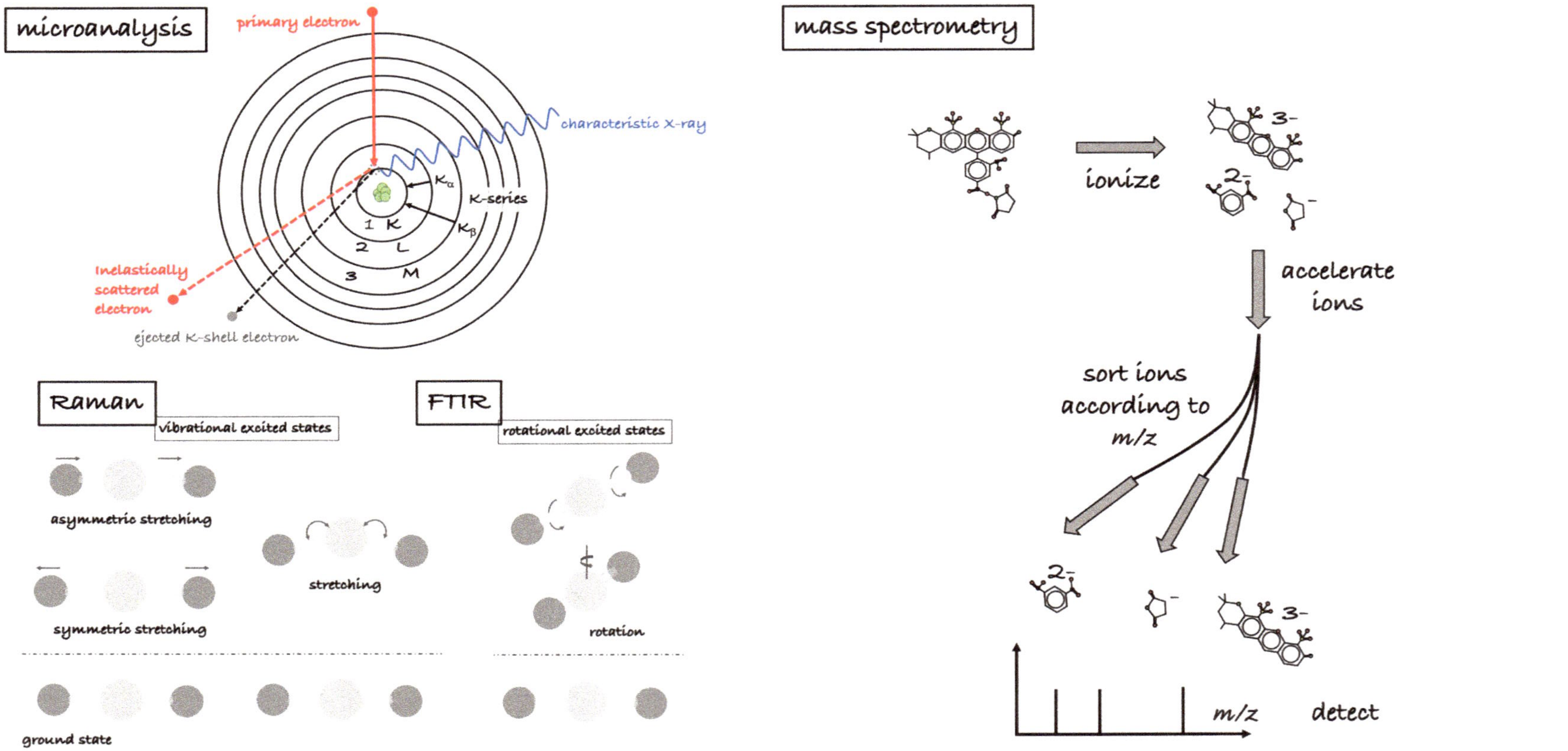

Figure 10.1 Chemical imaging – Principles. The main techniques in chemical imaging rely on very different principles: EDX/EDS microanalysis is based on the inelastic scattering of electrons which leads to the emission of element-specific characteristic X-rays. Raman and FTIR imaging rely on changes in vibrational and rotational molecular states. Mass spectrometry imaging requires molecules to be ionized, before being fractionated and detected according to their respective mass-to-charge ratio.

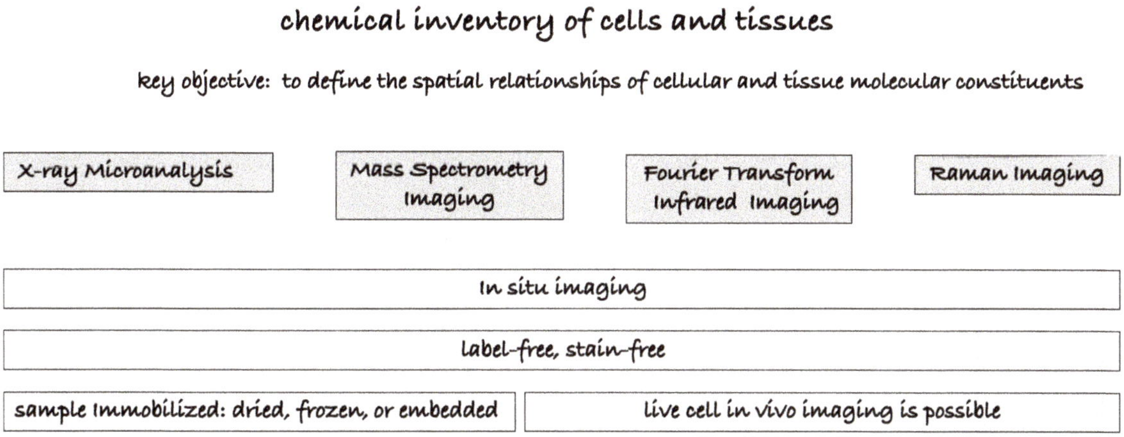

Figure 10.2 Imaging the chemical inventory of cells and tissues. The key objective of imaging the chemical inventory of cells and tissues is to identify molecular constituents and determine their spatial relationship inside their native cell and tissue context. The main techniques like X-ray microanalysis, Raman, and Fourier Transform InfraRed as well as mass spectrometry imaging are in in-situ imaging techniques that are label-free and stain-free (or minimally stained). The samples can be either immobilized (dried, frozen, or embedded) or live cell/tissue imaging is possible.

Table 10.1 Nobel Prizes involving chemical imaging.

Year	Laureate	Prize category	
1917	Charles Clover Barkla	Physics	For his discovery of the characteristic Röntgen radiation of the elements
1922	Francis William Aston	Chemistry	For his discovery, by means of his mass spectrograph, of isotopes, in a large number of non-radioactive elements and for his enunciation of the whole-number rule
1924	Karl Manne Georg Siegbahn	Physics	For his discoveries and research in the field of X-ray spectroscopy
1930	Sir Chandrasekhara Venkata Raman	Physics	For his work on the scattering of light and the discovery of the effect named after him
1989	Hans G. Dehmelt Wolfgang Paul	Physics	For the development of the ion trap technique
2002	John B. Fenn Koichi Tanaka	Chemistry	For their development of soft desorption ionization methods for mass spectrometric analyses of biological macromolecules

10.1 X-Ray Microanalysis: X-Ray Fluorescence Microscopy (XFM), Energy-Dispersive X-Ray Spectroscopy (EDX), Wavelength-Dispersive X-ray Spectroscopy (WDS)

X-ray fluorescence can yield information about the presence of elements. There are a variety of different techniques for elemental mapping, which share the same overall principle of X-ray fluorescence, but might differ in terms of radiation source, or the mode of detection and analysis. X-ray fluorescence can occur by irradiation with gamma rays, X-rays, or an electron (particle) beam, and is frequently available in scanning electron microscope setups as an additional chemical analysis capability.

The most frequently used techniques in X-ray microanalysis are Energy-Dispersive X-ray Spectroscopy (EDX) and wavelength dispersive spectroscopy (WDS) (Figure 10.3). Note that EDX is also known as EDS, but strictly speaking EDX refers to the technique, whereas EDS refers to the instrument used in EDX, namely an energy dispersive spectrometer. EDX distinguishes X-rays based on their energy, whereas wavelength dispersive spectrometers distinguish X-rays based on their wavelengths by using multiple crystals with specific lattice parameters in combination with multiple detectors to select wavelengths that are typical for an element.

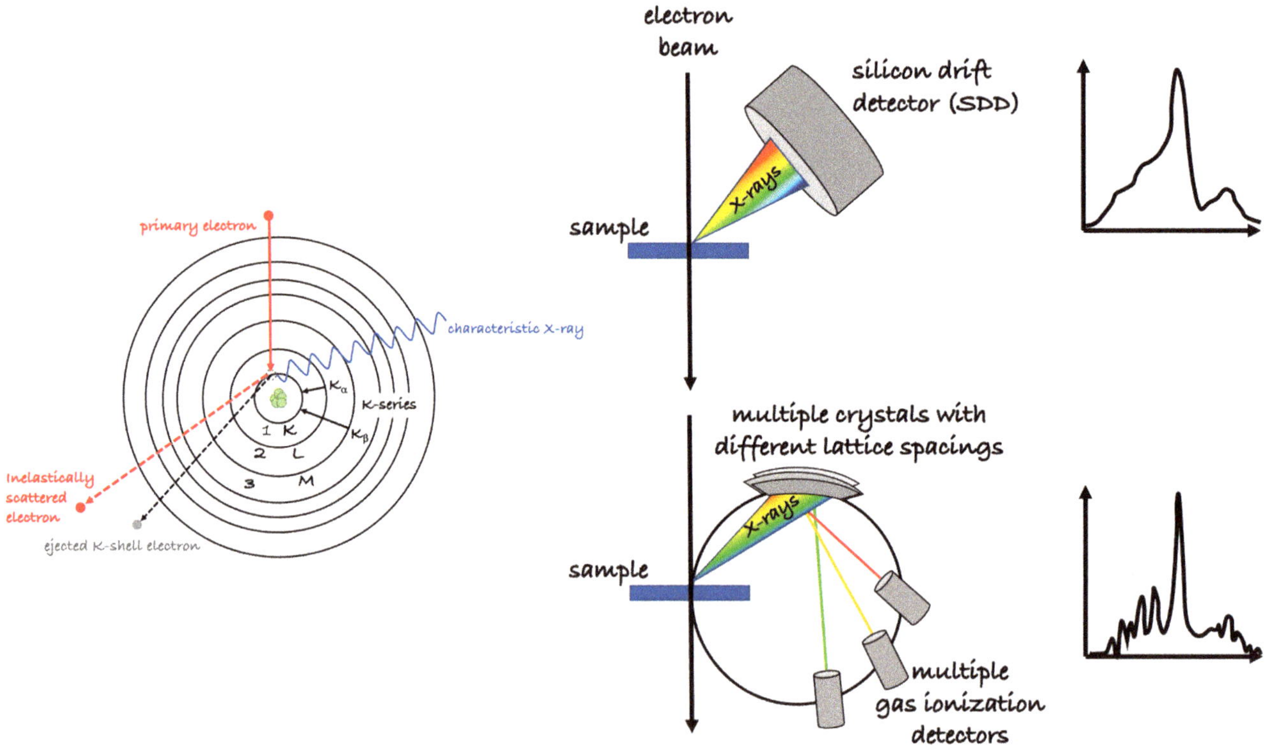

Figure 10.3 X-ray microanalysis: Energy-dispersive and wavelength-dispersive X-ray spectroscopy. Left: Both energy-dispersive X-ray spectroscopy (EDX) and wavelength-dispersive X-ray spectroscopy (WDS) rely on the inelastic scattering of an electron (of gamma/X-ray photon), which leads to ejection of an inner shell electron, which is then filled by an electron in the neighboring shell(s), which results in the emission of a characteristic X-ray signal. Right: EDX (top) and WDS (bottom) use different modes of detection of fluorescent X-rays, with EDX using a silicon drift detector, whereas WDS relies on multiple crystals with different lattice spacings and on multiple gas ionization detectors.

The underlying principle is the ionization of atoms by X-rays, i.e., by ejection of an inner orbital electron. This then results in an electron valence transition from an outer shell to an inner shell that is accompanied with the emission of a photon in the X-ray range.

As the first, second, and third shells are called K, L, M, respectively, the transition of electrons from the L (second) to the K (first) shell is known as a L→K transition or Kα, whereas a transition of electrons from the M (third) to the K (first) shell is known as a M→K transition or Kβ. Similarly, a transition of electrons from the M (third) to the L (second) shell is known as a M→L transition or Lα. The exact energy of the emitted photon leads to the identity of the element that was ionized, as the energy difference between she shells is characteristic for each type of element.

There are two different ways to detect X-ray fluorescence, either by energy-dispersive analysis or by wavelength-dispersive analysis. In the energy-dispersive analysis, the fluorescent X-rays enter a solid-state (semiconductor) detector (i.e., a Silicon Drift Detector; SDD), which converts the energy of the photons into electrical pulses, with a voltage that is proportional to the energy of the emitted photons (as a swarm of electron–hole pairs are generated). SDDs allow fast data acquisition and function even for low beam currents that are needed to study biological specimen. This set of electrical pulses is then processed by a multichannel analyzer (MCA) to produce a spectrum of the photons' energies.

For high quality data, the XFM/EDX setup needs to be operated under vacuum. Digital pulse processors are widely used in high-performance nuclear physics experiments and require substantial computer power. Another recent promising development for EDX are X-ray micro-calorimetry detectors, which measure the energy of single X-ray photons by means of a transition edge sensor. Figure 10.4 shows an example for EDX imaging, namely line profiles of extracellular metal deposits in a microbial biofilm of the anaerobe soil bacterium *Desulfovibrio vulgaris*, as well an extracellular high contrast feature that according to EDX imaging contains predominantly iron and sulfur, and in smaller amounts also phosphorus and oxygen.

In WDS, X-rays enter a diffraction grating-based monochromator with a crystalline core that allows wavelength analysis based on the angle of incidence and take-off in the crystal. The distances of different planes in a crystal correspond to different wavelengths of the X-rays for which

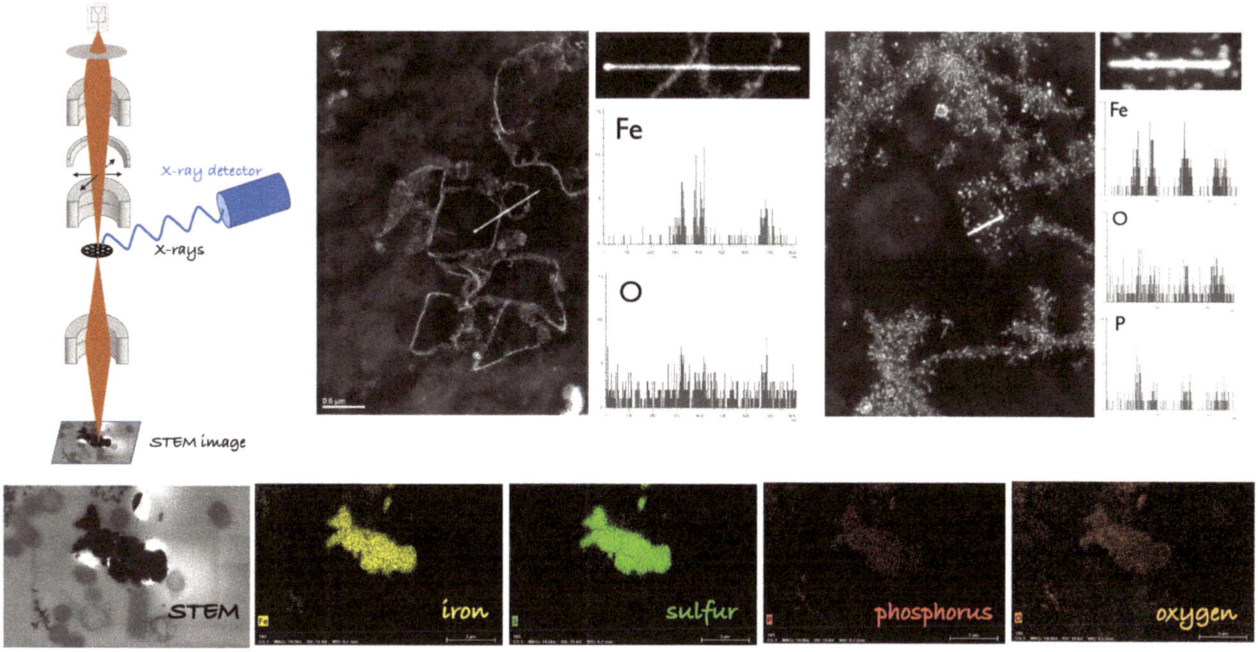

Figure 10.4 Energy-disperse X-ray spectroscopy imaging – Examples. This figure shows energy-dispersive X-ray spectroscopy (EDX) imaging of a microbial biofilm of the anaerobe soil bacterium *Desulfovibrio vulgaris*. Note high density microcrystals organized into membrane-like structures, which upon EDX imaging line scans shows these deposits as being composed of iron oxides and/or iron phosphates. A comparison of a similar biofilm shows large deposits that contain predominantly iron and sulfur, and in smaller amounts also phosphorus and oxygen.

Bragg's law of diffraction is satisfied. Each WDS-setup typically can only measure one X-ray wavelength at any given time, hence, it is most efficient to have multiple crystals, which act as monochromators, and multiple WDS detectors to detect multiple elements simultaneously. The single-wavelength signal from the monochromator, corresponding to a well-defined wavelength, is then detected, e.g., by a gas ionizing detector, which can count individual photons. Apart from gas-flow proportional counters and sealed gas detectors, scintillation counters and semiconductor detectors are also suitable if they have high pulse processing speeds.

Wavelength dispersive analysis can be done by simultaneous detection of up to 20 different wavelengths (with the equipment being very costly), or by sequential detection, essentially sweeping through the spectrum on wavelength band at the time. For faster data collection, one can choose a narrow band around the element of interest.

WDS analysis has a much higher spectral resolution compared to EDS, is often more sensitive and better suited for light elements such as Be, B, C, N, O, and F. However, it is easier obtain a full spectrum with EDS. EDS analysis allows qualitative analysis, meaning the detection of the presence or absence of a certain element, but only an estimate with respect to its quantity.

10.2 Raman Imaging

10.2.1 Overview

Photons with an energy in the visible light range can be absorbed by molecules and re-emitted at a slightly lower energy. The energy difference at discrete frequencies is transmitted to the quantized vibrational state of the chemical bonds resulting in the symmetric or asymmetric stretching and bending of atomic bonds in molecules, and thus in vibrational excited sub-states (Figure 10.5). This process is also known as the Raman effect or as Stokes Raman scattering. While this effect was known as early as 1928, with Raman being awarded the 1930 Nobel Prize in Physics, Raman effect-based imaging only become feasible in the 1990s.

As these frequencies are dependent on the type of chemical bonds (as dictated by quantum mechanics), a vibrational spectrum can be seen as a fingerprint of the molecules present in the sample. Such a spectrum is the result of the energy difference between absorbed and emitted photons in the visible light range or of the absorption of infrared photons, as will be discussed in the section on FTIR imaging.

Raman imaging is the acquisition of vibrational spectroscopic fingerprints or signatures for each pixel and allows

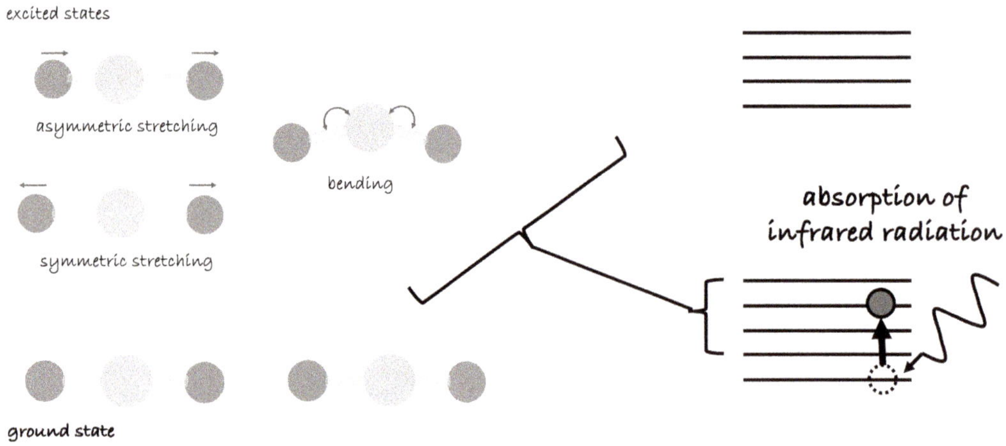

Figure 10.5 Vibrational states. Each electronic state has vibrational ground and excited sub-states, which reflects energy stored in the symmetric or asymmetric stretching and bending of atomic bonds in molecules. Those differences of energy lie at the heart of Raman (and also FTIR) imaging.

the detection of the presence (or absence) of certain molecules. One big advantage of Raman imaging is the fact that Raman imaging is label-free and does not require tedious and often destructive sample preparation steps.

Certain macromolecules, such as, e.g., cellulose or carotenoids, possess a characteristic Raman signal, and thus can be more easily identified, however in more general cases such as many subcellular structures, a precise prediction about the molecular constituents is not possible, in part due to the complexity of the spectrum and the possibility of Raman peaks having shifted due to the influence from the local environment. Therefore, the direct molecular interpretation of Raman shifts can be very challenging, and instead multivariate analysis is used to identify regions of self-similarity, and thus regions with presumably a similar molecular composition.

Spontaneous Raman scattering is inherently weak, typically a thousandfold weaker than Raleigh scattering, and hence the signal is very low. The resulting long data acquisition times limit the use of spontaneous Raman scattering. Furthermore, background fluorescence, as often encountered with high-powered lasers tend to drown out the much weaker Raman signal.

10.2.2 Theoretical Background

Raman scattering (also known as the Raman effect) refers to inelastic scattering of photons, including the absorption of photons by molecules, excitation of the molecule's vibrational energy state, and the emission of a photon with a slightly lower energy (at a wavelength that is longer and therefore red-shifted) (Figure 10.6).

While Raman scattering can occur over a larger range of the electromagnetic spectrum (including X-rays), photons in the visible light range are most relevant to the study of biologically relevant molecules and their vibrational bond excitation, and thus are used for bioimaging.

Molecules can undergo translational, rotational and vibrational motion, with vibrational motion referring to stretching and bending of chemical bonds, which in terms of energy is equivalent to infrared radiation of 5–3,500 cm^{-1}. Vibrational modes are quantized and can go from a ground state to an excited state either by absorption of infrared photons or by inelastic scattering of photons in the visible light range, which is also referred to Stokes Raman scattering (by analogy with Stokes shifts in fluorescence).

Raman scattering is equivalent to fluorescence in the sense that photons are absorbed by a molecule and re-emitted at a slightly longer wavelength. In non-resonant Raman scattering, the molecule absorbs a photon which results in the polarization of the molecule's electrons. The molecule is excited to a very short-lived unstable virtual excited state, which leads to the immediate emission of a photon at a slightly different energy, whereas in fluorescence absorption of the photon leads to the transition of an electron from a lower to a higher orbital, which is a longer-lived metastable state, from which the molecule relaxes to its ground state by emitting fluorescent light.

In Raman scattering the molecule can return to a different vibrational and rotational level of the ground state from which the molecule started, which means that the emitted photon can have either a longer wavelength, which is known as Stokes Raman scattering, or a shorter wavelength, which is known as Anti-Stokes Raman scattering (Figure 10.7).

In the case of Resonance Raman scattering, the excitation energy is close to an electron transition energy, which leads to a longer-lived state and thus a substantially

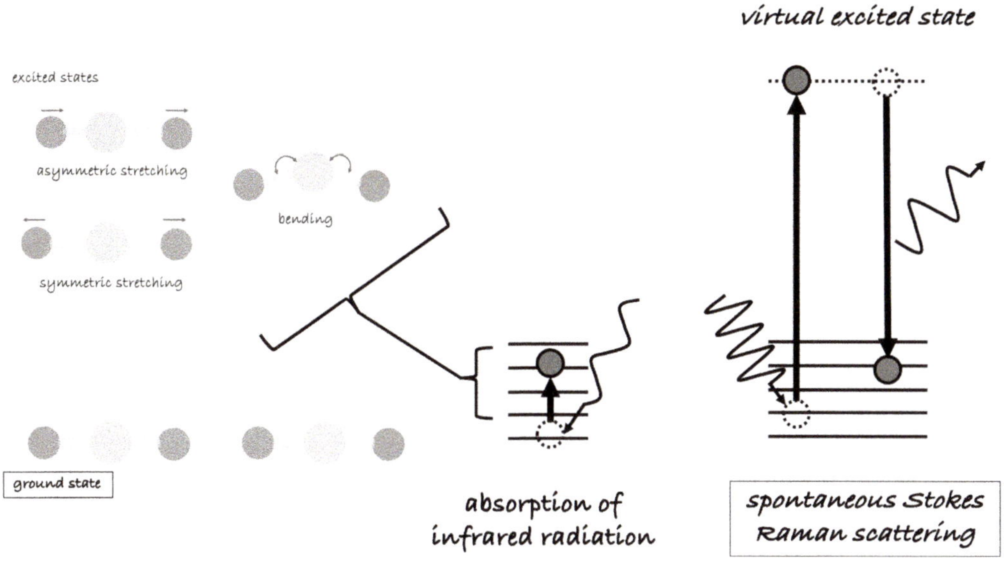

Figure 10.6 Raman scattering – Theoretical background. As vibrational modes are quantized, absorption of infrared photons or inelastic scattering of photons in the visible light range leads to emission of red-shifted photons. This known as spontaneous Stokes Raman scattering.

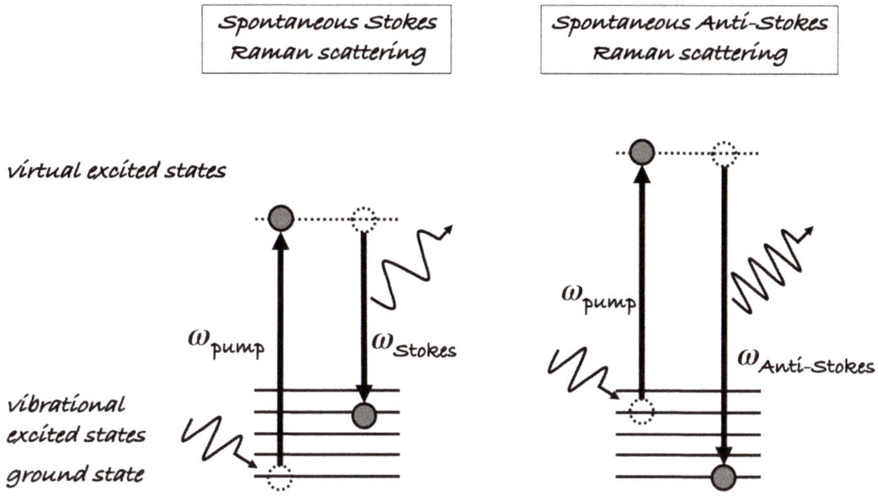

Figure 10.7 Spontaneous Stokes and Anti-Stokes Raman scattering. In spontaneous Stokes and Anti-Stokes Raman scattering the absorption of a photon results in the polarization of a molecule's electrons and thus to a very short-lived unstable virtual excited state. As a result, a photon is immediately emitted, and the electron returns to a ground state. However, in Raman scattering the molecule can return to a different vibrational level than from where it started, which means that the emitted photon can have a longer wavelength (Stokes Raman scattering) or a shorter wavelength (Anti-Stokes Raman scattering).

enhanced specific signal (with narrow peaks), but also to a fluorescence background signal that can drown out the Raman signal.

Most molecules that are excited by the absorption of a photon relax back to their ground state, and only a very small subset ends up in their first excited vibrational state. Hence, the signal one obtains for this effect is very small. Since spontaneous Raman scattering is a rare event, with only on in 1–10 million photons being affected, other approaches have been developed that boost the signal, such as coherent anti-Stokes Raman spectroscopy (CARS), stimulated Raman spectroscopy (SRS), and Resonance Raman spectroscopy (RRS), as well as surface-enhanced Raman spectroscopy (SERS) and tip-enhanced Raman spectroscopy (TERS).

Coherent Anti-Stokes Raman Spectroscopy

In Coherent Anti-Stokes Raman Spectroscopy (CARS), three laser beams are irradiating the sample, and together coherently drive the electron transitions and thus the Raman signal, instead of relying on the rather infrequent spontaneous transition of conventional Raman scattering. Of the three laser beams one is called the pump beam, a second one is called the Stokes beam and the third one is termed the probe beam. The interaction of these three beams generates a coherent optical signal at the anti-Stokes frequency and generate a strong signal when the frequency difference between the pump beam and the Stokes beam is equal to a Raman resonance in the molecule. To understand the CARS process, we need to assume the molecule in its lowest energy state (ground state) being excited by a photon of the pump beam to a virtual state, which is not an actual energy state the molecule can occupy. However, due to the simultaneous presence of the Stokes beam, the molecule can immediately relax from its virtual state to a vibrationally excited state, which is a real state the molecule can occupy. The Pump beam and the Stokes beam create a situation where the ground state and the vibrationally excited state coexist, the molecule exists in a coherent superposition of states.

When the probe beam photon now is absorbed, the system undergoes another transition to a virtual state (a state it cannot occupy), and thus must relax immediately to its ground state, thereby emitting a photon at the anti-Stokes frequency (blue-shifted) (Figure 10.8). Spontaneous Raman scattering yields a red-shifted signal and thus this process competes with fluorescence, which also yields red-shifted signals, whereas CARS produces a blue-shifted signal, and therefore cannot be confused with fluorescence that is always red-shifted with respect to the radiation source and which is a major source of background. CARS typically shortens data acquisition by a factor 10^5 compared to spontaneous Raman spectroscopy, causes less radiation damage due to tolerable laser powers, and allows for good tissue penetration. Also, CARS allows for 3D imaging as

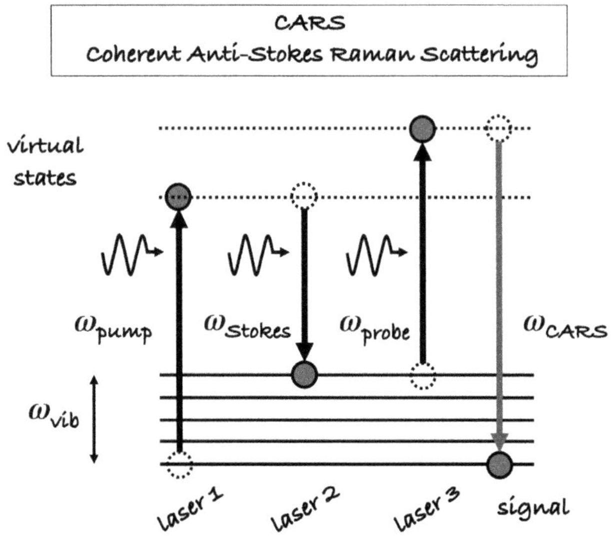

Figure 10.8 Coherent anti-Stokes Raman scattering. Coherent anti-Stokes Raman scattering (CARS) employs three laser beams: a pump beam (laser 1), a Stokes beam (laser 2), and a probe beam (laser 3). The molecule starts in its lowest energy state and is excited by a pump beam photon to a virtual state. With the help of the Stokes beam the molecule relaxes to a vibrationally excited state, from which the molecule is excited to another virtual state by the probe beam. This virtual state is very short-lived and thus the molecule relaxes back to its ground state, emitting a photon at the anti-Stokes frequency. As a result, CARS produces a blue-shifted signal that cannot be confused with a red-shifted fluorescence signal.

the CARS signal is nonlinear and only generated in the microscope's focal spot, where the laser intensity is highest.

However, CARS also has a few drawbacks, such as that the CARS signal is dominated by the most prominent constituents, is susceptible to incoherent background signals, and as a non-linear process requires rather exact experimental conditions, as small changes in the experimental setup can have huge consequences to the CARS signal. Consequently, it can be very difficult to interpret CARS spectra, as often peak assignment from the classical Raman literature do not match the CARS spectral data. CARS is an ideal technique if one probes for known substances in the sample, where only a narrow frequency band is considered. Such narrowing of the spectral band allows real-time imaging at video rate.

Stimulated Raman Spectroscopy

In stimulated Raman spectroscopy (SRS), two laser beams at slightly different wavelengths (also known as pump and Stokes beams) simultaneously irradiate the sample, hence a molecule absorbs photons of two different wavelengths (thus two different energies), which leads to the excitation of the molecule via the absorption of two photons from its lowest electronic energy level to a virtual state, from where it relaxes into vibrational state (Figure 10.9). With an appropriate energy difference of pump and Stokes photons, the probability for this stimulated Raman scattering increases by orders of magnitude. This approach is not unlike stimulated emission in fluorescence.

The pump beam is held at a constant frequency, whereas the Stokes laser beam scans a variety of frequencies, which leads to spectral fingerprints of the molecule. As a result, SRS increases the Raman signal by several orders of magnitude (up to a factor of 10^8), allowing much faster data acquisition. SRS is related to CARS but has only been around for about a decade. Just like it is the case for CARS, SRS does not suffer from autofluorescence interference and offers label-free chemical information. Unlike CARS, SRS spectra resemble spontaneous Raman Scattering spectra, which make analysis straightforward, and the signal is strictly dependent on the molecule concentration. When used for 3D imaging, tissue penetration depths of 100 μm is typical, up to 300–500 μm can be achieved for low-scattering tissues. If the tissue has been treated with the detergent Triton X-100 (TX-100), penetration can increase up to 1 mm.

There continues to be further variations in Raman imaging, such as RRS, where the laser wavelength is close to that of an electronic transition of the molecule, leading to a signal amplification. However, RRS requires highly powerful UV or X-ray lasers, which can cause photodegradation and can also induce fluorescence.

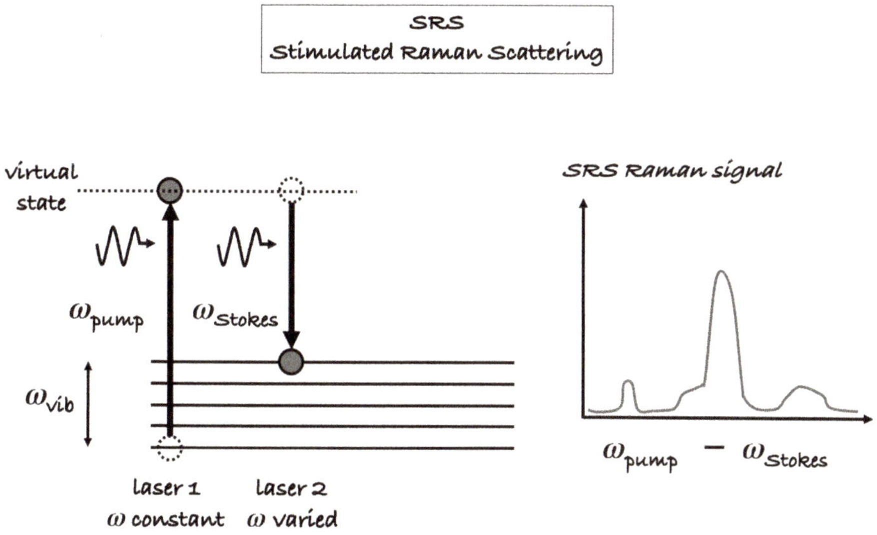

Figure 10.9 Stimulated Raman scattering. In stimulated Raman scattering (SRS), two lasers (pump beam and Stokes beam) simultaneously irradiate the sample, which leads to an excited state of the molecule from the ground state to a very short-lived virtual excited state from which the molecule relaxes back to a vibrational state. When the difference of the frequencies of the pump beam and the Stokes beam reaches specific values, the probability for stimulated Raman scattering increases by orders of magnitude. By holding the pump beam at a constant frequency and by scanning the Stokes laser beam through a variety of frequencies, one can obtain a spectral fingerprint of the molecules. The strong signal obtained in SRS allow much faster data acquisition.

Manhattan Raman Scattering (MARS) is yet another technique. MARS uses so-called carbon dyes and can be used for multiplex imaging, offering 14–24 different sets of signals that are distinguishable in Raman imaging, which compares well to fluorescence microscopy, which is limited to 5–6 different color tags (due to overlap of fluorescence emission spectra). Also, like it is the case for fluorescence optical techniques, STED-like techniques (using a donut-shaped laser for emission depletion) can enhance the resolution in Raman imaging.

Tip-Enhanced Raman Spectroscopy

Tip-enhanced Raman Spectroscopy (TERS) is a near-field imaging technique, that uses a pin probe with a very sharp gold tip, like a scanning probe microscope (Figure 10.10). Like in near-field scanning optical microscopy (NSOM), Raman scattering only occurs very close to the tip, allowing this approach to overcome the diffraction-limit and thus can provide very high-resolution data (in the tens of nanometer range). TERS is mostly dependent on the tip size and geometry. The fabrication of suitable gold or silver

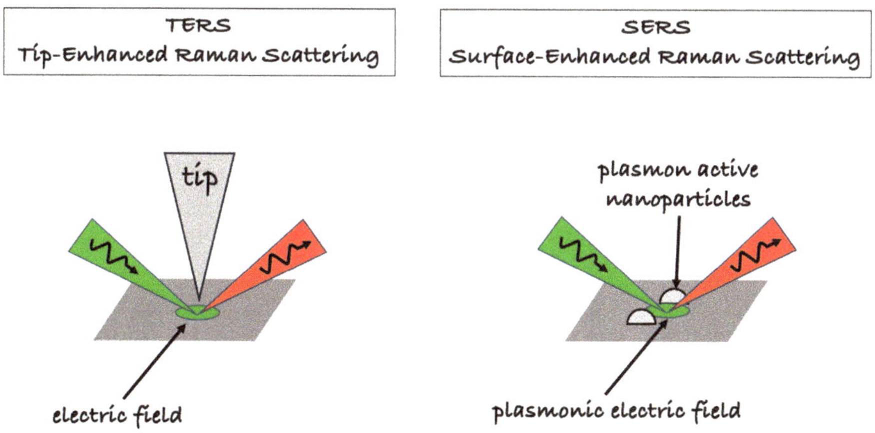

Figure 10.10 Tip-enhanced Raman scattering and surface-enhanced Raman scattering. Tip-enhanced Raman spectroscopy (TERS) uses a sharp gold tip (similar to a scanning probe) for near-field illumination, which results in strong, sharp Raman signal in the immediate environment of the tip. In the case of surface-enhanced Raman spectroscopy (SERS), collective electron charge oscillations in plasmon-active nanoparticles near the resonance frequency mediate the near-field illumination, resulting in high-resolution Raman scattering signals.

tips is challenging and not very reproducible. Once a working tip has been created, it is scanned over the sample in an atomic force microscope mode either with a wide spectrum at selected points or over a smaller spectral window where specific Raman signals are expected. Other types of plasmon-coupled structures, e.g., near-field geometry-tips with a narrow gap or a bowtie-geometry, have been successfully tested for TERS on pure, high-Raman-signal samples, but this type of Raman imaging requires more research before it can reach the maturity to become a routine bioimaging tool for real biological samples.

Surface Enhanced Raman Spectroscopy

SERS relies on nanoparticle exhibiting surface plasmon resonance. The exact mechanisms underlying SERS remain unclear, but according to electromagnetic theory, localized surface plasmons, collective electron charge oscillations in metallic nanoparticles (ideal are gold and silver) are excited by light, and exhibit at the resonance frequency a near-field illumination effect, with the field being highly localized to the nanoparticle and its immediate environment (Figure 10.10). The so-called chemical theory is an alternative to understand SERS and is based on the concepts of intermolecular and intramolecular charge transfers. SERS provides a signal that is several orders of magnitude stronger than spontaneous Raman scattering. Furthermore, the peaks often are sharper and fluorescence background is suppressed.

10.2.3 Experimental Design

Early on, Raman spectra have been recorded using scanning monochromator spectrometers, consisting of double or triple monochromators to sweep through the spectrum, and photomultiplier tubes or cooled charge-coupled device (CCD) array detectors for detection of the Raman signal. Optical filters that transmit the inelastically scattered Raman photons while blocking elastically scattered photons or unscattered photons have improved detection sensitivity and are used for high-resolution Raman imaging. As an experimental alternative, Fourier Transform (FT) Raman spectrometer, are used, in combination with a near-IR (NIR) laser (at 1,064 nm), which helps to minimize fluorescence, and a liquid nitrogen-cooled InGaAs or germanium-based solid-state detector.

Raman spectrum images are taken either in a raster scanning mode (pixel by pixel) or under flood-beam conditions, with images being recorded repeatedly in different spectral windows, using tunable lasers, rotating dielectric filters, acousto-optic or crystal tunable filters. Line mapping can be thought of as an intermediate between two modes, with an excitation laser beam being spread into a line with the help of a scanning mirror or cylindrical optics.

Like any far-field microscopy imaging approach, conventional Raman imaging is diffraction-limited imaging, and hence the highest achievable resolution corresponds to about half the wavelength of the Raman photons. In confocal Raman microscopes a pinhole blocks the out-of-focus light. Furthermore, Raman microspectroscopy has been combined with polarization microscopy to study the microfibril cellulose fiber orientation in plant cell walls (Figure 10.11).

Sensitivity and thus slow data acquisition is a challenge in Raman imaging not only with respect to temporal resolution, but also because photodamage of the sample stemming from extended high-power laser illumination can occur.

For stimulated Raman scattering (SRS) microscopy, the mode of signal detection is rather unique, as one measures the loss of the pump beam laser intensity, as each loss in the pump beam corresponds to a gain in the Stokes beam and thus the Raman signal. This loss of signal is best measured by applying a high-frequency modulation to one laser beam and detecting the modulation transfer to the other beam by using a radiofrequency (RF) lock-in amplifier, which shows high sensitivity and suppresses noise.

10.2.4 Data Analysis

One of the challenges in Raman imaging is that every pixel contains a full Raman spectrum or at least certain regions of the Raman spectrum, and thus does not represent a typical image that is based on colors, greyscale values or z-height. For 2D or 3D spatial dimension datasets, Raman images are often represented as hyperspectral cubes with the spectral component being an extra dimension. This representation can be very challenging to display or analyze, hence one goal of data analysis can be to reduce the complexity of the data, while retaining the information contained in the data. Since each pixel has a unique Raman signature, one goal for data analysis can be to create an image (via false color-coding) that reflects regions with similar Raman signatures (Figure 10.12).

This is an ideal case for multivariate analysis, either supervised, which requires a priori knowledge, calibration, and large training data sets (which can be difficult to obtain), or unsupervised that relies on self-similarity of the data sets, without a priori knowledge on how the spectra relate to the underlying molecules that are responsible for the Raman signatures in the first place. Multivariate analysis can then be performed using a variety of techniques including partial least square, discriminant analysis, principal component analysis, k-means cluster analysis,

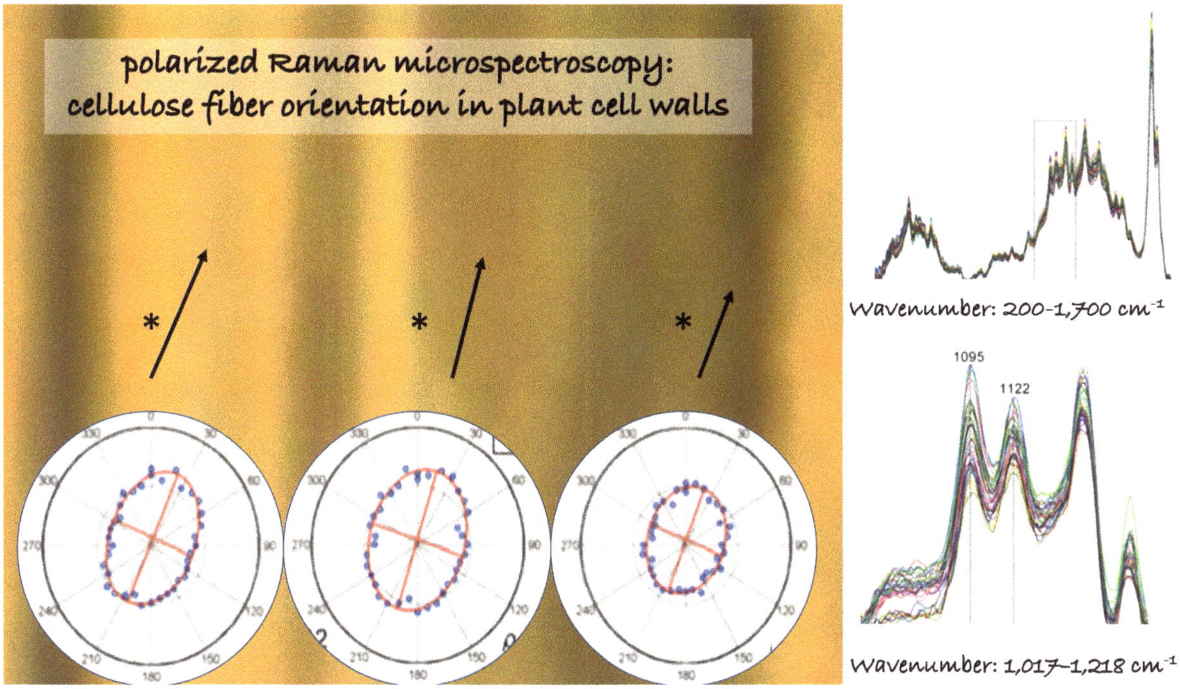

Figure 10.11 Polarized Raman microspectroscopy of plant cell wall. In this example, thin sections of plant cell walls were subjected to Raman microspectroscopic imaging, with the twist that polarized light was used. Analysis of the cellulose-specific Raman signal as a function of the light polarization angle allowed the determination of the net orientation of cellulose fibers in different sections of plant cell walls.

Figure 10.12 Analysis of Raman images. In Raman imaging, every pixel contains a Raman spectrum, and for this reason Raman images are often represented as hyperspectral cube with the spectral component being an extra dimension. Multivariate analysis, such as unsupervised *k*-means cluster analysis is one way to reduce the data complexity and to sort the data into categories of self-similarity, without a priori knowledge on how the spectra relate to the molecular composition.

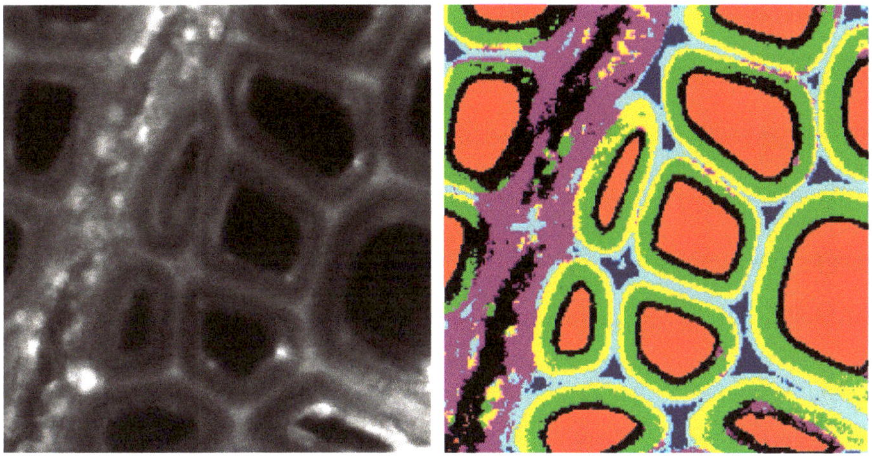

(agglomerative) hierarchical cluster analysis, divisive correlation cluster, vertex component analysis, and/or artificial neural networks.

10.3 Fourier-Transform Infrared (FTIR) Imaging

FTIR imaging allows label-free, non-destructive chemical mapping at a lateral resolution on the order of tens of micrometers. Interaction of molecules with mid-IR region radiation of 4,000–660 cm^{-1}, which corresponds to a wavelength of 2.5 μm to 15 μm (also known as the rock salt region of IR), results in changes in the dipole moments of the vibrational group in the molecules. To put it in simplistic terms, absorption of IR photons leads to an excitation of the molecular vibrational state, and thus to a stretching and bending of molecular bonds, particularly if the involved atoms have large differences in terms of electronegativity. For conventional Globar® (electrically heated glowing black-body broadband) illumination the typical resolution is 20–60 μm, which can be improved by nearly an order of magnitude (resolution up to ~5 μm) when the much brighter synchrotron IR radiation is used. Synchrotron-radiation FTIR imaging is still diffraction-limited, hence, further improvement in resolution would require near-field imaging technology.

The NIR range of the spectrum typically goes from 12,800 cm^{-1} to 4,000 cm^{-1} (780 nm to 2.5 μm), with some overtones of the fundamental vibrational states. However, absorption is one or two orders of magnitude lower in the NIR compared to the mid-IR region, and the line shapes tend to be much broader and more overlapping with one another. For these reasons, mid-IR is the preferred region for FTIR imaging. The far-IR region is below 200 cm^{-1} (>50 μm) and does not play any role in biological imaging.

It is customary in the field of IR to provide wavenumbers in cm^{-1}, instead of the wavelengths (typically in nm or μm), hence a typical IR-spectrum will show absorbance of IR (*Y*-axis) as a function of wavenumber (*X*-axis).

Absorption of IR photons lead to an excitation of the molecules' vibrational energy levels, with the frequency of the absorption peak being determined by the vibrational energy gap and the intensity of the absorption peak being determined by the change of dipole moment (and the possibility of transitions of energy levels). There can be multiple closely related absorption peaks, which reflects additional vibrational freedom of the molecule. The entire IR spectrum, the entity of absorption peaks, serves as a signature for a molecule, with most molecules being IR sensitive.

Early generation of IR spectrometers featured dispersive spectrometer, which included a radiation source, a detector, and a monochromator (such as a prism made of rock salt sodium chloride and narrow slits). The monochromator only allowed a narrow band of IR frequencies to interact with the sample. The light that passed through the sample was compared to a reference beam, and the relative absorbance at each wavenumber (frequency)/wavelength could be obtained. The entire IR spectrum was then recorded, by sweeping with the monochromator through the IR spectrum at small intervals. Apart from this being a slow process, the spectral resolution, the wavenumber accuracy, and the signal-to-noise ratio was rather low.

Newer generations of IR spectrometer, also known as FTIR spectrometers, abandoned monochromators altogether, and used instead the principle of interferometry and Fourier transform analysis of the interferogram to obtain an absorption spectrum. The advantages of FTIR over previous IR are speed (referred to as the Felgett advantage), sensitivity (referred to as the Jacquinot advantage), internal self-calibration by using a HeNe reference laser (referred to as the Connes advantage), as well as mechanical simplicity, and thus high accuracy, reproducibility, and reliability of IR measurements. Speed of data collection and spectral resolution are improved by a factor of ~10,000, with the signal-to-noise ratio being higher by a factor of ~100.

A Michelson interferometer lies at the core of FTIR spectrometers, where a beam of IR light is split into two beams, one being reflected by a stationary mirror and the other one being reflected by a mirror that can be moved. The two beams that have now taken two different paths are recombined and pass the sample before being detected. The differences of intensity of the two beams are measured as a function of the optical path difference (OPD) of the light, caused by a change in position of the movable mirror. If the OPD is a multiple of the wavelength of the IR light, the waves will interfere constructively, if OPD is a multiple of half a wavelength, the waves will cancel each other out. In between these two extremes there will be interference that leads to a signal between the maximum and the minimum, as a function of mirror position. This plot is known as an interferogram. Absorbance of the IR light by the sample modulates the interferogram, and this modulation can be extracted by Fourier analysis, leading to the corresponding IR light absorption spectrum (Figure 10.13) (note: an interferogram and a spectrum are mathematically related to one another via a Fourier transform). There are other optical geometries besides movable plane mirrors, such as cube corner reflectors, that serve the same purpose of creating an interferogram.

Apart from the interferometer, an FTIR instrument requires an IR radiation source which can be a glowing blackbody (sometimes referred to as a gray-body) thermal emission source, that is typically electrically heated to ~1,000–2,000 °C, also known as a Globar®. As an alternative, synchrotron radiation is much more desirable since it is collimated, coherent and much brighter than traditional thermal broadband sources. Instead of lenses, which would absorb IR light, the optics in IR imaging are reflective mirrors. Using an array of thermoelectrically cooled Mercury-Cadmium-Telluride (MCT) IR detectors (e.g., 64 × 64 or 128 × 128), raster images of the samples are being collected. MCT detectors show a fast response and possess an order of magnitude higher sensitivity than previous pyroelectric detectors.

One of the challenges for FTIR imaging of biological samples such as cells and tissues is that an IR spectrum of a cell is basically a linear combination of the spectra of all the biochemical constituents of a cell, including lipids, nucleic acids, and carbohydrates, in addition to other small molecule metabolites. Hence interpretation of the data is further complicated by the fact that each pixel of the image contains an entire IR spectrum (instead of a single value like intensity), hence, visualization and analysis (just like in Raman imaging) are very complicated. Instead of

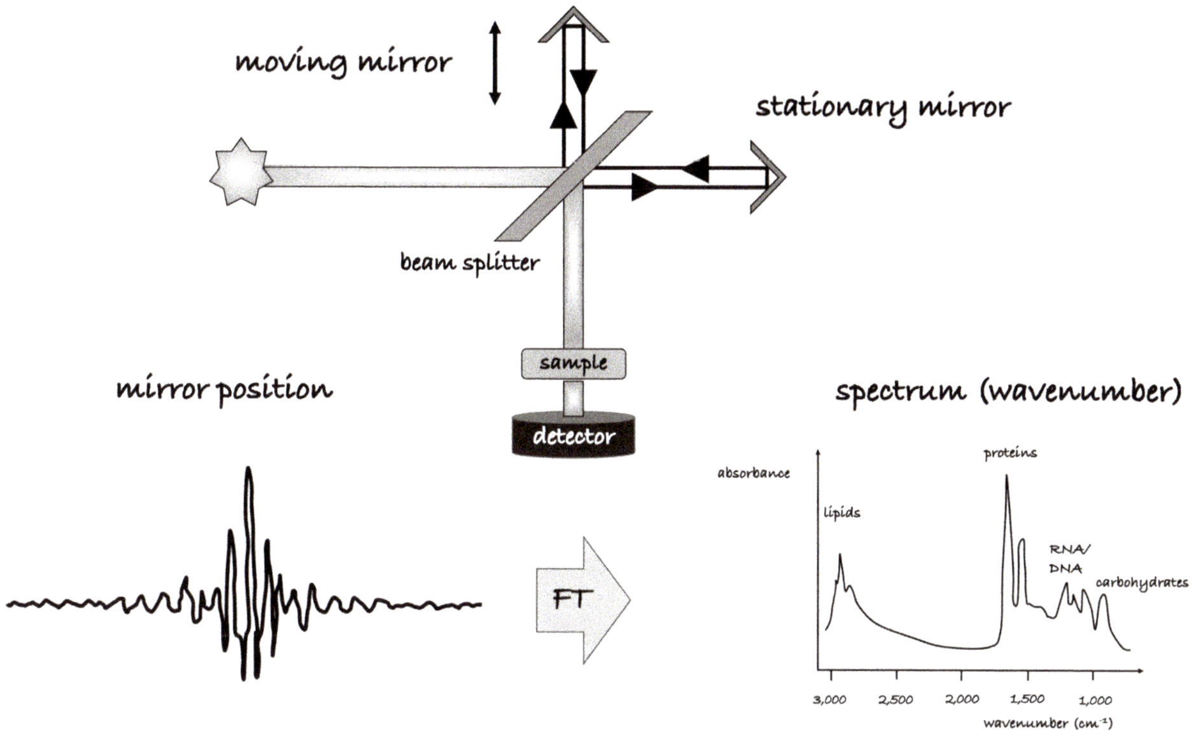

Figure 10.13 Fourier Transform Infrared Imaging. In Fourier transform infrared (FTIR) imaging one relies on interferometry to obtain an infrared spectrum since dispersive spectrometry takes too much time. In FTIR, an infrared beam is split and forced onto two different paths, one encountering a stationary mirror, whereas the other path involves a moving mirror. The two beams recombine before passing through the sample and encountering a detector. The optical path difference between the two beams lead to an interferogram with constructive and destructive interference as a function of mirror position. The sample further modulates this interference pattern and this modulation (and thus the molecular composition underlying this modulation) can be analyzed by a Fourier transform, resulting in an IR spectrum with an IR absorption signal as a function of wavenumbers.

considering the spectrum at each pixel, one looks for self-similarities in the image, based on multivariate statistical analysis, such as hierarchical cluster analysis or principal component analysis.

10.4 Mass Spectrometry

10.4.1 Overview

Mass spectrometry (MS) is an analytical tool to determine the molecular weight of atoms and molecules, and thus to obtain a spectrum of masses, which allows the identification of individual compounds, thus revealing the chemical composition of a sample. This is accomplished by putting a charge on the molecules, electrostatically propelling then into the mass analyzer, where the behavior of the ions in the electrostatic and magnetic fields of the mass spectrometer is being monitored. This can be as simple as monitoring the time of flight (TOF) of the ion through the mass analyzer to the detector (TOF), path differences of the secondary ions in the electrostatic and magnetic fields or energy differences as detected by radio frequency resonance differences (e.g., Orbitrap). The signal from ions according to their mass-to-charge ratio (m/z) is then analyzed by a computer, which compares the obtained spectrum with a reference databank for molecular identification.

Mass Spectrometry in Analytical Chemistry

For mass spectrometry used in traditional analytical chemistry, small sample volumes are typically injected directly into the vacuum of the instrument, or the mixture of molecules is separated into its various components via gas chromatography (GC) or high-performance liquid chromatography (HPLC), where the molecules interact with a column material, either in a gas phase or in a liquid phase, respectively. Different mass spectrometry approaches differ with respect to ionization, mass analysis and detection (Figure 10.14).

Mass Spectrometry Imaging (MSI)

While classical mass spectrometry is an analytical chemical technique of a bulk sample, and thus does not provide any spatial resolution, mass spectrometry can also be used for imaging by raster-imaging over a sample and collecting

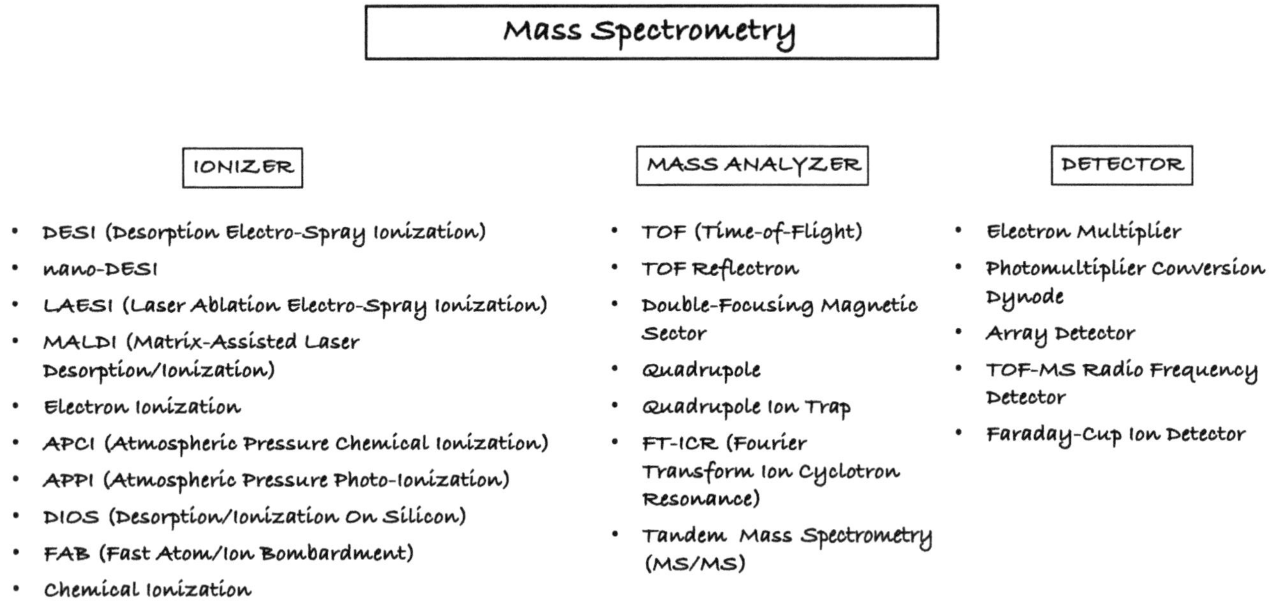

Figure 10.14 Mass spectrometry – Overview. In mass spectrometry there are different ways for ionization, including fast atom/ion bombardment (FAB), (nano-)desorption electrospray ionization (DESI), matrix-assisted laser desorption/ionization (MALDI) and other approaches. For mass analysis, choices are time-of-flight (TOF), TOF reflectron, double-focusing magnetic sector, quadrupole, quadrupole ion trap, Fourier transform ion cyclotron resonance as well as tandem mass spectrometry (also referred to as MS/MS). Which mass analyzer is chosen depends on the exact application. As for detectors, there are electron multiplier, photomultiplier conversion dynode, array, TOF-MS radio frequency, as well as Faraday-cup ion detectors.

mass spectrometry data for every pixel point examined. Hence, each pixel collected contains a mass spectrum of all the molecules present. As no label is required for mass spectrometry, many molecules can be detected simultaneously, whereas in fluorescence imaging only a few molecules can be detected simultaneously due to the limited spectrum, and the respective bandwidth of excitation and emission spectra.

For MSI the molecules are typically immobilized on a sample surface, and therefore molecules must be desorbed from that surface before entering the mass spectrometer. This is accomplished either directly by the bombardment of the molecules with fast atoms (Fast Atom Bombardment; FAB) or a primary ion beam that leads to the generation of secondary ions (Secondary Ion Mass Spectrometry, SIMS). Alternatively, a laser vaporizes a matrix in which the molecules are embedded (Matrix-Assisted Laser Desorption/Ionization; MALDI) or electrically charged droplets are sprayed onto the sample surface (Desorption Electro-Spray Ionization; DESI). FAB and SIMS require the sample to reside in a high vacuum, whereas both MALDI and DESI are compatible with an ambient pressure environment, although MALDI's sensitivity is higher when performed in a vacuum. When soft ionization approaches such MALDI and Electrospray Ionization (ESI) are used, intact molecules including small lipids and metabolites to proteins can be detected.

In terms of resolution, we must distinguish between spectral resolution (mass resolution) and spatial resolution (pixel location). Orbitrap and Fourier transform ion cyclotron resonance (FT-ICR) analyzers are both used for MALDI-MS and show a mass resolving power of up to ~0.2 Da. TOF analyzers have a high spectral (mass resolving) power with high-speed acquisition over a wide mass range and thus can be used for the detection of lipids, peptides, proteins, drugs, and metabolites. Quadrupole mass analyzers have the lowest resolution spectral power but excel in terms of sensitivity as well as selectivity and scan speed. Hybrid approaches are in use that combine a wide mass/charge ratio dynamic range with higher mass resolution through precursor ion isolation capabilities of quadrupoles, followed by collisional-induced fragmentation.

In terms of spatial resolution, resolution depends both on the diameter of the ionizing beam and on the lateral diffusion of the analyte during wet sample preparation. As a general guideline, the spatial resolution for SIMS is ~500 nm, up to ~25 μm for nanospray-DESI (nano-DESI) and ~5 μm for MALDI-MSI, but one may be limited by detector sensitivity, which means that only abundant analytes may be detected. Formalin-fixed, paraffin-embedded tissue samples can be dewaxed prior to MALDI-MSI analysis. Application of a digestive enzyme like trypsin to the tissue sample leads to peptides, which allows protein identification.

Since MS is based on determining the mass-to-charge ratio of ionized compounds, atoms or molecules need to be ionized for MS to be successful. If the molecule is already charged in solution, it needs to be transferred as a charged molecules to the gas phase. If the molecule was electrically neutral, ionization can be achieved by a variety of approaches discussed below: (1) The ejection (loss) of electrons as a result of the bombardment of molecule with an electron or ion beam, or the irradiation with ionizing far-UV light. This approach works well for hydrocarbons or other molecules that do not ionize easily otherwise. (2) The capture of electrons, which is effective for compounds with a high electron affinity such as halogenated molecules. (3) Protonation, which works well for amino acids and peptides where a proton can be easily added to their amine group. (4) Deprotonation which works well for phenols, carboxylic or sulfonic acids, which due to their acidic nature can easily lose a proton. (5) Cationization which works well for carbohydrates that can bind cations (other than protons), such as a sodium ion. SIMS uses electron loss-ionization and leads to a high degree of fragmentation, whereas MALDI and DESI are considered soft ionization techniques, which allows the detection of larger molecules.

Main Modes of Mass Spectrometry Imaging

There are three main ionization modes for MSI, with the first being secondary ion emission (SIMS), followed by electrospray ionization (DESI, nano-DESI) and MALDI. Based on these main types there are additional variations on these methods, such as laser desorption ionization (LDI), matrix-enhanced surface-assisted laser desorption/ionization (ME-SALDI), nanostructure initiator MS (NIMS) and laser ablation electrospray ionization (LAESI).

Secondary Ion Mass Spectrometry (SIMS)

SIMS provides information on the spatial distribution of elements and low-molecular weight compounds on solid surfaces and thin films by sputtering the surface of the sample with a focused primary ion beam (such as Cs^+, Ga^+, Ar^+, Xe^+, or In^+ beams, as well as cluster Au_n^{n+}, O_2^+, SF_5^+, C_n^+, C_{60}^+ ion beams), which leads to secondary ion emission from the surface at a depth of 1–2 nm and an area of a few nanometers (the lateral resolution depends on the primary ion beam size). Cluster ion beams tend to be more efficient for desorption and ionization of higher molecular weight organic compounds. Secondary ions are collected and analyzed by a mass spectrometer. SIMS is a highly sensitive technique, and typically detects ion species in the <1,000 Da range, thus detecting elements, lipids, small metabolites, toxins, and other pharmacological compounds. Since SIMS is destructive, a 3D volume can be built up by repeated SIMS imaging, slowly eroding the affected surface. SIMS imaging is carried out in a high vacuum to ensure secondary ions reach the detector.

SIMS imaging can be carried out in combination with different types of mass analyzers, such as sector, quadrupole as well as TOF mass analyzers, with TOF being the standard analyzer for SIMS since it is able to detect all generated secondary ions simultaneously. For detection, there are multiple ways, such as a Faraday cup, which measures the number of ions that hit a metal cup, electron multiplier, which offer high amplification of the signal, and/or microchannel plate (MCP) detector, which have lower amplification, but provide lateral resolution. Furthermore, it can be combined with a fluorescent screen to be recorded by a CCD camera.

Matrix Assisted Laser Desorption/Ionization – Time-of-Flight (MALDI-TOF)

MALDI-TOF MSI can yield spatial information (at 5–25 µm pixel size) about higher-molecular-weight compounds such as peptides and proteins (up to 100,000 Da). Unlike DESI, the sample needs to be prepared, with a low molecular weight organic compound (matrix) being deposited onto the sample. Some of the compounds will dissolve into the matrix and co-crystallize with it. There are a variety of challenges with respect to the matrix. For example, the matrix material dissolved in a solvent must be wet enough to extract the analyte from the tissue but not so wet that the analyte diffuses away from its original position. Furthermore, matrix crystal size should not be larger than the laser beam. Matrix crystallization may be affected by the surface composition of different tissues, including salts or lipids. Also, the matrix material is not uniformly efficient in extracting the analytes from the tissues, which means that the detected analyte of highest abundance in the MALDI-TOF experiment may not be the most abundant in the tissue, but simply reflect that it was more efficiently solubilized in the matrix than other components. Furthermore, the mode of depositing the matrix onto the sample, such as pneumatic spraying, acoustic deposition (ink jet printing), sublimation or brushing of finely crushed, powdered matrices may affect the success of the MALDI-TOF experiment.

A short (nanosecond) pulse of UV (or IR) irradiation will lead to the desorption and ionization of the analyte, followed by TOF analysis. The laser spot size plays an important role in terms of achievable spatial resolution in a MSI experiment, but other factors need to be considered, such as too small of a spot size might be too little analyte for the detection of a compound. In practical terms step sizes of 100–200 µm are often chosen, as a trade-off between resolution, area of coverage, data acquisition time and laser lifespan. For whole animal studies, even lower spatial resolution may be chosen.

Desorption Electrospray Ionization (DESI)

Desorption electrospray ionization mass spectrometry imaging (DESI-MSI) has the advantage that it can be performed under ambient atmospheric pressure condition, and hence (unlike in SIMS) no vacuum is needed. Electrosprayed charged solvent (most commonly water) droplets impact the surface of the sample and lead to the desorption of ions from the surface, which are then transferred into the mass spectrometer via an ion transfer line. This spray nozzle and ion transfer line setup is raster-scanned over the sample to create a spectrum at every pixel of the resulting image. There is no need for specific sample preparation steps, which means that DESI can be used for biological samples including living cells, tissues, or bacterial biofilms as long as they are flat to maintain the distance between droplet source and sample constant. Spatial resolution depends on the size of droplet source and its distance to the sample. Typically, the spatial resolution of DESI is 200–500 μm, whereas nano-DESI may yield <20 μm spatial resolution. In terms of spectral range, DESI-MSI is well-suited for small molecules such as lipids in a mass range of up to 1,500 Da. Figure 10.15 shows nano-DESI mass spectrometry imaging of two microbial communities (biofilms) that encounter one another, and the chemical signatures associated with the various regions of the biofilms and their interaction zone.

10.4.2 Historical Perspective

The history of mass spectrometry began in the 1880s with the discovery of so-called "canal rays" in gas discharge experiments. Canal rays, traveling from the positively charged anode through channels in a perforated cathode, could be deflected by electric and magnetic fields, and thus a mixture of gases could be separated according to their charge-to-mass ratio. Further improvement to the technique were made in the early 20th century, and so-called sector mass spectrometers (also known as calutrons: California University cyclotron) were used in the Atomic Bomb Manhattan Project to separate isotopes for uranium enrichment. In the 1950s and 1960s, ion trap technology was developed, which allows ions to be trapped inside the mass spectrometer, and consecutively leaving the trapping field according to their mass-to-charge ratio. For this accomplishment Hans G. Dehmelt and Wolfgang Paul were awarded part of the 1989 Nobel Prize in Physics. Until the 1980s, electron ionization (EI) was used for ionization,

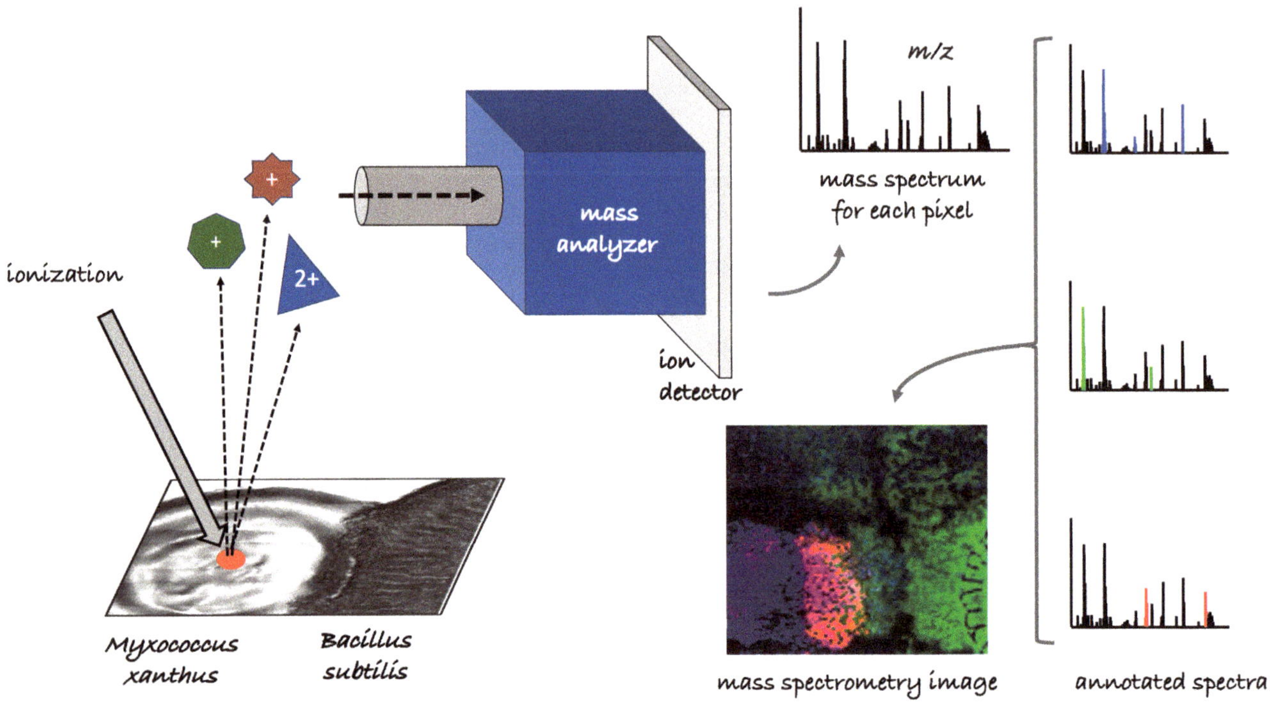

Figure 10.15 Mass spectrometry imaging. Mass spectrometry imaging (MSI) requires pixel by pixel raster scan ionization of a biological samples either in a vacuum or under ambient pressure conditions. The ionized molecules are then analyzed according to their mass-to-charge ratio before being detected. For each pixel there exists a mass spectrum, which needs to be analyzed. Signatures for certain components can be determined and color-coded. The color-coded pixels can then be displayed as a color mass spectrometry image.

which limited the use of mass spectrometry to molecules with a molecular weight of less than ~300 Da. The development of ESI and soft laser desorption allowed larger molecules to be detected and analyzed. The first experiments with ESI go back to the 1930s, with the first practical ESI being developed for mass spectrometry in the 1960s. ESI and MALDI, which was introduced in the late 1980s, have revolutionized biomolecular analysis of larger molecules, as these techniques offer high sensitivity (currently in the pico- to femtomole range) and a large mass range (currently up to ~70,000 Da and ~300,000 Da, respectively). The significance for soft ionization for the study of larger molecules by mass spectrometry was recognized in the 2002 Nobel Prize in Chemistry, awarded to Koichi Tanaka and John Bennet Fenn.

10.4.3 Instrumentation

A mass spectrometer consists of three components, namely an ionizer that creates and accelerates ions, a mass analyzer that separates the ions according to their mass-to-charge ratio and a detector system (one or multiple detectors) which will register the ion.

Ionizer

The creation of ions and their transport into the magnetic and/or electric field of the mass analyzer is the key for a successful mass spectrometry experiment. If a compound cannot be ionized, it simply will not show up in a mass spectrometry experiment, as there is no charge, which is needed for separation.

There are different ways to create ions, each has advantages and disadvantages (Figure 10.16): EI is a hard ionization technique, as it leads to a high degree of fragmentation of the molecules, which also leads to excellent mass spectra but is restricted to a low molecular weight of up to ~300–400 Da.

Soft ionization techniques, such as DESI and MALDI, result in little fragmentation of the molecule, and have extended the range of molecules that can be detected up to ~300,000 Da.

Ionizer: (Nano-)Desorption Electrospray Ionization DESI and nano-DESI are particularly well suited for chemical analysis of samples, containing proteins, peptides, carbohydrate, small oligonucleotides, secondary metabolites, and lipids, due to ionization at ambient pressure conditions. With the

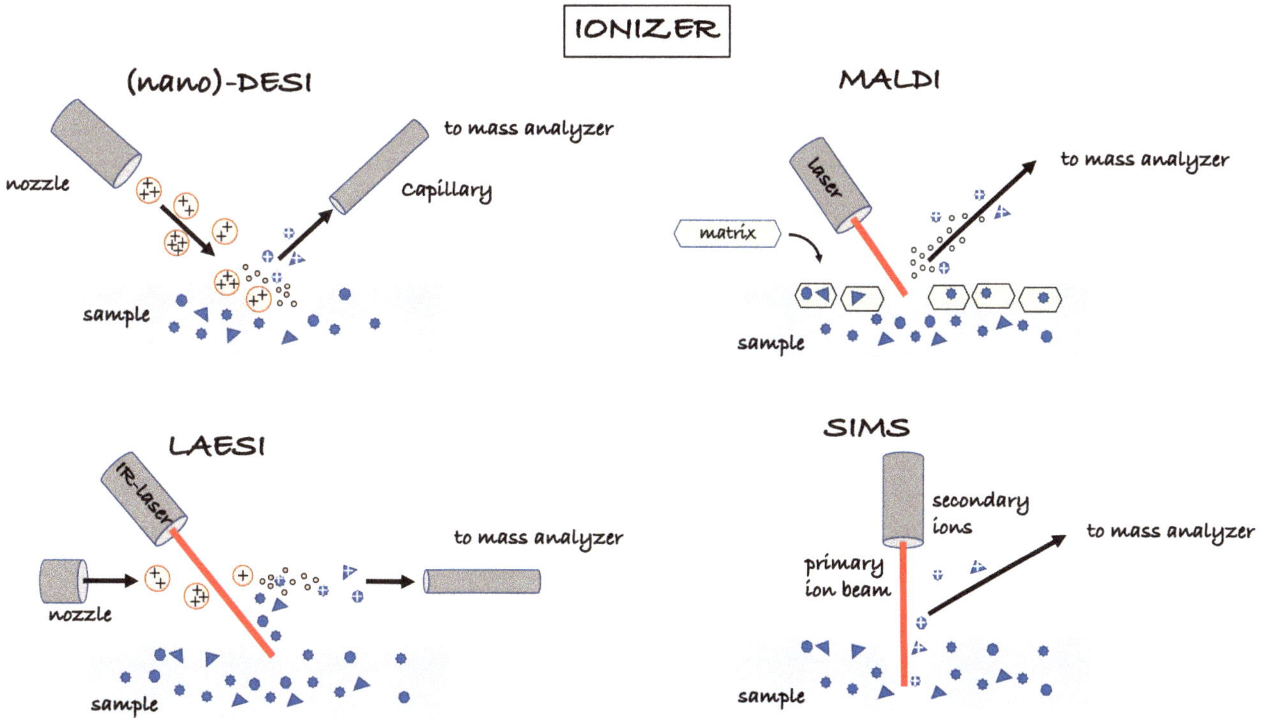

Figure 10.16 Mass spectrometry ionization. The ionization process is an important part of mass spectrometry as one can only mass-analyze and detect what has been ionized. There are multiple ways to ionize a sample ranging from hard ionization techniques like electron ionization as is used in secondary ion mass spectrometry (SIMS) to soft ionization techniques such as (nanospray) desorption electrospray ionization nano-DESI/DESI, laser-assisted electrospray ionization (LAESI) or matrix assisted desorption ionization (MALDI). Soft ionization leads to less fragmentation and allows detection of molecules with higher molecular weight.

sample not needing prior separation or any preparation (unlike MALDI), highly charged (nano-)electrospray droplets are sprayed onto the sample and desorb the analytes before they are being sucked through a capillary into the mass spectrometer for analysis. Hence single- as well as multiple-charged molecules are generated direct from a liquid solution, with multiple-charged molecules being advantageous in subsequent tandem mass spectrometry. A variety of solvents can be used in electrospray ionization, but typically a mixture of water and organic solvents works best for solubility and for protonation of the sample, whereas buffers and salts can reduce sensitivity. A complex sample mixture can be problematic for unambiguous molecule identification. Nano-DESI operates at low flow rates, works with 100× smaller sample volume as the capillary is placed next to the nano-electrospray nozzle, and allows for high sensitivity with higher tolerance to salt. In addition, (nano-) DESI is compatible with tandem mass analyzers such as ion traps and triple quadrupole instruments.

Ionizer: Matrix-Assisted Laser Desorption/Ionization The centerpiece in MALDI is a UV-absorbing matrix, typically consisting of weak organic acids, which is applied to the sample surface prior to imaging. The matrix material dissolves the analytes, which partition into the matrix layer upon its solidification.

While the exact mechanism of MALDI ionization is complex and still debated, it is thought that upon UV laser illumination, both matrix and analyte molecules are ejected into the gas phase. The ionization process is thought of being soft, meaning that molecules – unlike in harder ionization methods – do not get fragmented in the process, which makes conclusive identification easier. The development of appropriate UV lasers at the near UV emission wavelength have helped MALDI ionization significantly. Ionization of the analyte is thought to occur through proton transfer and cationization during the desorption process.

Among the advantages of MALDI is the fact that MALDI is suitable for the study of complex mixtures, allowing detection of a large mass range (up to ~300,000 Da). MALDI shows high sensitivity and soft ionization with little to no fragmentation, combined with a good tolerance to salt. However, molecules below 700 Da may not be detectable due to a high matrix signal background. MALDI is ideally suited for TOF mass analyzers, in part due to the pulsed nature of the laser desorption.

Ionizer: Laser Ablation Electro-Spray Ionization LAESI is a hybrid approach, combining elements of ESI and MALDI, as it is using a mid-IR laser and corresponding optics for analyte evaporation and electro-spray droplets for soft ionization. The advantage over MALDI is that the sample does not require any prior treatment, whereas the advantage over (nano-)DESI is that LAESI can ablate successive layers of the sample, thus yielding 3D information.

Ionizer: Electron Ionization EI, despite being a hard ionization technique that leads to high fragmentation, is still widely used for the analysis of small, hydrophobic, thermally stable molecules. Extensive fragmentation often leads to real-time identification of a compound, courtesy of existing large databases and fast data-processing. For EI, the sample resides inside a vacuum, and thus EI is well suited for the generation of secondary ions, which are used in SIMS.

Ionizer: Other Ionization Techniques Apart from the major three approaches (nano-DESI/DESI, MALDI, and SIMS) other ways for ionization have been developed: Atmospheric Pressure Chemical Ionization (APCI), which has some similarities but also significant differences to DESI as the droplets are not charged to begin with and the sample is thermically vaporized to generate ions through electron or proton transfer after collisions with the ionized solvent molecules, which results in single-charged analytes displaying no or little fragmentation. A closely related approach is Atmospheric Pressure Photoionization (APPI), which can be advantageous for thermally unstable analytes. Desorption/Ionization on Silicon (DIOS) is closely related to MALDI, but is a matrix-free approach, where pulsed laser desorption/ionization occurs on a UV-absorbing porous silicon surface. Likewise, Fast Atom/Ion Bombardment (FAB) shows similarities to MALDI in that it is considered a soft ionization source, but instead of pulsed laser evaporating a solid matrix, a continuous ion beam hits a liquid matrix. FAB is ~1,000 times less sensitive than MALDI.

Chemical ionization is related to EI but is not a widely used approach and when used is often restricted to cases where molecules, such as steroids, can be chemically modified with an electron-capturing functional group, resulting in high sensitivity and selectivity.

Mass Analyzer

Not all mass analyzers operate in the same way, with some separating ions in space, whereas other separating ions in time. Mass analyzers do not determine mass per se but a mass-to-charge ratio (m/z), with multiple charges being particularly common with ESI. Each analyzer type is characterized by its mass resolving power, mass accuracy, mass range, linear dynamic range (over which the ion signal is proportional to the analyte concentration), tandem analysis capabilities and data acquisition/scan speed.

Mass Analyzer: Time-of-Flight The simplest form of mass analyzer are the sector field mass analyzers, simply bending the path of the ions according to their mass (Figure 10.17). TOF analyzers use an electrical field to accelerate ions and measure the time before they reach the detector, with different masses reaching the detector at different times. However small differences in kinetic energy of the ions will broaden the peaks, but their highest peak position will allow identification. A TOF reflectron combines TOF technology with an electrostatic mirror and via its elongated flight path offers higher resolution compared to simple TOF instruments. Such instruments are also used in MS/MS (tandem mass spectrometry), where fragmentation results in differences in kinetic energies (also referred to as post-source decay), which is exploited for separation and analysis.

Mass Analyzer: Quadrupole Quadrupole mass analyzers have been used since the 1950s and are still the most common mass analyzers in current instruments, in part due to their lost cost. Given that they do not require a high vacuum for operation, quadrupole mass analyzers also interface well with nano-DESI ionization schemes. They can select for a range of mass/charge ratio at any given time by sweeping a radio-frequency quadrupole field through a broad spectrum of mass/charge ratios. Only ions of a specific m/z ratio will pass through whereas ions with a different m/z ratio and thus different frequency will not pass through (Figure 10.17).

Mass Analyzer: Magnetic Sector Magnetic sector mass analyzers use combination of static electrical fields and static magnetic fields to sort the ions spatially by forcing them on different trajectories, with each trajectory being detected independently by a different detector. Most modern sector mass analyzers are double-focusing devices, which focus the ion beams in terms of velocity and direction (Figure 10.17).

Mass Analyzer: Quadrupole Ion Traps and Fourier Transform Ion Cyclotron Resonance Building on the same principle as quadrupole mass analyzer, quadrupole ion traps, featuring a ring electrode and two hyperbolic endcap electrodes, use a three-dimensional quadrupole radio frequency field to trap ions and upon radio frequency sweeping sequentially eject them (Figure 10.17). Quadrupole ion traps have been successfully used for protein characterization, and they allow additional collision events that allows the analysis of additional fragments. They are compatible with (nano-)DESI as well as MALDI, yet their most important application has been in the characterization of proteolytic digests in liquid chromatography tandem mass spectrometry.

A popular quadrupole ion trap mass analyzer is the Orbitrap, widely used in proteomics and metabolomics, which is usually connected to liquid chromatography for analyte separation but can also be interfaced with GC and ambient ionization methods. Orbitraps are known for their high sensitivity, mass accuracy and dynamic range. Orbitraps are related to an earlier technology, the FT-ICR mass spectrometers, with ions being electrostatically forced onto an orbit around a central electrode that has the form of a spindle (Figure 10.17).

While orbiting around the central electrode, ions oscillate back and forth along its electrode axis, which forms a current in the surrounding detector plates. The frequencies of such oscillating, ion-induced image currents depend on the ions' mass/charge ratio and can be measured at high accuracy. By measuring the frequencies for about 0.5–1 second, high resolution mass spectra can be obtained via Fourier transformation.

Mass Analyzers: Summary of Characteristics All mass analyzers yield mass-to-charge ratios (m/z) rather than mass alone. They fall into several categories: Some mass analyzers, such as in TOF and double-focusing magnetic sector mass analyzers, measure a mass–charge (m/z) ratio directly by monitoring the ions' drift velocity or predict the ions' paths according to the Lorentz force that charged particles experience in a magnetic field. For TOF mass analyzers, ions must be delivered as a pulse to determine the time the ions need to reach the detector, which makes TOF ideal for pulsed ionization approaches such as MALDI. TOF-Reflectron mass analyzers help overcome the spread in velocity in an ensemble of ions due to small differences in kinetic energy.

Quadrupole mass analyzers are mass filters as they determine the m/z by monitoring the stability of ions' trajectories. During a systematic sweep of the electrostatic field (direct current) and radiofrequencies (RF), only ions of a certain m/z ratio will have stable trajectories for specific field combinations and thus reach the detector, with all other ions being lost in the process.

Yet other ways are taken by quadrupole ion traps and FT-ICR mass analyzers to determine m/z. They trap ions and store them using certain direct current and RF settings. In the case of quadrupole ion traps, changes in direct current and RF lead to the successive ejection of the ions from the trap to the detector. FT-ICR mass analyzers trap ions using RF resonance and force the ions on circular orbits. This results in specific cyclotron frequencies of the ions, which then can be detected by detection plates, and upon Fourier transformation such frequency measurements can yield m/z values.

There is no perfect mass analyzer that will work best for all applications, instead the various choices have their respective advantages and disadvantages (Figure 10.18). Double focusing magnetic sector mass analyzers yield classic mass spectra, with very high reproducibility, high sensitivity, high resolution, and high dynamic range. On the

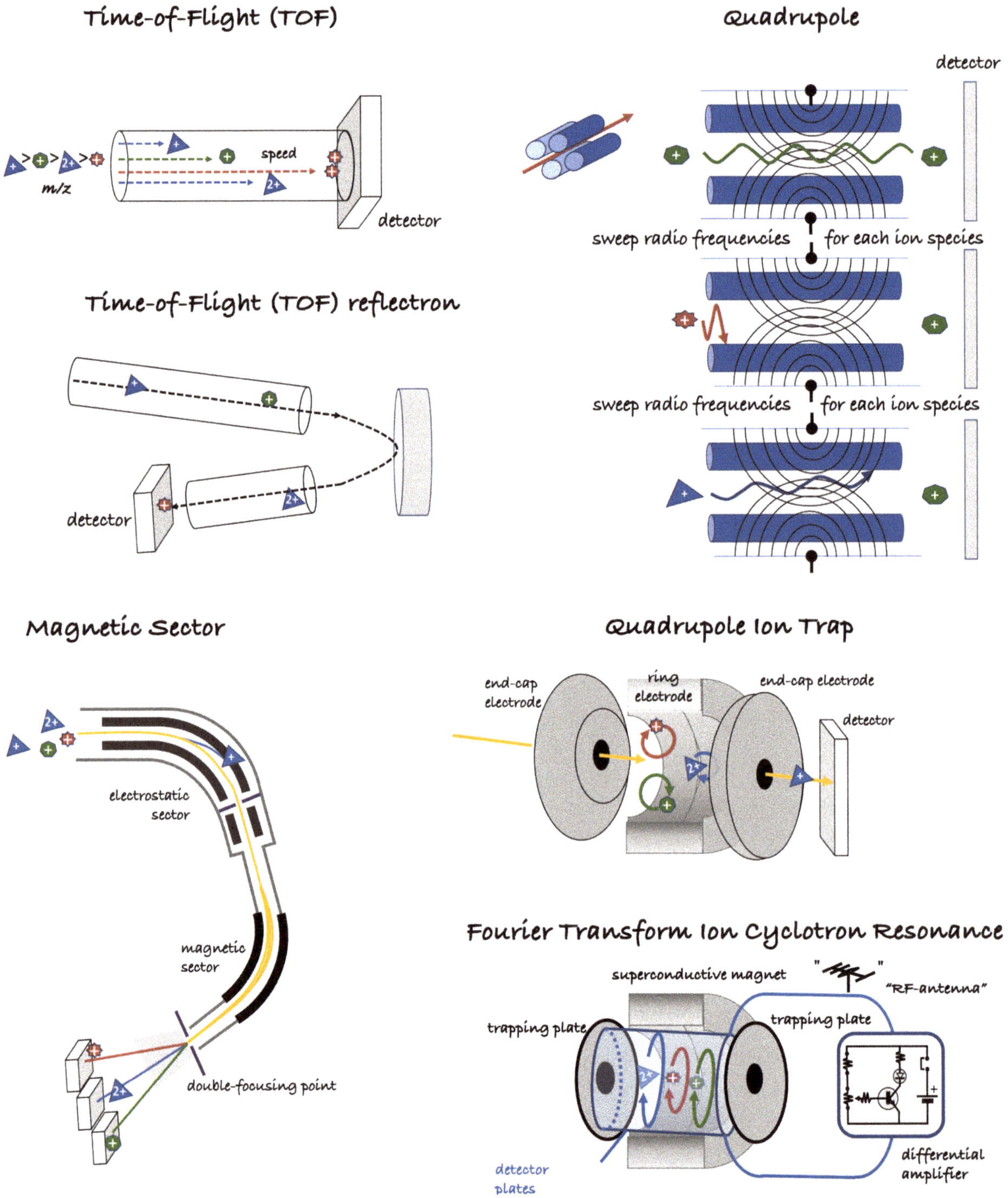

Figure 10.17 Time-of-flight and quadrupole mass analyzers. Time-of-flight (TOF) and time-of-flight reflectron mass analyzers separate ions (mass-to-charge ratio) according to their speed and thus arrival time at the detector. In quadrupole mass analyzers there is a sweep of radio frequencies. Certain frequencies will allow certain ions to pass through the quadrupole field, whereas other ion species are "filtered out." Each ion species is ejected from the quadrupole field and thus detected when sweeping with the appropriate radio frequency. Magnetic sector, quadrupole ion trap, and Fourier transform ion cyclotron resonance mass analyzers. Magnetic sector mass analyzers sort the ions spatially by forcing them on different trajectories, with each trajectory being detected independently by a different detector. Quadrupole ion traps mass analyzers use specific radio frequencies to successively release ions of a defined mas-to-charge ratio which are then monitored by a detector. Fourier transform ion cyclotron resonance mass analyzers measure a specific current in detector plates surrounding the central cavity, which indicates the ions' mass-to-charge ratio.

	TOF	TOF reflectron	Magnetic Sector	Quadrupole	Quadrupole Ion Trap	FT-ICR
ion supply	pulsed	pulsed	continuous	continuous	pulsed	pulsed
pressure	10^{-6} Torr	10^{-6} Torr	10^{-6} Torr	10^{-5} Torr	10^{-3} Torr	$<10^{-8}$ Torr
separation	drift velocity		ion path	ion trajectory stability		frequency
m/z range	<1 MDa	<10 kDa	<20 kDa	<4 kDa	<6 kDa	<30 kDa
accuracy	200 ppm	10 ppm	<5 ppm	100 ppm	100 ppm	<1 ppm
scan speed	milliseconds per scan		seconds per scan		seconds per scan	

Figure 10.18 Mass analyzer characteristics. The different mass analyzers differ in a variety of ways, such as how the ions are supplied (either as a pulse or a continuous stream), what vacuum pressures are needed for the technique to be able to work, the underlying mechanism for ion separation, the mass-to-charge range that can be analyzed, the accuracy by which the ions can be separated, as well as the scan speed by which the data can be obtained.

downside, they tend to be larger and more expensive compared to other mass analyzers, and they are not compatible with pulsed ionization methods such as MALDI, unlike TOF mass analyzers which are predestined for MALDI. The need for pulsed ion delivery may also be a disadvantage in some applications. TOF (and TOF-Reflectron) mass analyzers are the fastest mass analyzers with an extraordinarily high mass range that can be detected. Quadrupole mass analyzers are relatively small and low-cost instruments, which yield classical mass spectra with high reproducibility. Quadrupole mass analyzers work well for tandem mass spectrometry (MS/MS) due to low-energy collision-induced dissociation, but they are not well-suited for pulsed ionization approaches such as MALDI. Quadrupole ion traps are compact mass analyzers with high sensitivity, which allow multi-stage mass spectrometry (like in FT-ICR). Both, quadrupole ion traps and FT-ICR, rely on pulsed ion generation. One of the limitations for both quadrupole ion trap and FT-ICR is the poor dynamic range. However, unlike FT-ICR, quadrupole ion traps are compatible with poor vacuum conditions and thus well suited for liquid chromatography. FT-ICR has the highest mass resolution and is well suited for MS/MS, however since FT-ICR uses superconducting magnets and relies on very high vacuum conditions, FT-ICR instruments tend to be very expensive.

Mass Analyzer: Tandem Mass Spectrometry In tandem mass spectrometry multiple mass analyzers are used, i.e., three quadrupoles placed in series, allowing multiple rounds of mass spectrometry with fragmentation occurring between these rounds due to collision-induced dissociation (Figure 10.19). The term "tandem" refers to analysis in space, e.g., by consecutive analyzers, or in time with the same analyzer, e.g., of additional fragments. Each quadrupole has

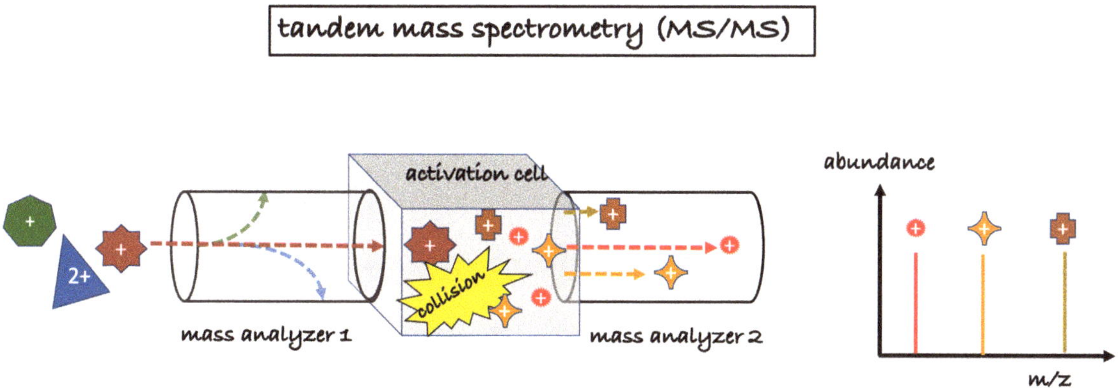

Figure 10.19 Tandem mass spectrometry. In tandem mass spectrometry, there are several mass analyzers, with a collision chamber in between where ions are further fragmented by colliding with collision gas. In the first mass analyzers only a small number of ions will be allowed to collide with the collision gas, which leads to fragmentation and detection by another mass analyzer. Changes of the quadrupole settings eventually allow an entire mass spectrum to be recorded.

a separate function: The first quadrupole selects an ion of interest, whereas the second quadrupole allows a collision of the ion with a collision gas, before a third quadrupole analyzes the fragments generated by the collision. Both the first and third quadrupoles are mass filters, allowing only a small subset of ions to reach the detector, but through changes at the quadrupole settings an entire spectrum can be collected eventually.

Tandem mass spectrometry is particularly useful for proteomics, where peptides obtained by digestion of proteins are identified. Fragments created by multiple collision energy and ionization modes show characteristic mass/charge ratios that can be identified and compared to a data base with nearly a million standard entries.

Detector

The detector records the arrival of the ion, either by the charge or the current it induces (Figure 10.20). The combination of mass analyzer settings and ion detection is what will produce a mass spectrum.

The most commonly used detector is an electron multiplier that closely resembles a traditional photomultiplier tube with a series of dynodes maintained at ever increasing potential, resulting in a cascade of electrons and thus a signal gain of a factor of up to 1,000,000. In the electron multiplier the ion hits the first dynode directly, which then leads to the emission of electrons. This design, while being sensitive, fast, and robust has a somewhat short lifetime. Photomultiplier Conversion Dynodes use a phosphorus screen where the ion signal is converted into a photon signal that is then detected by the photomultiplier. Photomultiplier conversion dynodes have a longer lifetime than electron multiplier and are equally sensitive and robust. Array detectors consist of a group of individual detectors that are aligned into an array. This allows the simultaneous detection of m/z differences without the need for scanning. Such detectors are used in combination with magnetic sector mass analyzers. Also, Faraday-Cup ion detectors are in use, but this type of detector is not very sensitive and does not offer much signal amplification, however it is tolerant to low vacuum pressure conditions. In Fourier Transform mass spectrometers the ions are detected in a different way, namely as an inductive current, produced between the outer shell and the inner spindle electrodes as the ions oscillate along the longitudinal axis of the spindle electrode.

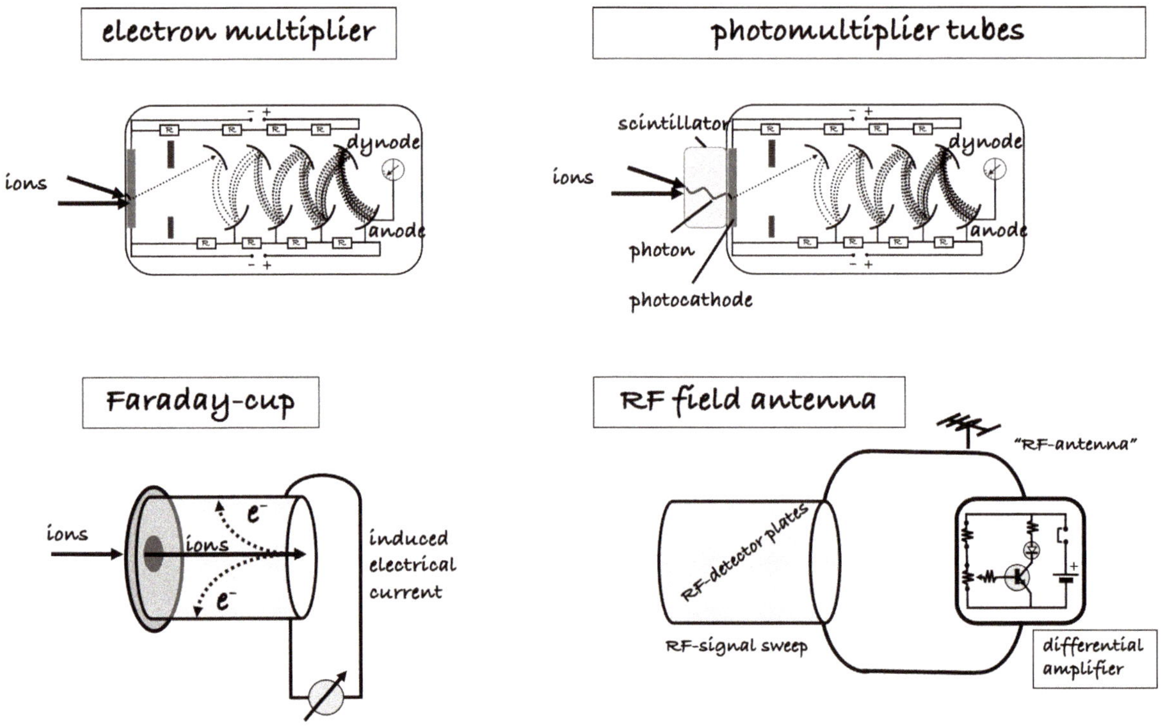

Figure 10.20 Mass spectrometry detectors. MS detectors can be based on very different detection mechanisms. Ions hitting an electron multiplier lead to the emission of secondary electrons and thus high amplification. Alternatively, photomultiplier conversion diodes will convert the ion signal into a photon signal that leads to signal amplification as is typical for photomultiplier tubes. Yet another way is to detect ions by the current they induce in a Faraday cup. The detection of an RF field of ions being forced on a resonance trajectory lies at the heart of FT-ICR MSI.

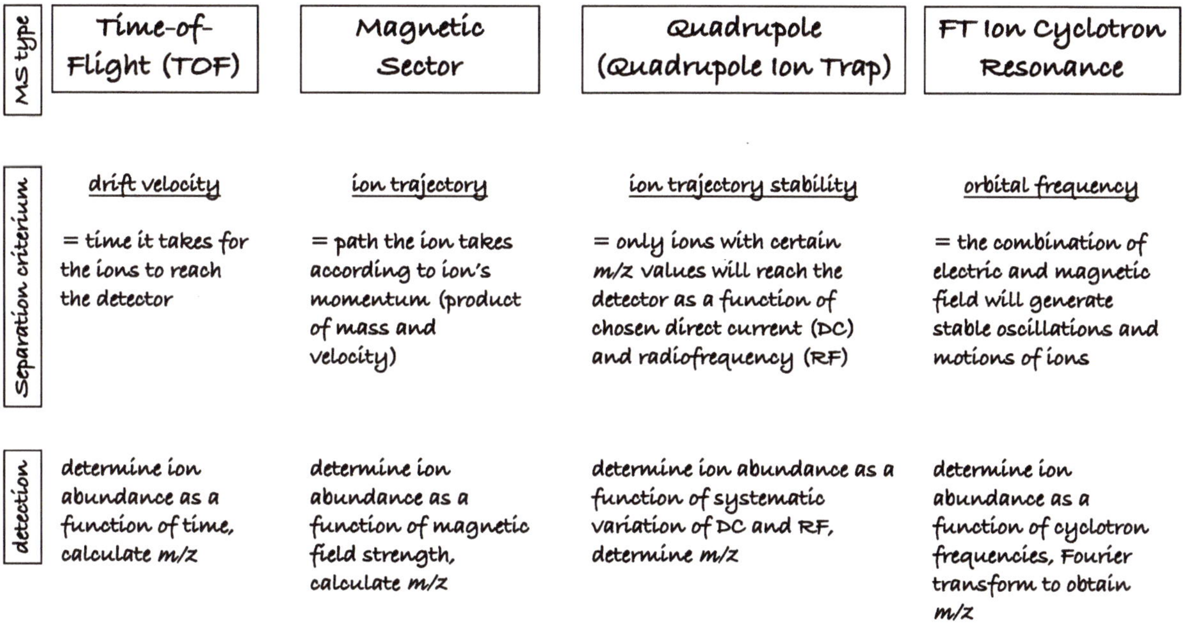

Figure 10.21 Analyzing mass spectrometry data. Different mass spectrometry techniques such as time-of-flight, magnetic sector, quadrupole, and quadrupole ion trap, as well as Fourier transform ion cyclotron resonance rely on different mechanisms for separating the different ions according to the mass-to-charge ratios. Also, their different mode of detection should be taken into consideration when interpreting the resulting mass spectrometry data.

Vacuum System

Just like it is the case for electron microscopes and ion beam microscopes, mass spectrometers require the maintenance of a high vacuum for delivering high quality spectra. Such high vacuum conditions are achieved by a combination of pumps, including a mechanical pump, also known as a roughing pump, that achieves 10^{-3} Torr (~1 mbar), before other pumping systems such as diffusion pumps, cryogenic pumps and turbomolecular pumps can be activated to achieve vacuum pressure conditions of less than 10^{-8} Torr.

10.4.4 Data Analysis

The most common way to present mass spectrometry data is to plot signal intensity as a function of the mass/charge ratio. However, for many mass spectrometry experiments the actual signal that is detected is not a mass/charge ratio, but differences in drift velocity, ion trajectory, ion trajectory stability or orbital frequency, and hence it is the detection of ion abundance as a function of time, as a function of magnetic field strength, as a function of direct current and radio frequency or as a function of cyclotron frequencies (with the additional step of a Fourier transform) that allows one to calculate the mass charge ratio (Figure 10.21). Some peaks may yield the mass of the intact analyte molecule, whereas other peaks represent fragments of the analyte molecule. It should be noted that many factors can affect signal intensity, such as the exact experimental conditions in terms of the types of separation, the types of ionization (positive or negative ionization), presence of buffer salt adducts, and other factors. Hence, it is often advisable to run a known standard under the same experimental conditions to unambiguously identify a suspected analyte. However, a fair amount of pre-processing is necessary when the raw data represents TOF arrival time, magnetic sector behavior, or productive quadrupole radio frequencies. Such signals need to be translated into a mass/charge (m/z) ratio, which then needs to be compared to existing databases for compound identification. To translate mass spectra for each raster pixel or voxel into images, certain regions or specific peaks of mass spectra need to be assigned to difference colors. This is already a form of interpretation as one needs to select what region in a spectrum or what specific peak to display in form of an image. The result can be a set of 2D or 3D images that are inherently very rich in information, and hence it may not be an understatement that while mass spectrometry may be a mature discipline, MSI is still in its early days with lots of room for improvement, particularly with respect to how all the rich information can be communicated.

11

Techniques – Tissue and Organ Medical Imaging

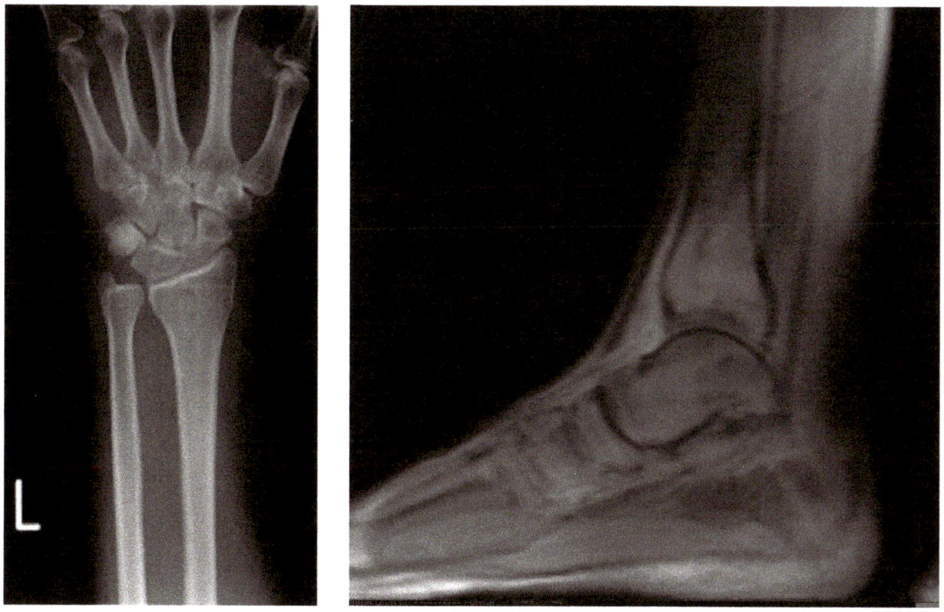

X-ray 2D image of a human hand and Magnetic Resonance Image of a human foot.

Techniques discussed:

- Positron Emission Tomography (PET)
- Computed (Axial) Tomography (CAT/CT)
- Magnetic Resonance Imaging (MRI)
- Medical Ultrasound
- Bioluminescence
- Optical Coherence Tomography (OCT)
- Histology/Histopathology/Histochemistry

The techniques discussed in this chapter belong to the category Medical Imaging and are frequently used in (pre-) clinical research and medical practice.

Medical Imaging and Bioimaging as disciplines have remarkably little interactions despite the vast overlap the two fields have, including challenges with respect to sensitivity, data resolution and volume complexity. Another reason for the separation of the two broad disciplines may be that some of the techniques, such as PET or ultrasound, have no counterpart on the macromolecular and cellular/tissue scale altogether. Also, while similar forms of radiation are being used, they are used in very different ways and/or at very different scales (e.g., MRI versus nuclear magnetic resonance [NMR] or CAT/CT versus X-ray microscopy tomography [XRMT]). Bioluminescence and OCT are optical imaging approaches, but they are used in very different ways compared to bioimaging. Histology, histopathology and histochemistry on the other hand have close counterparts in bioimaging but typically the scale of imaging is much bigger, as large regions of tissues are being studied. Many of these techniques target entire organs, whereas bioimaging focuses all the way from macromolecular complexes to the level of cells and small tissue portions (Figure 11.1). As bioimaging is starting to target 3D organ organization, the boundaries become more blurry, but organ imaging in bioimaging is restricted to small animal model systems, not human beings. These two imaging

Introduction to Biological Imaging, First Edition. Manfred Auer.

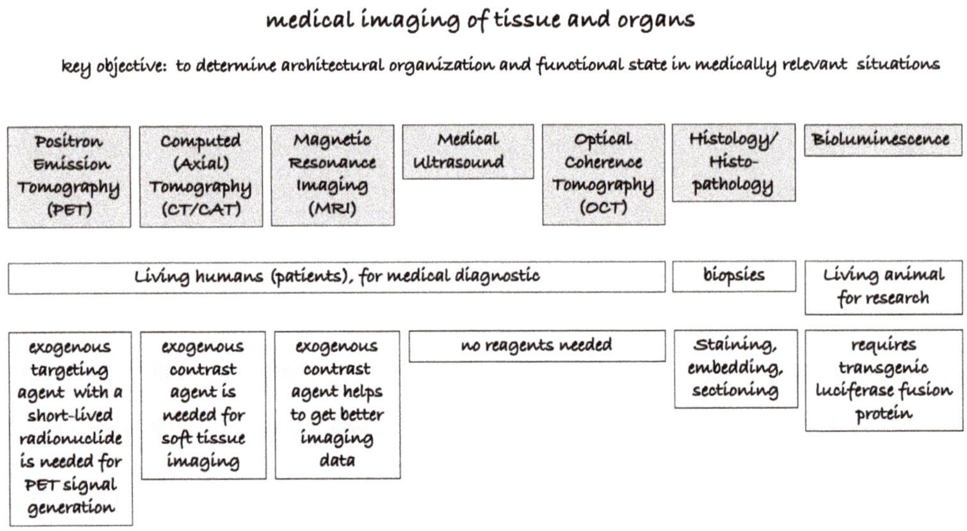

Figure 11.1 Overview of medical imaging of tissues and organs. Among the medical imaging techniques, computed tomography (CT), magnetic resonance imaging (MRI), and ultrasound are the most commonly used and widely available. CT imaging focuses on calcified tissues like bone or can be used in combination with exogenous contrasting reagents. MRI and ultrasound have their strength with soft tissues like many of the organs. Positron emission tomography (PET), while somewhat specialized and only offered in places where radioactive reagents with a short half-life are available, can play an important role in cancer diagnosis and in the detection brain diseases, including dementia. Optical Coherence Tomography is more of a niche technique predominantly used in ophthalmology to detect diseases of the retina and the optic nerve. Histology in history played a key role to understand the physiological function of tissues and organs. Histology and histopathology require biopsies (tissue samples) that undergo chemical fixation, staining, embedding, and sectioning prior to light microscopic imaging. The contemporary focus lies on pathological changes of organ and tissue histological structure for diagnosis of a large variety of diseases, including cancer. Bioluminescence requires genetic engineering of luciferase as a fusion protein and is therefore only used in preclinical animal model research.

Table 11.1 Nobel Prizes involving medical imaging.

Year	Laureate	Prize category	
1979	Allan M. Cormack Godfrey N. Hounsfield	Physiology/Medicine	For the development of computer assisted tomography
2003	Paul C. Lauterbur Sir Peter Mansfield	Physiology/Medicine	For their discoveries concerning magnetic resonance imaging

categories (medical imaging and bioimaging) have many things in common, which is why we discuss them here, albeit in a short and rather concise way. Given that all these imaging approaches face similar challenges, there is optimism that these two fields will further grow together and that each discipline will learn from one another. Two Nobel Prizes in Physiology/Medicine have been awarded, one for computer assisted tomography and one for magnetic resonance imaging (Table 11.1).

11.1 Positron Emission Tomography

PET is a functional imaging technique used in nuclear medicine, that shows biochemical and metabolic activity of an organ through the uptake of a metabolite analog that acts as a radiotracer (e.g., [^{18}F] fluorodeoxyglucose; 18F-FDG). PET is often combined with a structural imaging technique such as computed tomography (CT) to provide an organ-level reference frame in which the PET result can be interpreted.

The radioactive isotope (e.g., ^{18}F) is introduced by a small molecule (such as fluorodeoxyglucose, FDG), which is taken up by cells (and phosphorylated). The ^{18}F-labeled glucose is metabolically trapped inside the cells as it cannot be metabolized due to the replacement of the hydroxyl group by the fluorine atom at the carbon-2 position of the glucose ring. A high PET signal indicates tissues/organs that have a high uptake of glucose, which can be indicative for certain diseases such as cancer. The largest proportion of PET scans is carried out for the detection of metastases. Apart from cancer diagnosis, PET is also well-suited to monitor bone-related diseases as the radioactive isotope version of sodium fluoride (^{18}F-NaF; Na^{18}F), is rapidly absorbed by bone. ^{15}O is used in form of $H_2{}^{15}O$ or $CO^{15}O$ (CO_2) to study blood flow and for brain imaging. However, the short half-life of two minutes makes this form of imaging very challenging, as the radioisotope must be produced on site (at a cyclotron facility).

As brain cell metabolism relies on glucose, ^{18}F-FDG is an ideal radiotracer for studying brain activity (e.g., for visualizing seizure foci or for studying epilepsy), but ^{18}F can also be introduced to molecules that associate with amyloid-plaques, widely seen as a characteristics of Alzheimer disease (Figure 11.2). Likewise, other radiotracers can be synthesized that specifically bind to and thus recognize neuroreceptor subtypes, which is used in the study of diseases like schizophrenia, substance abuse or mood disorders. Other applications of PET in medical imaging include the study of bacterial infections, inflammation as well as pharmaco-kinetics and distribution of drug-candidates in pre-clinical animal studies.

PET imaging relies on the simultaneous detection in opposite directions of gamma-ray photons that form when the radiotracer-emitted positron annihilates with an electron of its immediate surroundings. A technique related to PET is single-photon emission computed tomography (SPECT), which uses radiotracers that emit gamma-rays instead of positrons. Both techniques rely on the detection of gamma-rays, however in SPECT single photons are detected, whereas in PET pairs of photons are detected, which means that PET has twice the signal and a better localization (thus higher resolution). The resolution for SPECT is about 6–10 cm, and thus lower than in PET (4–5 mm), however compared to PET, SPECT imaging has lower costs associated with it.

Radionuclides must be readily produced in a cyclotron nearby the PET imaging site, as some have half-lives as short as 2 minutes (^{15}O), 10 minutes (^{13}N), or 20 minutes (^{11}C) and they typically are incorporated into small molecule compounds to create a radiotracer. ^{18}F-FDG is one of the most commonly used radiotracers. With a half-life of 110 minutes, it is used for the vast majority of PET/PET-CT scans in oncology and neurology.

The radiotracer is injected into the blood circulation, and after an appropriate waiting period, in which the radiotracer is accumulated in its target organ, the patient is placed in the PET scanner. As the radioisotope decays, positrons are emitted in all directions and annihilate with an electron in close proximity (typically less than 1 mm) to produce a pair of gamma photons emitted in opposite directions. This pair of gamma photons hit the scintillator material in the PET scanner, and the resulting light is detected by photodetectors. Only pairs of photons, arriving at the same time, are recorded, other photons are presumed to be background and therefore they are ignored. Each of

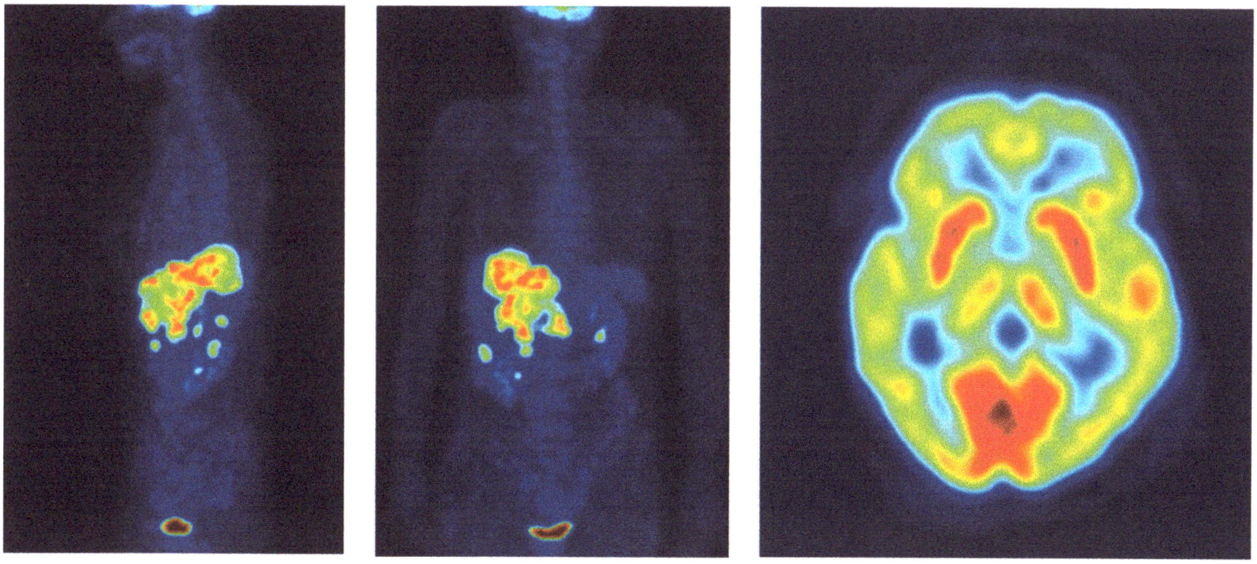

Figure 11.2 Positron Emission Tomography. *Source:* Alexandra Almonacid E. / Wikidoc / CC BY-SA 3.0. In positron emission tomography (PET) a radiotracer molecule will undergo radioactive decay, emitting a positron in the process. This positron will annihilate with an electron in its immediate environment leading to the formation of a pair of gamma-ray photons that will be emitted into opposite directions. Such coincidence events are detected via a scintillator-coupled PET detector and represent a line in space. Multiple rings of detectors can measure time differences between arriving photons, which helps to estimate the origin of the photon pair in 3D formation. 3D volumes can be reconstructed from the combination of such lines. Left and middle: ^{18}F-FDG whole human body scan; Right: human brain scan.

these coincidence events represent a line in space. Coincidence events can be grouped into projection images, which then can be combined to create a 3D volume, similar to reconstructing 3D volumes from projections in CT imaging. Due to the lower counting statistics, PET data has significantly more noise than CT.

Modern PET equipment has multiple rings of detectors, forming a detection cylinder, which can account for the time difference of detection of each photon of the photon-pair. This helps to estimate the center of emission of the photon pair along the coincidence line, and thus improves the resolution of the resulting 3D volume.

Ideally, PET is combined with CT or MRI imaging to provide anatomical background that helps interpreting the PET results.

11.2 Computed (Axial) Tomography

CT, formerly known as computed axial tomography (CAT), is a radiological diagnostic medical imaging tool that allows the non-invasive study of anatomical 3D structure and function of organs and tissues at sub-millimeter resolution. CT has its mathematical foundation in the Radon transform (in 1917) and its conceptional foundation in a US patent granted in 1963 to William H. Ohlendorf for a "radiant energy apparatus for investigating selected areas of interior objects obscured by dense material." The first commercially viable CT scanner was invented in 1972 by Godfrey Hounsfield. Both the physicist Allan M. Cormack and the electrical engineer Godfrey N. Hounsfield shared the 1979 Nobel Prize in Physiology or Medicine, for the development of computer-assisted tomography.

A typical CT scanner setup consists of an X-ray source, which produces a narrow X-ray beam that penetrates a patient before being detected by a row of digital detectors. Both the X-ray source as well as the detectors rotate around the patient. The resulting signal is then computer-processed to reveal a cross-sectional image (typically a 1–10 mm slice of the body). The patient is then shifted along the z-axis before another slice of image data is being recorded. A 3D volume is then built up by the stacking of successive slice, and further analyzed by 3D rendering and segmentation, not unlike what is done for electron tomograms or X-ray microscopy tomograms.

CT scans can identify injuries (bone fractures) and diseases of the abdomen, brain, heart, lungs, including tumors, excessive fluid formation or blood clots in connection with strokes, hemorrhage (Figure 11.3). While X-ray-dense structures like bone are readily visible, other structures may require a contrasting agent (often given intravenously), which can be iodine- or barium-based. The diagnostic value must be weighed against the risk of an increased dose of ionizing radiation (X-rays), as well as the allergenic or nephrotoxic potential of contrasting agents.

11.3 Magnetic Resonance Imaging (MRI)

MRI is a non-invasive medical imaging technique to reveal anatomical structures (particularly in soft tissues) as well as physiological processes. The theoretical background of interaction with matter and detection are similar to NMR imaging, and in short are based on atomic nuclei, being exposed to a strong magnetic field, to absorb radio frequency (RF) signals at a resonance frequency that affects nuclear spin polarization, most prominently of hydrogen atoms. MRI relies on a strong, homogenous magnetic field, which is often accomplished by liquid helium-cooled superconducting magnets (and shim coils), which is overlaid by gradient coils that alter the local magnetic field (resulting in a moving line scan). The RF system excites the tissue and detects the resulting NMR signal. The rate by which different tissues or blood relax to equilibrium state determines imaging contrast, but contrast reagents such as gadolinium chelates can further enhance imaging contrast. Gadolinium chelates have a water molecule in a chelating position which exchanges rapidly with water molecules in its surrounding. This affects magnetic resonance relaxation time.

In the 1970s, Paul Lauterbur at Stony Brook University (SUNY Stony Brook) and Peter Mansfield at the University of Nottingham developed the technique of MRI. They received the 2003 Nobel Prize in Physiology or Medicine for their discoveries concerning MRI.

In patients, typically a resolution of 200 μm to 3 mm can be accomplished, whereas in animal studies the resolution can be pushed to 50 μm. There are different modes of imaging, i.e., T1 relaxation (spin–lattice relaxation; along the static magnetic field) and T2 relaxation (spin–spin relaxation; transverse to the static magnetic field), which allows identification of low or high water-content. This difference is relevant for the detection of fatty tissue or edema/inflammation and allows discrimination between white matter and gray matter in the brain.

A whole variety of applications exist for MRI for medical diagnostics, including neurological cancers of the brain stem and the cerebellum (Figure 11.4), cardiovascular imaging (including myocardial ischemia, cardiomyopathies, myocarditis, and congenital heart disease), systemic muscle diseases, liver, pancreas, and bile duct diseases, as well as vascular diseases to evaluate the risk of stenosis (abnormal narrowing of arteries) or aneurysms (vessel wall rupture).

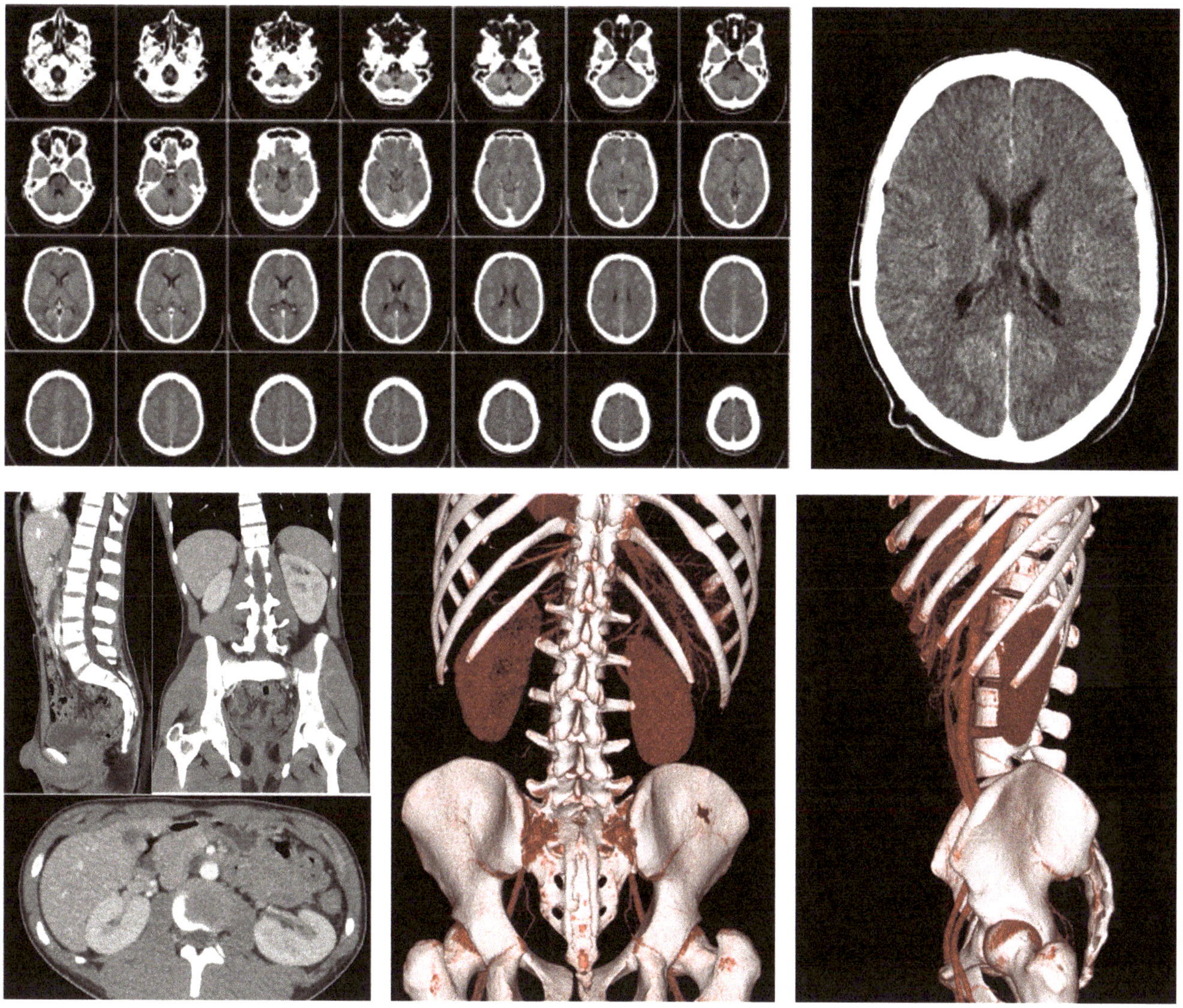

Figure 11.3 Computed tomography of a human brain and torso. *Source:* Uppsala University Hospital / Mikael Häggström / Wikipedia Commons / CC0 1.0, Mikael Häggström / Wikipedia Commons / CC0 1.0. Computed Tomography (CT) scan of a patient head (top) and torso (bottom). Note that bones show a strong contrast due to their calcium content, whereas soft tissues are more difficult to distinguish from one another; Bottom left: three 2D slices through a 3D volume in orthogonal orientation; Bottom middle and bottom right: 3D rendering of the skeletal organization, shown in different orientation.

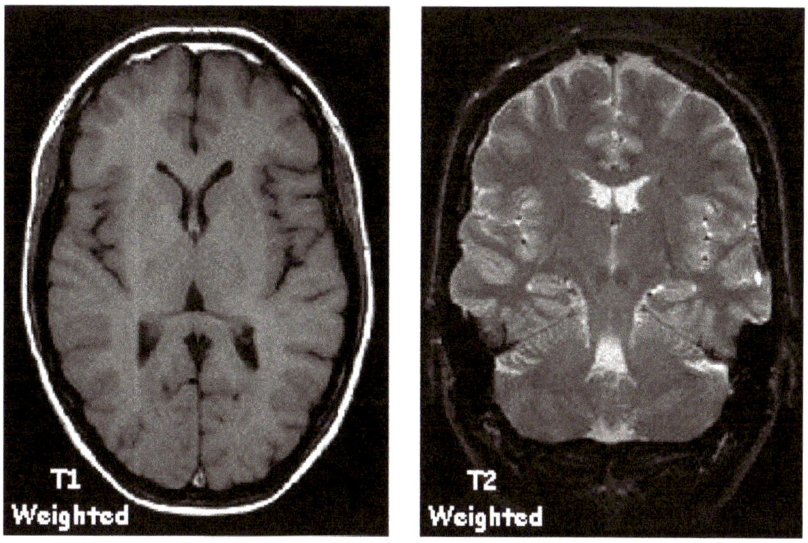

Figure 11.4 Magnetic Resonance Imaging. *Source:* KieranMaher / Wikipedia Commons / Public Domain. Cross-sectional T1-weighted and T2-weighted magnetic resonance images of a healthy human brain. Note that the cerebral spinal fluid appears dark in T1-weighted MRI head scans, whereas it would show up bright in T2-weighted MRI images.

11.4 Medical Ultrasound

Medical ultrasound is an imaging technique that uses ultrasound to examine non-invasively internal body structures, such as internal organs, blood vessels, muscle, joints, and tendons, and is of particular value in imaging the fetus during pregnancy. Different tissues reflect ultrasound waves differently, which leads to image contrast in so-called sonograms. In ultrasound sound waves at MHz frequencies and thus ~50–1,000-fold above the threshold of human hearing (at ~20 kHz) are used for imaging.

Unlike some other medical imaging devices, ultrasound equipment is compact (and thus portable), cheap and does not rely on ionizing radiation, and is therefore non-invasive with no long-term side effects and minimal discomfort. Further advantages of ultrasound imaging over other medical imaging approaches are the possibility to obtain "live"-images and to assess the mechanical properties (e.g., the stiffness) of a tissue/organ. Among its weaknesses is the difficulty of ultrasound to penetrate bone tissue, gas-filled compartments, and excessive body fat layers.

Transducers are typically applied to the outside of a patient's body with the help of a water-based gel to avoid total reflection by air. Sometimes transducers are placed directly into body cavities (e.g., vagina or rectum) or reside at the proximal end of a catheter, threaded into blood vessels, to provide better images.

Arc-shaped sound waves at frequencies between 1 and 18 MHz are produced by a piezoelectric transducer and scattered or reflected at tissue boundaries or by blood cells, where there is a change in acoustical impedance. The reflected portion of the sound is then detected by the piezoelectric transducer, which measures the intensity of the signal and the time delay of the echo with respect to the original signal, which in turn determines the depth from where the echo originated. As a result, we obtain an image of the ultrasound echo (Figure 11.5). A 2D images is formed by mechanical sweeping and rotating the transducer, and by accounting for this movement upon processing the reflected data to generate an image, which is a 2D representation of a slice of the body. 3D scans can be built up acquiring a series of 2D scan, but such 3D scans can be difficult to obtain for tissues undergoing movement. Movement such as the flow of blood can be visualized by using so-called Doppler ultrasonography, which is based on the Doppler effect, i.e., the change in frequency of the echo because of the movement (e.g., the blood flow). The choice of frequency is important with lower frequency usually means deeper penetration, whereas higher frequency allows higher resolution. Also, the assumption in sonography that sound travels at a constant speed in the body is not entirely correct as different tissues display different acoustical impedance, which further degrades image resolution. In medical sonography, typically multiple transducers are used simultaneously.

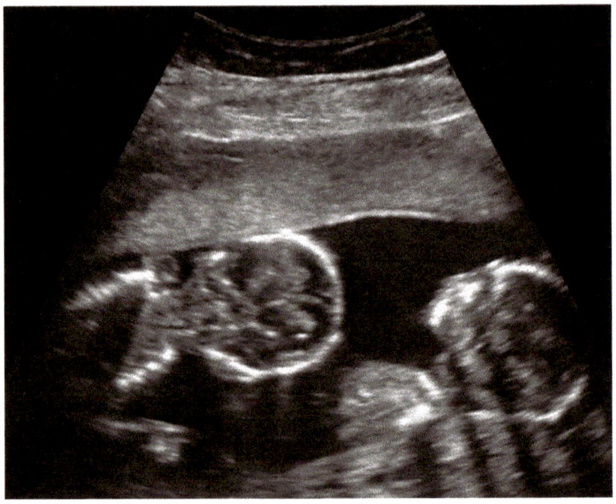

Figure 11.5 Ultrasound. *Source:* Mikael Häggström / Wikimedia Commons / CC0 1.0. Ultrasound imaging is frequently used to image fetuses inside the uterus during pregnancy due to its non-invasive nature that causes no long-term side effects.

There are several modes of ultrasound imaging. The simplest mode is the amplitude mode (A-mode), where a single transducer scans a line in the body with the echo being plotted as a function of depth. In the brightness mode (B-mode, also known as 2D-mode), a linear array of transducers simultaneously scans a plane in the body, resulting in a 2D image. In the C-mode, a particular depth of the body is selected from A-mode data, and a 2D plane (orthogonal to the B-mode plane) is obtained by manual (spiral) movement of the transducer. In the motion mode (M-mode), A-mode or B-mode scans are carried out with short pulsing of the ultrasound, which allows a video-like recording of organ boundaries. In the Doppler-mode one measures the frequency shift of the echo, caused by the movement of the reflecting object (blood flow). Pulsed wave Doppler ultrasound imaging also allows a measurement of the distance, as the time delay between the pulses and the received signal can be determined. The velocity information can then be visualized using color coding. In the pulse inversion mode, two successive pulses with opposite signs are emitted. The subtraction of the signal will lead to no contrast unless the reflecting object (such as gas bubbles) shows non-linear compressibility and thus stand out. In the harmonic mode, a deep penetrating fundamental frequency is emitted, and one detects a harmonic overtone echo. Encapsulated gaseous microbubbles, administered intravenously into the blood stream, enhance the contrast in ultrasound imaging and allow visualization of the organ's microvascular network. Ideally, such encapsulated microbubbles can be targeted specifically to certain locations (e.g., tumor tissue). Photoacoustic imaging (also known as optoacoustic imaging) is another form of ultrasound imaging, where ultrasound waves are generated when non-ionizing nanosecond laser light pulses are absorbed by the tissue. Such ultrasound waves are then detected by a Fabry Perot ultrasound sensor (ultrasonic transducer) and analyzed to produce images. Hemoglobin is particularly effective to produce a signal, with its absorption coefficient being dependent on its oxygen saturation status, which is why photoacoustic imaging is particularly useful for dynamic in-vivo monitoring of blood flow and blood oxygenation. It can be employed clinically for monitoring of tumor angiogenesis, functional brain imaging, as well as for the detection of skin melanoma (due to the strong absorption of melanin). Also, high contrast can be achieved by suitable exogenously delivered agents. The spatial resolution limit of ultrasound imaging for a 5 MHz signal is at ~0.3 mm.

11.5 Bioluminescence

Bioluminescence is a form of chemiluminescence, which has evolved independently several times. It has been found in many living beings, including bacteria, fungi, protozoa, invertebrates, including jellyfish, mollusca, crustaceans and insects, and vertebrate (i.e., ray-finned fish).

The underlying mechanism of the production and emission of light is the biochemical oxidation of the small molecule luciferin catalyzed by an enzyme called luciferase in the presence of molecular oxygen. Luciferases are rather diverse and therefore a variety of mechanisms exist, some requiring magnesium and ATP as co-factors.

For his work to obtain pure, crystalline luciferin and determine its chemical structure, the Japanese chemist Osamu Shimomura shared the 2008 Nobel Prize in Chemistry with Martin Chalfie and Roger Y. Tsien for their discovery and development of green fluorescent protein as a tool for biological research.

Luciferase systems can be used as reporters through the engineering of genetically encoded luciferase-fusion proteins, capable of producing a chemiluminescence signal. A variety of luciferase fusion proteins are commercially available, including firefly, sea pansy, and bacterial luciferase. While the former two require injection of D-luciferin or coelenterazine, respectively, the latter one usually uses the entire lux operon, which also encodes the enzymes making the substrate. Firefly luciferase emits at ~560 nm and is therefore red-shifted compared to the other two (with respective emission peaks at ~480 nm or ~490 nm), which makes it better-suited for in-vivo tissue work due to lower scattering of longer-wavelength light.

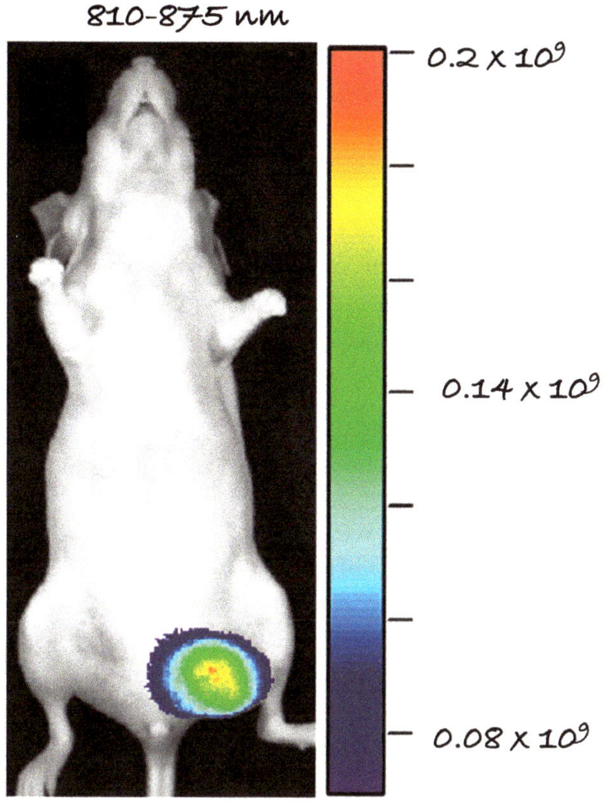

Figure 11.6 Bioluminescence. *Source:* Liat et al. (2010) / Springer Nature / CC BY 2.0. Bioluminescence is based on the oxidation of luciferin by oxygen, mediated by a luciferase protein introduced to mice by genetic engineering. Luciferin typically has to be injected prior to imaging.

For detection, ultrasensitive CCD cameras are needed, as the total amount of light emitted from bioluminescence is rather low. In a variation on the theme, induced metabolic bioluminescence can also visualize metabolic characteristics of tissues, to determine, e.g., lactate concentrations of tumors or brain metabolism (Figure 11.6).

11.6 Optical Coherence Tomography

OCT is a non-invasive medical imaging technique to study displacement of tissues with (sub-)micrometer resolution. OCT uses low-coherence light optical interferometry in the near-IR region. It has been successfully applied in the field of ophthalmology to image the retina, in otolaryngology to study the collagen-rich acellular tectorial membrane in animal models, in interventional cardiology to study coronary artery disease and in dermatology. Like in other interferometry approaches, the beam is split into a sample beam and a reference beam. It also typically includes a movable mirror. The interference signal is recorded as a function of mirror position (or timing of

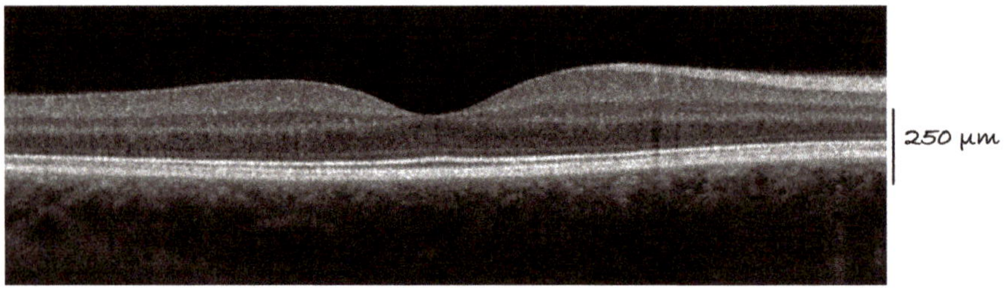

Figure 11.7 Optical coherence tomography. *Source:* Wies6014 / Wikimedia Commons / CC BY-SA 4.0. This image shows a cross-sectional slice of a spectral domain optical coherence tomogram taken of a healthy macula.

movement), which allows a determination of tissue displacement. Conceptionally one can think of OCT as an "optical ultrasound" technique. OCT provides instantaneous, direct images of tissue morphology/movement, without the need for prior sample preparation, close contact, or ionizing radiation (Figure 11.7).

11.7 Histology/Histopathology

While being discussed in more detail in Chapter 8, this section will serve as quick reminder, that optical white light microscopy is frequently used in medical imaging, either in the form of tissue biopsies, which are further processed into histochemical-stained sections, cell suspensions or smears (in medical microbiology, gynecology, and hematology). Histology, also referred to as microscopic anatomy or microanatomy, relies on optical microscopic imaging of tissues and cells, and can be performed on healthy or diseased tissue and cell samples. Histology gave us the division of animal cells into one of four categories (with respective further subclassifications): muscle tissue, connective tissue, nervous tissue, and epithelial tissue.

We call the imaging of diseased tissues histopathology, whereas the imaging of individual cells is known as cytopathology. There are a variety of stains, some of which go back many decades. There are some more specific stains such as Perl's Prussian Blue to visualize iron deposits or silver stains used prominently by Golgi and Cajal in their studies of the nervous system, Safranin, Congo Red, and many dozens other stains. However, the most frequently used stain is hematoxylin and eosin (also known as H&E stain), with hematoxylin staining cell nuclei blue, whereas the acidic stain eosin stains the remainder of the cell in various shades of pink (Figure 11.8).

In the case of antibodies that are targeted to certain proteins, carbohydrates, or lipids, one speaks of immunohistochemistry. Also, specific RNA and DNA sequences can be targeted and thus localized, which is termed in-situ hybridization.

In terms of sample preparation, typically punch biopsies (several millimeters to one centimeter in diameter) or other biopsies are chemically fixed in paraformaldehyde (e.g., formalin, which is a neutral-buffered 10% paraformaldehyde aqueous solution) or glutaraldehyde (depending

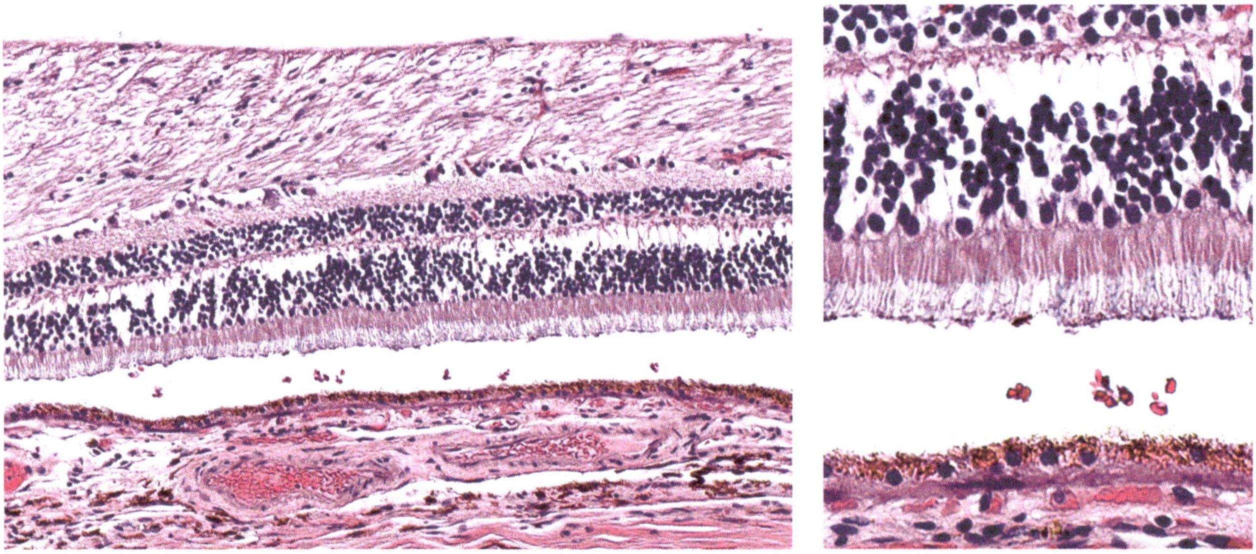

Figure 11.8 Histopathology. *Source:* Librepath / Wikipedia Commons / CC BY-SA 3.0. These images showing H&E-stained sections of the retina at intermediate and at high resolution, respectively.

on whether the samples will ultimately be studied by optical light microscopy or by electron microscopy). Alternatively, needle biopsies with diameters of less than 200 µm are “ultrarapidly” frozen, trimmed and sectioned in their frozen state. Larger samples can be frozen with prior exposure to cryo-protectants to minimize ice-crystal formation upon freezing. Optimal cutting temperature (OCT) compound (beside others) is a popular water-based embedding medium for cryostat sectioning and contains polyvinyl alcohols and polyethylene glycol compounds. Depending on the embedding medium, the tissue usually undergoes dehydration, infiltration and embedding into a wax, paraffin, or acrylic resin, which is then hardened prior to block trimming and sectioning for optical microscopy at thickness of 1–5 µm, using a microtome/vibratome, or at a thickness of 50–150 nm for electron microscopy, using an ultramicrotome. Frozen samples will be cut in their frozen state using a cryostat microtome/vibratome, and after thawing will display a higher affinity for antibodies in immunohistochemistry labeling than wax- or resin-embedded tissues samples.

Imaging slides with often multiple sections of millimeter to centimeter in dimension is a big challenge due the very large volume that need to be covered. The only way to deal with it in a digital imaging way has been to randomly select areas. However, a trained pathologist will take a glance at the entire tissue and use his expertise and experience to decide at lower resolution which areas to re-study at higher magnification and finally come to some diagnosis. Over the last decade, however, digital pathology has left its mark, and increasingly large fields of view at high resolution are being imaged automatically, followed by artificial intelligence-based (machine learning or more recently deep learning) automated analysis, which leads to a diagnosis built on the entire sample section and not on some randomly chosen region of interest.

12

The Future of Bioimaging

"Seeing is believing!" Few things are more powerful to convince skeptics than an image supporting the claims one makes. But there is more to images than just a visual argument for an otherwise foregone conclusion. Instead, if one were to speculate about the future of bioimaging, one might predict that images, particularly those recorded as part of large, systematic surveys, will increasingly become the source of new information and will lie at the center of biological discovery. In other areas of the biological sciences, particularly in its many -omics-based disciplines (such as genomics, transcriptomics, proteomics, metabolomics) gigantic datasets are being produced, with constituent components being named, categorized, and cataloged. Lists of alpha-numeric entries fill text string-based databases, which look and act more like data warehouses and all-to-often as data graveyards. Such data bases can be likened to telephone books, where all names, addresses and telephone numbers may be listed, yet there is little relationship between neighboring entries. The entries in such "White Pages" phone books can be grouped and sorted into different categories, maybe along with some pictures and illustrations, which is a step in the right direction but still only gets us to the level of the "Yellow Pages" phone book.

It seems fair to say that the organization of biological information is still stuck in the era of phone books, with each topic (cell type, disease, system) representing another city or town, some bigger and more populated with names and associated entries, some smaller and only sparsely filled with entries. Often there is little commonalities between these different towns and there is certainly little hope to mine such phone books for any information beyond what has already been logged in. It is a convenient tool to look up a phone number for a certain name, and maybe look up an associated address, but phone books do not offer much in terms of discovery of spatiotemporal relationships of their constituents. Clearly, in terms of information technology and how we organize data in other aspects of life, we have outlived phone books, and thus, if biology wants to outgrow its infancy and adolescence state of disconnected "one-off" discoveries, it will have to organize the information it produces in a much more efficient way.

Imaging is likely to play a key role in this maturation process, in part because imaging does not shy away from the heterogeneity of biological organization and its responses to perturbations/outside input. It is important to recognize the enormity of the task at hand, as biological function has many different aspects, which requires different experimental approaches. These different approaches provide information that somehow needs to be combined if one does not want to fall into the same trap as the six blind men that only got to touch one part of an elephant and came to very different conclusions of what an elephant looks like (Figure 12.1).

We must be aware and appreciative that different techniques map different aspects of a biological system and thus will provide complementary clues about the system that need to be combined (integrated) to do justice to the biological system's complexity.

Moreover, life happens at multiple scales, often spanning at least six orders of magnitude, which in terms of imaging requires the utilization of a large variety of imaging techniques, whose information content needs to be correlated and integrated.

I will discuss at the end what a biological information system (BIS) – the biological equivalent of a geospatial information system (GIS) – could look like and how it would revolutionize biology as a discipline and making biological research even more powerful and useful than it already is. I will attempt to make some predictions about the future of bioimaging, fully knowing (to quote the "baseball-playing philosopher" Yogi Berra) that "it is tough to make predictions, particularly about the future."

12.1 Future of Macromolecular Imaging

Since its inception in the early to the mid 20th century, X-ray crystallography was the dominant player and the gold standard in the structure determination of biological

Introduction to Biological Imaging, First Edition. Manfred Auer.

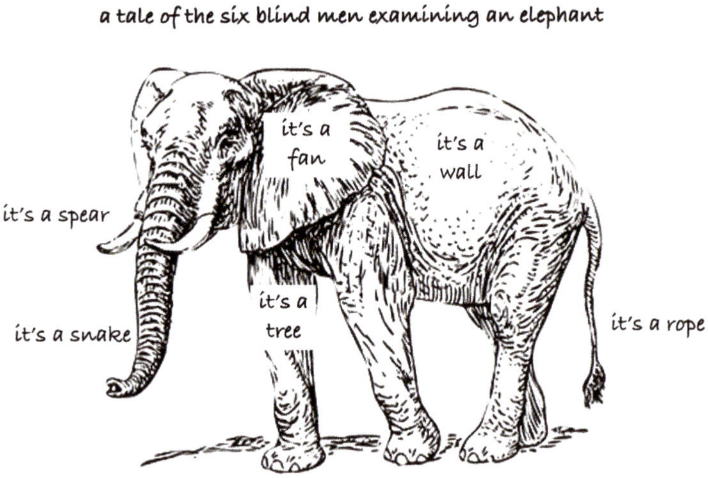

Figure 12.1 Seeing only part of the picture – Six blind men examining an elephant. When studying a biological system with different techniques, one needs to be aware what kind of information about the system the respective technique can deliver, and what its limitations are. Different techniques will yield different aspects of the biological system. Thus, to get a full picture and to recognize the elephant as a whole and not just parts of it, requires an integration of multiple modalities.

macromolecules, particularly proteins, multi-protein complexes as well as nucleic acid complexes. After its biggest theoretical problem of phasing was overcome, its only practical drawback was the need to grow large diffraction quality crystals. For a couple of decades, nuclear magnetic resonance (NMR) spectroscopy emerged as a rival technique for structure determination, but it remained the domain of smaller proteins and their study in solution. Cryo-electron microscopy slowly but steadily emerged as an alternative to structure determination, particularly when 2D crystalline and helical or icosahedral symmetry could be exploited, as has been frequently the case for membrane proteins and cytoskeletal protein assemblies or viruses, respectively.

Electron diffraction of very small micron-sized 3D crystals has also enjoyed increasing popularity and remains a growth area for macromolecular structure determination, as very small crystals are much easier to obtain than 3D crystals that are hundreds of micrometer-sized.

The last 10 years have seen cryo-electron microscopy (cryo-EM) in combination with single particle analysis to emerge as the dominant player for structure determination, as crystallization was no longer needed, proteins of low abundance and low concentration could be studied, and the sample does not even have to be homogeneous (although homogeneity, while no longer being a prerequisite, remains an advantage). Single particle cryo-EM will remain popular in the coming decade since it requires very little purified material applied to an electron microscopy support grid, with as little as some few thousand to ten thousands macromolecules being sufficient for a high-resolution 3D structure. The time it takes to reach atomic resolution has shrunk from decades or years to days or hours, hence the prediction that single particle cryo-EM will continue to be the method of choice for macromolecular structure determination does not seem that far-fetched.

However, one may dare to ask the question, how much longer structure determination of macromolecules will last. The argument goes as such:

First, as each structure takes less and less time to complete, a doctoral thesis may include many structures at atomic resolution, whereas years ago an intermediate resolution structure was more than sufficient to grant a doctoral degree. As sample heterogeneity can be dealt with and classification algorithms become better and better, one can envision a time when the samples do not even need to be purified or enriched anymore, one may simply break cells open and with sufficient dilution one may determine the structure of many particles simultaneously. However, such an approach if indeed realized, would open many more opportunities, as transient complexes formed in cells could be characterized this way.

Second, the number of laboratories/groups that have embarked on cryo-EM single particle analysis has risen sharply over the last few years, in part because data collection is largely automated, and large facilities already exist world-wide that produce data sets in a 24/7 manner, just like X-ray synchrotron facilities have over the last three decades. With high-throughput data collection in regional, national, and even international facilities further reducing the hurdle for each structure to be determined by cryo-EM, it reduces the threshold for universities to establish more single-particle cryo-EM groups. Furthermore, a large portion of groups that traditionally performed X-ray crystallography have entered the cryo-EM arena. So, while the number of groups to focus on structure determination by cryo-EM has sharply risen, the number of targets for structure determination has remained the same, or as I will argue below has declined. This is somewhat offset by the number of different states that can be imaged, including structures with inhibitors or activators bound, or assemblies where proteins undergo complex formation, but this line of argument has not rescued structural genomics (the 3D structure determination of every protein encoded in the genome) from its own success. In this field, structure prediction algorithms, particularly those that include deep learning-based approaches such as Alphafold/Alphafold2, RosettaTTAFold, OmegaFold, and ESM Metagenomic Atlas, have possibly made structure determination unnecessary, as indicated by their success in the three-decades-long annual CASP (Critical Assessment of Techniques for Protein Structure Prediction). It would seem likely that these successes in 3D structure prediction will also render cryo-EM single particle analysis studies obsolete.

Third, the actual number of targets has become smaller. Traditionally, the 3D-structure of a certain protein were solved from a variety of biological organisms, often bacterial proteins were easier to express, purify, and crystallize and thus the bacterial version(s) of a certain protein category was determined first, followed by versions of the protein expressed either in a eukaryotic expression system, such as fungi or insect cells, wherever large enough quantities for purification and crystallization could be produced. Hence, often the human version of the protein was determined last. Now, with very little material being needed and with funding pressures to be disease-relevant being at an all-time high, one may only aim for the human version, hence the need for all the other structures no longer exists.

Forth and lastly, while it is important to understand the mechanisms underlaying the biological processes in chemical (and thus atomic resolution detail), there is a growing appreciation that structure determination of purified proteins may not teach us much about disease mechanisms and possible route of intervention into pathogenesis. Not only will homology modeling, structure and structure-ligand prediction make the need for actual structure determination obsolete, it may be much faster to screen millions of possible small-molecule compounds and focus on the structure determination of a few ligand–protein complexes, once the compound has passed clinical trial toxicity and efficacy tests. After all, most small molecules never make it as an actual drug, not because they do not optimally bind to their target molecule, but because they fall through in clinical trials, typically due to toxicity. It is their interference in the function of other macromolecules inside cells and tissues that makes them toxic, which cannot be easily predicted by structure determination of the target protein. Also, although a minor concern, macromolecules when acting in the context of their native cell and tissue context may become part of larger transient complexes, which may alter their function and small-molecule-binding-behavior altogether.

In summary, while cryo-EM may win the day when it comes to what constitutes the method of choice for structure determination right now, it may be prudent to be concerned that over the next decade or two, the importance of the 3D structure determination of purified macromolecules and macromolecular complexes altogether may be on the decline, as with a limited number of targets of protein structures, set by the limited number of proteins in a genome, cryo-EM could become the victim of its own success

12.2 Future of (Sub)Cellular and Tissue Imaging

12.2.1 Light Microscopy Versus Electron Microscopy

Imaging of cells and tissues was for the longest time the domain of optical light microscopy, even since the first discovery in 1665 of cells in a plant tissue (thin slices of cork) by Robert Hooke, and of individual cells such as bacteria and protozoa by Antoni van Leeuwenhoek shortly afterwards, culminating in the fine-detailed drawings of brain tissue by Santiago Ramón y Cajal and Camillo Golgi, for which they shared the 1906 Nobel Prize in Physiology or Medicine. The second half of the 20th century saw a steady decline of optical microscopy as the major tool of discovery in cell biology due to the rise of ultrastructural analysis by transmission and electron microscopy, only to be revitalized by the widespread use of fluorescence light microscopy in the 1990s, courtesy of genetically engineered green fluorescent protein and its derivatives. Cellular electron microscopy began its retreat around this time, in part because it just seemed that cell biologist no longer needed the ultrastructural insights that electron microscopy could provide: They had seen what they needed to see in terms of organelles and cellular organization and could easily imagine the remainder. The excitement shifted from details in ultrastructural organization to the dynamic behavior in cells, something the electron microscope could not provide. The other reason electron microscopy fell out of favor had to do with the fact that many electron microscopy (EM) investigators stuck to the tried-and-(un)true conventional methods of sample preparation that involved (many hours-long) slow chemical fixation, heavy-metal staining, followed by room-temperature dehydration, resin-infiltration, resin-embedding, and resin-polymerization. Resin-embedded blocks needed to be trimmed and ultrathinly sectioned. 70–100 nm thin sections needed to be collected onto electron microscope grids with a support film, counterstained, and examined in the transmission electron microscope, where regions of interested needed to be identified at low magnification and resolution, only to finally take a high-resolution picture of the ultrastructure of interest. This represented a rather tiny part of the cell, typically not more than ~0.03–0.05% of a typical $10 \times 10 \times 10\,\mu m^3$ cell. Worse, the entire procedure took several days, possibly a week from the start to the end, and hence high throughput was out of the question (although the images taken yielded high content information).

While fluorescence microscopy was diffraction-limited and thus could only provide a ~300-fold lower resolution, the entire cell was in the field of view and could be studied in its dynamic behavior of in-vivo, without any sample preparation being needed. If phototoxicity could be kept to a minimum, fluorescence imaging was considered non-invasive and thus superior to electron microscopy, which was everything but non-invasive. However, fluorescence microscopy often lacks context and rather than providing the (ultra-)structural organization of everything, it provides localization information about certain constituents.

The resolution disadvantage of fluorescence optical imaging was overcome to a large degree in an impressive way in the first decade of the 21st century by the advent of superresolution microscopy. In the early 2000s, it seemed that cellular electron microscopy was a relic of the past, and indeed most electron microscopists (but not all) focused on cryo-EM of macromolecular machines.

12.2.2 Cryo-Preservation in EM Sample Preparation

Around the turn of the millennium, a number of factors contributed to the resurgence of electron microscopy: First, the embracement by a larger number of investigators regarding cryogenic sample preparation by either plunge-freezing of flat individual cells cultured on a microscope grid or by high-pressure freezing of cell aggregates/organoids and tissues. Cryogenic sample preparation overcame to a large degree the sample preparation artifacts associated with conventional chemical fixation/dehydration approaches. Second, the advent of 3D imaging in the form or electron tomography, which now allowed large macromolecular complexes or supramolecular machines to be visualized in 3D in their native cell and tissue context. Going three-dimensional was a big step forward, as before most of transition electron microscopy (TEM) had been two-dimensional. Going "cryogenic" in terms of sample preparation also vastly sped up the sample preparation protocols, as small cells (e.g., bacteria), organelles or the edge of flat cells could now be studied directly in their unstained, frozen-hydrated, closest-to-native state. However, the caveat was the thickness limitation of 500 nm to 1 μm, which excludes many of a cell biologist's most interesting targets. Also, according to the Crowther criterion, the thicker the volume to be studied by (cryo-)electron tomography the worse is the expected resolution for a fixed number of tilt series images. Given that the total dose tolerable by the sample remains limited, and the dose is already very low for each image, the total number of images (at smaller tilt increments) cannot easily increase for a now thicker specimen.

Cryo-sectioning was popular for a while in the field of cryo-electron tomography (cryo-ET) but the technical challenges for cryo-sectioning and transfer of frozen-hydrated sections into the microscope turned out to be formidable. Furthermore, compression artifacts were often observed, calling into question closest-to-native preservation.

12.2.3 FIB Milling Sample Preparation

Focused ion beam (FIB) milling techniques were adapted to cut thin frozen-hydrated lamella out from a frozen cell or tissue, and this is the current state-of-the-art of sample preparation for cryo-ET of larger cells and tissues. In some selected examples, the structures of interest such as inner ear hair cell stereocilia or isolated mitochondria could be visualized directly by cryo-ET as whole-mount samples. For FIB milling, choosing the volume of interest for lamella remains a challenge, and this approach also requires significant resources for lamella making, and transfer into a TEM, resources that most labs do not have access to.

12.2.4 Electron Tomography

The future of cryo-ET is likely going to be bright, particularly if the goal is to study macromolecular complexes in their native subcellular environment. Subvolume averaging techniques will help improve resolution and reduce macromolecular shape distortions due to the data anisotropy (which is the result of limitations in tilt angle during data collection and increased sample thickness upon data collection at high tilt angles).

Electron tomography of stained and resin-embedded samples will continue to play an important role in cell biology, if the goal is not to determine the exact macromolecular shape (3D structure) but to determine higher levels of subcellular 3D architectural organization of components that can still be confidently identified in the resin-section 3D volume, such as the cytoskeleton or adhesion complexes and others.

However, both resin- and cryo-electron tomography cannot overcome one fundamental limitation of TEM tomography, namely that the volume of interest that can be studied by this approach remains miniscule compared to the size of a typical eukaryotic cell (let alone a tissue), and hence the future of larger scale 3D architectural organization at nanometer resolution is more likely to lie in block surface scanning electron microscopy (SEM) approaches that are discussed further below.

12.2.5 Correlative Light and Electron Microscopy

Over the last two decades, both optical microscopy and electron microscopy approaches had their separate groups of followers. More recently, they are rightfully seen as complimentary, with fluorescence microscopy providing target specificity and possibly dynamic behavior whereas electron microscopy (both 2D and 3D data of cryogenically preserved samples), provides ultrastructural detail and cellular/tissue context. Some examples have been shown where both approaches have been successfully combined. However, in terms of correlative imaging the success rate has been painstakingly low, but when it was successful it was highly informative.

Correlative fluorescence light and electron microscopy (CLEM) imaging is certainly a method to watch out for, as there have been many advances to combine fluorescence and EM imaging. However, CLEM requires extensive expertise, and it remains to be seen whether CLEM will be adopted by the wider community. An area of active research is the quest for better photolabeling techniques and to find the EM-equivalent of green fluorescent protein (GFP), a genetically encoded probe that will produce a specific EM signal. Some significant steps have been taken, but this area of research remains far from mature. Among its challenges is the fact that not every electron-dense feature in a cell necessarily is the product of photoconversion but there can be other sources for electron stains in heavy metal-stained samples. One is tempted to draw a parallel to immunolabeling, where a variety of controls are needed to "trust" the photoconversion results, which means that unexpected results can be seen as suspicious.

12.2.6 Volume-SEM

Until recently, SEM was not unlike photography in the sense that it was not a true 3D imaging technique, just an 2D image of a 3D object. SEM intermittently played a crucial role in the understanding of cell biology using freeze-fracture and freeze-etching sample preparation techniques, which revealed 3D structural organization of organelles and supramolecular assemblies (such as the cytoskeleton) inside cells. However, SEM imaging (even in the case of freeze-fracture sample preparation) was confined to the "look from the outside" and while often providing "dramatic" views of entire cells and tissues, there was limited insight to be gained from such "outside" images.

This has slowly changed in the last two decades, as array tomography or automated tape-collecting ultramicrotome (ATUM) SEM, serial block face SEM, and focused ion beam SEM (FIBSEM)/dual beam SEM have become increasingly popular. While array tomography/ATUM is similar in concept to serial section transmission electron microscopy, it is typically more convenient to use SEM imaging and array tomography/automated when imaging large fields of view rather than using image mosaicking to stitch together tiles of TEM images (with the individual images slightly overlapping).

ATUM SEM has already been of great value in the study of brain connectomes with large fields of view being imaged at comparatively high spatial resolution. However, as ultrathin section ribbons need to cut, the axial resolution is limited to ~50–100 nm.

A factor of about two to three can be gained by using serial block face SEM, where ~30 nm ultrathin section can be shaved/sliced off a resin block. This is possible because one does not image the slice that has been shaved off but the surface of the block that now got freshly exposed due to the removal of a 30 nm layer of the resin block with a diamond knife. By repeating the cycle of shaving off a 30 nm section and imaging of the newly exposed block surface, a 3D volume can be built up at a ~30 nm axial resolution.

If one uses a FIB instead of a diamond knife to remove that resin-block surface layer, one can gain another factor of about six. It is possible to build up a 3D volume at a step size of 3.5–5 nm, which is about the average size of a protein. So, it would seem that ATUM SEM, Serial Block Face SEM and FIBSEM have a bright future ahead of them, as they will increasingly produce large 3D volumes of cells and tissues of $50\,\mu m \times 50\,\mu m \times 50\,\mu m$ at a pixel size of 3.5–5 nm.

In comparison, mosaic TEM imaging of intermediate fields of view to $200\,\mu m \times 200\,\mu m$ at 2 nm pixel size is feasible and can yield spectacular 2D insight into biological processes such as organotypic cultures. Unfortunately, such a large mosaic 2D image then is still represents only a tiny (100 nm thin) sliver of the sample.

12.2.7 Helium Ion Microscopy

Helium Ion Microscopy (HeIM) has many similarities to SEM but has a larger focal depth, which means that for the typical "from-the-outside" view of a biological sample the entire 3D object can now be in focus. Also, the helium ion beam is very bright and can be focused to a smaller spot size, which means that HeIM can accomplish higher resolution than SEM. Furthermore, specimen charging is not an issue, as it can easily be dealt with using an electron flood beam for charge compensation. This means that the object does not have to be electrically conductive, and thus no metal or carbon-coating is necessary. The higher resolution, longer focal length, better contrast, lack of charging (which means that there is no need for carbon or platinum coating) makes HeIM superior to SEM, and possibly the method of choice for conventional 2D images of 3D objects. The advantage of HeIM for 3D imaging of block surfaces (as done in serial block face SEM or FIBSEM) is less clear. While the helium bombardment still produces secondary electrons when interacting with the target volume, the backscattered electron (BSE) signal (important for block face imaging) is missing. HeIM can be easily combined with SIMS (secondary ion mass spectrometry), thus there may be additional information available when using the combination approach. The future application of HeIM is promising, but given the high price tag on the instrument, its embracement beyond some enthusiastic early-adopter groups by the wide cell biology community remains to be seen.

12.2.8 Cryo-Soft-X-Ray Microscopy Tomography

Cryo Soft X-ray Microscope Tomography (cryo-XRMT) has developed over the last two decades into a mature discipline and offers a resolution that is in between the diffraction-limited optical microscopy and electron microscopy. A variety of samples has been successfully imaged in a high throughput manner with minimal sample preparation requirements (apart from freezing). Cryo-XRMT can also be readily combined with fluorescence microscopy, which makes this approach very powerful, as the volume data from both techniques can be readily correlated. Furthermore, given that a full 180° rotation is possible during data collection, the resulting resolution of the 3D reconstruction is isotropic. Despite the bright X-ray beam afforded by synchrotron radiation, damage to the sample in its frozen-hydrated state is minimal, courtesy of the immobilization of free radicals in the frozen sample, and the imaging in the "water window" of the soft X-ray part of the electromagnetic spectrum.

While the resolution is currently limited to 50–60 nm, further advances in the technology of zone plates needed for focusing of the X-rays may improve resolution by a factor of two. Cryo soft-XRMT is a very promising technique despite the limited access that cell biologists will have to such a synchrotron X-ray microscopy facility. However, the biggest limitation, and one that may be difficult to overcome, is that for such high resolution XRMT imaging data, the sample thickness size is limited of ~15 μm diameter. This means that while this approach works well for prokaryotic and individual eukaryotic cells, it will not extend to organotypic cell cultures or tissues that are often a factor of 4–20 times bigger.

12.2.9 Hard-X-Ray Microscopy Tomography

Hard X-ray microscope tomography (XRMT) can image sample of a broad range of scales and resolution. It is sometimes also referred to as micro-CT (computed tomography), but in micro-CT there is typically no effort made to refocus the X-rays once they have penetrated the sample, and the image is recorded with flat panel X-ray detectors. In XRMT, a zone plate is used to act like an objective lens and to refocus the X-ray beam that has passed through the sample. Commercial setups, which also have the option of a flat panel X-ray detector to image large specimen (up to 200 mm/20 cm in size) at coarser resolution, allow the imaging of millimeter-sized samples (e.g., entire zebrafish larvae or organs like a mouse) at voxel sizes of up to 40 nm and at ~500 nm resolution, which corresponds well to the resolution limit of diffraction-limited fluorescence microscopy. Another commercial X-ray microscope instrument version can even yield 50 nm resolution, but to accomplish this resolution limit, the sample is restricted to (or needs to be trimmed to) ~65 μm in diameter.

Tissues (or even organs) that have been subjected to heavy metal staining and thus have become opaque to optical microscopy can still be studied by XRMT and their 3D tissue organization can be revealed at a resolution that is comparable to diffraction-limited optical imaging. Individual cells and certain prominent organelles like the inner ear sensory epithelial hair bundle can be distinguished in X-ray microscopy tomograms. While this is an impressive achievement in itself, what makes hard-XRMT so valuable is that it seems like the ideal bridging technology between optical imaging and electron microscopy imaging. The ability to study small animals, and their organs, to identify 3D tissue organization, and to correlate fluorescence microscopy to the XRMT signal and to identify regions of interest with cellular precision makes XRMT uniquely qualified to play a dominant role in the future of multiscale imaging.

The future of subcellular, cellular and tissue imaging will likely be multiscale and multimodal, with a variety of optical imaging techniques yielding information about overall morphology, reporter molecule localization and chemical identity, which is then connected to ultrastructural imaging by EM via XRMT. The targets of the future in cell biology will be tissues and organs, which means that techniques of the future will need to be able to image larger fields or views/volumes, thicker tissues and possibly even organs, ideally in-situ. From an optical microscopy point of view, emphasis will increasingly be placed in light sheet and multiphoton approaches that allow deeper penetration into tissues, and as well as (hyper-)spectral imaging. There will be an increasing need for time-series, which puts additional demands on the fluorophores to be specific, bright, robust, and resistant to photobleaching.

Such advances in imaging for cells and tissues will prompt further developments on the data analysis side to keep up with the increased production of terabyte-sized datasets, and with increased quantitative volumetric analysis. Also, conceptionally new ways will need to be found to integrate the information beyond a simple correlative approach between two neighboring techniques in this multimodal pipeline, maybe at the model rather than raw imaging data level.

12.3 Future of Chemical Imaging

Information about the chemical composition can be obtained from a variety of imaging techniques, including X-ray microanalysis, vibrational spectroscopic imaging such as Raman and Fourier Transform InfraRed (FTIR) imaging, as well as mass spectrometry imaging. Some of the advantages of vibrational spectroscopy-based imaging techniques such as FTIR and Raman imaging are that samples are label-free, do not require much sample preparation and can be imaged non-destructively, however FTIR and Raman do not show the specificity of NMR spectroscopy, which can identify (macro-)molecular identity, at least at high concentration and homogeneity.

With respect to Raman imaging, spatial localization and speed of data acquisition can be improved, e.g., by resorting to surface-enhanced Raman spectroscopic (SERS) imaging, coherent anti-Stokes Raman scattering (CARS) or stimulated Raman spectroscopy (SRS), or by combining Raman with near field imaging using atomic force microscopy (AFM). While bright sources, including powerful lasers and synchrotron radiation do exist, access to such bright beams is limited, hindering throughput and thus progress for the larger biological community.

Finally, better data extraction techniques are needed for the elucidation of more and different kinds of information from an image: We need user-friendly multivariate analysis tools and hyperspectral image deconvolution and analysis. However, there some fundamental issues that need to get resolved before chemical imaging can reach its full potential: In the absence of a dominant peak like cellulose in plant cell walls, the spectra can be very broad and do not uniquely reflect one chemical signature that could be easily attributed to a few chemicals. Using a known substance as a standard has been long-standing practice in spectroscopy, as one could compare the experimental spectrum with the spectrum of the known substance. The difficulty arises when going from a spectrum of a few known components to a spectrum of many components, where at least some of which are unknown, as these compounds will affect the shape of the spectrum, where peak profiles are already rather broad. Chemometric techniques such as factor analysis, least square fitting, principal component analysis and even neural networks needs extensive training data of known composition (ground truth), otherwise they can only determine regions of self-similarities, and thus address the homogeneity/heterogeneity of the system, and not its actual underlying chemical inventory.

12.4 Future of Medical Imaging

As mentioned before, medical imaging is a field entirely in its own right and is only treated here tangentially as a field related to, but distinct from bioimaging (i.e., the imaging of biological samples with no direct diagnostic or therapeutic ambitions typically in the context of basic science biological research). However, since many of the concepts underlying these two fields are highly similar, and the techniques used have many commonalities, it comes as no surprise that they share current and future imaging trends. Machine Learning (and particularly Deep Learning) artificial intelligence is becoming increasingly powerful for semi-automated processing and analysis of image data, particularly with respect to segmentation. Datasets are increasingly stored in cloud-based repositories, which allows wide access to the image data and thus empowers patients and other healthcare providers for further follow-up analysis. As image data becomes increasingly mobile and can be securely stored on distributed servers, image data can be accessed by anybody around the world if proper access is given, which empowers telemedicine, and allows remote diagnosis by an expert in some distant city or another country.

Datasets in medical imaging are becoming increasingly 3D in nature, which will require further improvements in the visualization of such 3D data (including the use of virtual reality and augmented reality) for image-guided intervention (surgery).

Digital Pathology has emerged as a promising future trend in medical imaging, where machine learning and deep learning can presently support or in the future even replace a human expert to come up with a medical diagnosis for most histopathological image results. Artificial intelligence-based approaches will rival or even surpass humans in terms of speed of analysis and possibly even accuracy of diagnosis.

Multiplexing is another recent development worth watching. Multiplexing relies on optical imaging of tissue sections, which undergo many cycles of immunohistochemical labeling with fluorescence reporter-molecule conjugated antibodies, whole-slide (or region-of-interest) imaging and photobleaching, also known as tissue cyclic immunofluorescence (t-CyCIF). Each cycle features a different antibody and the photobleaching ensures that there is no carry-over of fluorescence from a previous round of labeling. Alternatively, metals or other molecules can be conjugated to the antibodies which are then read out by mass spectrometry imaging. This information is then typically overlaid with a conventional H&E stain of formalin-fixed paraffin-embedded (FFPE) samples, routinely used in histology and pathology.

The Human Tumor Atlas network project is an example for current and future large scale multimodal imaging approaches that are currently underway, where H&E histology, multiplexed CyCIF and multiplexed GeoMx RNA expression (transcriptomics) are performed in parallel on consecutive serial sections.

12.5 Future of Image Processing and Analysis

While this book is focused on the technological aspects of data acquisition in bioimaging and only scratches the surface for image processing and analysis, it may well be the computational aspects that have the greatest potential for improvement in the coming years and decades. They will likely dominate progress in the field of bioimaging for years to come. Both sample preparation and computational analysis are the unsung hero of biological imaging, presumably due to the fact that biology traditionally had little overlap with computer science and its many subdisciplines, such as image restoration, visualization, computer vision and bioimage informatics.

Unfortunately, biologists in their training rarely come in contact with computer science. Creating images seems intuitive and like an endpoint in itself. Hence, the focus in bioimaging traditionally was on operating increasingly complicated instruments to create better-quality images rather than getting the maximum amount of information out of the images recorded.

As "seeing is believing," the goal has been to visualize an expected experimental outcome, and to create images that best exemplify a desired result, and if needed to select for images that can serve as confirmation or proof that a biological conclusion was justified.

In other words, the aim of imaging has been to confirm a conclusion and not to assess heterogeneity and/or to seek quantitative information, and thus to become the source of discovery. Obtaining information that wasn't obvious to the naked eye, was way down on the list of importance, which also may be owed to the relative ignorance of both biologists and computer scientists about each other's field. The situation is different from astrophysics and cosmology, where physicists owing to their training are much closer in spirit to computer scientists. Hence, it should come as no surprise that many of the more recent breakthroughs in biological imaging (like multiscale, multimodal imaging or adaptive optics) had been adopted in the field of astrophysics and cosmology field for quite some time.

Also, in terms of the organization of science, cosmology and astrophysics are leaps ahead of biological sciences (including bioimaging), as theoretical physicists, imaging experts, image analysis experts, and imaging data scientists working as a multidisciplinary team have been the norm for decades in cosmology. Still today in many biological disciplines, the scientific model is predominantly based on single individual investigators or very small teams of (two or three) investigators. Imagine what would be possible if teams of dozens of experts could be brought together on a single topic, as has been the case for cosmology for a long time.

Traditionally, biologists have had a conflicted relationship to image processing, image analysis experts and (large) data scientists, a situation that has changed to some extent over the last decade. When both sides (biologists and computer scientists – and even applied mathematicians) have learned to communicate with one another, progress has been enormous and thus it seems safe to predict that the computer science aspect of bioimaging will be the single most important with respect to future impact.

The visualization of 2D and 3D images by computer graphics has come a long way since the humble beginnings in the 1950s and 1960s with the light pen and Ivan Sutherland's revolutionary Sketchpad software. The company of Evans and Sutherland, being the first commercial source of computers dedicated to 3D visualization, later were joined by and then replaced by Silicon Graphics Computer Systems (SGI), before home computers with their much lower price tag started to become powerful enough to carry out 3D-rendering-tasks.

From a graphical user interface (GUI) to dedicated graphics processing units/graphic cards to head-mounted devices for stereoscopic viewing, hardware evolved rapidly. What used to take a supercomputer a fair amount of time to render now is done in real-time on a desktop machine or even a laptop computer. From a hardware point of view, computer graphics are mature, and therefore, future developments may be somewhat mundane, such as improved processor speed and increased memory, allowing even faster processing and display of larger volumes.

Many software advances were made, which is even more impressive, if one compares today's packages with the early days when only simple geometrical objects could be drawn. Among the many things that have improved are hidden surface determination, shading, texture mapping, bump and normal mapping, specular highlighting and reflection, as well as ray tracing. While many visualization packages now offer photorealistic rendering of models and 3D image data, going from 3D data to 3D models is still a rather complicated procedure, typically requiring denoising, segmentation, annotation, and manual model building steps.

It would seem like a much-needed growth area for computer graphics to automatically turn 3D image maps into volumetric model objects that can be quantified with respect to geometric/volumetric properties, such as size, volume, surface area, but also spatiotemporal relationships between cellular components, including vicinity, distances, and distribution.

Automated volumetric model building for automatically segmented volume data ideally would result in resolution-faithful yet simplified and somewhat abstracted versions of these often-complex densities: For example, actin filaments could be modeled as rope-like structures with an idealized average geometry, microtubules on the other hand could be represented as narrow hollow tubes, while mitochondria appear as wide hollow double-walled tubes with invaginations of the inner tube.

Cell–cell adhesion complexes could be represented as two connected round or elliptical rafts each sitting in the plasma membrane of adjacent cells, where the key parameter to note would be the surface area covered as this may indicate the strength of local cell–cell adhesion.

Once the segmented densities become volumetric model objects, they could serve as the base for real-time fly-through animations and/or exploded view representations that show the spatial relationship of the parts of a complex assembly, and how the assembly can be put together by the isolated parts. This trick of taking complex machineries apart in a mechanical drawing goes back to the Renaissance, even though the term "Exploded View Drawing" wasn't coined until the middle of the 20th century. Often, exploded lines indicate the path of how the components need to be moved in order fit together into the complex assembly (Figure 12.2).

If one could combine the ability to walk in real time through a 3D volume (e.g., in the model space) and to warp space (such in the exploded view drawings), one could explore in real time such 3D volume, not unlike walking through a big city with all its main roads and back alleys. No areal map can ever substitute for walking through the city and to be immersed in the 3D space. Again, simplified yet resolution-faithful volumetric model building, based on density segmentation, would be a crucial first step in this vision of immersive visualization. With such models being built, immersive visualization and virtual reality manipulation of the object space would be very powerful tools for better understanding the 3D volumes of cells and tissues. One key to success may be model simplification and feature abstraction as not to overwhelm our visual sense.

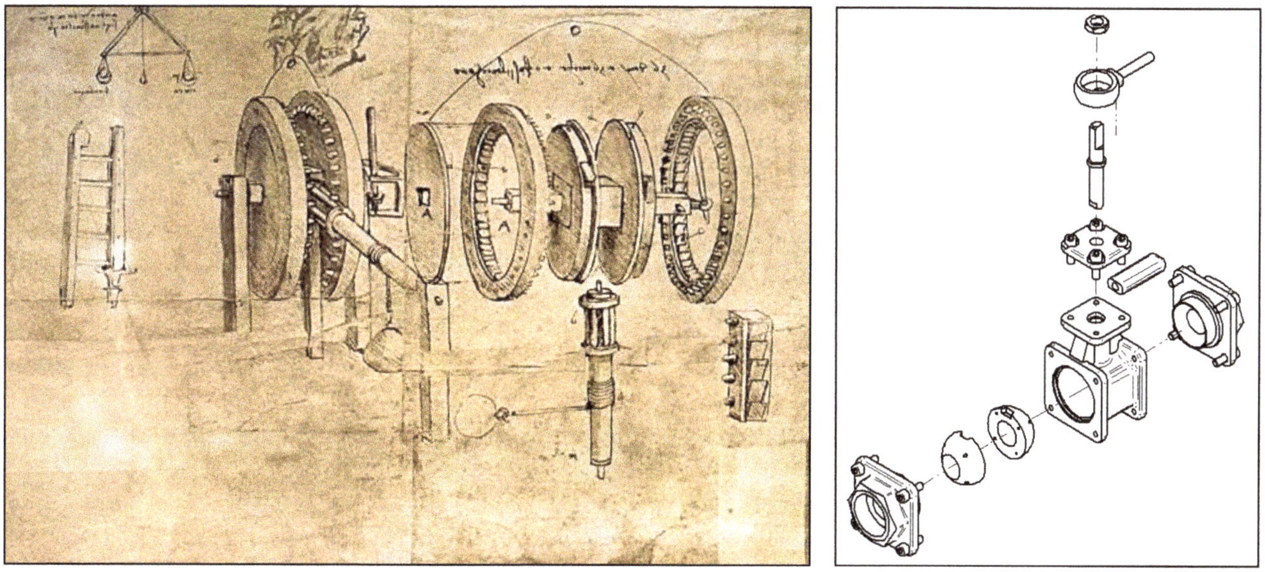

Figure 12.2 Exploded view of a mechanical machine in the renaissance. *Source:* John Edgar Park / CC BY 3.0. The concept of exploded view as a pictorial representation of how mechanical machines are put together from individual parts dates back about 6 centuries to the Renaissance, including an exploded view drawing from Leonardo da Vinci (left). The term "exploded-view drawing" emerged in the 1940s and was first defined in 1965. Exploded-view drawings shows the spatial relationship or order of assembly of various parts, typically depicted from above and in a diagonal manner (right). The parts are separated by distance as if a small explosion occurred in the center of the machine that pushes parts away from one another.

Apart from such interactive visual exploration of 3D volumetric data, one key objective going forward is to enable quantitative analysis of the features of interest. Automation is certainly high on everybody's wish list, as datasets become increasingly larger, more complex, and higher throughput. Since many steps are needed to convert original data into information, manual image processing, feature extraction, feature annotation and quantitative analysis become less and less feasible for large volume data.

The world of computer packages for basic image processing and image restoration, segmentation, annotation is fragmented into many specialized tools, some of which may only work for ideal conditions. A potential user must look through the literature, may ask friends or colleagues for advice, what package to use for which step of the analysis, only to then trying to figure out from tutorial webpages or instruction videos how to best use each package. A consolidation of analysis tools into fewer, but more multifaceted packages that use standardized input/output data formats and standardized procedures to carry out a variety of tasks would be desirable. In the past, getting the data converted into the right format often has been a significant hurdle in developing new image processing capabilities. Now, tools exist that can convert basically any image format into any other image format.

While some online forums already exist where a novice may be able to get help, a concerted effort would be helpful to provide a help portal for potential/novice users and experts alike. While several open-source point and click software such as ImageJ, Fiji, CellProfiler, Icy, and others exist, some investigators prefer to still write their own routines, using Scikit-image, MATLAB and other using computational libraries and scripts. At the very least, such routines should be made available to the broader community, e.g., in form of plugins for ImageJ.

Automated segmentation persists as a problem, but supervised and unsupervised Machine Learning, and particularly Deep Learning, have become a dominant force, and likely will be increasingly powerful for segmentation and annotation of features of interest. Apart from visualization/computer graphics, image processing and computer vision/image analysis, another field that will be increasingly more important is that of Bioimage Informatics. Among its tasks is how to deal with image storage in data repositories and to capture and warehouse not just the image data, but also all the metadata that accompanies the image data, from specimen information and sample preparation details to imaging conditions and microscope settings, as well as parameters used in image processing, data segmentation, annotation, and (quantitative) analysis. Controlled vocabularies are necessary to keep track of the vast amount of data, with a key goal to ensure that such data repositories and databases do not become data graveyards. The Open Microscopy Environment (OME) project with its OMERO platform has developed a secure, central data repository, where image data can be viewed, organized, analyzed, and shared from anywhere in the world on any platform, as long as there is internet access. In addition, OMERO supports over 150 image formats.

The Protein Data Bank for many decades now has been the repository for macromolecular structures (mostly atomic models) as determined by X-ray crystallography, NMR spectroscopy and cryo-EM. The Electron Microscopy Data Bank (EMDB) was developed to deposit medium resolution EM data. Other databases/repositories exist such as the UCSD Cell-Centered Database, the JCB Data Viewer, the ASCB CELL Image Library or the Edingburgh Mouse Atlas of Gene Expression (EMAGE), to name a few. This is an area of continued effort and research, which will become increasingly more important as larger and larger datasets are being produced as part of several systematic surveys, e.g., by the Human Cell Atlas initiative or the Human Tumor Atlas Network.

The future of image processing and image analysis will lie in the multiscale analysis (from macromolecules to in-situ imaging of tissues and organs), multimodal analysis (using many imaging techniques, each of which contributing unique information regarding scale, resolution, and type of information) and ultimately in the integration of information derived from multiple imaging modes and multiple scales, and to make the leap from voxels to biological insight.

12.6 Future of Multiscale Imaging

One of the vastly underestimated tasks in biological imaging, particularly when attempting to image a sample across multiple scales, is to find the region of interest at low magnification for imaging at high magnification. A small animal like zebrafish larvae or mouse embryo, small organs like the inner ear cochlea or tissue biopsies can easily be millimeter(s) in size, whereas the resolution one would like to image is in the 2–200 nm range.

This means that any attempt to image a cube of 2 mm side length at 2 nm resolution (e.g., in a large volume SEM) would require 1,000,000 × 1,000,000 × 1,000,000 million (or 10^{18} or 1 quintillion) voxels, even at 200 nm resolution the task would still be 10,000 × 10,000 × 10,000 (or 10^{12} or 1 trillion) voxels. Even at 8-bit per voxel, thus would amount to 1 EB (exabyte) or 1 TB (terabyte) of information, respectively. Even if an imaging device could produce such images, the amount of storage of such data, let alone the processing, would be prohibitive (Figure 12.3).

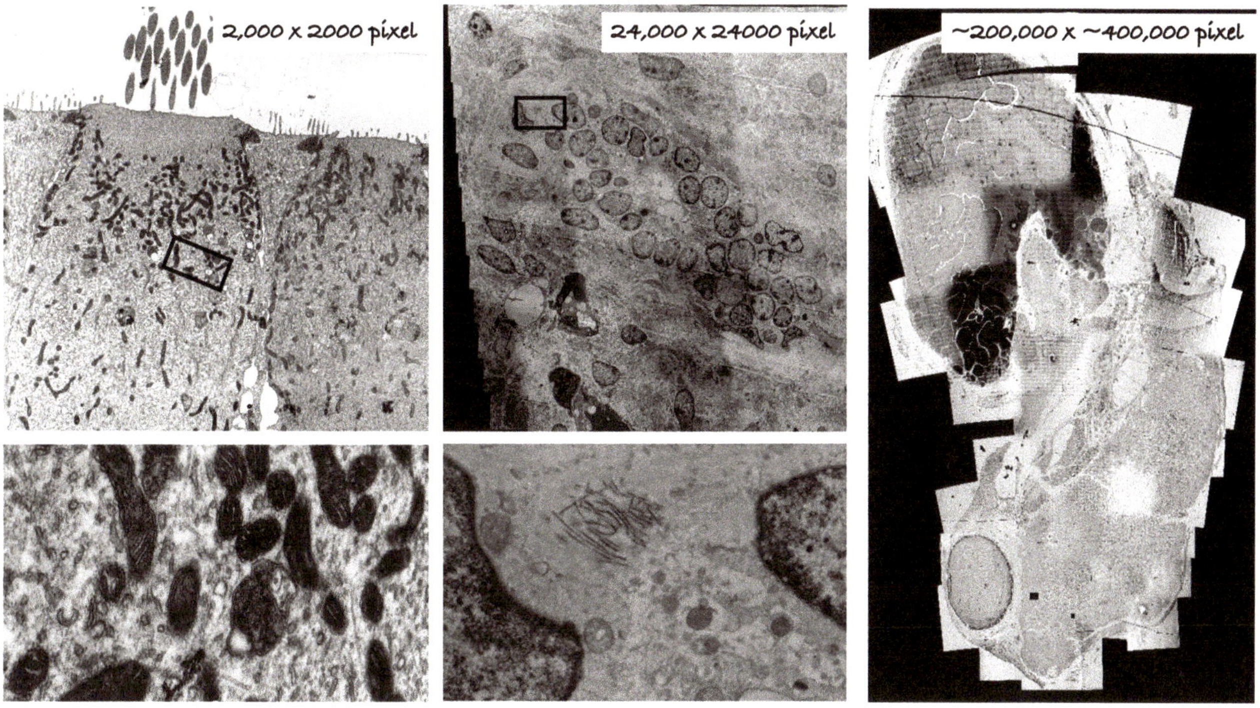

Figure 12.3 Multiscale imaging: Hair cell, mammary gland tissue, and zebrafish larvae. Left: 2,000 by 2,000 pixels image (4 MB at 8 bit) of a 100 nm thin section of an inner ear hair cell, note in the close-up view (bottom) the wealth of information that even a small region of the picture has, including cytoskeletal filaments, vesicles, endoplasmic reticulum, vesicles, and mitochondria. Middle: 24,000 by 24,000 pixels montage image (576 MB at 8 bit) of a 100 nm thin section of a mammary gland tissue with dozens of cells. Note that in the close-up view extracellular collagen strands can be readily recognized. Right: ~200,000 × ~400,000 pixels montage image (80 GB at 8 bit) of a 100 nm thin section of a zebrafish larvae head region. Note that 3,000–5,000 more sections of 100 nm thickness would need to be imaged as a montage before the entire head region would be covered, which would bring the total amount of data to hundreds of terabytes of data.

At the current moment, there are several attempts to bridge adjacent scales and levels of complexity. In the macromolecular imaging world, a variety of structural biology techniques are being used to determine the structure of individual proteins, including X-ray crystallography, NMR spectroscopy and cryo-EM.

However, with increased size and complexity comes compositional and conformational heterogeneity, and thus many macromolecular machines in their cell context can no longer be expected to reside in a unique state that can be determined by implicit or explicit averaging. Some macromolecular or supramolecular complexes may only be transient, complicating classification and thus ultimately leading to lower-resolution structures, due to the smaller number of particle views for each class-averages of particles. Into such lower resolution envelopes one can still dock higher resolution structures, provided there is enough additional information such as knowledge about the location and interaction of proteins in such a complex. Before the recent resolution-revolution, this hybrid approach of fitting higher resolution structures into lower-resolution envelopes has been used many times in the field of cryo-EM, in a time when cryo-EM was still the field of "blobology." A similar situation has emerged in the field of cryo-tomography, where subvolume averaging now can yield envelopes to which known high-resolution structures can be fitted.

Going one level up in size and complexity to the world of subcellular sceneries and organelles, this is the world where cryo-ET rules the day. Reconstructions of entire organelles such as mitochondria have served as the envelopes into which the 3D structure of the F-ATPase could be fitted. Studying the ATPase in its native mitochondrial environment revealed an unexpected organization of proton gradient-utilizing, ATP generating complex, which in turn may be the reason for the high curvature of the mitochondrial cristae and most likely have mechanistic implications of protein complex function. Other organelles and their protein constituents have been studied including stereocilia, which are membrane enclosed protrusions of the apical hair cell membrane surface, and which assemble into the so-called hair bundle that is crucial to the mechanoelectrical transduction of sound. While the resolution of the data was too low fit individual structures into the resulting cryo-ET density map, it was possible to build a (simplified) volumetric model of the actin bundle with its individual actin filaments and its cross-connectors. Again, there were surprises in the overall organization of the actin filaments, including systematic bending of the actin bundle, as well, as a compaction and twisting of the actin filaments in the so-called rootlet region at the stereocilia base that anchors the actin-bundle in the cuticular plate.

Subcellular sceneries need to be placed into the context of entire cells. Our work regarding the imaging of the lateral wall of outer hair cells (OHCs) may serve as an example: OHCs are crucial in the amplification of sound in the OHCs of the mammalian cochlea through a mechanism known as electromotility, where voltage changes across a membrane drive a 5% elongation of the cell plasma membrane of OHCs (which are ~100 μm in length). Some of the players in this process are known, or at least suspected, however, the mechanism for electromotility remains unclear. Our electron tomographic reconstructions of high-pressure frozen, freeze-substituted, and resin-embedded samples revealed an unexpected 3D organization of the lateral wall region and formerly unknown connections between the cortical actin lattice and the subsurface cisternae (SSC), as well as a regular protein pattern in the SSC, that led us to propose an entirely different mechanism for this cell-wide phenomenon of electromotility, despite not knowing the molecular identity of its machinery's components.

How cellular organization affects tissue organization can be illustrated by some of our other work on human breast cancer cells grown in an organotypic 3D cell culture system. Depending on the cell subtypes cultured, cells form either growth-arrested acini (S1 cells) or malignant (T4) cell aggregates with metastatic potential. Under certain experimental conditions, such aggressive T4 tumor cell aggregates can be avoided, and the phenotype can be reverted to a growth-arrested acini (T4-reverted), which in its cytoskeletal organization remarkably resembles a pre-malignant phenotype that we had also characterized using large volume SEM (in combination with six additional imaging techniques, each of which provided unique information about the system). Large volume SEM not only revealed unusual finger-like protrusions of the apical membrane surface, which mediates a loose (uncommitted) but nevertheless close contact between adjacent cells, but also deep invaginations into and tunnels through the cell nucleus, with cytoskeletal filaments residing within, which have physical connections to the nuclear membranes and cell–cell adhesion sites. Such connectivity is of uttermost significance, as it implies that the cell nucleus is directly, mechanically reading out the tension state of the cell, which in turn may suggest a mechanism to go from a premalignant senescent state to a malignant proliferative and migratory cellular state. Hence, a change in the cytoskeletal 3D architecture from a highly regular and organized structure to a more disheveled organization, may underlie the mechanism of transformation to malignancy.

Moving up one or two steps of scale and complexity, one can ask the question of how cells assemble into tissues that form organs, which in turn create an entire organism. Both zebrafish larvae and mouse embryos have been used for some time as model systems for embryogenesis and tissue and organ development. Some impressive results have been at Howard Hughes Medical Institute Janella Farm Research Campus. Using a suite of optical microscopy techniques, they studied the spatiotemporal organization of cells inside developing zebrafish and mouse embryos, tracked the motion of each cell, and recorded each cell division. By color-coding cells according to their final tissue destination, they were able to create a dynamic fate map for any individual mouse embryo studied. Also, they were able to map clusters of cell division to the sites of tissue growth. Furthermore, they were able to combine multiple datasets, each showing some variability in the development of an individual embryo. As a result of their analysis, they were able to determine a probability for each cell to end up of with a particular fate, and thus instead of obtaining a dynamic fate map for an individual cell they were able to generate a dynamic cellular atlas of zebrafish and mouse embryonic development based on statistical fate and tissue morphogenesis maps. This truly remarkable accomplishment required multiple optical imaging techniques, including interferometric photoactivation localization microscopy, lattice light sheet microscopy, structured illumination microscopy (SIMView), light sheet microscopy and multifocal microscopy. However, it should be noted that these imaging techniques are variations on a theme, and not entirely different imaging approaches, while in the strict sense being multimodal, the scale of imaging was cellular, albeit at a very large field of view.

To be clear, with each dataset for each embryo being 10 TB, multi-view image registration (as samples were simultaneously imaged from four different directions), deconvolution, automated cell tracking and lineaging, automated cell division detection, as well as accurate long-term cell flow mapping and the spatiotemporal registration of multiple embryos were far from trivial tasks. It seems certain that landmark studies like this will guide us into the future where datasets will be increasingly larger in size and higher in complexity.

Now, if we imagine adding to this study the subcellular and even macromolecular imaging levels, as we might want to study the cytoskeletal organization inside developing embryos and the role they play for cell differentiation, with all the previous information given, it should be clear that such detailed studies would require the selection of a smaller field of view for subcellular higher-resolution 3D imaging. One can consider any place to be as good as any other, and hence one could randomly pick a field of view, and declare the volume chosen for higher-resolution imaging to be representative of what is happening in the entire sample. But this assumption has as much truth to it than randomly picking a 3×3 block portion of any city and declaring that the rest of the city looks just the same.

So, one needs to find a way to find a promising region at low resolution within a large field of view and somehow mark that region for higher resolution imaging studies. One of the challenges between toggling between a large field of view at low resolution and small field of view at high resolution is that the former lacks details while the latter lacks context. Hence, multiple data maps at different scale and resolution may be helpful to bridge these two worlds, just as one uses multiple scale representations of geospatial maps to navigate when traveling.

Optical microscopy and in particular fluorescence light microscopy can reveal the dynamic properties of a biological system and when imaging a few selected macromolecular constituents, the complexity of the systems is vastly reduced. Hence, one can follow the dynamics and pick a time point when the biology is then fixed in place and time (e.g., by chemical fixation or freezing).

Going from the optical microscopy overview of tissue architecture straight to electron microscopy can be extremely challenging as heavy-metal staining during sample preparation turns the sample typically black, and one typically loses the landmarks that allowed orientation in a tissue. Furthermore, even if location in *XY* can be established, determining how deep one will need to cut/mill into the tissue to get to the region of interest is far from trivial, and often requires the cutting and evaluation of many sections or block surfaces at different *Z*-height. This is very time consuming as one needs to be careful not to cut/mill too deep into the tissue and missing the region of interest altogether.

Hard X-ray microscopy tomography (XRMT) appears to be an ideal technology to bridge the gap between optical microscopy and electron microscopy (particularly dual beam SEM). Hard X-rays can easily penetrate heavy metal-stained, optically opaque samples, and provide a 3D map of tissue organization, which can be overlayed with fluorescence maps to determine the region of interest. The XRMT map then serves as a starting point for ion beam milling or sectioning to get to the region of interest, followed by large volume FIBSEM imaging (Figure 12.4).

How other imaging approaches such as chemical imaging can be worked into the multiscale imaging process depends on whether destructive or non-destructive imaging approaches are used. Non-destructive chemical imaging approaches such as FTIR imaging and Raman imaging can be easily integrated in the workflow as part of the optical imaging, whereas for other techniques such as mass spectrometry imaging it is less intuitive how such destructive imaging approaches can be included in the workflow.

Possibly, one could aim for a serial section approach, where one alternates between imaging of some section with non-destructive approaches, imaging of the adjacent section using a destructive mass spectrometry imaging approach.

12.7 Future of Multimodal Imaging – Correlative Imaging

One of the areas in cell biological imaging that is becoming increasingly important and successful is correlative light and electron microscopy (CLEM). With fluorescence microscopy one can locate the positions of the targeted (macro-)molecule in a cell, and with superresolution fluorescence light microscopy such localization has a high degree of precision, but unless such macromolecules form a filament or an otherwise interesting pattern, it is hard to make profound conclusions from the localization information alone. What is missing is contextual information, some ultrastructural/architectural landmarks to which such localization signals can be mapped to. This is the strength of electron microscopy that provides an ultrastructural framework, and thus a "lay of the land," but it cannot reveal the position of individual proteins, many of which look the same at intermediate to low resolution, and thus cannot be identified by their size or shape. An exception are a few selected proteins, which are known to form assemblies, such as actin filaments, intermediate filaments or microtubules with a characteristic diameter.

For the longest time, immunolocalization was an attempt to overcome this weakness, typically by using a gold particle attached to either a primary antibody or a secondary antibody. Primary antibodies are often precious and cannot be obtained in quantities large enough for gold conjugation reactions, recovery, repurification and reconcentration of the conjugated antibody. For this reason, the gold particle typically was conjugated to a secondary antibody, which in turn recognizes the primary antibody, however as a result, the distance of the gold particle (which is the only part of this entire labeling reagent that is visible in the electron microscope) can come to lie anywhere with a 24 nm-radius

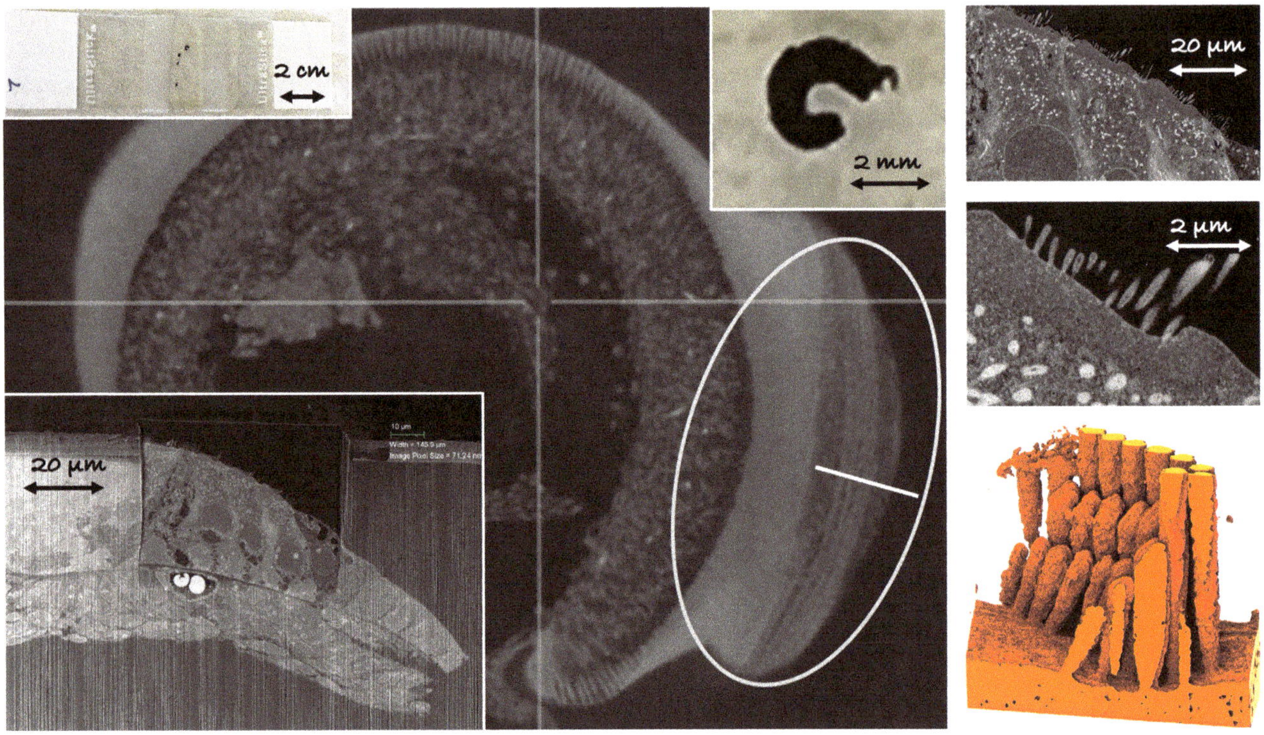

Figure 12.4 Multiscale, multimodal imaging of mouse cochlea. A heavy metal-stained, millimeter-sized inner ear cochlea sample is opaque to optical imaging. However, tissue organization can be determined by hard-X-ray microscope tomography, which allows precise subsequent ion milling for high resolution (5–10 nm) FIBSEM imaging of hair bundles. Note that this multimodal imaging approach allows a seamless transition in scale of size orders of magnitude in a single sample.

circle around the epitope. Hence there is great uncertainty of where the actual antigen epitope was residing.

Pre-embedding labeling procedures have the advantage that the epitope is more freely available and retains its antigenicity, but often result in poor sample preservation, including extraction due to the use of mild detergent for membrane penetration. Post-embedding labeling approaches on the other hand usually lead to better preservation, but epitopes are often buried, and thus are not accessible, or they have lost much of their antigenic potential, which also means that they are not recognized by the primary antibodies. Steric hindrance prevents antibodies to recognize an epitope in the immediate vicinity of an antigen-site that has already bound an antibody. Typically, the chance to recognize an epitope by post-embedding immunolabeling is between 1% and 5%. Even in the best-case documented scenario of a freely accessible epitope, chances for labeling did not exceed 20%, which means that only abundant epitopes will yield a convincing signal, as false positive results due to non-specific binding cannot be totally ruled out either.

Another approach, known as photoconversion, has been explored to turn the immediate surrounding of a photobleachable fluorophore with the help of (singlet) oxygen into a diaminobenzidine precipitate (polymer). Upon exposure to osmium tetroxide solutions this precipitate will turn electron-dense and thus will appear dark in the EM images due to the high accumulation of the heavy element osmium. The fluorophore could be a small organic (synthetic) molecule such as fluorescein and its derivative fluorescein-5-isothiocyanate (FITC) or one of the many genetically encoded fluorescent proteins. Some of the earlier fluorescent proteins such as GFP and yellow fluorescent protein (YFP) do not photoconvert well, whereas others like cyan fluorescent protein (CFP) do. One of the challenges however has been that even relatively mild chemical fixation destroyed the fluorescent signal prior to photoconversion. The same problem also generally prevents the retention of the fluorescence throughout resin-EM sample preservation, even though some fluorescent protein derivatives have been reported to withstand chemical fixation and are thus an attractive candidate for future correlative imaging studies. Small organic synthetic fluorescent dyes can be bound to small-molecules that can traverse the cell membranes and can recognize a genetically encoded tag (such as used in the SNAP-tag labeling approach). Their fluorescent signal can be preserved through resin-embedding or photoconverted into a highly localized heavy metal precipitate. This approach seems to be particular promising, as long as other sources of how such precipitates can form can be ruled out. The metal does not necessarily need to be osmium, which is often used a general stain, but other metal precipitate like silver or gold might be of great value as these could also be uniquely identified via elemental mapping techniques such as energy-dispersive X-ray spectroscopy (EDS) imaging or secondary ion mass spectrometry (SIMS).

Both synthetic small molecule dyes and fluorescent proteins that are compatible with superresolution imaging also are very promising. Being able to pinpoint the location of a fluorophore with high precision by superresolution fluorescence light microscopy and imaging the same area by electron microscopy for ultrastructural context holds great promise.

Another approach that holds great promise for the future is to image the sample at liquid nitrogen temperature using cryo-fluorescence light microscopy of thin sections of frozen-hydrated cryo-lamella, which had been ion beam-milled from high-pressure frozen cell or tissue samples. Cryo-fluorescence imaging is then followed by cryo-TEM 2D imaging or cryo-ET. Efforts to combine both fluorescence microscopy and electron microscopy into one instrument have been attempted but have not met with much success, likely due to the challenges in engineering and microscope design for such a hybrid instrument. Furthermore, success rate for correlative light-electron imaging has been limited and the technical challenges for lamella making, low-temperature fluorescence and TEM imaging are significant. It is therefore not clear whether this approach will find a wide following, and thus remain the domain of a few highly specialized labs (Figure 12.5).

For any techniques to gain wide acceptance in the field, and thus to find many followers, they need to be simple enough that laboratory members at the technician-, predoc-, and postdoc-level can carry out the workflow with instruments, that need to be readily available and/or easily accessible for operation. If a technique is too complex and/or will only work in a fraction of all the experiment, most cell biology investigators will shy away from it and seek alternative approaches, even if such alternatives only constitute a compromise compared to what one might be able like to get otherwise. Hence, user-friendliness and the ability for a wide swath of labs and investigators at different levels of skills to master the necessary techniques might be key components for the success of a imaging techniques, as very few labs will be able to dedicate staff-level personnel to assist in data collection and analysis.

12.8 Future of Information Integration – Multiscale, Multimodal, and Integrated

As discussed in the previous section, correlative imaging comes with many challenges: for example, sample preparation that is needed for conventional electron microscopy tends to destroy the fluorescent signal. While the fluorescent signal can be collected prior to EM sample preparation, the chemical fixation destroys the fluorescent signal and heavy metal staining turns the sample black, and thus opaque to light. In other words, when samples are prepared for EM, all references to cell and tissue signature/hallmarks are lost, which makes it very difficult to correlate fluorescence localization signal with cellular ultrastructural organization.

goal of multimodal imaging: combine different types of information

- putting the localization of (macro-)molecule into an architectural context
- ask whether cellular distribution of (macro-)molecule is random, clustered, organized into filamentous structures, is associated with certain organelles or co-localized with other known (macro-)molecules

past, present, and future strategies:

<u>immunolocalization in EM</u>

- distance label-epitope <24 nm
- pre-/post-embedding
- preservation of ultrastructure, antigenicity and accessibility
- challenge: only 1-5% of epitopes recognized, false positive

<u>fluorescent imaging and photoconversion of photo-bleachable fluorophore, EM</u>

- synthetic fluorophore (extrinsic FP)
- CFP (GFP/YFP) (chemical fixation is problematic)
- diaminobenzidine (DAB) precipitate (Os, Ag, Au) enhancement, challenge: unrelated metal deposits -> detection of specific metals by EDX or SIMS?

<u>correlative FLM/EM (CLEM)</u>

- CLEM (diffraction limited, resin sections)
- cryo-superresolution fluorescence light microscopy of cryo-FIB lamella followed by cryo-electron tomography

Figure 12.5 Correlative light and electron microscopy imaging. The goal of CLEM imaging is to combine different types of information, such as the localization of macromolecules and cellular ultrastructure.

An alternative to stain in EM is cryo-EM imaging, however high-resolution imaging of frozen-hydrated samples at liquid nitrogen temperature, localizing a signal in *X*, *Y*, and *Z* in a 3D tissue volume and selecting that volume for cryo-EM imaging is far from trivial. Requiring in-detail knowledge in multiple imaging disciplines typically goes far beyond the level that a typical university core facility can provide. Additional challenges arise due to differences in resolution and scale that can differ between these two different techniques by two orders of magnitude.

Furthermore, most microscopists tend to be highly knowledgeable about one imaging technique, but not necessarily possess expertise in multiple imaging techniques, which in turn reduces the success rate for correlative imaging. However, sparse success rate for any approach/workflow makes it somewhat unlikely that this approach will find wide acceptance broader community of cell biologists/cell microscopists. There is huge potential for imaging approaches beyond fluorescence imaging, such as chemical imaging, which in its various incarnations have their own sample preparation requirements.

Given all the hurdles listed, one may question whether CLEM is just too complex and thus whether it will be widely adopted. Perhaps a better way to combine information from different imaging modalities at different scales and resolution levels is to integrate the information obtained at the model level rather than trying to correlating individual data sets collected from the same sample.

As each imaging technique will allow certain aspects of the systems to be identified, each model represents unique aspects of information. Rather than correlating datasets, the proposal is to allow integration to happen in the model space, as it is currently done in geospatial information systems (GISs), such as web-based or app-based maps applications. In such applications, information about topology and surface features from satellite imaging or aerial photography/video is brought together with multiscale model representation such as road grids and other transportation systems. Onto this model other kinds of information are mapped, such as traffic data which is derived from various sources such as traffic monitoring cameras, highway toll stations and cell phone movement data. Yet another level of this model space may be retail stores, restaurants, coffee shops, each of which with its own unique opening hours, menus, or customer recommendations.

By moving to the model space and by mapping all data onto simplified representations of reality (such as the road grid, which can change in its level of details as one zooms in and out), there are all kinds of data beyond just imaging data that can be integrated in this manner. One of the advantages of such a model space-based rather than data space-based approach is that there is no need to image the exact same sample by different modalities, instead each imaging method is just required to image closely related/matched systems, with each system/specimen likely displaying some heterogeneity. Rather than obtaining one sample that can be imaged with two modalities, it may be better to image an ensemble of samples, each with its own technique, and to determine (and to record) the level of similarity and/or heterogeneity of the system under investigation. This information (i.e., its information robustness) will also become part of the model.

In an integrated approach, no technique needs to make any compromises with respect to optimal sample preparation and imaging. Now, a key aspect and currently heavily underutilized is the quantification of volumetric properties and the rigorous use of statistics, as it will be this information that informs and allows the creation of volumetric models and the generation of a prototypic model that does not exactly match any of the recorded data sets but is the result of information integration and averaging.

Such a prototypic model will be the consensus product of all quantitative volumetric model properties, with the models being derived from the actual (segmented and annotated) imaging data.

These prototypic models will be at the core of a map-centered "biospatial" information system, the biological equivalent of a GIS. Each biological system will require the generation of its own database, and each database will provide spatiotemporal model information that can be queried for volumetric properties. We will be able to inquire with such a GIS to show all instances where the distance between two or multiple objects, the size, length, diameter, volumes, surface areas or branching patterns deviate from certain defined values. It will be in the true sense of the word data mining as it will allow us to unearth hidden patterns that were not inputted explicitly into the database.

Skeletonization in combination with graph theory or some other mathematical approaches will allow us to simplify the sceneries and to conduct mathematical statistical inquiries, e.g., to assess the degree of similarities and differences between biological systems and to compared healthy versus diseased tissue or cellular state. Such simplified models, e.g., of the cytoskeleton, may also become a starting point for (finite element and otherwise) simulation for example of the mechanical properties of a cell that result from differences in cytoskeleton organization. Such differences in mechanical tension/load may ultimately underlie decision making of a cell whether to stay in a senescent state, or enter a state of proliferation and migration, or a premalignant state.

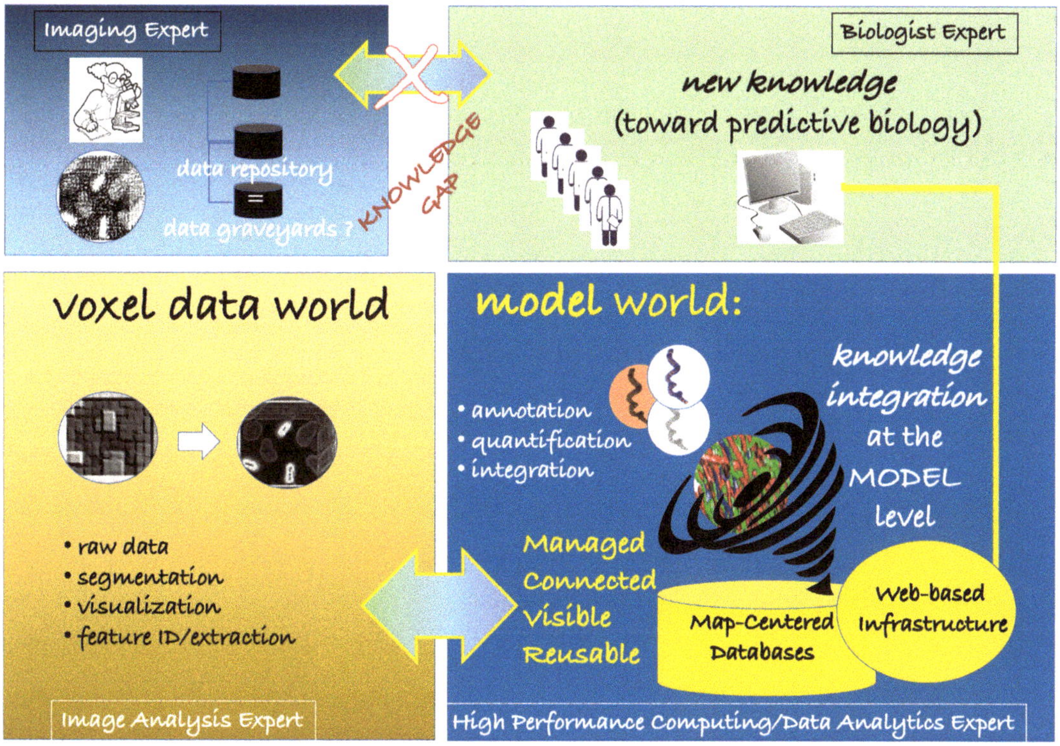

Figure 12.6 Multiscale, multimodal integrated bioimaging. The scientific community is divided into highly specialized groups, with some being focused mostly on the biology, whereas others are experts on the technical aspects of image data creation, image analysis or data-analytics. Biology experts are rarely imaging experts and vice versa, and thus imaging studies are carried out in specialized imaging facilities or as transient collaborations between biologists and imaging experts. Frequently, biology experts are not fully aware of the instrument capabilities and imaging experts do not necessarily know much about the biology of the system they are supposed to image. So, they turn over the images to the biologists, who will then try to make sense of the images or in many cases just pick the image that best support their hypothesis. The image data, once collected, are typically stored on local hard drives in biologist's lab, and most of the images will never be analyzed again. In more systematic imaging surveys, images are stored in image data repositories, which often serve as data graveyards rather than data warehouses. In this age of large-scale imaging, more image data is created than can be analyzed, with data collection taking hours to days, whereas image data analysis may take weeks to months. However, there is so much more information in the images, if only they are adequately processed and analyzed, which typically requires an image analysis expert. Both image acquisition expert and image analysis expert typically deal with voxel data, whereas the biology expert lives in the data model world. Hence, one key objective is to gain knowledge from the image data, e.g., by data annotation, data quantification, and data integration. Such models may provide new knowledge to the biology experts and help them refine their hypotheses.

The ultimate future of bioimaging, will lie in the analysis (Figure 12.6). Perhaps the most difficult part commences when 2D, 3D, 4D, and multidimensional datasets have already been generated: The challenge arises to turn pixel, voxel or hypercubic information into actual biological knowledge and derive meaning from the imaging data and thus to go 'beyond the pretty pictures".

Index

Note: Italic page numbers refer to figure and Bold page numbers reference to tables.

Introduction to Biological Imaging, First Edition. Manfred Auer.

d

t